PEDIATRIC NURSING

An Introductory Text

sixth edition

Barbara Pledg

PEDIATRIC NURSING

An Introductory Text
sixth edition

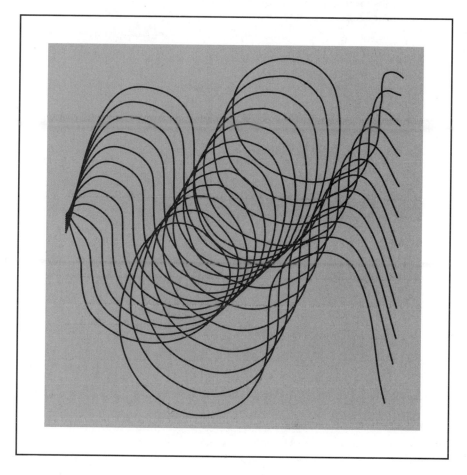

ELEANOR DUMONT THOMPSON, MS, RN, ATR
Mental Health Clinician, Portsmouth Regional Hospital, Portsmouth, New Hampshire
Art Therapist, Silverman and Associates, Inc., Plaistow, New Hampshire

JEAN WEILER ASHWILL, MSN, RN, CPNP
Associate Professor of Nursing, Maternal-Child Coordinator
Tarrant County Junior College, Fort Worth, Texas

W.B. SAUNDERS COMPANY
A Division of Harcourt Brace & Company
Philadelphia / London / Toronto / Montreal / Sydney / Tokyo

W.B. SAUNDERS COMPANY
A Division of
Harcourt Brace & Company

The Curtis Center
Independence Square West
Philadelphia, Pennsylvania 19106

Library of Congress Cataloging-in-Publication Data

Thompson, Eleanor Dumont.
Pediatric nursing: an introductory text /
Eleanor Dumont Thompson, Jean Weiler Ashwill.—6th ed.

p.   cm

Includes bibliographical references and index.

ISBN 0–7216–3125–8

1. Pediatric nursing.   I. Ashwill, Jean Weiler.   II. Title.

[DNLM: 1. Pediatric Nursing.   WY 159 T469p]

RJ245.T475 1992

610.73′62—dc20

DNLM/DLC   92-3579

Listed here is the latest translated edition of this book together with the language of the translation and the publisher:

Spanish (4th Edition)—Nueva Editorial Interamericana S.A., Mexico City, Mexico

Editor: Ilze S. Rader
Designer: Bill Donnelly
Cover Designer: Ellen Bodner-Zanolle
Production Manager: Ken Neimeister
Manuscript Editor: Wynette Kommer
Illustration Specialist: Lisa Lambert
Indexer: Nancy Newman

PEDIATRIC NURSING: AN INTRODUCTORY TEXT, Sixth Edition   ISBN 0–7216–3125–8

Printed in the United States of America.

Last digit is the print number: 9   8   7   6   5   4   3

To my grandson, Chad Porell.

Eleanor Thompson

To my husband, Vince, and my children Vin, Amy, and Heidi, who bring love, joy, support, and laughter to my life. To my Mother, who has always been a source of love and encouragement.

Jean Ashwill

PREFACE

The sixth edition of *Pediatric Nursing: An Introductory Text* has been updated, and rewritten in some areas, to provide the novice pediatric nursing student with the fundamental knowledge needed to practice in a pediatric setting. The integrity of previous editions has been retained because of the positive response this book has received from faculty and students in the past. The framework is growth and development, and the focus is nursing intervention.

Every chapter has been revised; many new illustrations, tables, and photographs have been added. Each chapter is accompanied by Terms, Objectives, and Study Questions and ends with References and a Bibliography.

Nursing Briefs continue throughout the book, and a new feature called Communication Alert has been added. The student is given examples of application of communication skills in the pediatric setting. New subject matter includes burns, care of the family of the hospitalized child, and bronchiolitis with attention paid to the respiratory syncytial virus. The care of the family as well as the child is emphasized throughout the book. The NANDA-approved nursing diagnoses have been added to the Appendix. Nursing diagnosis has been added to several sections in the book.

As I have updated this edition, I have been guided in content and development by my experience in the specialty of pediatrics. I hope students will find the information to be clearly presented and easily understood. I hope my love of pediatrics, the children, their families, and the nurses who work in this area is reflected in my writing.

Jean Ashwill

ACKNOWLEDGMENTS

My work on this book, building on the previous five editions by Eleanor Thompson, would not have been possible without the support and input from many people. I want to thank friends and colleagues who listened and supported me when the job seemed overwhelming. Special thanks to Emily McKinney, Carol Schieffer, and Kay Willis. My editor, Ilze Rader, was supportive, creative, and ever calm as deadlines became closer and closer. Likewise, Marie Thomas' help was just a phone call away.

I appreciate all the children and families who were photographed for this book. They included members of my family, friends, and staff, children and families from Cook–Fort Worth Children's Hospital and North Hills Medical Center, both in Fort Worth, Texas. Cathy White at Cook–Fort Worth Children's Hospital and Michele Duskin at North Hills Medical Center assisted in providing me with many new clinical pictures. Both were professional and most helpful in obtaining the particular pictures needed. My brother, Bill Weiler, spent many hours taking and retaking pictures to meet the deadlines and needs of the book. My sister-in-law, Vickie Ashwill, traveled the roads of Texas to capture nieces and nephews in their particular growth and development poses. My friends and colleagues Jean Smith, M.S., R.N., and Jackie Rowe, M.S.N., R.N., obliged me with pictures of their grandchildren to meet a particular need. Thanks to my friend Peggy Rigilano, M.S.N., R.N., who shared her children through pictures. Mary Sexton, the public services librarian at Tarrant County Junior College, provided many hours of research and aided me in retrieval of numerous references.

Sharon Odozynski, R.N., and Susan Zappa, R.N., provided information in the areas of diabetes and hematology. Emily McKinney, M.S.N, R.N., provided information and review in the area of the newborn infant. I thank the following persons, who reviewed chapters within the book, for their thoughtful and objective comments:

Susan Burkett, R.N., M.S.N., P.N.P., C.P.N.
Wrennah Gabbert, R.N., M.S.N., C.E.N.
Susan Haase, R.N., B.S.N.
Joy Zajac, M.S.N., R.N.

all from the Cook–Fort Worth Children's Medical Center, and Marianne Kay Kindsfater, R.N., B.S., from Central Community College, Kearney, Nebraska.

Finally, I am grateful for all the nurses and student nurses who have had an impact on what I know and believe about pediatric nursing. A special thanks to my husband, who has listened and kept things in perspective throughout this project. Finally, to my children who have made growth and development come alive and who bring such joy to my life.

J.A.

CONTENTS

PEDIATRIC NURSING

An Introductory Text

sixth edition

C H A P T E R 1 _____

Chapter Outline

THEN AND NOW
    Cultural Influences
    Advances
THE CHILDREN'S BUREAU
WHITE HOUSE CONFERENCES
FEDERAL PROGRAMS AFFECTING CHILDREN
CURRENT TRENDS
ROLE OF THE PEDIATRIC NURSE
THE NURSING PROCESS
    The Care Plan

Objectives

Upon completion and mastery of Chapter 1, the student will be able to
- Define or identify the vocabulary terms listed.
- List four historical developments that have affected the care of children.
- Contrast present-day concepts and attitudes of child care with those of the early 19th century.
- Identify the role of the pediatric nurse.
- Discuss current trends in pediatrics and the effect they will have on nursing care.
- Discuss the use of the nursing process in pediatrics.

CHILD HEALTH EVOLUTION

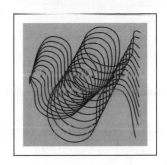

Terms

Children's Charter (6)
DRGs (7)
Fair Labor Standards Act (6)
infanticide (3)
Jacobi (3)
pediatrics (3)
UNICEF (6)
White House Conference on Children and Youth (4)
WIC (7)
World Health Organization (6)

Then and Now

Pediatrics is defined as the branch of medicine that deals with children and their development and care, and with the diseases of childhood and their treatment. The word is derived from the Greek *pais, paidos*, child + *iatreia*, cure. Abraham Jacobi (1830–1919) is known as the father of pediatrics because of his many contributions to the field. The emergence of pediatric nursing as a specialty paralleled the establishment of departments of pediatrics in medical schools, the founding of children's hospitals, and the development of separate units for children in foundling homes and general hospitals.

In the middle ages the concept of childhood did not exist. Infancy lasted until about the age of 7 years, at which time the child was assimilated into the adult world. Paintings of this era depict children wearing adult clothes and wigs. Most children did not attend school. Childhood became a separate growth stage only when large numbers of people entered the middle class and leisure time increased. Because infants were surviving longer, parents were willing to become more invested in them.

Today we no longer consider the child a "miniature adult." Childhood has become a separate phase of life, which is characterized by schooling in Western society. Children's rights are protected by laws and customs. As youths have been freed from the labor of farms and factories, adolescence as a separate entity has also emerged. It is important to see children as composed of physical, intellectual, emotional, and spiritual natures and to relate to them as whole or biopsychosocial individuals.

As the organic causes of death and disability are reduced, we turn to improving the quality of care by helping provide an environment for optimal growth and development. Child experts in these fields, such as Erikson, Bowlby, and Piaget, are now well known in the health care fields.

Cultural Influences

Methods of child care have varied throughout history. The culture of a society has a strong influence on standards of child care. Many primitive tribes were nomads. Strong children survived, while the weak were left to die. This practice of *infanticide* (French and Latin *infans*, infant + *caedere*, to kill) helped ensure the safety of the group. As tribes achieved permanent locations, more attention could be given to children, but frequently they were still valued in terms of their productivity. Certain peoples such as the Egyptians and

Greeks were quite advanced in their attitudes. The famous Greek physician Hippocrates (460–370 B.C.) wrote of illnesses that were peculiar to children. Christianity had considerable impact on child care. In the early 17th century several children's asylums were founded by St. Vincent de Paul. Many of these eventually became hospitals, although their original concern was for the abandoned. In the United States, numerous homeless children were cared for by the Children's Aid Society founded in New York City in 1853. In 1855 the first pediatric hospital in the United States, The Children's Hospital of Philadelphia, was founded.

NURSING BRIEF ▷ ▷ ▷ ▷ ▷ ▷ ▷ ▷
Cultural beliefs today, as in the past, affect how a family perceives health and illness. Holistic nursing includes being alert for cultural diversity and incorporating this information into nursing care plans.

Advances

Many advances have been made in medical and surgical techniques through the years. For instance, children with heart problems are now treated by a pediatric cardiologist. Much of the complex surgery required by the newborn infant with a congenital defect is provided by the pediatric surgeon. Emotional problems are managed by pediatric psychiatrists. Many hospital laboratories now are better equipped to test pediatric specimens. Congenital and heritable defects have become of increasing importance. Chromosomal studies and biochemical screening have made identification and family counseling more significant than ever. The field of perinatal biology has advanced to the forefront of pediatric medicine. The medical profession and allied agencies work as a team for the total well-being of the patient. Children with defects previously thought to be incompatible with life are taken to special diagnostic and treatment centers where they receive expert attention.

THE CHILDREN'S BUREAU

Lillian Wald, a nurse who was interested in the welfare of children, is credited with suggesting the establishment of a federal children's bureau. She and Florence Kelley, an ardent foe of child labor, were jointly responsible for the far-reaching conception of a children's bureau. The first White House Conference on Children and Youth was held in 1909. It resulted in 15 recommendations, the most important of which called for the formation of a Children's Bureau as the first national activity directed toward child welfare (Cone, 1979).

Once the Children's Bureau was established, it focused on the problems of infant mortality. This study was followed by one that dealt with maternal mortality. These investigations gave great impetus to drives for improvement in maternal and child health (Table 1–1). Another early effort was made in the area of birth registration. This study eventually led to birth registrations in all states.

NURSING BRIEF ▷ ▷ ▷ ▷ ▷ ▷ ▷ ▷
Today the Children's Bureau is administered under the auspices of the Department of Health and Human Services.

In the 1930s, the Children's Bureau began to investigate the effects of the economic Depression on children. It found that the health and nutrition of children throughout the nation were declining because of the great increase in poverty. As a result of the research done in this area, hot lunch programs were established in many schools.

During the Depression, many adolescents found home life unbearable because of unemployment. Great numbers of young people wandered throughout the country in search of work. Since there was none to be found, they were not welcome in most communities. In 1933, the chief of the Bureau made suggestions that led to the establishment of the Civilian Conservation Corps. These work camps provided opportunities for training in a wholesome environment, and they proved very successful.

Throughout this period the Children's Bureau had been observing the conditions under which children were forced to work. Their reports were appalling. A description of 13 and 14 year old children working in coal mines was particularly vivid (Bradbury and Oettinger, 1962):

> Black coal dust is everywhere, covering the windows and filling the air and lungs of the workers. The slate is sharp so that slate pickers

Table 1–1. LEADING CAUSES OF DEATH BY AGE GROUP IN THE UNITED STATES

RANK ORDER IN 1987	CAUSES OF DEATH AND AGE
	Under 1 Year—All Causes
1	Congenital anomalies
2	Sudden infant death syndrome
3	Disorders relating to short gestation and unspecified low birth weight
4	Respiratory distress syndrome
5	Neonate affected by maternal complications of pregnancy
6	Accidents and adverse effects
7	Infections specific to the perinatal period
8	Neonate affected by complications of placenta, cord, and membranes
9	Intrauterine hypoxia and birth asphyxia
10	Pneumonia and influenza
	1 to 4 Years—All Causes
1	Accidents and adverse effects (motor vehicle accidents; all other accidents and adverse effects)
2	Congenital anomalies
3	Malignant neoplasms, including neoplasms of lymphatic and hematopoietic tissues
4	Homicide and legal intervention
5	Diseases of heart
6	Pneumonia and influenza
7	Meningitis
8	Certain conditions originating in the perinatal period
9	Human immunodeficiency virus infection
10	Septicemia
	5 to 14 Years—All Causes
1	Accidents and adverse effects (motor vehicle accidents; all other accidents and adverse effects)
2	Malignant neoplasms, including neoplasms of lymphatic and hematopoietic tissues
3	Congenital anomalies
4	Homicide and legal intervention
5	Diseases of heart
6	Suicide
7	Chronic obstructive pulmonary diseases and allied conditions
8	Pneumonia and influenza
9	Benign neoplasms, carcinoma in situ, and neoplasms of uncertain behavior and of unspecified nature
10	Cerebrovascular diseases
	15 to 24 Years—All Causes
1	Accidents and adverse effects (motor vehicle accidents; all other accidents and adverse effects)
2	Homicide and legal intervention
3	Suicide
4	Malignant neoplasms, including neoplasms of lymphatic and hematopoietic tissues
5	Diseases of heart
6	Congenital anomalies
7	Human immunodeficiency virus infection
8	Pneumonia and influenza
9	Cerebrovascular diseases
10	Chronic obstructive pulmonary diseases and allied conditions

Adapted from National Center for Health Statistics (1989). Advance report of final mortality statistics, 1987. *Monthly Vital Statistics Report* (Suppl.) 38:5.

often cut or bruise their hands; the coal is carried down the chute in water and this means sore and swollen hands for the pickers. The first few weeks after the boy begins to work his fingers bleed almost continuously and are called "red tops" by the older boys.

In one community, 64 per cent of the children less than 16 years of age worked regularly standing in cold, damp, and drafty sheds, doing wet, dirty, and sometimes unsanitary and dangerous work. School attendance was sporadic. A child was considered well educated if he or she finished eighth grade.

These studies paved the way for a federal government law that controls child labor. The *Fair Labor Standards Act* passed in 1938 established a general minimum working age of 16 years and a minimum working age of 18 years for jobs considered hazardous. More importantly, this act paved the way for the establishment of national minimum standards for child labor and provided a means for enforcement (Fig. 1–1).

NURSING BRIEF ▷ ▷ ▷ ▷ ▷ ▷ ▷ ▷ ▷
Two international organizations concerned with children are the United Nations Children's Fund (UNICEF) and the World Health Organization (WHO).

WHITE HOUSE CONFERENCES

The first White House Conference on Children and Youth was convened by President Theodore Roosevelt in 1909. A similar conference now gathers every 10 years.

In the White House Conference on Child Health and Protection (1930), the famous *Children's Charter* was drawn up. This is considered to be one of the most important documents in child care history. It lists 19 statements relative to needs of children in the areas of education, health, welfare, and protection. This declaration has been widely distributed throughout the world.

The 1980 White House Conference on Families focused on involving the states at the grass roots level. A series of statewide hearings was held in an attempt to identify the most pressing problems

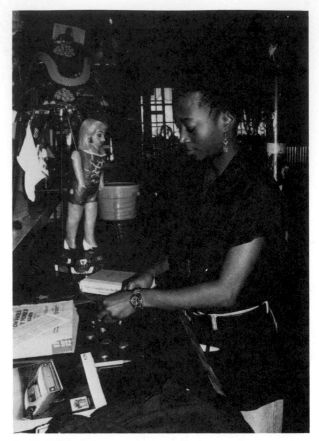

▲ FIGURE 1–1

The Fair Labor Standards Act of 1938 stipulates a minimum working age of 16 years. (Courtesy of Vickie Ashwill.)

of families in the various localities. An enormous range of viewpoints on many subjects was shared, and specific recommendations were made. All participants had the common concern of *strengthening and supporting the American family*.

Because there are no permanent members of these conferences and the members have very little authority, it is almost impossible to implement the recommendations that come out of these meetings.

NURSING BRIEF ▷ ▷ ▷ ▷ ▷ ▷ ▷ ▷ ▷
The American Academy of Pediatrics (AAP), made up of pediatricians nationwide, has established its position of leadership in setting health standards for children.

FEDERAL PROGRAMS AFFECTING CHILDREN

In the past 25 years, child health care has been affected by several federal programs. In 1965, Medicaid and the Children and Youth Project were formed to provide care to children in low-income and inaccessible areas. Both these programs remain viable today, although they have been affected by budget cuts. The Special Supplemental Food Program for Women, Infants, and Children (WIC) was formed in 1966. This program provides nutritious food and nutrition education to low-income, pregnant, postpartum, and lactating women and their children. The National School Lunch Act and Child Nutrition Act passed in 1966 also provide meals, either free or at a reduced rate, for low-income children. In 1982, the Missing Children Act was passed, which has established a national clearing house for missing children.

Table 1–2 summarizes the federal programs affecting maternal-child care.

CURRENT TRENDS

Probably one of the greatest effects on health care in the 1980s was the establishment of the Medicare system of payment for hospital stay based on a patient's diagnosis-related groups

Table 1–2. SUMMARY OF FEDERAL PROGRAMS AFFECTING MATERNAL-CHILD HEALTH

NAME	YEAR	COMMENT
Social Security	1935	Provides matching state and federal funds for maternal and child care and for crippled children, supports preventive health programs (immunizations, screenings)
Fair Labor Standards Act	1938	Establishes minimum working age of 16 years
Maternal-Child Health Infant Care Project	1963	Effort to decrease infant and child mortality
Children and Youth Project	1965	Targets low-income and less accessible children requiring health care
Medicaid EPSDT	1965	Early and periodic screening, diagnosis, and treatment (EPSDT) for poor children
Crippled Children's Service	1965	Services to handicapped children under 21 years
WIC	1965	Supplemental food program for low-income women, infants, and children (WIC)
Head Start	1965	Assists disadvantaged preschool children, increases educational skills
National School Lunch Act and Child Nutrition Act	1966	Provides reduced or free meals to low-income families
Education for All Handicapped Children	1975	P.L. 94–142, free public education for all handicapped children ages 3–21 years; provides necessary supportive services
CMHCs (Community Mental Health Centers)	1982	Attempt to increase availability of mental health centers to low-income families
Missing Children's Act	1982	Nationwide clearing-house for missing children (National Crime Information Computer)

(DRGs). This system also affected the private sector, since many third-party insurance companies are developing prospective payments of their own. These changes have led to shorter hospital stays, more acutely ill children, and an increased need for discharge teaching and home health care. Health promotion has become a priority; many conditions that were once treated by inpatient care are now treated in clinics, day surgery, and other ambulatory settings. Chronically ill children are living to become adults and, therefore, need increased support services. Preterm infants who once could not survive are living and requiring highly technical support in neonatal intensive care units. Organ transplants have become more common and give rise to questions about expense, availability, and complications. As technology increases, nurses are faced with many legal and ethical questions concerning quality of care, patient rights, and the role of the health care worker.

ROLE OF THE PEDIATRIC NURSE

The pediatric nurse may serve in a variety of roles, some of which are depicted in Table 1–3. Health promotion and anticipatory guidance continue to play an important role in pediatrics. The nurse working in pediatrics participates with other members of the health care team, as well as the family, in providing care. The nurse must be able to give competent, skillful care to the child while maintaining a caring, holistic attitude. This can be a challenge in a system that is experiencing a shortage of nursing personnel.

Because of the rapid changes taking place in

Table 1–3. CURRENT PEDIATRIC NURSING SETTINGS	
Community nurse	Home nurse
School nurse	Hospital nurse
Camp nurse	Critical care unit nurse
Office nurse	Children's long-term care
Day care nurse	facility nurse

health care today, it is the nurse's responsibility constantly to update knowledge. As the role of the pediatric nurse expands, the issue of accountability becomes essential. Nurses also have a responsibility to the community and to their profession. Involvement in the community and in their professional organizations not only is encouraged but also is necessary for continued growth.

THE NURSING PROCESS

The nursing process is a method of problem solving that incorporates five steps; assessment, diagnosis, planning, intervention, and evaluation. This process can be used in giving care throughout a patient's lifespan. In pediatrics, both the child and the family are the focus of the nursing process.

The assessment phase is the data-gathering step. Nursing diagnoses describe actual or potential health problems that nurses, by virtue of their education and experience, are capable and licensed to treat (Gordon, 1987). Those diagnoses approved by the North American Nursing Diagnosis Association (NANDA) are listed in Appendix B. In the planning phase, the nurse develops patient goals and assigns their priority. Interventions (nursing orders) give direction for nursing care. The focus is on the care required to prevent, reduce, or eliminate the problem or to promote health. In the implementation phase, the nurse provides nursing care, continues data collection, and documents the child's responses. The evaluation phase appraises the changes experienced by the child in relation to achievement of the goals.

The Care Plan

A nursing care plan provides individualized guidelines for care of the child. It serves as a communication tool between members of the health care team. Care plans usually consists of nursing diagnosis, patient goals, and interventions. Care plans should be reviewed and updated daily. Nursing care plans appear throughout this text to illustrate treatment of selected illnesses.

References

Bradbury, D., and Oettinger, K. (1962). *Five Decades of Action for Children.* Washington, D.C., Children's Bureau, Department of Health, Education, and Welfare.

Cone, T. (1979). *History of American Pediatrics.* Boston, Little, Brown and Company.

Gordon, M. (1987). *Nursing Diagnosis, Process and Application.* New York, McGraw-Hill.

Grad, R. (1989). National Commission acts on behalf of children. *Am. J. Maternal/Child Nurs.* July/August.

Health Division, Children's Defense Fund. (1990). *Maternal and Infant Health: Key Data, Special Report One.* Washington, D.C.

Stahlman, M. (1990). Ethical issues in the nursery: Priorities versus limits. *J. Pediatr.* Feb., pp. 167–170.

Swartz, M. (1990). Infant mortality: Agenda for the 1990s. *J. Pediatr. Health Care* 4:169–174.

Wegman, M. (1989). Annual Summary of Vital Statistics—1988. *Pediatrics* 84:943–955.

Bibliography

Carpenito, L. J. (1989). *Nursing Diagnosis: Application to Clinical Practice*, 3rd ed. Philadelphia, J. B. Lippincott.

STUDY QUESTIONS

1. Define the following: infanticide; pediatrics; pediatrician; Children's Charter; Fair Labor Standards Act; UNICEF.
2. How often does the White House Conference on Children and Youth convene?
3. Contrast present-day concepts and attitudes of child care with those of the early 19th century.
4. What weaknesses exist in the family unit today? What can we as nurses do to help strengthen them?
5. Compare the role of the pediatric nurse with that of a nurse working on an adult medical-surgical unit.
6. Explain the use of the nursing process in pediatrics.

C H A P T E R   2 _____

Chapter Outline

HEREDITY AND THE DEVELOPING CHILD
Karyotypes
Genetic Counseling and Research
ADVANCES IN PERINATOLOGY
GROWTH AND DEVELOPMENT
Clarification of Terms
Characteristics of Growth and Development
GROWTH STANDARDS
FACTORS THAT INFLUENCE GROWTH AND DEVELOPMENT
Hereditary Traits
Nationality and Race
Ordinal Position
Sex
Environment
The Family
THEORIES OF DEVELOPMENT
Psychosocial Development
Cognitive Development
Moral Development
NURSING IMPLICATIONS OF GROWTH AND DEVELOPMENT

Objectives

Upon completion and mastery of Chapter 2, the student will be able to
- Define or identify the vocabulary words listed.
- List the stages of development from the newborn period to adolescence.
- Describe characteristics of growth and development.
- Read a growth chart.
- List six factors that influence growth and development.
- Demonstrate an understanding of the influence of the family on the developing child.
- Identify four growth and development theorists.
- Describe the predictable physical changes that take place in normal growth and development.
- Explain why nurses must have an understanding of growth and development.

GROWING CHILDREN AND THEIR FAMILIES

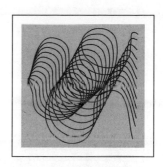

Terms

cephalocaudal (16)
cognition (20)
development (16)
Erikson (21)
growth (16)
Maslow (21)
maturation (16)
metabolic rate (16)
ossification (17)
proximodistal (16)

Heredity and the Developing Child

Most of us understand that something that is inherited is received from one's ancestors. It may be money or a desired heirloom. It is also possible to inherit physical traits and sometimes even a disorder such as hemophilia. A person's sex and all the person's inherited characteristics are determined at the moment of conception, when the male sperm cell unites with the female ovum. There are 23 pairs of chromosomes, 22 autosomes (chromosomes common to both sexes), and 1 pair of sex chromosomes (XX in females and XY in males). Modern cytogenetics (*cyto*, cell + *genetic*, origin) has led to the identification of chromosomes as bearers of *genes* and of *DNA* as the key molecule of the gene. Like chromosomes, genes are paired. Although matching genes in a pair of

chromosomes have the same basic function, they do not act with equal power. Some are *dominant*, others *recessive*. If a gene is recessive, its instructions are overpowered if it is matched with a dominant gene. If, however, a child inherits two recessive genes (one from each parent), the particular characteristics associated with them will prevail. When any two members of a pair of genes carry the same genetic instructions, the person carrying those genes is said to be *homozygous* for that particular trait. When the two genes in a pair carry different instructions, the person is *heterozygous* for the trait. One member of a heterozygous pair of genes will be the dominant gene.

The concept of dominant and recessive genes is important in studying birth defects, because some parents who carry defective genes can have normal children or children who are carriers but are not affected themselves. It also explains how outwardly normal parents can give birth to a baby with a defect. An individual's particular set of genes is known as a *genotype*. Researchers have localized many genes to specific chromosomes. This is termed *gene mapping*. Such new techniques make an *accurate family health history more vital than ever*.

Karyotypes

Geneticists are able to photograph the nuclei of human cells and to enlarge them enough that one can see the 46 chromosomes. These are cut from the picture, matched in pairs, and grouped from large to small. The result is called a *karyogram* (*karyo*, nucleus + *gram*, chart). The karyogram of

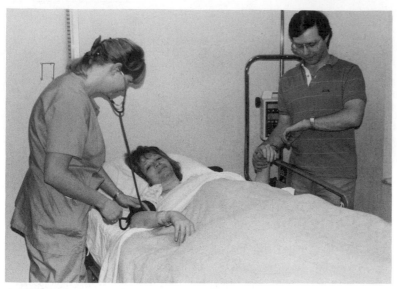

▲ **FIGURE 2–1**

Preparing for a healthy baby includes genetic counseling, good prenatal care, and family involvement. (Courtesy of HCA North Hills Medical Center, Fort Worth, Texas.)

a normal individual shows 22 pairs of chromosomes called *autosomes*. These chromosomes, which are alike in both male and female, direct the development of the individual. An example of an autosomal defect is *Down syndrome*, also known as trisomy 21 because patients have a third number 21 chromosome in most of the cells in their bodies (Fig. 2–2).

The remaining pair of chromosomes are *sex chromosomes*. These differ in male and female, determining sex and secondary sexual characteristics. Defects in sex chromosomes are more prevalent than those in autosomes and account for a greater variety of abnormal conditions. The Y chromosome is small and apparently carries only the genes for masculinity. The X chromosome is much larger and carries the female genes plus many others essential to life, such as those that direct various aspects of metabolism, blood formation, color blindness, and defense against bacteria. Omissions and duplications of chromosomes can occur during *meiosis* (the cell division seen only in sex cells, in which the chromosomes divide in half before the cell divides in two). When a piece of a chromosome, or an entire one, becomes joined to another chromosome, or when broken segments exchange places, the abnormality is termed a *translocation*. When the genes that cause a specific condition are known to be carried on the sex chromosomes, the disorder is *sex-linked*.

Mutations or mistakes in the DNA of a specific gene are not completely understood. Once a gene becomes abnormal, the defect is repeated whenever the chromosome on which it appears reproduces itself during normal cell division. Radiation in the form of x-rays, radium, atomic energy, and isotopes is known to cause mutations. Since a defect may not appear for generations, the amount of radiation a person can safely be exposed to is difficult to determine. New gene mutations also occur. A mutation of a gene that directs the production of an enzyme can result in a disruption in the orderly process of metabolism. These biochemical disorders are termed *inborn errors of metabolism*. Without proper direction of the enzymes, harmful chemical products accumulate in the system. Some examples of inherited pathological conditions discussed in this text are cystic fibrosis, sickle cell anemia, and hemophilia. If a genetic mistake affects only an unimportant link in the metabolism

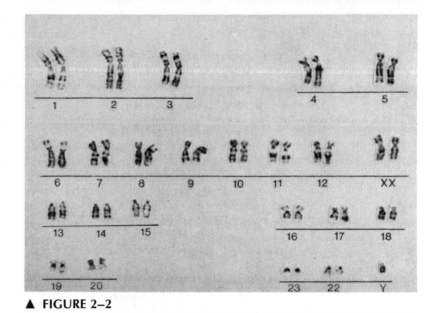

▲ FIGURE 2–2

Karyotype of a patient with Down syndrome (47,XX +21). (From Hacker, N. F., and Moore, J. G. [1986]. *Essentials of Obstetrics and Gynecology*. Philadelphia, W. B. Saunders Company.)

chain or if the body otherwise compensates, no abnormal symptoms may occur even though a gene is defective.

Genetic Counseling and Research

As researchers gather more knowledge concerning the mysteries of the gene, they are able to discover more ways to prevent and treat genetic mishaps. The role of the *genetic counselor* has broadened and taken on greater importance in recent years. Genetic counseling has been described as "the process by which patients or relatives at risk of a disorder that may be hereditary are advised of the consequences of the disorder, the probability of developing and transmitting it, and of the ways in which this may be prevented or ameliorated" (Harper, 1984). Patterns of inheritance are known for hundreds of specific birth defects. Counselors often can suggest laboratory tests to determine whether prospective parents are carriers. A list of genetic counseling services can be obtained from The National Foundation/March of Dimes.

In specific genetic disorders in which a precise enzyme or protein is missing, it is often possible to supply the necessary factor. For example, clotting agents may be given to hemophiliacs and pancreatic enzymes to those afflicted with cystic fibrosis. In other disorders, eliminating the offending substance can correct the problem. This is seen in PKU (phenylketonuria), in which the elimination of foods high in phenylalanine can prevent brain damage.

Medical researchers believe that we are on the threshold of important breakthroughs in this large group of disorders. For example, the gene associated with cystic fibrosis (CF) has been identified recently. It is now possible to identify healthy individuals who carry the CF trait, although there is no consensus among geneticists regarding widespread screening for CF carriers at this time (Caskey and associates, 1989). As biochemists learn to create some of these vital factors in laboratories, and as the genetic code is further deciphered, it is hoped that we may learn how to send messages to the nuclei of cells and supply the minute amount of DNA needed to correct the mistake. Other physicians anticipate the development of

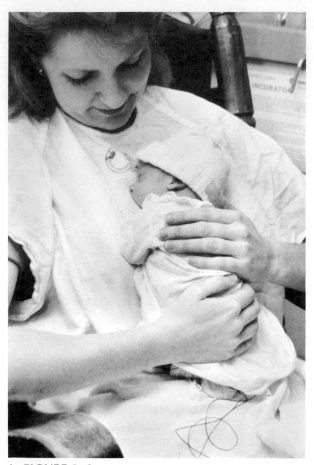

▲ **FIGURE 2–3**

Not all inherited diseases are present at birth. Awareness of a family disease can alert the physician to the need for early testing of an infant. (Courtesy of Cook–Fort Worth Children's Medical Center, Fort Worth, Texas.)

long-lasting enzymes that the patient could take perhaps once a year.

ADVANCES IN PERINATOLOGY

The quality of the uterine environment is as important to the fetus as the quality of genetic makeup. If the fetus inherits a susceptibility to a seemingly harmless drug or minor pathogenic organism, great harm can ensue. Certain chemicals and radiation are also known *teratogens*— agents or factors that cause the production of physical defects in the developing embryo. These substances are hard to pinpoint, as the defect may not be apparent for several months after delivery. The offenders are most harmful during the first weeks after conception, before a mother is aware that she is pregnant. It is thought that many disorders are *multifactorial.* Cleft lip or palate, clubfoot, congenital dislocation of the hip, spina bifida, hydrocephalus, and pyloric stenosis are defects now thought to be multifactorial in origin.

It is now possible to directly monitor a fetus and to measure the amount of oxygen concentration in the blood of the unborn child. Both these procedures tend to be done late in pregnancy. Ultrasound sends sound beams into body tissues to determine early pregnancy, multiple fetuses, fetal growth, location and size of the placenta, and certain malformations.

Intrauterine diagnosis has also been greatly facilitated through *amniocentesis*—a procedure in which amniotic fluid is withdrawn from the womb for the purpose of examining fetal cells (Fig. 2–4). Certain types of retardation such as Down syndrome and Tay-Sachs disease can be determined, as well as Rh-negative blood problems. Amniocentesis can also enable the physician to determine the sex of the baby, which assumes importance in sex-linked disorders. It is also possible to diagnose spina bifida (open spine) and anencephaly (absence of the brain) by testing for elevation of a certain fetal protein, alpha-fetoprotein (AFP). This procedure can be augmented by ultrasonography.

Growth and Development

Growth generally refers to the process that results in increases in size, whereas development refers to increases in complexity of form or function. Growth is *orderly* and proceeds from the simple to the more complex. Although orderly, it is uneven at times. Growth "spurts" are often followed by plateaus. The periods of most rapid growth occur during infancy and adolescence. The *rate* of growth varies with the individual child. Each has a timetable that revolves around established norms. Siblings within a family will vary in growth and development. Growth and development are measurable and can be observed and studied. This is done by comparing height,

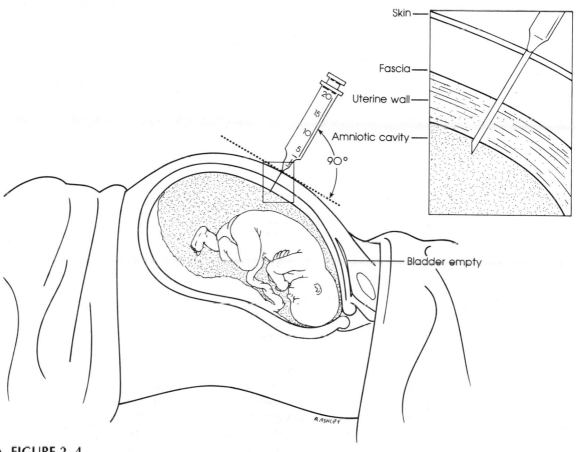

▲ FIGURE 2–4

Amniocentesis. Amniotic fluid is drawn by needle from within the amniotic sac. Cells from the fetus are in the fluid; analysis of these cells can indicate certain genetic disorders. (From Burroughs, A. [1986]. Maternity Nursing, 5th ed. Philadelphia, W. B. Saunders Company.)

weight, increase in vocabulary, physical skills, and other parameters. There are variations in growth within the systems and subsystems, for not all parts mature at the same time. Skeletal growth approximates whole body growth, whereas the brain, lymph, and reproductive tissues follow distinct and individual sequences.

Clarification of Terms

The stages of growth and development that are referred to throughout this text are as follows:

Prenatal life	Conception to birth
Newborn infant or neonate	Birth to 4 weeks
Infant	4 weeks to 1 year
Toddler	1 to 3 years
Preschool	3 to 6 years
School age	6 to 12 years
Adolescence	12 to 21 years

Growth refers to an increase in physical size, measured in inches or centimeters and pounds or kilograms. *Development* refers to a progressive increase in the function of the body. The two are inseparable. *Maturation* (*maturus*, ripe) refers to the total way in which a person grows and develops, as dictated by inheritance. Although independent of environment, the timing of maturation may be affected by it.

KEY TERMS IN CHILD DEVELOPMENT

Growth refers to an increase in physical size, measured in pounds or kilograms.

Development refers to a progressive increase in the function of the body (baby's ability to digest solids as he or she matures).

Maturation refers to the total way in which a person grows and develops, as dictated by inheritance.

Directional Patterns. Directional patterns are fundamental to the growth of all humans. *Cephalocaudal development* proceeds from head to toe (Fig. 2–5). The infant is able to raise the head before she or he can sit and gains control of the trunk

before walking. The second pattern is *proximodistal,* or inner to outer. Development proceeds from the center of the body to the periphery. These patterns occur bilaterally. Development also proceeds from the *general* to the *specific.* The infant grasps with the hands before pinching with the fingers.

Characteristics of Growth and Development

Height, Weight, Body Proportions

Height. The newborn infant at birth has an average length of about 20 inches (50 centimeters). Linear growth is caused mainly by skeletal growth. Growth fluctuates throughout life until maturity is reached. Infancy and puberty are both rapid growth periods. Height is generally a family trait, although there are exceptions. Good nutrition and general good health are instrumental in promoting linear growth. Height is measured during each well-child conference (see page 39 for procedure).

Weight. Weight is another very good index of health. The average newborn infant weighs seven pounds (3.25 kg). The quality of the uterine environment has a bearing on weight. Birth weight usually doubles by 5 to 6 months of age and triples by 1 year of age. After the first year, weight gain levels off to approximately 4 to 6 pounds (1.81 to 2.72 kg) per year until the pubertal growth spurt. Weight is determined at each office visit. A marked increase or decrease requires further investigation.

Body Proportions. Body proportions differ greatly in the child and adult. The head is the fastest growing portion of the body during fetal life. During infancy the trunk grows rapidly, and during childhood growth of the legs becomes the predominant feature. At adolescence, characteristic male and female proportions develop as childhood fat disappears. Alterations in proportions in the size of head, trunk, and extremities are characteristic of certain disturbances. Routine measurements of head and chest circumferences are important indices of health. Head circumference need not be taken routinely after 3 years of age.

Metabolic Rate. The metabolic rate in children is higher than in adults. Infants require more calories, minerals, vitamins, and fluid in proportion to weight and height than do adults. Higher metabolic rates are accompanied by increased heat

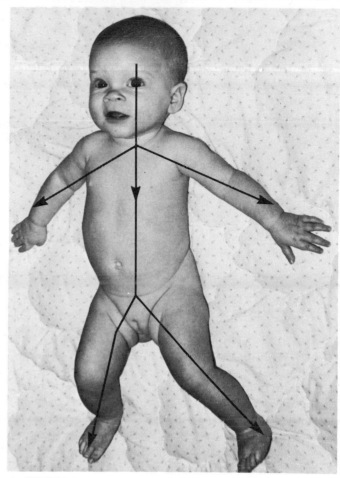

▲ FIGURE 2–5

The development of muscular control proceeds from head to foot (cephalocaudal) and from the center of the body to its periphery. (From Foster, R., Hunsberger, M., and Anderson, J. J. [1989]. Family-Centered Nursing Care of Children. Philadelphia, W. B. Saunders Company.)

production and increased waste products. The body surface area of young children is far greater in relation to body weight than that of the adult. The young child loses relatively more fluid from the pulmonary and integumentary systems.

Bone Growth. Bone growth provides one of the best indicators of biological age. "Bone age" can be determined by x ray films. In the fetus, bones begin as connective tissue, which later is converted to cartilage. Through *ossification*, cartilage is converted to bone. The maturity and rate of bone growth vary within individuals; however, the pro-

gression remains the same. Growth of the long bones continues until *epiphyseal fusion*. Bone is constantly being synthesized and reabsorbed. In children, bone synthesis is greater than the destruction of bone. Calcium reserves are stored in the ends of the long bones.

Critical Periods. There appear to be certain periods when environmental events or stimuli have their maximal effect on the child's development. The embryo, for example, is adversely affected during times of rapid cell division. Certain viruses, drugs, and other agents are known to cause congenital anomalies during the first 3 months following conception. It is believed that these sensitive periods also apply to factors such as bonding, developing a sense of trust during the first year of life, learning readiness, and others. Most research in this area has been done with animals, and questions have been raised as to its application in humans.

Integration of Skills. As the child learns new skills, they are combined with those previously mastered. For instance, the child who is learning to walk may sit, pull himself up to a table by grasping it with his hands, balance himself, and take a cautious step. Tomorrow he may take three steps! Children connect and perfect each skill in preparation for learning a more complex one.

Growth Standards

Growth is measured in dimensions such as height, weight, volume, and thickness of tissues. Measurement alone, without any standard of comparison, would limit interpretation of the data. Data have been collected and standards have been developed that make it possible (1) to compare the measurement for any one child with those for other children of the same age and sex, and ideally race, and (2) to compare that child's present measurements with the former rate of growth and pattern of progress. *Length* indicates horizontal measurement; it is used before a child can stand. *Height* is measured with the child standing. Some pointers in reading and interpreting growth charts follow.

1. Children who are in good health tend to follow a *consistent* pattern of growth.

2. At any age there are wide individual differences in measured values.

3. Percentile charts are customarily divided into seven percentile levels designated by lines. These lines generally are labeled: 97th, 90th, 75th, 50th, 25th, 10th and 3rd, or 95th, 90th, 75th, 50th, 25th, 10th, and 5th.

4. The median (middle), or 50th percentile, is designated by a solid black line. Percentile levels show the extent to which a child's measurements deviate from the 50th percentile or middle measurement. A child whose weight falls in the 75th

percentile line is 1 percentile *above* the median. A child whose height is at the 25th percentile is 1 percentile *below* the median.

5. A difference of 2 or more percentile levels between height and weight may suggest an underweight or overweight condition and indicates the need for further investigation.

6. Deviations of 2 or more percentile levels from an established growth pattern require further evaluation.

It is important to note that a child below the 10th percentile may be normal if the child has shown regular growth in height and weight and has a growth pattern that is comparable with that of the general population. Likewise, children whose height and weight fall in the 75th percentile may need further evaluation if this constitutes a major change from previous measurements (previously was in the 25th percentile). See Appendix F for examples of growth charts.

Factors That Influence Growth and Development

Growth and development are influenced by many factors, such as heredity, nationality, race, ordinal position in the family, sex, environment, and the family (Fig. 2–6).

Hereditary Traits. Characteristics derived from our ancestors are determined at the time of conception by countless *genes* within each chromosome. Each gene is made up of a chemical substance called *DNA*, which plays an important part in determining inherited characteristics. Examples of these inherited traits are the color of eyes and hair and physical resemblances within families.

Nationality and Race. Many ideas about physical differences between people of various nationalities and races have changed in our age of common environment and customs. For instance, persons of Japanese origin were once thought of as being short of stature. However, children of Japanese origin living in America are found to be comparable in height to other children in the United States.

Ethnic differences affect many areas, including speech, food preferences, family structure, reli-

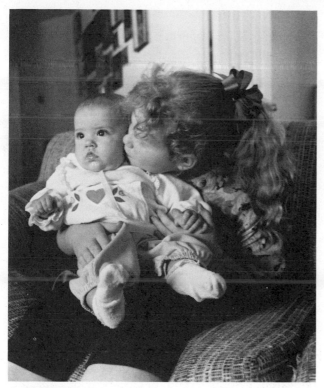

▲ FIGURE 2–6

Children who are secure and loved can direct their energies toward positive development. (Courtesy of Vickie Ashwill.)

gious orientation, and moral code. Ascertaining cultural beliefs and practices is important when collecting data for nursing assessment.

Ordinal Position. Whether the child is the youngest, middle, or oldest in the family has a bearing on development. The youngest and middle children learn from their older brothers and sisters. The motor development of the youngest in a family may be prolonged, as this one tends to be babied by the others in the family. The only child tends to mature faster intellectually, but, like the youngest child, is apt to be slower in motor development, as a lot is done for her or him. None of the above is an absolute, however, and individual variances abound.

Sex. The male infant weighs more and is longer than the female. He grows and develops at a different rate. Parents often treat boys differently from girls by providing sex-appropriate toys and play and by differences in expectations.

Environment. The physical condition of the newborn infant is influenced by the prenatal environment. The health of the mother at the time of conception and the amount and quality of her diet during pregnancy are important for proper fetal development. Infections or diseases may lead to malformations of the fetus. A healthy and strong newborn baby can adapt easily to the surroundings.

The home greatly influences the infant's physical and emotional growth and development. If a family is financially strained by an added member and the parents are unable to provide nourishing foods and suitable housing, the infant is directly affected. An uneducated mother may not know the proper methods of cooking foods to preserve their nutritional value. Immunizations and other medical attention may be neglected. In addition, the baby senses tension within the family and is affected by it.

In contrast, when the surroundings are secure and stable and the infant is made to feel wanted and loved, energies can be directed toward positive development. Most environments are neither completely positive nor completely negative but fall somewhere between.

Intelligence plays an important role in social and mental development. Potential intellect is believed to be inherited but to be greatly affected by environment. These and other factors are closely related and dependent on one another in their effect on growth and development. They make each person unique. If a child is ill, physically or emotionally, the developmental processes may be slowed.

The Family. Today's family is very different from that of the past. Because of changes in women's roles in society, more women are employed. The 1990s find the majority of women with children under 6 years of age employed outside the home (Breslow and associates, 1990). Between 1959 and 1985, the number of female-headed households with children more than tripled, while families with adult males present rose less than 10 per cent (Fig. 2–7) (Ellwood, 1988). The traditional roles of the mother and father have changed, with many parents sharing both child care and household duties. The family is also very mobile, therefore eliminating many of their support systems and causing the children to change schools.

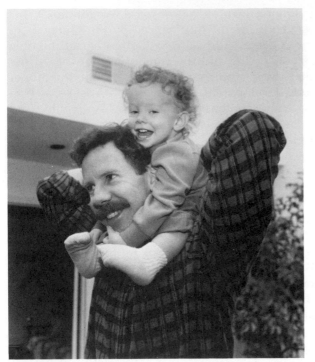

▲ **FIGURE 2–7**

Divorce, separation, death, and pregnancies outside of marriage create many one-parent families. Single parent fathers are no longer uncommon. (Courtesy of Vickie Ashwill.)

As the family changes, so does the child. Children may be raised by one parent, by a relative, or in a foster home. Many children live in poverty and lack proper nutrition and health care. The current supply of child care is short of the demands that will be put on it during this decade.

The home into which a child is born influences the child's entire life. Poverty is less detrimental to a child in a home where there is love and affection than in a home where there is discord and rejection. Each person brings to the role of parent certain attitudes about parenting based on his or her life experiences. A knowledge of growth and development can help the parent set realistic goals for the child and self.

The effect of the family will greatly outlast concerns of health care systems. It is imperative that we take advantage of its strengths while attending to its weaknesses.

Theories of Development

Psychosocial Development

Although no one group of theories can explain all human behavior, each can make a useful contribution to it. Many experts have devoted their lives to understanding why children and families behave as they do. Some, called *systems theorists*, believe everyone in the family or system is affected by each of its members. This theory focuses on the interrelatedness of the various persons as opposed to an analysis of an individual in the group. The nurse relating to the systems theory would focus on caring for the child by caring for the whole family. The family is seen as protector, educator, resource, and health provider for the child. In turn, the child's health is seen as having an impact on each individual member and the family as a whole.

Many see human development as a composite of various theories. Maslow's hierarchy of needs is depicted in Figure 2–8, and the developmental theories of Erikson, Freud, Kohlberg, Sullivan, and Piaget are presented in Table 2–1. Other theorists are briefly contrasted within appropriate chapters, in particular how portions of their theory relate to the age group being discussed. Theories provide a framework for the practitioner, but it must be emphasized that human beings are not a gathering of isolated parts, even though these parts need to be analyzed for research purposes.

Cognitive Development

Cognition refers to one's intellectual ability. Children are born with inherited potential, but this must be developed. There are a number of theories as to how learning takes place, with some disagreement as to the roles or importance of inner drives or needs or environmental stimuli. The

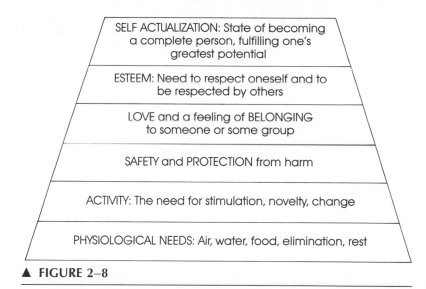

▲ **FIGURE 2–8**

Maslow's hierarchy of basic needs.

Table 2–1. THE DEVELOPMENTAL THEORIES OF ERIKSON, FREUD, KOHLBERG, SULLIVAN, AND PIAGET

	ERIKSON	FREUD	KOHLBERG	SULLIVAN	PIAGET (INTELLECTUAL DEVELOPMENT)
Infancy					
	Trust/mistrust Getting Tolerating frustration in small doses Recognizing mother as distinct from others and self	Orality— understanding the world by exploration with the mouth		Security, patterns of emotional response, organization of sensation	Sensorimotor stage (birth to 2 years)— at birth, responses limited to reflexes; begins to relate to outside events; concerned by sensations and actions that affect directly
Early Childhood					
	Autonomy/shame and doubt Trying out own powers of speech Beginning acceptance of reality vs. pleasure principle	Anality—learning to give and take		Mastery of space and objects	Preoperational (2 to 7 years)—child is still egocentric; thinks everyone sees world as he or she does Preconceptual (2 to 4 years)—forms general concepts, not capable of reasoning yet

Table continued on following page

Table 2–1. THE DEVELOPMENTAL THEORIES OF ERIKSON, FREUD, KOHLBERG, SULLIVAN, AND PIAGET *Continued*

	ERIKSON	FREUD	KOHLBERG	SULLIVAN	PIAGET (INTELLECTUAL DEVELOPMENT)
Late Childhood					
	Initiative/guilt Questioning Exploring own body and environment Differentiation of sexes	Phallic/oedipal phase—becoming aware of self as sexual being	Preconventional or pre-moral morality—rules are absolute; breaking rules results in punishment (4 to 7 years)	Speech and conscious need for playmates, interpersonal communication	Preceptual (4 to 7 years)—capable of some reasoning; but can concentrate on only one aspect of a situation at a time
School Age					
	Industry/inferiority Learning to win recognition by producing things Exploring, collecting Learning to relate to own sex	Latency—focusing on peer relations, learning to live in groups and to achieve	Conventional morality—rules are created for the benefit of all; adhering to rules is the right thing to do (7 to 11 years)	Chumship, one to one relationship, self-esteem, compassion (homosexuality)	Concrete operations (7 to 11 years)—reasoning is logical, but limited to own experience; understands cause and effect
Adolescence					
	Identity/role diffusion Moving toward heterosexuality Selecting vocation Beginning separation from family Integrating personality (altruism, etc.)	Genitality	Principled morality (autonomous stage) (12 years on)—acceptance of right or wrong on basis of own perceptions of world and personal conscience	Capacity to love, empathy, partnership (heterosexuality)	Formal operational stage (11 to 16 years)—acquires ability to develop abstract concepts; oriented to problem solving

development of logical thinking and conceptual understanding is a complex process. One outstanding authority on cognitive development was Jean Piaget, a Swiss psychologist. He proposed that intellectual maturity is attained through four orderly and distinct stages of development, all of which are interrelated. These are sensorimotor (up to 2 years), preoperational (2 to 7 years), concrete operations (7 to 11 years), and formal operations (11 to 16 years). The ages are approximate and each stage builds upon the preceding one.

Piaget felt that intelligence consists of interaction and coping with the environment. Babies begin their interaction by reflex response. As they grow older, their use of symbolism (particularly language) increases. This gradually shifts to a here and now orientation (concrete operations) and finally to a fully abstract comprehension of the world (formal operations). Current theorists have identified inconsistencies in Piaget's theories; however, he was an important pioneer in the study of intelligence.

Moral Development

Lawrence Kohlberg is one of the leading theorists of moral development. Kohlberg's theory is described in three levels, with two stages at each level. In the preconventional phase, children operate on a level of obedience to parental authority, and behavior is driven by a wish for avoidance of punishment. At the conventional level, the child is interested in pleasing others, and there is a need to maintain social order in society by maintaining law and order. At the postconventional level is development of moral principles that can be used to solve complex moral and ethical dilemmas. Children reach these stages at various ages. It is believed that most children begin to develop the stages of the postconventional level only in adolescence and do not attain this stage until adulthood.

NURSING IMPLICATIONS OF GROWTH AND DEVELOPMENT

An understanding of growth and development and its predictable nature encompassing individual variation has value in the nursing process. Such knowledge provides the basis for the nurse's anticipatory guidance to parents. For example, the nurse who knows when the infant is likely to crawl begins to expand teaching on safety precautions. The nurse also incorporates these precautions into nursing care plans in the hospital. Age-appropriate care cannot be administered when one does not have an understanding of growth and development. As the nurse explains various aspects of child care to families, the importance of individual differences is stressed. Parents tend to compare their children's development and behavior with those of other children and with information in popular magazine articles. This may relieve their anxiety or cause them to impose impossible expectations and standards. In addition, many parents had very poor role models who influenced their own experiences as children. Lack of knowledge concerning parenting can be recognized by the nurse and suitable interventions begun.

The nurse who understands that children are born with their own individual temperament and "style of behavior" can help frustrated parents cope with a newborn baby who has difficulty settling into the new environment. It can be determined by specific procedures whether an infant is merely on her own timetable or whether a variation from normal is evident. The nurse recognizes when to intervene in order to prevent disease. For example, a brief visit with a caretaker may reveal that the child's immunizations are not up to date. Abnormalities can be avoided by education of the expectant mother. Other threats to health may likewise be anticipated. Knowing that specific diseases are prevalent in certain age groups, the nurse maintains a high level of suspicion when interacting with these patients. This approach, based on knowledge, experience, and effective communication, helps ensure a higher level of family care.

The nurse must understand how to provide nursing care to children of various ages so that their physical, mental, emotional, and spiritual development is enhanced according to their specific needs and comprehension.

References

Breslow, L., et al. (1990). *Annual Review of Public Health*, 11, p. 198, Annual Reviews Inc.

Caskey, C. T., et al. (1989). *The American Society of Human Genetics Statement on Cystic Fibrosis Screening*. November.

Ellwood, D. T. (1988). *Poor Support: Poverty in the American Family*. New York, Basic Books.

Harper, P. (1984). *Practical Genetic Counseling*. Bristol, United Kingdom, John Wright & Sons Ltd.

STUDY QUESTIONS

1. What factors contribute to the formation of a child's psychosocial development?
2. Why is a knowledge of growth and development essential for nurses caring for children and their families?
3. List four characteristics of growth and development and provide an example of each characteristic.
4. Discuss the statement "Development occurs at different rates for various parts of the body." Give examples.
5. Of what importance are child growth and development theories to the nurse?
6. What is the purpose of a growth chart?

CHAPTER 3 _____

Chapter Outline

HEALTH CARE DELIVERY
SAFETY MEASURES
    Transporting, Positioning, and Restraining the
      Child
THE CHILD'S REACTION TO HOSPITALIZATION
THE FAMILY'S REACTION TO HOSPITALIZATION
HOSPITAL ADMISSION
ASSESSMENT OF THE CHILD
    Pulse and Respiration
    Blood Pressure
    Temperature
    Weight
    Height
    Head Circumference
PEDIATRIC PROCEDURES
    Sponge Bath to Reduce Fever
    Collection of Urine Specimens
    Collection of Stool Specimens
    Collection of Blood Specimens
LUMBAR PUNCTURE
ADMINISTERING MEDICATIONS
PRINCIPLES OF FLUID BALANCE IN CHILDREN
PROCEDURES TO ASSIST NUTRITION,
    DIGESTION, AND ELIMINATION
    Gastrostomy
    Enema
CARE OF THE CHILD WITH A TRACHEOSTOMY
OXYGEN THERAPY FOR CHILDREN
    General Safety Considerations
    Methods of Administration
ADAPTING PROCEDURES RELATED TO SURGERY
THE CHILD WITH A CONTAGIOUS DISEASE
DISCHARGE PLANNING
THE CHILD IN PAIN
FACING DEATH WITH CHILD AND FAMILY

Objectives

Upon completion and mastery of Chapter 3, the
student will be able to
- Define the vocabulary terms listed.
- Describe the physical facilities of a children's
  unit and their significance to the patient's
  adjustment to hospitalization.
- List five safety measures applicable to the care of
  the hospitalized child.
- Describe how illness affects the child and family.
- Discuss three measures the nurse can take to
  make hospitalization less threatening for the
  child.
- Contrast the administration of medicines to
  children and adults.
- Discuss two precautions necessary when a child
  is receiving parenteral fluids, and the rationale
  for each precaution.
- Briefly summarize what impact a life-threatening
  illness has on a 4 year old patient and the family,
  including types of positive nursing support.
- Demonstrate taking an infant's vital signs.
- Describe the collection of urine from an infant.
- Describe the preferred sites for intramuscular
  injections in infants and small children.
- Plan care for a child who is in enteric isolation.
- Discuss the various pain behaviors of the
  different developmental stages.

HEALTH CARE ADAPTATIONS FOR CHILDREN AND THEIR FAMILIES

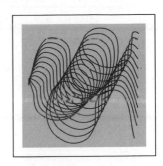

Terms

Broviac catheter (53)
BSA (45)
heparin lock (53)
lumbar puncture (44)
nomogram (45)
palpation (36)
pediatric nurse practitioner (25)
urine collection (40)

Health Care Delivery

Outpatient Clinics

Most large hospitals today have well-organized outpatient facilities and satellite clinics for preventive medicine and care of the child who is ill. Although substantial socioeconomic differences are still involved in the receipt of routine preventive services, Medicaid and other such programs have made these services available to more low-income families. Within clinics there may be specialty areas (particularly at children's facilities) such as cardiac clinics, orthopedic clinics, and so on, where the student can observe and assist. In some institutions information is distributed and brief lessons are given to waiting parents.

In many cities a group of pediatricians practice in an office removed from the hospital, which aids in the distribution of health services and provides evening and weekend health coverage. In some offices the pediatricians or their nurses are available at certain hours of each day to answer telephone inquiries.

The *pediatric nurse practitioner* may visit patients in the home, give routine physical examinations at the clinic, and otherwise assist the physician so that a higher quality of individual care may be attained. This nurse frequently is the primary contact person for children in the health care system. Another area of outpatient care is the *pediatric research center*, such as the one at St. Jude's Hospital in Memphis, Tennessee; this type of institution offers highly specialized care for patients with particular disorders, often at little or no expense to the patient.

Elective outpatient surgery for patients with uncomplicated conditions such as a hernia repair is also being done. Among the advantages of same-day surgery are a reduction of cross-infection, hospital costs, and bed use. Outpatient clinics also eliminate the need to separate the child from the family, and thus the possibility of hospital trauma is avoided. In this type of program, careful preparation must be given, and assurance must be obtained that the child's home environment is adequate to meet recovery needs.

The attitude of nurses, receptionists, and other personnel in outpatient departments can make the difference between an atmosphere that is warm and kindly and one in which the patient is made to feel dehumanized. As more and more medical care occurs in outpatient clinics, there will be an even greater reduction in the number of children who require hospitalization. It is expected that, for many, their only exposure to medical personnel will be through brief clinic appointments. It is our responsibility to make the encounters positive ones for patients and families.

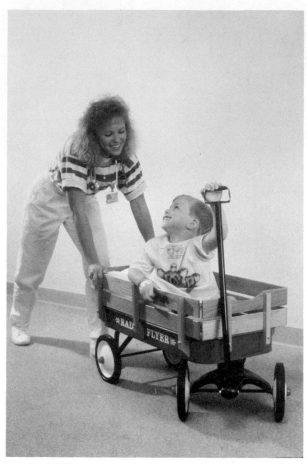

▲ FIGURE 3–1

Children feel anxious when they are in new surroundings. The nurse's taking a child for a ride in a wagon (a familiar object) can lessen the anxiety. (Courtesy of Cook–Fort Worth Children's Medical Center, Fort Worth, Texas.)

Home Care

Since hospitalizations are now briefer for most children, the choice is not either hospital or home care but a combination of the two. They are becoming interdependent. Technical improvements and research in specific disease entities are also helping advance the movement to home care (e.g., cryoprecipitate for hemophiliacs, Broviac catheters for chemotherapy, heparin locks, glucometers, and so on). Home care, however, is not merely a matter of supplying appliances and nursing care but includes assessment of the total needs of children and their families. Families need to be linked to a wide variety of network services. This ideally involves a team approach headed by the physician or medical center.

The hospice concept for children is also under way and has helped families who have needed its service. Local and national support groups for specific problems afford opportunities for families to share and support one another and to learn from others' successes and failures. Special groups and camps for children with chronic illnesses are also well established. Group therapy for children under stress is equally important in preventing mental health problems (e.g., groups for children whose parents are divorced; Alateen). These and other programs not only have the potential for improving life for the child and family but may help reduce the high cost of medical care.

The Children's Unit (Fig. 3–2)

The student nurse may find the first day on the children's unit confusing because it is noisy and cluttered—it differs in many respects from adult divisions. The pediatric unit or hospital is designed to meet the needs of children and their parents. A cheerful, casual atmosphere helps bridge the gap between home and hospital and is in keeping with the child's emotional as well as physical needs. Patients often wear their own clothing while they are hospitalized, and nurses wear colorful smocks or pastel uniforms. Colored bedspreads and wagons or strollers for transportation are also more homelike.

The physical structure of the division includes furniture of the proper height for the child, soundproof ceilings, and color schemes with eye appeal. All invasive or traumatic procedures are done in the treatment room. In this way, the child's room remains a safe place, and the other children are not disturbed or frightened by the proceedings. Some hospitals have a schoolroom. When this is not available, it is necessary for the teacher to visit each child individually in her or his room. Today's modern general hospitals have separate waiting rooms for children. This is more relaxing for parents, since they don't have to worry about whether their child is disturbing adult patients, and it is less frightening to the child.

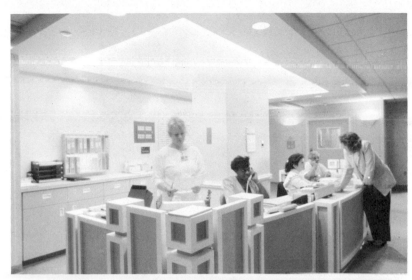

▲ **FIGURE 3–2**

The pediatric unit is a busy place. Note the low desk and colorful uniforms of the nurses and staff. This says to the child, "We want you to feel comfortable with us." (Courtesy of Cook–Fort Worth Children's Medical Center, Fort Worth, Texas.)

Most pediatric departments include a playroom in their structural plan. It is generally large and light in color. Bulletin boards and blackboards are

COMMUNICATION ALERT ▶ ▶ ▶ ▶ ▶
Always meet children at their eye level. Figures towering over them can be frightening to children.

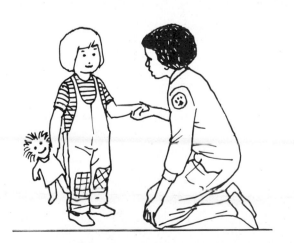

within reach of the patients. Mobiles may be suspended from the ceiling. Some playrooms are equipped with a fish aquarium and blossoming plants because children love living things. A variety of toys suitable for different age groups is available. This room may be under the supervision of a play therapist or nursery school teacher. Parents usually enjoy taking their children to the playroom and observing the various activities. The nurse assisting should allow each child freedom to develop independently and should avoid excessive demands or partiality. Further discussion on the value of play to the child is found in Chapter 11.

Some children are not able to be taken to the playroom because of their physical condition. In such cases the nurse should provide a comfortable chair for the patient's parent so that he or she will be able to cuddle or read to the child according to needs and state of health.

Mealtimes on the children's unit differ from those on adult divisions. Patients whose conditions permit may be served together around small tables. This provides a homelike setting and offers the child a satisfying social experience.

The daily routine also differs widely for obvious

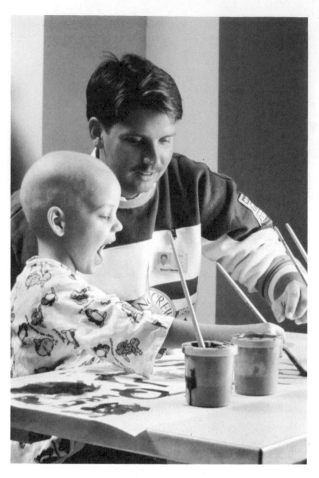

▲ FIGURE 3–3

The child life therapist plays an important role in the care of the ill child. Through play, role playing, art, and other modalities, children can express their feelings. (Courtesy of Cook–Fort Worth Children's Medical Center, Fort Worth, Texas.)

reasons. Although rigid schedules should be discouraged, children benefit from a certain amount of routine. Meals, rest, and play are carried out at approximately the same time each day. *Primary nursing,* in which one specific nurse cares for the child, promotes further security. Visiting hours on the pediatric unit are usually very liberal. Parents are encouraged to stay with the child whenever possible, and most hospitals provide beds for parents.

SAFETY MEASURES

The nurse must be especially conscious of safety measures on the children's division. By demonstrating concern about safety regulations, nurses not only reduce unnecessary accidents but also set a good example for the parents of children who are placed in their care. Although the physical layout of each institution cannot be altered by

personnel, many simple safety measures must be carried out by the entire hospital team. The following measures apply to the children's unit.

Do

1. Keep cribsides up at all times when the patient is unattended in bed.

2. Place a hand on the infant or child's back or abdomen when you turn your back to the child (Fig. 3–4).

3. Wash your hands before and after caring for each patient.

4. Identify child by Identiband, not room number or name.

5. Check wheelchairs and stretchers before placing patients in them.

6. Place cribs so that children cannot reach sockets and appliances.

7. Inspect toys for sharp edges and removable parts.

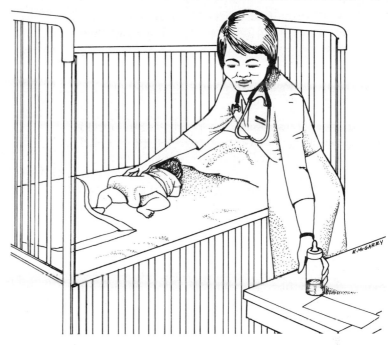

▲ FIGURE 3–4

Maintain hand contact if you must turn your back on the infant or toddler. If you need equipment that is out of reach, raise the side of the crib before leaving the infant or child.

8. Apply restraints correctly to prevent constriction of a part.

9. Keep medications and solutions out of reach of the child.

10. Lock the medication room when not in use.

11. Identify the patient properly before giving medications.

12. Keep powder, lotions, tissues, Chucks, disposable diapers, safety pins, and so on, out of infant's reach.

13. Check thermometers for breakage before inserting, and remain with the patient while taking temperature.

14. Prevent cross-infection. Diapers, toys, and materials that belong in one patient's unit should not be borrowed for another patient's use.

15. Take proper precautions when oxygen is in use.

16. Handle infants and small children carefully. Use elevators rather than stairs. Walk at the child's pace.

17. Locate fire exits and extinguishers on your unit and learn how to use them properly. Become familiar with your hospital fire manual.

18. Protect children from entering the treatment room, elevator, utility rooms, and stairwells.

19. Restrain children when they are in a highchair.

Do Not

1. Do not prop nursing bottles or force-feed small children. There is a danger of choking, which may cause lung disease or sudden death.

2. Do not allow ambulatory patients to use wheelchairs or stretchers as toys.

3. Do not leave a child unattended in the bathtub.

4. Do not leave an active child in a walker, feeding table, or highchair unattended.

5. Do not leave small children out of their cribs unattended in their rooms.

6. Do not leave medications at the bedside.

7. Do not leave a child unattended in an infant seat if it is placed on any area above the floor.

Many other safety measures must be carried out as each student becomes more familiar with the hazards of individual units. The nurse must use the eyes to see with, not just to look at, and then must take the necessary precautions.

Transporting, Positioning, and Restraining the Child

The means by which the child is transported within the unit and to other parts of the hospital depends on age, level of consciousness, and how far one has to travel. Older children are transported in the same way as adults. Younger children are often transported in their cribs, in a wagon or wheelchair, or on a stretcher. The side rails on a stretcher are raised during transport. Ensure that the patient's identification band is secured before leaving the division. A notation is made about where the child is being taken and for what purpose. When a child is being transferred permanently, as from the intensive care unit (ICU) to a private room, the primary nurse should visit beforehand and meet the family.

Figure 3–5 depicts three safe methods for holding a baby. Head and back support are necessary for young infants. The movements of small children are often random and uncoordinated; therefore, they must be held securely. The football hold is useful when one hand needs to be free, such as for bathing the baby's head.

Restraints are used to immobilize a child for diagnostic and therapeutic procedures and for safety. Restraint may be accomplished by holding the child or using some type of physical device. Restraint should be used only when other measures have failed and *never as punishment*. Table 3–1 describes some restraints for children.

THE CHILD'S REACTION TO HOSPITALIZATION

How a child reacts to hospitalization depends on age, preparation, previous illness-related experiences, support of family and health professionals, and the child's emotional status. Three major stresses have an impact on children when they are hospitalized: separation, loss of control, and bodily injury. These reactions are detailed according to age in each growth and development chapter.

The nurse must determine how hospitalization can become a time of growth rather than a negative experience. This can be accomplished through several nursing interventions, which include

1. Explain all procedures.
2. Include parents in care of child.
3. Encourage parents to stay with child.
4. Maintain routines and rituals of home.

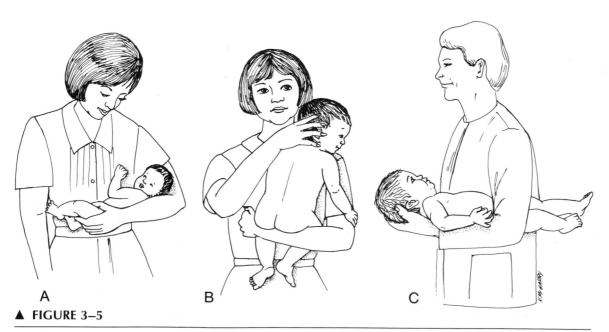

▲ **FIGURE 3–5**

A, The cradle position. *B,* The upright position. *C,* The football position.

Table 3-1. PROTECTING AND RESTRAINING CHILDREN

TYPE	USE
Enclosed crib	Prevents older infants and toddlers from falling or climbing out of the crib
Highchair restraint	Prevents older infants and toddlers from climbing out of chair. Even when restrained, the child should never be left alone in a highchair. The tray is not protection; be sure that the restraint is fastened.
Clove hitch arm and leg restraint	Immobilizes extremities. Must be applied correctly so that it does not tighten. Pad under the restraint with gauze, washcloth, or opened ABD. Attach restraint to frame of bed. Range of motion of extremities
Mummy restraint	Immobilizes an infant or small child for a short time while a procedure is performed or child is examined. Arms and legs are secured so the child cannot wiggle free
Elbow restraint	Keeps child from reaching face or head. Covers most of arm. Must be correct size and positioned so that it does not rub against axilla or wrist
Jacket restraint	Keep child flat in bed or safe in a highchair. Tied in the back of the child and to frame of bed. Mainly used to keep children in the supine position after surgery

5. Encourage parents to bring familiar objects from home (stuffed animal, blanket, doll).

6. If parents cannot stay with child, provide flexible visiting hours. Encourage them to call, leave photographs.

7. Perform all invasive procedures in the treatment room, to maintain the child's room as a safe place.

8. Provide for a consistent caretaker when possible.

9. Comfort the child after traumatic procedures if the parent is not present to care for the child.

10. Provide age-related diversional activities.

THE FAMILY'S REACTION TO HOSPITALIZATION

When a child is hospitalized, the whole family is affected. Parents may initially feel guilty, helpless, and anxious. Parents often blame themselves for the child's illness because they did not recognize early symptoms of a disease, delayed treatment, or were behind in preventive care. Parents seldom are the direct cause of a child's hospital admission. Even in cases of child abuse, nothing is gained by blaming the parents. The nurse must realize that developing a trusting relationship with the parents is often at the center of helping the child. This can be done only if the nurse remains objective and empathetic. The nurse listens, acknowledges feelings, and supports the family.

Parents also may experience fear related to the unknown. They may be unfamiliar with the hospital setting, procedures, treatments, and the disease itself.

Hospitalization may cause financial problems for the family. This is especially true in long-term illness and treatment. In addition to the obvious expense of the hospital and doctor, families often have the added costs of travel, lodging, food, and missed work. The nurse must be aware of these needs and make the appropriate referrals.

As with the child, the nurse assesses the family's needs and develops interventions to meet these needs. Some of the interventions include

1. Assist parents in obtaining information concerning the condition of the child and the treatment plan (written and verbal).

2. Orient the family to the hospital.

3. Explain all procedures.

4. Refer as needed to social services to assist in areas of medical expenses, food, and lodging.

5. Listen to parents' concerns and clarify information.

6. Involve parents in care of the child.

7. Provide for rooming-in.

8. Reinforce positive parenting.

Siblings are also affected when a family member is hospitalized. They may experience anger, resentment, jealousy, and guilt. Suddenly attention is focused on the sick family member, and siblings may feel neglected. Routines are changed, members are separated, and the needs of the siblings may not receive the attention they require. Siblings may feel resentment which can lead to guilt over resenting someone who is ill. The nurse can assist the parents in identifying and meeting the needs of the siblings.

1. Keep siblings informed of the child's illness and progress.

2. Allow siblings to visit the hospitalized child.

3. Encourage siblings to provide their pictures and cards and to call.

4. Allow older siblings to assist with care of the ill child if she or he is comfortable in doing so.

Hospital Admission

Psychological Aspects

As a member of the nursing team, a nurse is often called upon to admit new patients. As well as knowing how to do the procedure skillfully, the nurse must be prepared to meet the emotional needs of those involved. The impression given, whether good or bad, will definitely affect the patient's adjustment. The inexperienced student may be nervous and frightened. After completing the admission procedure, the student should stop for just a moment and recall any anxiety and realize that the parents and child are equally upset. The student will never have to do that procedure for the first time again, but almost every admission will bring contact with parents and a child undergoing an experience that is unfamiliar to them. Empathy in dealing with the fears of the child and parents makes the admission procedure stimulating rather than merely a task to be completed.

> **COMMUNICATION ALERT ▶ ▶ ▶ ▶ ▶**
> Use of the third person can help a child express feelings. The nurse might say, "Sometimes when I am in a new place, I feel afraid." The child can either agree, disagree, or remain silent. Silence might indicate agreement but that the child is still unable to express feelings.

A child must be prepared for hospitalization. If possible, a tour of the pediatric unit by the parents and child before admission is advisable and will enable the parents to meet the people who will be caring for their child. Children and their families are often overwhelmed by the size of the institution and the fear of becoming lost.

Between the ages of 1 and 3 years, the child is very worried about being separated from the parents. After age 3, children may become more fearful about what is going to happen to them. Parents should try to be as matter of fact about this new experience as possible. Unless they have been hospitalized before, children can only try to imagine what will happen to them. It is not necessary to go into much detail, since children's imaginations are great, and giving information that is beyond their understanding may create unnecessary fears. It would seem logical to dwell on the more pleasant aspects, but not to the extent of saying that hospitalization will involve no discomforts. For example, one might mention that meals will be served on a tray, that baths will be taken from a basin at the bedside, and that the child will be with other children. The fact that there is a buzzer to call the nurse if necessary may add to the child's sense of security. The parents may plan with the child what favorite toy or book to bring to the hospital.

Perhaps more important than explaining certain occurrences is listening to the patients and encouraging questions. Parents should prepare them a few days, but not weeks, in advance and never lure them to the hospital by pretending that it is someplace else. In emergency situations there is little time for such preparation. The entire medical team must try to give added emotional support to the child in such cases.

The nurse prepares the equipment for the admission procedure in advance. This will save time and will increase secure feelings. Once the technical details are attended to, the nurse concentrates on the approach to the patient and the family. The initial greeting should show warmth and friendliness. Smile and introduce yourself.

Some hospitals allow the patient to be taken to the playroom for a short time before going to the room. When the mother tells you the child's name, associate it with someone you know who has the same name. This will help you remember it. It creates a much warmer feeling to speak of "John" or "Susy" than "your little boy" or "your daughter."

When the child and parents are taken to the child's room, introduce them to the other children present. The mother is seated comfortably. Explain the admission procedure carefully. Avoid discussing information in front of the child that he or she will not understand. The mother is encouraged to do as much for her child as possible, e.g., remove clothes. Try not to appear rushed. A matter-of-fact attitude must be maintained regardless of the patient's condition. A soft voice and quiet approach are less frightening to the child. If the nurse looks anxious, it will merely cause unnecessary worry for everyone concerned. A nurse may look troubled even though this apprehension has nothing to do with the patient involved. Take one step at a time. Calmness is catching. The nurse remains available to answer questions that might arise. When there is a good relationship between mother and nurse, the child benefits from a higher level of care.

Pediatric Nursing Care Plan

Developing the pediatric nursing care plan is similar to developing an adult care plan. The care plan is the result of the nursing process. It states specifically what is to be done for each child and keeps the focus on the child, not on the condition or the therapy. An established list of accepted *nursing diagnoses* is available and in use in many hospitals (see Appendix B). These serve as a standard for organizing data collection. They also serve as a vehicle by which one nurse can communicate with another. Assessing the child includes a knowledge of growth and developmental processes. It also includes evaluating the primary caretaker who has a direct role in the safety and maintenance of the child's health. Nursing care plans are guides that need continual evaluation to determine whether the goals for the individual child are being met. In some hospitals, a comprehensive view of patient care can be found in the Kardex (Fig. 3–6).

ASSESSMENT OF THE CHILD

Pulse and Respiration

When the nurse counts the pulse, the wave of blood is felt as it is forced through the artery. The pulse rate varies considerably in different children of the same age and size (Table 3–2). The pulse rate and respiratory rate of the newborn infant are high but both pulse and respiratory rates gradually slow down with age until adult values are reached.

The pulse may be counted at any of the peripheral pulse points. However, an apical pulse is recommended for infants and small children. The apical pulse is heard through a stethoscope at the apex of the heart. The nurse counts the rate for 1 full minute. Figure 3–7 shows the location of the pulses.

The respirations of the infant are counted by observing the movement of the abdominal wall, because respirations are primarily abdominal at this time. The rate is counted for 1 full minute because respirations tend to be irregular during infancy. The child's respirations are measured in

KARDEX

NAME **Scott Weiler** ROOM **409** DIAGNOSIS **Diarrhea (Shigella)**

AGE **6 months** DOCTOR **Small** ALLERGIES **None**

DIET **N P O** ACTIVITY **May be held** TYPE OF BED **Crib**

IV FLUID **D_5 NS** PUMP IN USE **yes** TUBING CHANGED **1/17/92**

ISOLATION **yes** TYPE **Enteric** RESPIRATORY THERAPY ————

X-RAY	LABORATORY	SURGERY
	1/18 UA CBC	

TREATMENTS	TIME	DATE	MEDICATIONS	TIME
Stool Flow Sheet				
Strict Intake & Output		1/17	Ampicillin 240 mg IV	08-14-20-02
PRN		PRN		
		1/17	Acetaminophen 80 mg fever ↑ 101° p/o	q 4 hr. PRN

▲ **Figure 3–6**

The Kardex.

Table 3–2. AVERAGE PULSE RATES AT REST

AGE	LOWER LIMITS OF NORMAL		AVERAGE		UPPER LIMITS OF NORMAL	
Neonate	70/min		125/min		190/min	
1–11 months	80		120		160	
2 years	80		110		130	
4 years	80		100		120	
6 years	75		100		115	
8 years	70		90		110	
10 years	70		90		110	
	Girls	*Boys*	*Girls*	*Boys*	*Girls*	*Boys*
12 years	70	65	90	85	110	105
14 years	65	60	85	80	105	100
16 years	60	55	80	75	100	95
18 years	55	50	75	70	95	90

From Behrman, R., and Vaughan, V. (1987). *Nelson Textbook of Pediatrics,* 12th ed. Philadelphia, W. B. Saunders Company.

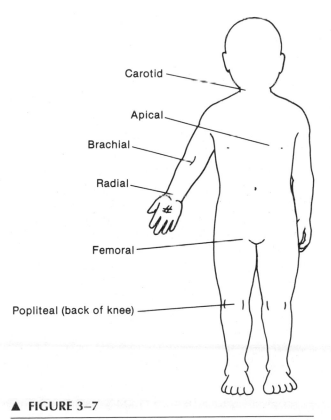

Carotid

Apical

Brachial

Radial

Femoral

Popliteal (back of knee)

▲ FIGURE 3–7

Location of pulses.

the same way as in the adult. Table 3–3 shows normal respiratory rates for children.

Blood Pressure

Blood pressure is defined as the pressure of the blood on the walls of the arteries. It is an index to elasticity of arterial walls, peripheral vascular resistance, efficiency of the heart as a pump, and blood volume. Blood pressure may be measured at the brachial, radial, popliteal, dorsalis pedis, or posterior tibial arteries (Fig. 3–8).

Table 3–3. NORMAL RESPIRATORY RANGES FOR CHILDREN

AGE	RATE
Birth to 1 month	30–40
1 month to 1 year	26–40
1–2 years	20–30
2–6 years	20–30
6–10 years	18–24
Adolescent	16–24

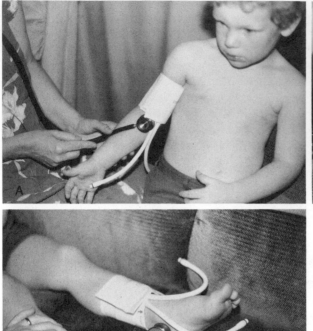

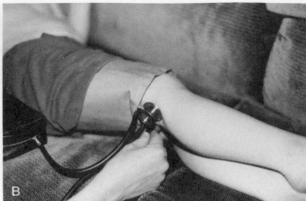

▲ **FIGURE 3–8**

Common sites for measuring blood pressure in children. *A*, Brachial artery. *B*, Popliteal artery. *C*, Posterior tibial artery.

There are several old and new methods for measuring blood pressure in infants and children.

1. Auscultation. Measure as for an adult, using the pediatric stethoscope and cuff. Use the correct size. The cuff should be long enough to encircle the extremity. It should cover two thirds of the upper arm. The following sizes are suggested: birth to 1 year—1½ inches; 2 to 8 years—3 inches; 8 to 12 years—4 inches. Pressure is normally higher in the lower extremities. The American Heart Association designates the muffled tone as the most accurate index of diastolic pressure but recommends recording both that and the final distinct sound as the complete record: thus, 120/80/78. Nurses should clarify this with the physician or the institution employed to ensure uniformity. To determine *pulse pressure,* subtract the diastolic reading from the systolic. This usually varies from 20 to 50 mm Hg. Widening pulse pressure may be a sign of increased intracranial pressure.

2. Palpation. One of the oldest methods. Apply the cuff and inflate above the expected pressure.

Place the fingers over the brachial or radial artery. Record the systolic pressure as the point where the pulse reappears. Diastolic pressure is unobtainable. This is useful in neonates.

3. Ultrasonographic (Doppler) measurement. Noninvasive blood pressure monitoring that ultrasonically detects motion of the arterial wall. A transducer with an attached cuff is secured over an artery, usually the brachial, femoral, or popliteal. The cuff is inflated above systolic pressure and then gradually reduced. The transducer transmits vascular sounds, and measurement is by digital readout. Both systolic and diastolic pressure are recorded. An accurate reading can be obtained only if the child's arm is held still. If the reading shows a major change from the child's baseline blood pressure, the measurement should be repeated because the machines are sensitive to movement.

Some hospitals require blood pressure readings for all children and others only for older children. The width of the cuff should cover approximately two thirds of the extremity used. Thigh readings average 10 to 20 mm Hg higher than those taken in the arm. A cuff that is not the correct size will cause an error in measurement.

Blood pressure is lower in children than in adults. The child's blood pressure may be affected by time of day, age, sex, exercise, pain, medication, and emotion.

The nurse explains what is about to occur, e.g., "This will hug your arm and feel tight for a few seconds." The child is allowed to examine the sphygmomanometer and cuff. An age-appropriate explanation of the procedure is given to the child. The reading should be rechecked if a significant change or abnormal numbers are obtained. Abnormal readings are charted and reported to the appropriate charge person.

Temperature

Temperature can be measured orally, in the axilla, or rectally. A rectal temperature may be preferred for the infant and small child who cannot hold a thermometer in the mouth without danger of biting it. Because taking a rectal temperature is traumatic to children, some institutions use only axillary temperatures for children who are not seriously ill. Research is ongoing in this area, as measurement accuracy and temperature differences are examined. If a rectal temperature is to be taken, it should be done last because it may make the child cry, which influences the pulse, respirations, and blood pressure. Table 3–4 shows normal temperature ranges.

Rectal Temperature. Place the child in a comfortable position, either on the side with knees slightly flexed or on the stomach. Infants may be in the supine position with their legs held around the ankles. Insert the lubricated thermometer a *maximum* of 1 inch into the rectum and leave it there for 3 to 5 minutes. Rectal temperatures are contraindicated in children who have had rectal surgery or are receiving chemotherapy.

Oral Temperature. The procedure is the same as for adults.

Axillary Temperature. The thermometer is held in the axilla with the child's arm pressed close to the body. Hold the thermometer in place for 3 minutes.

Tympanic Temperature. Some hospitals have introduced the use of the infrared tympanic thermometer. Advantages include rapid results, easier to use than conventional thermometers, decreased exposure to infections, patient preference, and elimination of inaccurate oral readings that may be affected by eating, drinking, or smoking (Newbold, 1991).

Body temperature does not remain at 37°C (98.6°F), and slight variations are considered normal. Rectal temperatures are slightly higher than oral, and axillary temperatures slightly lower than oral, but not the full degree Fahrenheit that was once thought. When recording temperatures, the nurse notes the route used. If the reading is abnormal, the appropriate charge person should be notified. Managing fever in children is depicted in Nursing Care Plan 3–1.

Weight

Weight must be recorded accurately on admission. The weight of a patient provides a means of determining progress and also is necessary to determine the dosage of certain medications. The way in which the nurse weighs the child depends on the age.

The infant is weighed completely naked in a warm room. A fresh diaper or scale paper is placed on the scale. This prevents cross-contamination, i.e., the spread of germs from one infant to another. The scale is balanced to compensate for the weight of the diaper. There are various ways of balancing scales; the nurse should request specific instruction for the particular scale used. The infant is placed gently on the scale. The nurse's left hand

Table 3–4. NORMAL TEMPERATURE RANGES FOR CHILDREN

METHOD	RANGE
Oral	36.4–37.4°C (97.6–99.3°F)
Rectal	37.0–37.8°C (98.6–100.0°F)
Axillary	35.8–36.6°C (96.6–98.0°F)

NURSING CARE PLAN 3–1

THE CHILD WITH A FEVER

Nursing Diagnosis	Goals/Outcome Criteria	Nursing Interventions
Fluid volume deficit, potential for dehydration due to increased metabolic rate	Child will not become dehydrated Child will show no signs of dehydration, as evidenced by good skin turgor, moist mucous membranes, and no weight loss	Increase fluid intake Offer juice, water, popsicles, yogurt, as age-appropriate Monitor for dehydration Monitor intake and output
Comfort, alterations in, fever	Child's temperature will be within normal range Child's temperature will be between 36.5 and 37.4°C (97.4 and 99.4°F)	Administer *tepid* sponge bath for fever of 40.0°C (104.0°F) Assess vital signs prior to sponge bath for baseline data Retake vital signs 30 minutes after procedure Cover with light clothing and cover Prevent shivering Administer antipyretic medications according to physician's instructions
Injury, potential for, seizure	Child will not injure self Child will show no signs of injury, as evidenced by the absence of bruising, aspiration, or breaks in the skin	Keep side rails up Observe child frequently Remain with child if tub bath is given Pad side rails

is held slightly above the infant to make sure that she or he does not fall. The nurse regulates the weights with the right hand. The scale should be read when the infant is lying still. If the mother is present, she may distract the patient by waving or speaking softly. Once the exact weight is determined, the infant is removed from the scale, wrapped in a blanket, and given to the mother to soothe. Record the weight immediately. The scale paper is disposed of in the proper receptacle. An unsoiled diaper is returned to the patient's unit. Digital pediatric scales that provide readouts in pounds and grams are used in many institutions. They do not require the regulation of weights.

The older child is weighed in the same manner as an adult. A paper towel is placed on the scale for the patient to stand on. The patient is generally weighed in a hospital gown. The shoes are removed. If the child is unable to stand on the scales, it may be necessary for the nurse to hold the child and read the combined weights. The nurse then gets weighed and subtracts the weight from the combined weight to obtain that of the patient. Occasionally, a child is weighed who is wearing a cast. The nurse records this as, for example, weight 34 pounds with cast on right arm.

Other Observations. The child who has been undressed for weighing is observed for such objective symptoms as skin coloring, abrasions, rash, swelling, facial expressions (fear, pain, fatigue), discharge from nose or ears, dyspnea, condition

NURSING CARE PLAN 3–1 *Continued*

THE CHILD WITH A FEVER

Nursing Diagnosis	Goals/Outcome Criteria	Nursing Interventions
Knowledge deficit, parent	Parent will understand and verbalize the cause and treatment of fever	Explain nature of fever (not always bad); too vigorous control may mask signs of illness
		Emphasize removal of clothes when child has fever
		Explain that degree of fever does not always reflect the severity of disease; call physician if child looks sick or acts different
	Parent will demonstrate ability to read a thermometer	Demonstrate how to read a thermometer
	Parent will verbalize understanding of potential for seizure	Discuss with parent potential for seizure
	Parent will verbalize understanding of care during a seizure	Discuss with parent care of child during seizure
		a. Remain with child and assist to side-lying position
		b. Do not restrain movements, and loosen tight clothing
		c. Do not put anything in child's mouth

of joints, odor of breath, condition of teeth, coughing, or other unusual abnormalities or markings.

Height

The older child's height is measured at the time of weighing. The infant must be measured while lying on a flat surface alongside a metal tape measure or yardstick. The knees should be pressed flat on the table. Measure from the top of the head to the heels and record. Place head in the midline.

Head Circumference

Head circumference should be measured on all children under 36 months of age and on children with neurological defects. Place a steel or paper tape around the head from slightly above the eyebrows and pinnae of the ears to the occipital prominence of the skull. See Figure 3–9 for procedure.

PEDIATRIC PROCEDURES

Sponge Bath to Reduce Fever*

Tepid baths may be given in a tub or in the child's bed. The child should not be permitted to

---

*A table of Celsius (centigrade) and Fahrenheit temperature equivalents appears in the back of the book

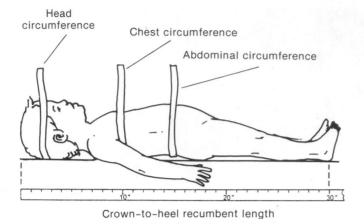

Head circumference

Chest circumference

Abdominal circumference

Crown-to-heel recumbent length

▲ FIGURE 3–9

Crown-to-heel recumbent measurements.

shiver, because shivering will produce heat and a temperature increase. The bath is given for 20 to 30 minutes. Alcohol should never be added to the water as it reduces the heat too rapidly and can be absorbed.

PROCEDURE ▶ ▶ ▶ ▶ ▶ ▶ ▶ ▶ ▶

Equipment. Basin of tepid water, three facecloths, towel, two bath blankets, waterproof sheet.

1. Assemble the equipment at the bedside. Explain the procedure to the patient.

2. Screen the child. Take and record temperature, pulse, and respiration.

3. Cover the patient with a bath blanket or sheet. Fanfold bedclothes to the foot of the bed. Place a waterproof sheet and bath blanket beneath the patient.

4. Remove the pillow from the bed. Remove patient's gown.

5. Wash the patient's face and neck with tepid water.

6. Lift the corner of the bath blanket and bathe the child's body, part by part. Use long strokes. Expose one area of the body at a time.

7. Place moist, folded cloths over blood vessels that lie close to the skin (underarms and groin).

8. Turn the patient and repeat the procedure, beginning with the neck, and going to shoulders, back, and so forth.

9. Check color and pulse to be sure that the child is tolerating the procedure well.

10. If the child begins to shiver, the water temperature should be raised. If shivering continues, stop the bath.

11. When the bath is completed, pat the skin dry and cover the patient with only a sheet.

12. Remove the waterproof sheet and blanket. Replace the hospital gown. An infant may merely be placed on a large turkish towel, covered by a receiving blanket.

13. Arrange pillows and bedding for the patient's comfort.

14. Take the patient's temperature within 30 minutes of the time the procedure ended, and record. If the temperature has not started to go down, check to see if the procedure should be repeated. Note: The temperature is not expected to drop to normal but merely to a more reasonable level.

15. Chart: Time procedure began, length of time administered, untoward reactions, patient's temperature before and after procedure.

Collection of Urine Specimens

A urine specimen is obtained from the newly admitted patient (Table 3–5). Certain general prin-

Table 3–5. AVERAGE DAILY EXCRETION OF URINE		
AGE	FLUID OUNCES	CUBIC CENTIMETERS
First and second days	1–2	30–60
Third to tenth day	3–10	100–300
Tenth day to 2 months	9–15	250–450
2 months to 1 year	14–17	400–500
1–3 years	17–20	500–600
3–5 years	20–24	600–700
5–8 years	22–34	650–1000
8–14 years	27–47	800–1400

ciples are observed regarding the collection of specimens:

PROCEDURE ▶ ▶ ▶ ▶ ▶ ▶ ▶ ▶ ▶

1. Explain the procedure to the patient (age-appropriate).
2. Wash hands.
3. Use a clean container or apply a urine collection bag (Fig. 3–10).
4. If a bag is used, secure diaper over bag.
5. Check bag every 20 to 30 minutes. Figure 3–11 shows recovery of the specimen.
6. Label all specimens clearly and attach the proper laboratory slip.
7. Record in nurse's notes.

Clean Catch. Special sterile containers are available for clean catch specimens; follow the directions of the manufacturer. All require cleansing of the perineum. Cleanse the perineum with a soap or antiseptic, wiping from front to back. Repeat twice and follow with sterile water to prevent contamination of the specimen. After the urine stream has started, the midstream specimen should be caught in the sterile container, being careful not to contaminate the container. Infants and young children may have a sterile urine bag applied. The specimen should be taken immediately to the laboratory for testing as bacteria accumulate at room temperature.

Catheterization. Obtaining specimens by means of a catheter is seldom indicated in pediatric patients. When required, catheterization is the same as for adults, except that the size of the catheter is usually an 8 or 10 Foley. When required for surgical patients, the catheter may be inserted once the child has been anesthetized. This is less traumatic for children, who are usually frightened by this procedure.

Collecting a 24-Hour Urine Specimen. At times a 24-hour urine specimen may be requested to determine the rate of urine production and to measure the excretion of specific chemicals from the body. This requires close supervision by the nurses on each shift to maintain accuracy of the test, as lost specimens necessitate restarting the test. Problems can arise if the collection device does not adhere to the skin properly; therefore, the nurse must be alert for this occurrence. Diversions suitable to the child's age are employed. Certain tests require that chemicals be added to the bedside collection receptacle. It is important to clarify this before the procedure is begun. A sign is attached to the infant's crib to alert personnel of a 24-hour urine collection.

Determining the Specific Gravity of Urine. The nurse may be asked to measure the specific gravity of the urine. The normal range is 1.005 to 1.030.

PROCEDURE ▶ ▶ ▶ ▶ ▶ ▶ ▶ ▶ ▶

Equipment. Urinometer and urine specimen.

1. Fill the test tube three fourths full of urine.
2. Insert the bobbin of the urinometer. Spin it gently to be sure that it is not touching the sides of the container.
3. Take the reading from the bottom of the meniscus.
4. Record results.

Refractometers are also used for this purpose in some hospitals. Urine can be obtained from some infants' diapers by means of a syringe without a needle. Only a few drops of urine are required.

Albumin Determination. The nurse working in a doctor's office or clinic also may be requested to

For Girls

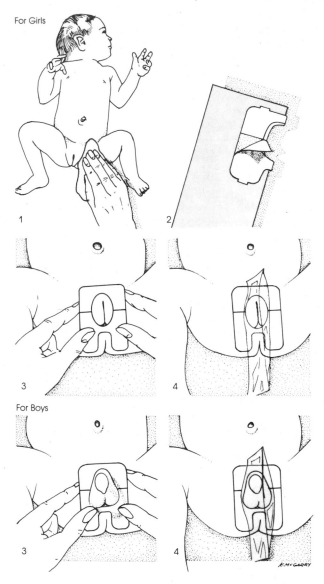

For Boys

▲ FIGURE 3–10

Applying newborn and pediatric urine collectors. Two key points are (a) Skin must be clean and perfectly dry. Avoid oils, baby powders, and lotion soaps that may leave a residue on the skin and interfere with the ability of the adhesive to stick. (b) Application must begin on the tiny area of skin between the anus and genitals. The narrow "bridge" on the adhesive patch keeps feces from contaminating the specimen and helps position the collector correctly. (Courtesy of Hollister Incorporated, Libertyville, Illinois.)

1. With child on her back, spread legs and wash each skinfold in the genital area. A gentle bath soap is best. Do not use a scrub soap solution; it may leave a residue that interferes with adhesion. Wash the anus last. Rinse and dry. For boys, wash the scrotum first, then the penis; wash the anus last. Allow a few moments for air drying.

2. Remove protective paper from the bottom half of the adhesive patch. Most persons find it easier to keep the top half of the adhesive covered with paper until the bottom part has been applied to the skin. With a very active boy, you may want to keep all the paper in place until you have fitted the collector over the genitals.

3. For girls, stretch the perineum to separate the skin folds and expose the vagina. When applying adhesive to the skin, be sure to start at the narrow bridge of skin separating the vagina from the anus. Work outward from this point. For boys, begin between the anus and the base of the scrotum.

4. Press adhesive firmly against the skin and avoid wrinkles. When the bottom part is in place, remove paper from the upper portion of the adhesive patch. Work upward to complete application.

(Courtesy of Hollister Incorporated, Libertyville, Illinois.)

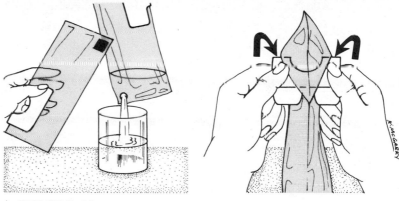

▲ **FIGURE 3–11**

Recovering the specimen. You can drain the urine bag collector into a *clean* beaker or specimen bottle by removing the tab in the lower corner, or you can seal the specimen inside the collector itself by folding the sticky adhesive sides together. Then place the collector with specimen into a paper or plastic cup.

test urine for albumin, i.e., protein. Normally little or no albumin is found in the urine of a healthy child. Reagent strips especially intended for this purpose are available. The nurse dips the end of the strip into urine and compares the strip with a special color chart. Specific instructions accompany test materials.

Collection of Stool Specimens

Stool specimens from older children are obtained as for an adult. This is embarrassing for most children, who are turned off by the suggestion. The ambulatory child can use a bedpan placed beneath a toilet seat. It is difficult for a child to tell the nurse that the sample has been collected. The nurse can acknowledge these feelings by giving the child permission to express them without being critical, e.g., "I know this must be embarrassing for you. It is for grown-ups too, but we need this because. . . ."

PROCEDURE   ▶ ▶ ▶ ▶ ▶ ▶ ▶ ▶ ▶

1. A stool specimen can be obtained from the infant directly from the diaper if it has not been contaminated by urine.

2. A rectal swab may also be ordered.

3. Some specimens must be sent to the laboratory while they are warm.

4. The specimen is labeled properly and the laboratory slip is attached.

5. The nurse charts the time, color, amount, and consistency of the stool; the purpose for which it was collected, i.e., blood, ova, parasites, bacteria; and any related information.

Collection of Blood Specimens

Blood specimens are generally collected by the laboratory technician or a specially trained nurse. The antecubital fossa is a common site in children older than 2 years of age. Another site is the dorsum of the hand or foot. The external jugular vein can be used in infants when other sites have not worked. The femoral vein may be used when other sites have been exhausted.

Positioning the Child. Positioning the pediatric patient for blood drawings is extremely important. The nurse is often asked to assist in these procedures. Figures 3–12 and 3–13 depict how to position the patient for jugular and femoral venipuncture. Both the jugular and the femoral veins are large; therefore, the patient is checked frequently

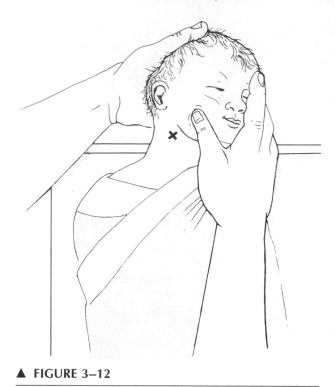

▲ FIGURE 3–12

An infant positioned for jugular venipuncture.

to ensure that there is no bleeding. The child is soothed accordingly, as crying and thrashing may precipitate oozing. The nurse charts the site utilized, the name of the blood test, and any untoward developments.

LUMBAR PUNCTURE

The nurse sometimes assists the physician with a lumbar puncture, which is also referred to as a "spinal tap." It is done to obtain spinal fluid for diagnosis and treatment. Disposable lumbar puncture sets are available.

Normal spinal fluid is clear, like water. The pressure ranges from 60 to 180 mm Hg. It is somewhat lower in infants. The procedure for children is essentially the same as for adults. The main difference lies in the patient's ability to cooperate with positioning.

PROCEDURE ▶ ▶ ▶ ▶ ▶ ▶ ▶ ▶ ▶

1. The nurse explains that the child must lie quietly and that there will be help in doing this.
2. The nurse explains that sensations during a

lumbar puncture include a cool feeling when the skin is cleansed and a feeling of pressure when the needle is inserted.

3. The patient lies on the side with the back parallel to the side of the treatment table. The knees are flexed and the head is brought down close to the flexed knees. The nurse can keep the child in this position by placing the child's head in the crook of one arm and the knees in the crook of the other arm. The nurse then clasps hands together at the front of the child and leans forward, gently placing his or her chest against the patient (Fig. 3–14). Infants may be placed in the sitting position. The way in which the child is held can directly affect the success of the procedure.

4. When the puncture is completed, a sterile Band-Aid is placed over the injection site and the child is comforted.

5. The site should be checked for any drainage or redness.

6. Monitor vital signs according to the procedure of the hospital.

7. Specimens are labeled and taken to the laboratory with the appropriate requisition form.

8. Children do not usually suffer from headaches following a lumbar puncture and may play

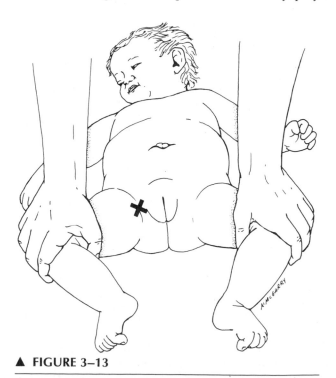

▲ FIGURE 3–13

An infant positioned for femoral venipuncture. This provides exposure of the groin area.

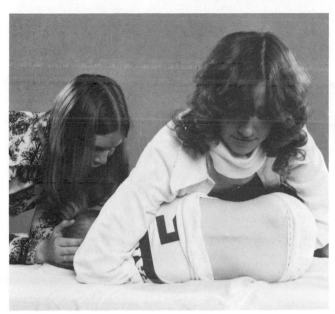

▲ **FIGURE 3–14**

A child positioned for a lumbar puncture. Although the nurse may appear to be placing her weight on the child, the weight is actually placed on her elbows. If the parents are present during this procedure, they can provide emotional support for the child. (From Foster, R., Hunsberger, M., and Anderson, J. J. (1989). *Family-Centered Nursing Care of Children*. Philadelphia, W. B. Saunders Company.)

quietly after the procedure unless ordered otherwise.

9. The nurse charts the date and time of the lumbar puncture and the name of the attending physician. Also charted are the amount of fluid obtained; its character, e.g., cloudy or bloody; whether or not specimens were sent to the laboratory; and the reaction of the patient to the procedure.

10. The nurse cleans and restocks the treatment room.

Administering Medications

Variations in Children

The responsibility for giving medications to children is a serious one. Although the full description of technical details in administering drugs is be-

yond the scope of this text, the following considerations and hazards applicable to pediatric patients are pertinent.

More than half the drugs currently on the market are unsuitable for children because of their toxicity or because of lack of information of their effect on pediatric patients. Children are smaller than adults and their medications have to be adapted to their size and age. For instance, a student nurse who takes one adult aspirin receives 5 grains. A mother who gives her 3 year old child one baby aspirin is administering 1¼ grains, which is only one fourth the dose taken by the nurse. Neonates and preterms are in particular jeopardy because of the immaturity of their body systems. In these patients simply adjusting the dosage is insufficient. Drugs must be individualized and tailored to a multitude of factors (Fig. 3–15). Appendix A lists commonly used pediatric drugs.

Most pediatric medications are prescribed in milligrams per kilogram of body weight per 24 hours. A hospital drug formulary is usually available on the unit to enable the nurse to determine the safety of a particular dose. If there is any question, one should also consult with another nurse, the physician who wrote the order, the hospital pharmacist, or the shift supervisor.

The nurse should always ask whether the calculated dose makes sense. It is also helpful to remember that children usually receive small doses and amounts, and if either of these is large, the nurse should recheck.

At times the physician needs to calculate a particular dosage of a medication for a certain child. One method, calculation by body surface area, is now considered to be the most accurate. In this method a *nomogram* is used (Fig. 3–16). The child's height is located on the left scale and weight on the right scale. A line is drawn between the two points. The point at which the line transsects the surface area (SA) gives the body surface area (BSA). If the patient is roughly of average size, the surface area also can be estimated from the weight alone using the enclosed area. The results are inserted into a formula. The average adult body surface area is approximately 1.7 square meters.

Body surface area:

$$\frac{\text{BSA (child)}}{\text{BSA (adult)}} \times \text{average adult dose} = \text{child's dose}$$

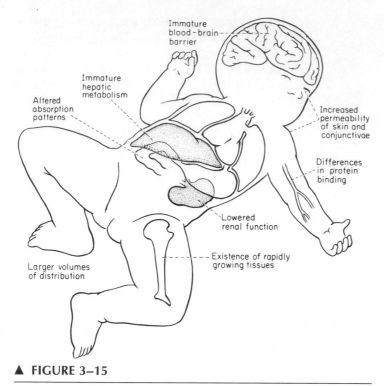

Immature
blood-brain-
barrier

Immature
hepatic
metabolism

Altered
absorption
patterns

Increased
permeability
of skin and
conjunctivae

Differences
in protein
binding

Lowered
renal function

Existence of rapidly
growing tissues

Larger volumes
of distribution

▲ FIGURE 3–15

Some of the multiple factors that modify drug disposition in the newborn infant. (Adapted from Hirata, T.: In Smith, D. [ed.] [1977]. *Introduction to Clinical Pediatrics*, 2nd ed. Philadelphia, W. B. Saunders Company.)

Besides knowing the correct amount and route of a drug, the nurse must also be aware of the toxic side effects that might occur. The absorption, distribution, metabolism, and excretion of drugs differ substantially in children, who also react more quickly and violently to medication. Drug reactions are therefore not as predictable as in adult patients. The impact of a drug upon normal growth and development must be considered. Drug circulars must be read carefully to determine suitability of a particular drug for children. *Drugs should be given only by the route indicated.* Double check with another nurse if using calculated dosages or for any drug or dosage that may give reason for concern. (Some hospitals specify double checking for Lanoxin, insulin, heparin, and certain other drugs.) **The child should be correctly identified by using the hospital identification band. The nurse must always know what medications the patient is receiving, whether or not the nurse administers them personally.**

See Table 3–6 for further considerations about pediatric medications.

Oral Medications

The administration of medication by mouth is preferred in children but is not always possible because of vomiting, malabsorption, or refusal. Children younger than 5 years of age find it difficult to swallow tablets or capsules, so many pediatric medications are available in liquid, suspension, or chewable tablets. Only scored tablets should be divided. Suspensions must be fully shaken before use.

Capsules may have to be emptied and the powder disguised in a pleasant-tasting medium. This is also necessary when the medication is bitter or

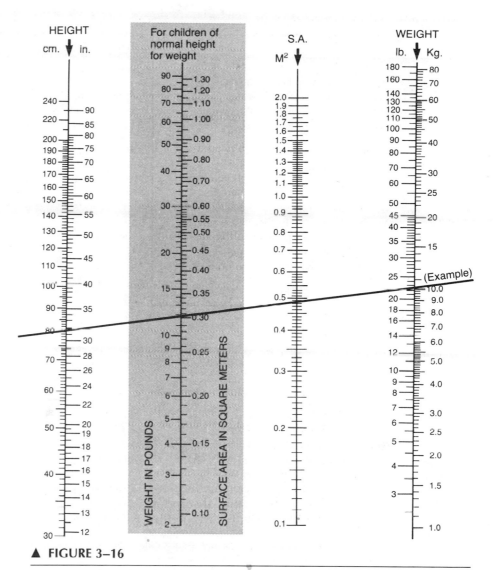

▲ **FIGURE 3–16**

Nomogram for calculating body surface area. The surface area is indicated at the intersection of a straight line connecting the height and weight column with the surface area column; if the patient is of roughly average size, it is determined by the weight alone (enclosed area). (Nomogram modified from data of E. Boyd by C. D. West. From Behrman, R., and Vaughan, V. [1987]. *Nelson Textbook of Pediatrics,* 13th ed. Philadelphia, W. B. Saunders Company.)

Table 3–6. SELECTED CONSIDERATIONS IN GIVING MEDICATIONS TO CHILDREN

AGE	CONSIDERATIONS
Infant	Apply bib
	Support and elevate head and shoulders
	Plastic disposable syringe is accurate and safe for oral medications
	Depress chin with thumb to open mouth
	Slowly insert medication along the side of the infant's mouth; this will help prevent gagging
	Allow time for swallowing
	The preferred sites for IM injections are the lateral and anterior aspects of the thighs
	Avoid use of buttocks, as gluteal muscles are undeveloped in infants; danger of injury to sciatic nerve
	As a rule of thumb give no more than 1 ml of solution in a single site; if in doubt, confer with another nurse or physician
	Soothe infant
Toddler	May require help of another person
	May require some type of restraint if no assistance is available
	Let child explore an empty medicine cup
	Explain reasons for medication
	Crush tablets if not chewable variety
	If cooperative, child may hold medicine cup
	Allow child to drink at own pace
	When giving medications IM, carry out injection quickly and gently
	Be prepared to find that resistive behavior will be at its peak, particularly kicking, crying, and thrashing about
	Be prepared to be surprised, as some toddlers are very cooperative
Preschool	Chewable tablets and liquids are preferred
	Regression in pill taking may be seen
	Watch for loose teeth that could be swallowed
	Avoid prolonged reasoning
	Involve parents if appropriate
	Provide puppet play to help child express frustrations concerning injections
	Praise child following procedure
School Age	Can take pills and capsules; instruct child to place pill near back of tongue and immediately swallow water
	Emphasize swallowing of fluid to distract child from swallowing of pill
	Some children will continue to have a difficult time swallowing pills, and other forms of the medication should be explored (many come in suspensions); never ridicule child
	Children can be unpredictable from day to day in their cooperation; allow more time for the giving of pediatric medications
	Always ascertain that child is fully awake (particularly after nap time and during night shift)
	Always inform child of what you are about to do
	Remain with fearful child after procedure until composure is regained
	When this is not possible or appears prolonged, enlist help of auxiliary personnel
Adolescent	Prepare patient with explanations suitable to understanding
	Always ensure privacy
	Teach adolescent what side effects to report
	Identify adolescents on contraceptives to avoid drug interactions (may have been too embarrassed to provide information during history or may be attempting to keep secret from significant others)
	Remain with patient until medicine is consumed (particularly if the patient has a behavioral disorder)
	Anticipate mood swings in compliance
	Consider possibility of adolescent addiction (drugs, alcohol) even though this may not be presenting problem; many medications would be altered by such conditions

otherwise unpalatable. Cherry syrup or jelly may be used. Use of important sources of nutrients such as orange juice for this purpose is discouraged because the child may develop a distaste for them. Never refer to the medication as "candy." Administer medication slowly, especially if the child is crying. *Elevate the patient's head and shoulders to prevent aspiration.* Toddlers may attempt to push the medicine cup away. In anticipation of this the child is held in the nurse's lap in a semi-sitting position with hands restrained (Fig. 3–17). "Chasers" of water, fruit juice, or carbonated beverage are appreciated. In choosing a chaser, the patient's age and diet are considered.

If a nasogastric tube is in place, test for proper placement of the tube before pouring medication into the funnel. Administer a small amount of

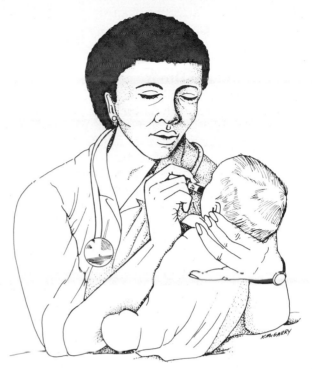

▲ **FIGURE 3–18**

Medications can be administered to the infant using an oral syringe. The head of the infant must be elevated when oral medications are given.

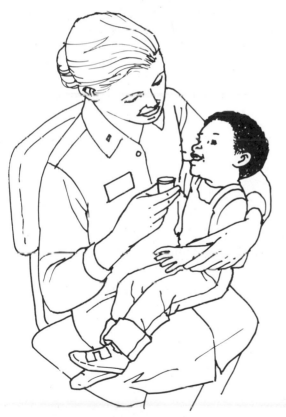

▲ **FIGURE 3–17**

The cup method of administering medication. The nurse may hold the child on the lap and restrain the child's hands as shown to prevent spilling of the medication.

water afterward to cleanse the tube. Record the procedure on the intake and output sheet.

For infants an oral syringe is an excellent device for measuring small quantities (Fig. 3–18). It is easily transported, and medication can be given directly from the syringe. Inspect for rough edges before using it. Place the syringe midway back at the side of the mouth. An empty nipple also may be used. Apply a bib to an infant before performing the procedure. Do not place medication in a bottle of juice or water; if some of the contents are refused, there is no way to determine how much of the drug was consumed. A plastic medicine dropper is useful and may be provided with the medication by the drug manufacturer. Use only for the medication specified, as these droppers are not intended for measuring other liquids. A drug ordered in teaspoons should be measured in milliliters to ensure accuracy (5 ml = 1 teaspoon). When administering medications in pediatric units, it is particularly important to keep the medicine cart or tray in sight at all times, so that a child does not take or play with any medications.

Nose, Ear, and Eye Drops

Except for a few differences, the principles of administering nose, ear, and eye drops to children are essentially the same as for adults. Infants and small children may need to be restrained. If restraint is necessary, a second person can help or a mummy restraint can be used. Warm all medications to room temperature. Explain the procedure to the child in age-appropriate detail.

Nose Drops. To administer nose drops, first wipe mucus from the nose with a tissue. Position the infant or child lying flat with head over the edge of a pillow. Encircle the child's cheeks and chin with your left arm, to hold the head steady. Instill the drops with the right hand. Keep the child in this position with head back for 1 minute to allow the drops to reach the proper area.

After instilling the drops, chart the time, name of medication, strength, number of drops instilled, how child tolerated the procedure, and untoward reactions.

Ear Drops. The doctor may prescribe a drug to be instilled into the ear to relieve pain. Ear drops should be warmed to room temperature before instilling. The infant and young child may need to be restrained during this procedure. Cooperation may be gained through the use of games and the involvement of parents. In the child under 3 years of age, the infected ear is drawn down and back to straighten the canal, and the correct number of drops is instilled. In the older child, the earlobe is pulled up and back to obtain a straight canal. The patient remains supine for a few minutes to permit the fluid to be absorbed. The nurse charts the following: time, name of drug, number of drops administered, the area (right or left ear), untoward reactions, and whether or not the patient obtained relief.

The area in front of the ear may be gently massaged to aid in the entry of the drops into the ear canal. A cotton pledget may be placed in the canal to prevent leakage of medication; however, this should be loose enough to allow for drainage.

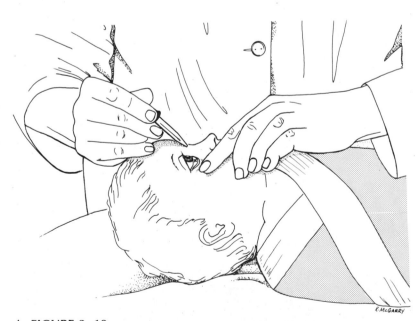

▲ **FIGURE 3–19**

Technique of instilling eye drops. The eye drops should fall in the center of the lower conjunctival sac, never directly on the eyeball. Put pressure on the lacrimal gland to prevent systemic absorption.

Eye Drops. Ophthalmic medication is administered to a child in the same manner as for the adult. Ascertain which eye requires treatment: O.D., right eye; O.S., left eye; O.U., both eyes. The child should be either supine or in the sitting position (Fig. 3–19). The infant and small child may need to be restrained.

With the thumb and index finger, use gentle pressure in opposite directions to open the eye. Instruct the child to "look up." Supporting the hand on the patient's forehead, instill the medication into the center of the lower lid (conjunctival sac). Instruct the child to close the eye but not to squeeze it, as this could expel some of the solution. Infants may clench their eyes shut. When this happens, the drops can be placed in the nasal corner where the lids meet. When the child opens the lids, the medication flows onto the conjunctiva.

Ointment is applied into the same conjunctival sac as the eye drops. Excess ointment may be wiped outward with a tissue.

Intramuscular Injections

The recommended injection site for children under 3 years of age is the vastus lateralis. It is the largest muscle mass in infants and small children and has few major nerves and blood vessels. After age 3 the ventrogluteal site may be used. The dorsogluteal site should not be used in any child who has not been walking for at least 2 years, and it is generally avoided in children under 6 years of age. The deltoid is also avoided in children under 6 years, and it should be used only for very small amounts of medication. Figure 3 20 shows the location of preferred injection sites.

The size of the syringe and needle to be used depends on several factors: size of the child, amount of medication to be given, amount of muscle tissue available, and the viscosity of the medication. A 25- to 27-gauge needle with a 0.5 to 1 inch length is usually used.

The nurse should anticipate some protest from children in regard to injections. Whenever possible, a second nurse should assist to distract the child and restrain the patient when necessary. If a parent chooses to be present, he or she should not be asked to restrain the child but rather should be there for distraction before and comforting after the procedure. The nurse should remain with the child until the child is calm and can focus attention on more pleasant things.

> **COMMUNICATION ALERT ► ► ► ► ►**
> When children ask if a procedure will hurt, the nurse should be truthful. The nurse might say, "Some children say it feels a little like a mosquito bite. I want you to tell me what you think after we are finished."

Intravenous Medications

Medications given by the intravenous (IV) route are being administered routinely in pediatric patients. Some drugs are effective only if given by this method. The medication is also absorbed more rapidly, which is of value. It is also less traumatic for the child to receive some medications, such as pain medications and antibiotics, intravenously rather than intramuscularly. The nurse assesses the IV site carefully for infiltration, inflammation, and patency, particularly prior to the administration of medication.

Compatibility is always checked between the fluid that is infusing and the medication to be given. If two drugs are ordered to be given at the same time, compatibility must be checked again. Medication is never administered via blood products.

Intravenous fluids given to children should be administered through a continuous infusion pump to prevent fluid overload. Medications may be added directly to the IV bag or bottle. More often medications are added to the Soluset (calibrated burette) or are given by precision-controlled syringe pumps. The precision-controlled syringe pump, sometimes called an auto-syringe, allows a small amount of fluid to be given over a specified period of time. Although the use of this equipment provides a safety factor, the nurse must remember that it is a machine and is subject to failing. For this reason, children receiving intravenous fluids must be observed closely. The "piggyback" method is also used in children. In general, antibiotics should infuse within 1 hour.

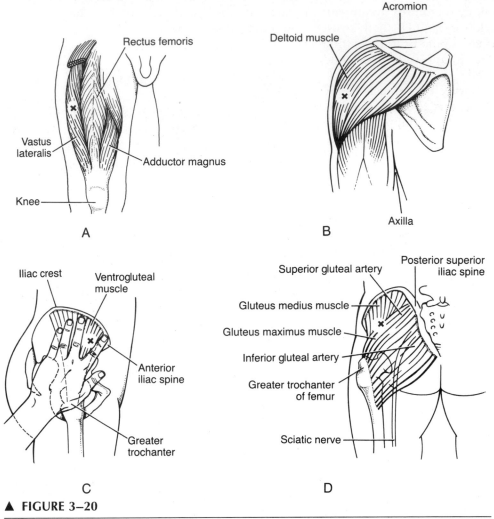

▲ **FIGURE 3–20**

Injection sites. *A, Vastus lateralis site,* in the midthird of the thigh. It is found by dividing the thigh into thirds from the greater trochanter to just above the knee. The area of insertion within the midthird of the thigh is found midway between imaginary lines midanteriorly and midlaterally. *B, Deltoid site,* in the lower part of the upper third of the deltoid. The site of insertion is midway between the acromion and the axilla on the lateral surface of the arm. *C, Ventrogluteal site.* Place the palm on the greater trochanter and the index finger on the anterior iliac spine (this may be facilitated by the flexion of the thigh at the hip). The middle finger is extended along the iliac crest as far as possible, forming a triangle. The injection is given in the center of the triangle, or V, formed by the hand, with the needle directed slightly upward toward the iliac crest. *D, Gluteal region.* Injection is given into the gluteus medius. The site is found by locating the greater trochanter and posterior iliac spine. Draw an imaginary line between these two points and inject above the line into the gluteus medius. (From Foster, R., Hunsberger, M., and Anderson, J. J. [1989]. *Family-Centered Nursing Care of Children,* Philadelphia, W. B. Saunders Company.)

Long-Term Venous Access

The heparin lock is usually used as an alternative for a keep-open infusion when long-term access is needed for administration of medication. The needle remains in place and is flushed with heparin according to the protocol of the hospital.

Indwelling central venous catheters (Broviac or Hickman catheters) and implantable infusion ports (MediPort, Port-A-Cath) are other methods of obtaining long-term venous access. Medications, chemotherapy, IV fluids, and blood products can be given through the catheter. The child and the parents are taught how to care for the catheter at home. There is a varied approach to care of these catheters, and each institution will provide this information.

Rectal Medications

Some drugs come in the form of suppositories, e.g., aspirin and glycerin. Children's suppositories are long and thin in comparison with the cone-shaped types administered to adults. The nurse, wearing a rubber glove or finger cot, inserts the lubricated suppository well beyond the anal sphincter about half as far as the forefinger will reach. The nurse applies pressure to the anus by gently holding the buttocks together until the patient's desire to expel the suppository subsides.

Principles of Fluid Balance in Children

Infants and small children have different *proportions of body water and body fat* than do adults (Fig. 3–21), and the water needs and water losses of the infant, per unit of body weight, are greater. In children under 2 years of age, *surface area* is particularly important in fluid and electrolyte balance because more water is lost through the skin than through the kidneys. The surface area of the infant is two to three times greater than that of the adult in proportion to body volume or body weight. *Metabolic rate and heat production* are also two to three times greater in infants per kilogram of body weight. This produces more *waste products,* which must be diluted in order to be excreted. It also stimulates respiration, which causes greater evaporation through the lungs. Compared with adults, a greater percentage of body water of children under age 2 years is contained in the *extracellular compartment.*

Fluid turnover is rapid and *dehydration* occurs more quickly in infants than in adults. The infant cannot survive as long as the adult can in the presence of continued water depletion. A sick infant does not adapt as rapidly to *shifts in intake and output* because the *kidneys lack maturity.* They are less able to concentrate urine and require more water than an adult's kidneys to excrete a given amount of solute. Disturbances of the gastrointestinal tract frequently lead to vomiting and diarrhea. Electrolyte balance depends on fluid balance and cardiovascular, renal, adrenal, pituitary, parathyroid, and pulmonary regulatory mechanisms. Many of these mechanisms are maturing in the developing child and are unable to react to full capacity under the stress of illness.

NURSING BRIEF ▷ ▷ ▷ ▷ ▷ ▷ ▷ ▷
One way of determining fluid loss in infants is to weigh the dry diaper, mark the weight on the outside of the diaper, and then weigh the wet diaper. This includes both urine and liquid stools.

Oral Fluids

Whenever possible, fluids are given by mouth. It is the most natural and satisfactory method. The nurse must use her ingenuity to encourage the sick child to take enough fluids because the patient may refuse food and water and cannot understand their relation to recovery. The infant and small child become dehydrated more quickly than does the adult. Toddlers and infants are not capable of drinking by themselves. The busy nurse must find time to offer fluids and must be patient and gently persistent. Liquids are offered frequently and in small amounts. Brightly colored containers and drinking straws may be a help. The nurse keeps an accurate record of the patient's intake and output. The doctor cannot determine whether a child requires intravenous fluids with a partially completed chart. *One cannot overemphasize the im-*

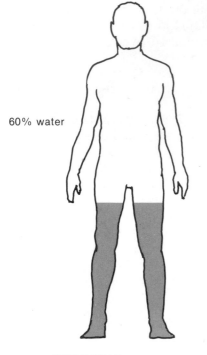
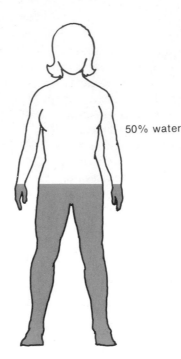
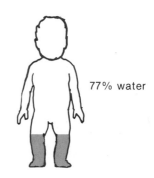

ADULT MALE

60% water
48% intracellular
15% extracellular
40% fats and solids

ADULT FEMALE

50% water
35% intracellular
15% extracellular
50% fats and solids

INFANT

77% water
48% intracellular
29% extracellular
23% fats and solids

▲ FIGURE 3–21

Average body weight composition. Water (particularly extracellular water) makes up a larger percentage of an infant's total body weight than of an adult's. Because extracellular water is lost first when water loss occurs in illness, trauma, or environmental stress, the infant is extremely susceptible to fluid and electrolyte imbalances.

portance of this particular responsibility on the pediatric unit.

Some common clear liquid fluids used to replace fluid lost are popsicles, decarbonated cola or ginger ale, gelatin water, and the glucose-electrolyte oral solutions (Lytren, Pedialyte). Milk is not included because of the curding that occurs when it combines with renin in the stomach.

Parenteral Fluids

Parenteral (*para*, beside or apart from + *enteron*, intestine) fluids are those given by some route other than the digestive tract. This is necessary when sickness is accompanied by vomiting or loss of consciousness or when the gastrointestinal system requires rest. Use of parenteral fluids is important in severe cases of vomiting and diarrhea in which the loss of excessive water and electrolytes will lead to death if untreated. It also provides a means for the safe and effective administration of selective parenteral medications. Solutions given parenterally must be sterile to prevent a general or local infection. The nurse must be aware of the importance of parenteral therapy and the problems that might arise.

The infant or child receiving parenteral fluids needs the nurse's warmth and affection. Babies miss being held and are also deprived of the pleasures they receive from sucking. The doctor may recommend that a pacifier be used, if it is not contraindicated. Older children need suitable diversions and company. All children receiving parenteral fluids are charted for intake and output.

Fluids Given by Vein. Intravenous infusion presents certain problems in pediatric patients. The procedure is more complicated and dangerous in infants and small children and is more taxing psychologically. The infant's veins are small and hard to locate. Often the veins of the scalp are used, which requires shaving the head. The baby must be effectively restrained to prevent the needle from becoming dislodged. When fluids are given intravenously, regardless of the site, the infant must be *closely observed*. Fluids given by vein are passing into a closed space that can be distended only to a certain point without serious difficulties. If the circulation becomes overloaded with fluid that is infused too rapidly, cardiac failure can result. The flow of a solution can become disturbed when an infant cries or wiggles.

The nurse should observe the child for these changes:

1. **Increase in the rate of flow of a solution**
2. **Swelling at the insertion site**
3. **Decrease or stopping of dripping**
4. **Low volume in the bottle, bag, or Soluset**
5. **Pain or redness at the insertion site**
6. **Moisture at the site or on the dressing covering the site**

A special hourly chart is kept on infants who are being given fluids by vein. The nurse charts such information as time, name and amount of the solution, amount absorbed, number of drops per minute, amount of fluid remaining in the bottle, and condition of site.

Modern adapting devices are used to improve the accuracy and safety of IV fluids. In the past it was difficult to slow down an IV infusion to 4 to 6 drops per minute without stopping the flow completely. The "mini" or "micro" drop decreases the size of the drop and allows the patient to receive 50 to 60 "mini" or "micro" drops per cubic centimeter rather than the usual 15 drops from the standard setup. Another device uses a graduated control chamber, which is attached to the IV bottle to ensure that the child does not receive too much fluid too fast. Most hospitals are also using parenteral fluid regulators such as the IVAC pump

to monitor infusions. An alarm sounds when difficulties arise. Such safeguards, nevertheless, do not replace close observation and charting by the nurse.

Total Parenteral Nutrition (TPN)

Intravenous alimentation (IVA) solutions are complex combinations of crystalline amino acids, dextrose, vitamins, trace minerals, and electrolytes. Conditions other than low birth weight that may require its use include severe burns, chronic intestinal obstruction, intractable diarrhea, irradiation, and other life-threatening maladies. Although the beginning student would not be given total responsibility for the child receiving TPN, all nursing personnel must be alert to the fact that this is not just the usual superficial vein infusion.

A Silastic catheter is passed directly into the superior vena cava by way of the jugular or subclavian vein using careful surgical technique. It is secured in place. A Millipore filter is attached to filter out bacteria and minimize contamination. An IV pump monitors the flow. The patient receiving TPN requires careful supervision and evaluation. Complications of this therapy can be serious and are related to both the catheter and the metabolism of the infusate. Contamination via catheter or solution is particularly dangerous because infectious organisms have direct access to body circulation. Thrombosis, dislodgement of the catheter, and *extravasation* (the escape of fluid into surrounding tissue) can occur. *Metabolic* complications include hyperglycemia due to the high glucose content of the solution, osmotic diuresis, dehydration, and *azotemia* (the presence of nitrogenous bodies in the blood). Home hyperalimentation is now being successfully utilized for selected children. This requires specific instruction and demonstrations by specialty teams. Continuous support and supervision are vital to success. The parents' insurance coverage requires investigation, as home hyperalimentation is costly.

Peripheral vein hyperalimentation may be used for short-term therapy or as a supplement to intravenous alimentation. More diluted solutions are used. Infiltration must be avoided, as severe tissue sloughing due to dextrose irritation may occur. Since hyperalimentation provides no fatty acids, solutions such as Intralipid 10 per cent may be ordered; this is administered via a peripheral line.

Procedures to Assist Nutrition, Digestion, and Elimination

Gastrostomy

A gastrostomy (*gastro,* stomach + *stoma,* opening) is made for the purpose of introducing food directly into the stomach through the abdominal wall. This is done by means of a surgically placed tube or button. It is used in patients who cannot have food by mouth because of anomalies or corrosive strictures of the esophagus or who are severely debilitated or in coma.

GASTROSTOMY TUBE FEEDING

PROCEDURE ▶ ▶ ▶ ▶ ▶ ▶ ▶ ▶ ▶

Equipment. Tray with warmed formula, funnel or syringe barrel, syringe for aspiration, 15 to 30 ml of water to flush tube as ordered.

Note: Equipment should be sterile for premature and newborn infants.

1. Position child comfortably, either flat or with head slightly elevated if not contraindicated. Provide pacifier to relax baby.

2. Check residual stomach contents by attaching syringe to gastrostomy tube and aspirating. If amount of residual is large (10 to 25 ml for neonates, over 50 ml for older children), replace residual and decrease present formula by equal amount or delay feeding for a short time. (This may vary according to the pediatrician's protocol.) Overloading the stomach can cause reflux and increases the danger of aspiration. If residual continues or increases, report this to the physician.

3. Attach syringe barrel (if not already present for continuous elevation) to gastrostomy tube. Fill with formula. Remove clamp. (This prevents air from entering the stomach and causing distention.)

4. Elevate receptacle. Allow formula to flow slowly by gravity—force should not be used.

5. Continue to add formula to the syringe before it empties completely. The feeding should take 15 to 20 minutes to complete.

6. Clamp the tube as the final formula or water is passing through the lower part of the syringe. (*Note:* In infants some physicians may prefer that the gastrostomy tube remain open at all times to produce a safety valve in the event that the baby vomits. In such cases the tube is elevated above the patient's body.)

7. Whenever possible, hold the patient quietly after feeding. Reposition in Fowler's position or on right side to promote gastric emptying.

8. Record the type (gastrostomy feeding), the amount given, the amount and characteristics of residual, and how the patient tolerated the procedure. If the patient is on measured fluids, record on intake and output section.

GASTROSTOMY BUTTON FEEDING

PROCEDURE ▶ ▶ ▶ ▶ ▶ ▶ ▶ ▶ ▶

Equipment. Tray with warmed formula, bolus feeding tube, 60-ml catheter tip syringe, water.

1. Twist the feeding button a full circle. (The button is correctly positioned when it turns easily.)

2. Attach the syringe to the feeding tube and purge the tube. Clamp the tube to prevent the fluid from escaping.

3. Attach the feeding tube to the button by holding one of the wings securely and pushing the end of the feeding tube into the button.

4. Open the clamp until the fluid begins to flow. Allow 15 to 20 minutes for the feeding.

5. Flush with water.

6. Remove the feeding tube by firmly grasping the wing of the button and withdrawing the tube.

7. Snap the attached plug into the lumen of the button (Huth, M., and O'Brien, M., 1987).

In both the tube and button, skin care is a concern. Special attention should be paid to the area under the wings of the button. To prevent this, the wings are periodically rotated; if breakdown does occur, the button is changed to one that has a longer shaft. The area around the stoma should be cleansed frequently with mild soap and water. If a dressing is used, it should be kept dry (Huth, M., and O'Brien, M., 1987).

Enema

Administering an enema to a child is essentially the same as to an adult; however, the amount, type, and pressure of the solution require modifications. An isotonic solution is used with children instead of tap water. Tap water is hypotonic and can cause a rapid fluid shift and overload. Commercial enemas are available specifically for children. Always be certain you know what type of solution is intended. This is an invasive procedure for the patient; therefore, careful age-appropriate explanations are necessary. Other invasive procedures related to the gastrointestinal tract include barium enema, intestinal biopsy, endoscopy, and colonoscopy. These are performed by the gastroenterologist. It is important to allow children to express all concerns in regard to these tests and for the nurse to give feedback to physicians concerning the difference in behavior between children who were well prepared and those who did not benefit from preparation.

PROCEDURE ▶ ▶ ▶ ▶ ▶ ▶ ▶ ▶ ▶

Equipment. Disposable irrigation bag with connecting tube and clamp. For smaller amounts, funnel or Asepto syringe and pitcher, No. 10 to 12 French catheter, saline solution (1 teaspoon of salt to 1 pint of water), lubricant, toilet paper, rubber sheet, incontinent pad, bedpan with cover, extra diapers.

1. Assemble the equipment and take it to the bedside.
2. Place the rubber sheet and incontinent pad beneath child.
3. Pad the bedpan with a diaper. Place the child's pillow under the head and back.
4. Place the child on the bedpan. Restrain the legs by a diaper brought under the bedpan and

pinned over the legs. Older children are positioned in the same manner as adults are.
5. Allow the solution to run through the tubing to warm it and to expel air.
6. Insert the tube 1.5 to 4 inches into the rectum, depending upon the age of the child.
7. Administer the prescribed amount of fluid, which will be from 150 to 750 ml, depending upon the age of the child. The temperature of the solution should range from 37.8 to 40.6°C (100 to 105°F).
8. Hold the irrigating bag not more than 18 inches above the level of the patient's hips. The solution should run slowly without pressure. Clamp the tubing at intervals.
9. Remain with the patient while the enema is being expelled. Small children may use the pot chair.
10. Remove the bedpan and pillow. Cleanse the buttocks.
11. Remove the rubber sheet and incontinent pad.
12. Apply a clean diaper. Check to see if a stool specimen is desired.
13. Chart: time of procedure; name, amount, and temperature of solution used; amount and character of results; untoward reactions.

Aftercare of Equipment. Empty and cleanse the bedpan. Discard disposable enema setup and tubing.

Oil Retention Enema. When giving an oil retention enema, use the prescribed amount, generally 60 to 100 ml of oil at 37.8°C (100°F). Apply gentle pressure over the anal area to prevent the oil from being expelled. A cleansing enema (saline) generally follows within one half to three quarters of an hour.

CARE OF THE CHILD WITH A TRACHEOSTOMY

A tracheostomy is a surgical procedure in which an opening is made in the trachea to enable the patient to breathe. This artificial airway may be used in emergency situations, may be an elective procedure, or may be combined with mechanical ventilation. Some of the childhood conditions that may require tracheostomy are acute laryngotracheobronchitis, epiglottitis, head injury, burns, and any condition in which the patient is unconscious or debilitated for an extended period. Nursing care is indispensable to the survival of the patient, as blockage of the tube by mucus or other secretions can lead to suffocation. In many hospitals the patient is placed in the intensive care unit immediately following surgery, because this is a critical period requiring frequent suctioning and very close observation. When the child's condition stabilizes, she or he is transferred to a regular unit.

The child is placed in an area of high visibility. Infants and small children communicate their needs by crying. The tracheostomy prohibits vocalization. Whenever possible one person is assigned to the child and to work with the parents. Reinforce preoperative teaching. Explain what has happened in an age-appropriate manner. For example, "You were having a lot of trouble breathing. This operation called a tracheostomy helps you breathe easier. A small opening has been made in your neck. A hollow tube was inserted to keep the area open. It is frightening not to be able to speak. When you are better the hole will close by itself and your voice will return." An explanation of suction might be, "We have to keep the area in your neck open. This tube goes into the throat and clears it." Demonstrate use of suction in a glass of water. Prepare the child for the unfamiliar sound. "You might feel like gagging, but afterwards you will feel better. I know this is difficult for you and I'm sorry there is no easier way." Another approach is to make up a story involving the child's favorite toy, which goes to the repair shop because the toy is having trouble breathing.

The nursing care of the child with a tracheostomy is a significant responsibility. The anatomical differences between children and adults and the small child's inability to communicate through writing increase the need for close observation. Toddlers often have short, stubby necks that become easily irritated. It may be helpful to place a reminder on the intercom at the clerk's desk or in other suitable areas indicating that this patient cannot cry or speak. The nurse's touch and quiet voice and the presence of significant others promote security in the child.

Room temperature should be comfortably warm. Added moisture and humidity are provided by the use of a mist tent, a special tracheostomy collar, or direct attachment to a mechanical ventilator. This is necessary because the nose and mouth no longer warm and moisten the inspired air. Provide adequate fluids.

Maintaining *patency* of the tracheostomy tube is of utmost importance. Plastic or Silastic tubes are generally used, as they are flexible and reduce crust formation. They are lightweight and disposable, and most do not have inner cannulas. Cuffed tubes are not usually necessary in infants and small children, as their air passages are smaller and the tracheostomy tube provides a sufficient seal. The surgeon chooses a tracheostomy tube that is appropriate for the size of the patient's neck and condition.

Suctioning and Changing Tubes

Selection of a suction catheter by the nurse is of importance. Choose one that will not completely block the tube during suctioning. The diameter should be approximately one half that of the tracheostomy tube. Measure the length of the tracheostomy tube (use an extra one) and pass the suction catheter only the measured length to prevent trauma to the mucosa. A small amount of sterile isotonic saline (0.5 to 2 ml) can be injected into the tube prior to suctioning to aid in loosening secretions and crusts. Check your agency for the accepted procedure. Suction is not applied as the catheter is introduced. Withdraw the catheter while rotating and applying suction by covering the port on the catheter with the thumb.

Suctioning is done at intervals (three to four times daily) and when there are signs of secretions in the airway. This may include coughing, noisy breathing, or a bubbling sound. The child should be allowed to rest for about a minute between suctioning. Aseptic technique must be used. Nurses should be aware of any variations in this procedure that might be unique to the agency in which they are working.

PROCEDURE ▶ ▶ ▶ ▶ ▶ ▶ ▶ ▶ ▶

Equipment. Sterile tracheostomy tube, twill tape, scissors, sterile cotton-tipped applicators, sterile water, hydrogen peroxide, sterile dressing or Telfa pad, sterile suctioning catheters, sterile gloves, sterile saline.

1. Use sterile technique when suctioning or changing the tube.

2. Instill 0.5 to 2 ml of normal saline into the trachea before suctioning to loosen secretions. (The amount instilled depends upon the size of the child.)

3. Lubricate the tube with sterile saline and insert the catheter without applying suction.

4. Withdraw the catheter in a continuous rotating motion while applying suction (5 seconds in infant, 10 to 15 seconds in older children).

5. Allow the child to rest. Some children may need a few breaths via a resuscitation bag.

6. Clear the catheter with sterile water between insertions.

7. Discard the suction tube and gloves after each use. Water should also be discarded to prevent growth of *Pseudomonas* in the standing water.

The tracheal stoma is treated as a surgical wound. Keep the area free of secretions and exudate to minimize the risk of infection. Cotton-tipped applicators dipped in half-strength hydrogen peroxide can be used to remove crusted mucus. Rinse by dipping in sterile water. Tapes around the child's neck should be snug, but loose enough to insert one finger easily. Place the knot to the side of the neck. Assess the condition of the skin beneath the tape. Change the tape as necessary. Two people should be used for this procedure, one to hold the cannula and the other to change the tape. When feeding the infant, cover the tracheostomy with a bib or moist piece of gauze to prevent aspiration of food particles.

The nurse observes the patient for such symptoms as restlessness, rising pulse rate, fatigue, apathy, dyspnea, sternal retractions, pallor, cyanosis, and inflammation or drainage around the incision. Possible complications include tracheoesophageal fistula, stenosis, tracheal ischemia, infection, atelectasis, cannula occlusion, and accidental extubation. Baseline assessment of the patient is done on each shift and prior to suctioning. The patient's mental status, respirations, pulse rate and rhythm, and chest sounds are of particular importance. Accurate recording of observations is essential to evaluation. The time and frequency of suctioning, the character of secretions, the relief afforded the patient, the patient's behavior, the appearance of the wound, and other pertinent data are recorded.

A sterile hemostat is kept at the bedside for emergency use. Accidental *extubation* or expulsion of the tube, although uncommon, can occur from severe coughing if the tapes are too loose. Patency of the airway is maintained by spreading the edges of the wound with the sterile clamp until a duplicate tube is inserted. An extra tracheostomy tube and the equipment needed for its replacement are always kept in a visible, easily reached area at the bedside for use in such emergencies. As the child's condition improves, he or she is weaned from the tube. The opening will gradually close by granulation. Children whose tubes must remain in place longer require periodic tube change.

Additional nursing measures include frequent change of position, the use of arm restraints, oral feedings unless contraindicated, and careful bathing to prevent water from entering the tube. Range of motion exercises are a must for long-term patients, and, in acute cases, arm restraints are removed one at a time to allow for passive exercises. The diet is ordered by the physician. Although patients initially may have nothing by mouth (NPO), as their conditions improve they progress to a soft or normal diet. Fowler's position is preferred during feedings. Older children can cooperate by holding the head flexed with chin down. This decreases swallowing difficulties, as the esophagus opens and the airway narrows.

Some patients are discharged with a tracheostomy (Fig. 3–22). This should be anticipated, and instruction and demonstration for the parents should be begun early. Parents who are comfortable with the procedure during hospitalization will feel more secure when the child returns home. It is advisable that the parents spend one night with the child before discharge. Information about parent groups and visiting nurse and other referrals are made prior to discharge.

OXYGEN THERAPY FOR CHILDREN

General Safety Considerations

It is important that all equipment used for oxygen therapy be inspected periodically to determine

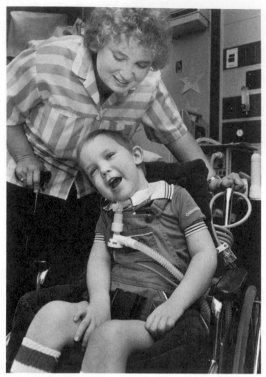

▲ **FIGURE 3–22**

The acuity levels of discharged patients necessitate careful instruction of caregivers. This child is returning home with a tracheostomy in place. (Courtesy of Blank Memorial Hospital for Children, Des Moines, Iowa.)

Prolonged exposure to high oxygen concentrations can be toxic to some body tissues, e.g., the retina in preterm babies and the lungs in the general population but particularly in children with pulmonary diseases such as asthma or cystic fibrosis. It is therefore necessary to measure oxygen content at regular intervals with an *oxygen analyzer*. This is usually done by the respiratory department; however, the nurse needs to ensure that the procedure is carried out on the assigned patients. Readings should be obtained close to the child's head. The amount of oxygen administered will depend on the child's arterial oxygen concentration. Frequent blood gas determinations (PO_2 and PCO_2) will assure safe and accurate therapy. Noninvasive techniques that measure blood oxygen tension via the skin are available. One example is the oximeter.

Oxygen is a dry gas and requires the addition of moisture to prevent irritation of the respiratory tree. *Oxygen therapy should be terminated gradually.* This allows the patient to adjust to *ambient* (environmental) oxygen. Slowly reduce liter flow, open air vents in incubators, or open zippers in the oxygen tent. Constantly monitor the child's response. An increase in restlessness and an increase in pulse and respirations indicate that the child is not tolerating withdrawal from the oxygen-enriched environment.

that materials are intact and that no pieces are missing. Keep combustible materials and potential sources of fire away from oxygen equipment. These materials are essentially the same as for adults; however, for the child friction toys are also to be avoided. Nylon or wool blankets are not to be used. Know where the nearest fire extinguisher is located. Alert parents to the presence of no smoking signs.

Infection control is extremely important. It is imperative that cross-infection via unclean equipment be prevented. Humidifiers and nebulizers, which are warm and moist, serve as an excellent medium for the growth of disease-producing organisms. Although most masks, tents, and cannulas that come into direct contact with the child are disposable, other pieces of mechanical equipment cannot be discarded. *They require periodic cleansing if therapy is extended and terminal cleaning according to product direction.*

Methods of Administration

Oxygen is administered to pediatric patients as age-appropriate via Isolette, nasal cannula, mask, hood, or tent (Table 3–7). Regardless of the method used, the child is observed frequently to determine the effectiveness of the oxygen. *The desired goals include decreased restlessness and improved breathing, vital signs, and color.* The highest concentrations of oxygen are delivered by way of a plastic hood. Warmed, humidified oxygen is delivered directly over the child's head. It may be used in an incubator or warming unit.

Oxygen tents are available from various manufacturers. The directions for the specific apparatus should be closely followed. Before assembling the tent, carefully examine the plastic for tears. Tents consist of a plastic canopy suspended from an overhead rod that is attached to a cabinet containing a machine. When adjusted, the machine reg-

Table 3–7. SELECTED CONSIDERATIONS FOR THE CHILD RECEIVING OXYGEN

AGE	COMMENTS

General Considerations: Signs of respiratory distress include an increase in pulse and respiration, restlessness, flaring nares, intercostal and substernal retractions, and cyanosis. In addition, children with dyspnea frequently vomit, which increases the danger of aspiration. Maintain a clear airway by suctioning if needed. Organize nursing care so that interruptions are kept at a minimum. Observe children carefully, as your vision may be obstructed by mist, and young children are unable to verbalize their needs.

Neonate
Oxygen may be provided via hood, which may be used in incubator or warming unit
May be provided via Isolette; keep sleeves closed to decrease oxygen loss
Oxygen needs to be warmed to prevent neonatal stress from cold
Analyze concentration carefully to avoid retrolental fibroplasia or pulmonary disease
Parents are primary focus of preparations; help develop good parenting skills and self-confidence in their ability to care for the child who is ill

Infant
Nose may need to be suctioned by bulb syringe to remove mucus
May benefit from use of infant seat; secure seat to bedframe, watch for slumping in seat
Make sure cribsides are up; a canopy often gives the illusion of safety
Avoid the use of baby oil, A and D ointment, Vaseline or other oil- or alcohol-based substances
Anticipate stranger anxiety at around 8 months; baby clings to parents, turns away from nurse
An extremely irritable baby may benefit from comforting in parent's lap, followed by sleeping in tent; clarify at report time.
Frequently children can be removed from oxygen for bathing and eating; determine before proceeding

Toddler
Anticipate that a toddler will be distressed by a tent
Anticipate regression
A restless and fussy child may pull tent and covers apart
Toddler cannot tell nurse if tent is "too hot" or "too cold"
Change clothing and bed linen when damp
May be comforted by transitional object such as blanket
Parents may have suggestions as to how to keep child happy in tent

Preschool
Tent plastic distorts view
Because thought processes are immature in preschool children, reality and fantasy are inseparable
Prepare child for all procedures to decrease fear
Anticipate that child will feel lonely and isolated
Will enjoy stories, puppets, dramatic play
An extremely restless and anxious child may benefit from holding parent's hand through small opening in zippers
Helpful if child can be out of tent for meals and can eat with peers

School Age
School children usually are less frightened by tent; fears center around body mutilation and loss of control
Preparation information continues to focus on what the child will see, hear, feel, and be expected to do
Child may benefit from writing a story about the experience; nurse reviews story with child and clarifies misconceptions; posting story on unit affirms child's self-esteem and mastery (always ask permission to post)
Allow child to make realistic choices before, during, and after procedures
Draw "what it feels like to be in a tent," discuss

Adolescent
Needs more time to process information, needs to know the results of blood studies and other tests
Nurse remains available to the patient to answer questions as they arise
Trust is extremely important as adolescent attempts to move beyond the nuclear family
Anticipate problems of being restricted by apparatus
May feel "weird" when visited by peers, wavers between feeling self-confident and feeling ineffective
Reiterate no smoking and other safety precautions with patient and peers
Include patient in therapy, may be able to manage own oxygen needs
Review safe use of oxygen in the home if required for comfort and survival

ulates the ventilation and temperature of the tent and may also provide increased humidity in connection with the oxygen flow. Following are several general recommendations for the use of tents:

1. Prepare bed and place bath blanket, rubber sheet, or absorbent pad over the mattress.

2. Select the tent according to the age and size of the patient. This information will need to be ascertained prior to admission for patients in acute respiratory distress.

3. Bring the canopy and control unit to the bedside; extend the overhead bar and fold tent out along the bar.

4. Plug in control cabinet and turn on unit. If there is a ventilation control on the refrigerator unit, set this halfway between low and high or according to the manufacturer's instructions.

5. Connect tubing to oxygen flow meter and flush tent with oxygen for 2 minutes. Reset flow meter to prescribed number of liters. Another method is to allow oxygen to flow at 15 liters for about 30 minutes. Analyze the concentration.

6. Maintain a tight canopy. Provide nursing care through zippered openings; organize nursing care. Oxygen loss is greater at the bottom of the tent, as oxygen is heavier than air. The front of the tent may be secured with bath blanket or sheet.

7. Tent temperature is adjusted to 17.8 to 21.1°C (64 to 70°F). The patient should not appear too warm or too cold. Dress the child according to body temperature.

8. Inspect connecting tubes periodically for kinks, loose connections, or faulty apparatus. A hissing sound can be heard as oxygen passes through the tubing if lines are patent. This may also be tested by holding one finger over the end momentarily.

9. Empty condensation reservoir as needed.

10. Refill distilled water jar as appropriate.

11. Select toys that retard absorption and will not produce static electricity.

ADAPTING PROCEDURES RELATED TO SURGERY

The child is particularly fearful of surgery and requires both physical and psychological preparation at the patient's level of understanding. Listening to the child is especially valuable in clarification of misunderstandings. Ask the child to point to the operative site on a body outline. "Show me what they are going to fix." Explain anesthesia and allow the child to play with a mask (Fig. 3–23). Children and adults need reassurance that

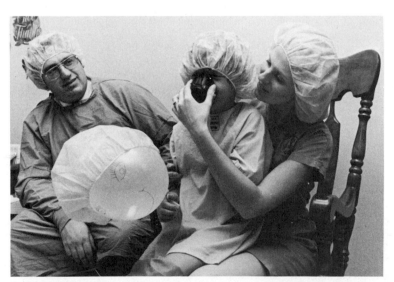

▲ **FIGURE 3–23**

Preparing the child for the sights and sounds of surgery. (Courtesy of Blank Memorial Hospital for Children, Des Moines, Iowa.)

they will not awake during surgery. Nursing interventions following surgery are aimed at assisting the child to master a threatening situation and minimizing physical and psychological complications. (See index for nursing care principles for specific surgery.)

Tables 3-8 and 3-9 summarize preparation for surgery and postoperative care.

THE CHILD WITH A CONTAGIOUS DISEASE

Any patient who is suspected of having a contagious disease must be isolated until a definite diagnosis has been established. A pediatric hospital will have an isolation unit for this purpose. The smaller children's division of a general hospital may not have these facilities. The nurse admitting the patient must take certain precautions. The purpose of medical aseptic technique is to prevent the spread of the disease to the nurse and others. *Proper handwashing* cannot be overemphasized.

The patient is placed in a private room. All unnecessary furnishings are removed before the patient's arrival. Place an ample supply of paper towels and soap near the sink. Attach a paper bag to the bed for the patient to use as a wastebasket. Equipment for daily patient care is placed in the unit. This includes thermometer, bath equipment, bedpan, urinal, tissues, and linen. Such equipment remains there until the patient is discharged, when it will be treated by terminal disinfection. Disposable equipment is discarded in the proper receptacle. Linen is changed daily. An ample supply of gowns, masks, and gloves saves much time and energy. A clean area is prepared according to hospital procedure. The floor is always considered contaminated. Anything that touches the floor must be discarded. Toys are tied to the bed with a short tape and must be washable.

In taking the blood pressure, the patient's arm and the bed are protected by a clean gown or sheet to prevent contamination of the sphygmomanometer. Built-in wall units reduce the danger of contamination. When a flashlight, otoscope, or ophthalmoscope is used, it is protected by a technique paper. Any part that comes in direct contact with the patient must be disinfected. All the specimens that leave the room are placed in a clean outer container according to hospital procedure. Trays necessary for general unit use are not brought into the patient's room. Remove the necessary articles, place them on a smaller paper tray, and carry the tray to the bedside.

Medical Asepsis

The purpose of medical aseptic technique is to prevent the spread of infection from one child to another or from the child to the nurse. A person or object is considered *contaminated* if it has touched the infected patient or any equipment that has come in contact with the patient. People or articles that have not had any contact with the patient are considered *clean*.

Articles that have come in direct contact with the patient must be *disinfected* before they can be used by others. When something is disinfected, microorganisms in or on it are killed by physical or chemical means. The autoclave, which uses steam under pressure, is considered very effective in killing most germs when the article is adequately exposed and sterilized for the proper length of time. However, some materials, e.g., the glass clinical thermometer, would be destroyed if autoclaved. A chemical disinfectant must be used instead. Before soaking an article in a disinfectant, the nurse must be sure that it has been properly washed in soap and water and rinsed. The strength of the disinfecting solution is generally determined by the hospital pharmacist and is dispensed to the units in suitable containers. Seventy per cent alcohol is an example of one type used. The article must be totally submerged and must remain in the solution for a *suitable length of time*. It is extremely important that articles in chemical solutions be marked with the time at which they are to be removed. If the nurse fails to do this, an unsuspecting person may assume that items are clean and may remove them before they are properly sterilized. Use disposable items, such as diapers, tissues, needles, suction catheters, syringes, thermometers, suture sets, dishes, nursing bottles, and utensils, whenever possible. They should be double-bagged and disposed of according to hospital procedure.

Table 3–8. PREPARATION OF THE CHILD FOR SURGERY

PROCEDURE	ADULT	CHILD	MODIFICATION
Consent	Yes	Yes	Parent or legal guardian
Blood work	Yes	Yes	Age-appropriate restraint
Urinalysis	Yes	Yes	Age-appropriate collection (U-bag)
			Assist schoool child
			Age-appropriate instructions
Evaluate for respiratory infection, nutritional status	Yes	Yes	Use more objective observations in infants and toddlers because of their limited verbal skills
Allergies	Yes	Yes	Indicate clearly on chart
NPO	Yes	Yes	Increase fluids prior to NPO
			Length of time may vary with age and type of surgery (6–12 hours)
			If surgery is late, place appropriate notice on child: "Do not feed me"
			Remove goodies from bedside stand
			No gum
			Supervise hungry ambulatory patients carefully
Vital signs	Yes	Yes	Approach child carefully, explain, demonstrate
Void before surgery	Yes	Preferred	Not always possible in infants and toddlers
Bath	Yes	Yes	Hospital gown; may wear underwear or pajama bottoms depending on age, type of surgery
Identification	Yes	Yes	Identiband
Teeth	Yes	Yes	Check for loose teeth, orthodontic appliance
Skin prep	Yes	Possible	May be done in OR
Nails	Yes	Yes	Trim, remove nail polish
Glasses or contact lenses	Yes	Yes	Have children and adolescents remove glasses and contact lenses
Enemas	Possible	Possible	Not routine
Transportation	Yes	Yes	Crib or stretcher
			Parents may accompany to OR door
Emotional preparation	Yes	Yes	Preoperative tour
			Group and individual puppet play
			Body drawings of parts involved
			Play selected by child as mode of expression
			Support parents during surgery
Sedation	Yes	Yes	Usually 20 minutes prior to surgery
Record all pertinent data	Yes	Yes	Essentially the same with pediatric modifications as indicated by the preceding

Table 3–9. SUMMARY OF POSTOPERATIVE CARE OF THE CHILD

PROCEDURE	ADULT	CHILD	MODIFICATION
Return from recovery room	Yes	Yes	Notify parents (parents may be allowed in recovery room)
			Smaller patients generally in crib
			Age-appropriate safety precautions
Note general condition, alertness	Yes	Yes	Infant and toddler cannot verbalize fear or pain
Vital signs	Yes	Yes	Every 15–30 minutes until stable
			Blood pressure reading is sometimes omitted for infant
Evaluate for shock	Yes	Yes	Essentially same
Assess operative site for bleeding, dressing intactness	Yes	Yes	Essentially same
			Elevate casted extremities
			Circle drainage
Restraints	Possible	Probable	May be necessary to protect IV line
			Remove periodically for range of motion
Connect dependent drainage (urinary catheter, Levin tubes, oxygen)	Yes	Yes	Prepare child for sight and noises of equipment, draw pictures to clarify purpose
Position patient	Yes	Yes	Abdomen or side unless contraindicated, no pillow
IVs	Yes	Yes	Should have pediatric adapting device (infusion pump)
			Monitor rate meticulously, as infants and small children respond quickly to fluid shifts
			Measure and record intake and output
Assess elimination	Yes	Yes	Bowel and bladder
Relief of pain	Yes	Yes	Hold, comfort small children unless contraindicated
			Be sensitive to behavioral changes such as increase in irritability, crying, regression, nail biting, passivity, withdrawal
			Administer pain relievers
			Involve parents in care
			Provide transitional object such as blanket, favorite toy, pacifier
			Be aware of transcultural considerations that provide familiarity and comfort
NPO	Yes	Yes	Until fully awake
			Babies are started on clear fluids by bottle unless contraindicated
			Avoid brown or red liquids, which may be confused with old or fresh blood
			Monitor bowel sounds
Consider diet	Yes	Yes	Advance from clear to full liquids to soft to regular diet
Observe for complications	Yes	Yes	Turn, cough, deep breathe, dangle feet, early ambulation; less of a problem in children
			Splint operative site with hands when child coughs

Used needles are not recapped and are placed in a properly labeled puncture-proof container. These special containers should be available in each patient room as well as other areas where disposal is likely.

Throughout this text, emphasis is placed on the role of the nurse in preparing a safe environment for the child and parents. Of all dangers in our surroundings, none is more serious than disease-bearing organisms. The nurse must understand the importance of protecting self and others from the isolated patient. This is accomplished by specific procedures such as cleaning and disinfecting clothing, bedding, excreta, and hospital equipment. While doing this, the nurse must not, however, forget that the patient is the primary concern. As the student's confidence increases with repetition of the details of isolation, the approach to the patient and the patient's problems also will be more effective.

Isolation precautions are presented in Table 3–10.

Preventing the Transmission of Infection

Universal Precautions. Because a history and physical examination cannot identify all patients infected with the human immunodeficiency virus (HIV) or other blood-borne pathogens, blood and body fluid precautions are used for all patients. Gloves should be worn for contact with blood or blood-containing fluids (see Table 3–10).

Respiratory Infections. These include most common childhood diseases. Precautions must be taken against discharges from the eyes, nose, throat, and ears. Caregivers wear a mask and hands must washed after touching the child or potentially contaminated articles and before taking care of another patient. Floors are damp-mopped to control dust.

Wound Infections. Organisms leave through the wound and may enter the body of the nurse through breaks in the skin, particularly of the hands. Germs may also become air-borne when a wound is dressed. An infected wound is kept covered. To handle the dressing, a nurse wears disposable gloves. The contaminated dressings are disposed of according to institution procedure.

Articles of clothing and bed linen that come in contact with the wound are treated as "precaution" linen. The nurse wears a gown if soiling is likely and gloves when changing a dressing. Hands must be washed after touching the patient and before contact with another patient. Floors are damp-mopped to control dust.

Skin Infections. If the lesions cannot be covered, the patient is isolated, and bedding, clothes, and dishes are disinfected. The nurse wears a gown and gloves.

Digestive Infections. Precautionary measures are taken against all discharges from the mouth, stomach, and intestinal tract. Dishes, toilet articles, bedding, and clothing are considered contaminated. Stools may require added disinfection in some diseases. The gown and glove technique is employed.

Genital Infections. The danger of this type of infection lies in the discharge coming in contact with the mucous membranes of the well person. The conjunctiva of the eye is particularly susceptible to infections from the same germs that invade the genitals. Soiled dressings are disposed of according to hospital policy. Precautions should be used when handling clothing, bedding, dishes, and toilet facilities. The gown and glove technique is used.

Specific Techniques

Handwashing. Handwashing is the most important barrier against transmission of disease. Hands should be washed before and after contact with every patient. Contact with a patient in isolation only increases the importance of the procedure.

Mask Technique. A supply of disposable masks is kept outside the patient's room. A fresh one should be donned each time the nurse enters the room. A mask is used once and discarded. It should never be allowed to hang around the neck and then be placed back over the face. It should cover the nose and mouth and should be changed at least once every hour. Do not touch a mask once it is in place. Remove it after the gown when leaving the unit, and do not touch the part that comes in contact with the face. Discard the mask in the room. Authorities disagree as to the effec-

Table 3–10. ISOLATION PRECAUTIONS

TYPES AND EXAMPLES[†]	PURPOSE	PRIVATE ROOM	ARTICLES
Universal (applies to all people regardless of known health status) Hepatitis B HIV and other blood-borne pathogens Includes blood, semen, vaginal secretions; and cerebrospinal, pleural, synovial, peritoneal, pericardial, and amniotic fluid	To prevent infections that are transmitted by direct or indirect contact with infected blood or body fluids	Yes, if patient hygiene is poor *Gowns and gloves* for direct contact	*Hands must be washed after touching the patient or potentially contaminated articles and blood or body fluids and before taking care of another patient* *Avoid needle puncture injury* Articles contaminated with infective material should be discarded or bagged and labeled before being sent for decontamination and reprocessing Clean blood spills promptly with solution of 5.25% sodium hypochlorite diluted 1:10 with water
Strict Herpes zoster Varicella (chickenpox)	To prevent transmission of highly contagious organisms by both air and contact	Yes; *gowns, masks, and gloves;* door closed	Discard or wrap before being sent for decontamination and reprocessing Bags are labeled or color-designated to denote contaminated articles or infectious waste *Hands must be washed after touching the patient or potentially contaminated articles and before taking care of another patient*
Contact Acute respiratory diseases in infants and young children: croup, bronchitis, bronchiolitis caused by various viruses, colds, viral pneumonia Conjunctivitis, gonococcal in newborn Eczema vaccinatum Herpes simplex Impetigo Influenza, in infants and young children Multiple resistant bacterial infection or colonization, i.e., *Pneumococcus* resistant to penicillin Pediculosis Pharyngitis Rubella, congenital or other Scabies Skin wound or burn infection, including those infected with *Staphylococcus aureus* or group A streptococci	To prevent spread of highly transmissible diseases that do not warrant strict isolation, spread mainly by close or direct contact	Yes; during outbreaks, children with the same respiratory problem may share the same room *Masks, gowns,* and *gloves* for direct contact	As above

Table continued on following page

Table 3–10. ISOLATION PRECAUTIONS Continued

TYPES AND EXAMPLES*	PURPOSE	PRIVATE ROOM	ARTICLES
Respiratory Epiglottitis (*Haemophilus influenzae*) Measles Meningitis (*H. influenzae*, meningococcal) Mumps Pertussis Pneumonia *H. influenzae*)	To prevent air-borne infection by droplets that are coughed, sneezed, or exhaled and are transmitted over a short distance	Yes; door closed; masks	As above
Enteric Coxsackievirus Diarrhea Encephalitis Gastrointestinal upsets Hepatitis (viral, type A) Meningitis (viral) Typhoid fever	To prevent transmission of infection by pathogens in feces	Yes; *gowns and gloves* for direct contact	Articles contaminated with infective material should be discarded or bagged and labeled before being sent for decontamination and reprocessing *Hands must be washed after touching the patient or potentially contaminated articles before taking care of another patient*
Drainage/Secretion Precautions Minor or limited: burn infection, wound infection, abscess, decubitus ulcer, skin infection Conjunctivitis	To prevent infections transmitted by direct or indirect contact with purulent material or drainage from an infected body site	Desirable, but not necessary; *gowns and gloves* for direct contact	Same as above

*The examples cited are not intended to be all-inclusive. Data are adapted from the CDC Guidelines for Isolation Precautions in Hospitals, HHS Publication No. (CDC) 83–8314. Specific diseases are listed alphabetically in this publication and more detailed information is provided.

tiveness of the use of masks, so nurses follow the procedures of the hospital in which they are employed.

Gown Technique. The nurse wears a gown to protect clothing from contamination when giving direct care to the child in isolation. If this were not done, organisms causing disease would be carried on the uniform, and the nurse would also endanger the health of other patients. Sweaters should not be worn in isolation. The nurse must be particularly conscientious on the children's unit, since small children need to be held for feedings and comforting and the nurse's relationship with the child is very direct. Paper disposable gowns are now widely used. The gown is used once and discarded in a plastic isolation laundry bag held by a ringstand. When the gown is put on, it is lapped over in the back (right side over left). When removing the gown, untie the waist strings, wash your hands, untie the neckband, and discard. Rewash hands. Use technique papers to open door; discard these in the patient's room. Close the door of the room. The nurse's shoes are always a source of contamination, and hands need thorough washing after touching them. Contaminated linen and trash are double bagged and disposed of according to hospital procedure.

Toys. Toys must be washable. They may be kept in a special cloth bag tied to the patient's crib so that they will not drop to the floor. The string of the bag is kept short, so that it will not become twisted around the child's neck. Since there is no satisfactory method of disinfecting books, reading should be limited to magazines or materials that are not highly prized by the owner. In highly communicable diseases, reading material is destroyed during terminal disinfection of the unit.

Education of the Family. Visitors are usually restricted to members of the immediate family. This information is posted on the patient's door. Family members should wear gowns and possibly masks while in the patient's room. Articles brought to the patient must be washable or disposable. After the visitor's gown has been removed and deposited in the laundry hamper, the hands must be washed. Do not allow visitors to take articles from the room.

Education of family members is ongoing. Factors to be emphasized include the necessity for immunizing children, proper care of food (particularly perishables), the importance of using pasteurized milk, proper cooking of meats, cleanliness in food preparation, and the importance of handwashing. Review the ways in which infectious diseases are spread. Other modes of transmission, such as crowded living conditions, insects and rodents, and sandbox hazards may also be topics to explore.

DISCHARGE PLANNING

Preparation for the patient's discharge ideally begins on admission, for the goal of hospitalization is to return a more healthy and happy child to the parents. Good physical care of the patient's disease is basic, but not enough. The nurse must also consider the emotional growth of the child and the education of the patient and family. This should provide a positive learning experience for all involved.

If a patient will require specific home treatment, such as hyperalimentation, colostomy care,

crutches, special diet, or insulin therapy, instructions should be given to the parents gradually throughout their child's hospitalization. The instructions should be written so that they may be referred to as needed. If older children are to administer any treatments to themselves, they will need careful explanations and supervision until both they and the parents are confident that the procedure will be carried out correctly at home. This may require home health care services.

Parents also must be prepared for behavioral problems that may arise following hospitalization. Severe stress will be obvious during the patient's stay and will require in-service care and professional follow-up. In guiding the parents, the following suggestions may prove helpful.

1. Recognize that after hospitalization the child may display such behaviors as clinging, regression in bowel and bladder control, aggression, fears, nightmares, and negativism.
2. Allow the child to become a participating family member as soon as possible. Return former family responsibilities within the limits of the present abilities.
3. Try not to make the child the center of attention because of the illness. Praise accomplishments unrelated to it.
4. Be kind, firm, and consistent when the child misbehaves.
5. Be truthful so that the child continues to trust you.
6. Provide suitable play materials such as clay, paints, and doctor and nurse kits. Allow free play.
7. Listen to the child and clear up any misconceptions about the illness.
8. Do not leave the child alone for a long period or overnight until a sense of security is regained.
9. Allow the child to visit hospital staff upon return for routine clinic visits.

Whenever possible, parents should be given at least one day's notice of their child's discharge from the hospital so that they can make necessary arrangements. This is particularly important if both parents work or when transportation is a problem. The physician writes the discharge order. The approximate hour of dismissal is relayed to the parents. The child is weighed and dressed, and all personal belongings are collected. Parents are given a written return appointment card when indicated. They are informed of any new habits the patient may have acquired during hospitalization. Necessary medications or materials that the parents have paid for are rendered.

Most hospitals have a special discharge sheet that provides the family with written instructions regarding medications, diet, activity, and any other special precautions or procedure the child may need. The nurse prepares the discharge sheet, reviews it with the parent to determine understanding, and then has the parent sign the sheet. A copy is given to the parent and a copy retained on the patient's chart. Parents sign a release form and visit the hospital business office according to hospital procedure. In most cases this is done on the way out. The nursing student tells the nurse in charge that he or she is leaving the unit with the patient. According to condition, the child is placed in a hospital wagon, wheelchair, or stretcher and accompanies the family to the exit. The nurse assists the patient into the car as needed. Some hospitals require that parents have car seats for infants and small children before they can be discharged from the hospital. Families without car seats are provided with them either on a permanent or loan basis. Charting includes time of departure, and with whom, patient's behavior (smiling, alert, crying), method of transportation from the division, patient's weight, and any instructions or medications given to the patient or parents.

NURSING BRIEF ▶ ▶ ▶ ▶ ▶ ▶ ▶ ▶
Discharge planning includes the identification and follow-up of children who may be at risk for child abuse, neglect, poverty, or a number of other conditions associated with their health problem or family lifestyle.

THE CHILD IN PAIN

Pain in children has long been a topic of much research. We now know that children of all ages experience pain. The developmental stage of the child affects the expected response to pain (Nursing Care Plan 3–2).

Facing Death With Child and Family

Facing death with a child and the family is not an easy task, but it can be rewarding. Nurses who do become involved with dying patients often express a sense of gratitude to have had the privilege of the experience. This is an area where rules fall short and patience becomes stretched. It can be tiring, discouraging, and sad and requires a profound look at acceptance.

NURSING BRIEF ▶ ▶ ▶ ▶ ▶ ▶ ▶ ▶
"Death, like birth, is a part of the natural order of things. It happens sooner for some, later for others" (Leukemia Society of America, Inc.).

Self-Exploration

One of, if not the, most important preparations for dealing with the dying patient is self-exploration. Our own attitudes about life and death affect our nursing practice. Our attitudes and emotions may be buried deep within us and can form barriers in effective communication unless they are recognized and released. How we have or have not dealt with our own losses affects our present lives and our ability to relate to patients. Nurses must recognize that *coping is an active and ongoing process.* At times we will need to lovingly detach ourselves from the patients and their families in order to be revitalized. We must find constructive outlets such as exercise and music to help maintain our equilibrium. An active support system consisting of nonjudgmental people who are not threatened by natural expressions of emotions is crucial. Proper channeling of these feelings can be a valuable part of our empathetic response to others.

NURSING BRIEF ▶ ▶ ▶ ▶ ▶ ▶ ▶ ▶
A long illness threatens a child's independence. Do not contribute to this by overprotection.

Child's Reaction to Death

Each child, like each adult, approaches death in an individual way, drawing on limited experience (Table 3–11). Nurses must become well acquainted

NURSING CARE PLAN 3–2
A CHILD IN PAIN

Nursing Diagnosis	Goals/Outcome Criteria	Nursing Interventions
Comfort, alteration in, related to pain	Patient will demonstrate a decrease in pain, as evidenced by a. vocalizing decreased pain b. nonverbal signs (relaxed body position, decreased crying, sleeping) c. vital signs within normal limits	Assess and record signs of pain in child (verbal and nonverbal) Use an assessment tool or other measurements of pain Distraction techniques (visitors, games, stories) Relaxation techniques Administer analgesics Encourage parents to stay with child Assess vital signs Adjust the environment (temperature, lighting, noise) Reposition Medicate before painful procedures Involve the older child in problem-solving for solutions
Anxiety, related to pain	Child will show a decrease in anxiety by 1. verbalizing decreased anxiety 2. decreased crying 3. interacting with staff 4. participating in activities	Assign a consistent caregiver Involve parents in care of child Explain all procedures to child Follow home rituals when possible Allow the older child some control Reassure preschool children that they are not to blame for illness and are not being punished

Table 3–11. CHILDREN'S CONCEPTS OF DEATH

AGE	CONCEPT
Infant–Toddler	Little understanding of death Fear and anxiety over separation
Preschooler	Something that happens to others Not permanent Curious about dead flowers and animals Magical thinking Feel ''bad thoughts'' may come true, harbor guilt Death is reversible Won't happen to them
Early School Years	Death is final Feel they might die but only in the distant future May understand death as a ''person'' Death is universal Suspect parents will die ''someday'' Fear of mutilation
Preadolescent–Adolescent	Able to understand death in a logical manner Understand it is universal Understand it is permanent Fear of disfigurement and isolation from peers

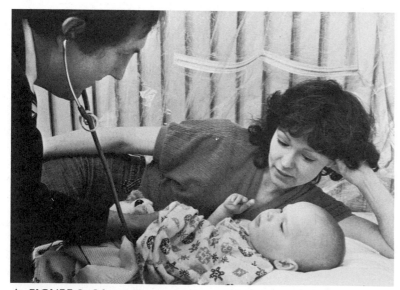

▲ **FIGURE 3–24**

Close contact between caregivers and family is of great importance for a child who has a potentially life-threatening disease. (Courtesy of Blank Memorial Hospital for Children, Des Moines, Iowa.)

with patients and view them within the context of the family and social culture. Their anxiety often centers about symptoms. They fear that the treatments necessary to alleviate their problem may be painful, as indeed some of them are. Their sense of trust is in a precarious balance. It is very important that nurses be honest and inform them of what they are about to do and why it is necessary. This is done in terms that they will understand. Encourage expression of feelings, e.g., "You seem angry." Allow sufficient time for a response. It is important that children be allowed to have as much control over what happens to them as possible. This is fostered by including them in decisions that concern their welfare (Fig. 3–24). Do not, however, offer a choice when there is none. Children often communicate symbolically. *Listen* to what they are saying to you, to their toys, and to other children. Provide crayons and paper.

NURSING BRIEF ▷ ▷ ▷ ▷ ▷ ▷ ▷ ▷ ▷
Brothers and sisters often feel neglected and lonely. They are frustrated because they are unable to comfort their parents and loved ones.

Although age is a factor, the child's cognitive development rather than chronological age per se affects the response to death. Children younger than 5 years of age are mainly concerned with separation from their parents and abandonment. (Even adults are threatened by thoughts of dying alone.) Preschool children respond to questions concerning death by relying on their experience and by turning to fantasy. They may believe death is reversible or that they are in some way responsible. Children do not develop a realistic conception of death as a permanent biological process until the age of 9 or 10 years. Dying adolescents are faced with conflicts between their treatment regimens and their need to establish independence from their parents and conformity with their peers. This leads to anger and resentment, which are frequently displaced onto hospital staff members. An atmosphere of acceptance and nonjudgmental listening allow patients freedom to ventilate their hostility in a nonthreatening environment.

Child's Awareness of Condition

Surprising as it may seem, many investigators have shown that terminally ill children are gener-

ally aware of their condition even when careful concealment has been advocated. This is reflected in their drawings and play and can be detected through psychological testing. Failure to be honest with children leaves them to suffer alone, unable to express fears and sadness or even to say good-bye. "It is better to address the issue of the seriousness of the child's illness from the time of diagnosis. In this way, energy that would be wasted in maintaining a deceit can be applied to the real problem of living with a life-threatening illness" (Spinetta and colleagues, 1983).

Stages of Dying

The stages of dying as detailed by Kubler-Ross (1969)—denial, anger, bargaining, depression, and acceptance—can be applied to parents and siblings as well as the sick child. (Nurses also may respond with similar feelings.) It is important to accept and support each participant at whatever stage has been reached and not to try to direct progress. Be available and denote your availability. Parents are encouraged to assist in the care of their child. It is therapeutic for children to be in their own surroundings whenever possible. Siblings involved in the patient's care feel less neglected, and the necessary sacrifices they make become more meaningful. Discussions before death allow them to make amends for their hostilities toward the sick child (Petrillo and Sanger, 1980). The family's religious associations can be a source of strength and support, as can caring neighbors and friends. Statistics show a high correlation between the death of a child and divorce. Nurses should try to be alert to signs of tension between parents so that suitable intervention may be established. It is important to realize that each parent grieves in his or her own time and way, often making it impossible for spouses to be supportive of each other. The suppression of strong feelings of guilt, helplessness, and outrage can be devastating. The father may be easily overlooked because of his absence during the day or because of a need to conceal his emotions from others.

NURSING BRIEF ▷ ▷ ▷ ▷ ▷ ▷ ▷ ▷ ▷
Grandparents, teachers, and friends are also grieving. Be alert for all significant others.

References

Huth, M., and O'Brien, M. (1987). The gastrostomy feeding button. *Pediatr. Nurs.* 13:241–245.

Kubler-Ross, E. (1969). *On Death and Dying.* New York, The Macmillan Company.

Marlow, D., and Redding, B. (1988). *Pediatric Nursing,* 6th ed. Philadelphia, W. B. Saunders Company.

Newbold, J. (1991). Evaluation of a new infrared tympanic thermometer: A comparison of three brands. *J. Pediatr. Nurs.* 6:281–283.

Petrillo, M., and Sanger, S. (1980). *Emotional Care of Hospitalized Children: An Environmental Approach,* 2nd ed. Philadelphia, J. B. Lippincott Company.

Spinetta, J., et al. (1983). *Emotional Aspects of Childhood Leukemia.* New York, Leukemia Society of America, Inc.

Bibliography

American Academy of Pediatrics (1988). *Report of the Committee on Infectious Diseases,* 21st ed. Elk Grove Village, IL.

Behrman, R., and Vaughan, V. (1987). *Nelson Textbook of Pediatrics,* 13th ed. Philadelphia, W. B. Saunders Company.

Bombeck, E. (1989). *I Want to Grow Hair, I Want to Grow Up, I Want to Go to Boise.* New York, Harper & Row.

Foster, R., Hunsberger, M., and Anderson, J. J. (1989). *Family-Centered Nursing Care of Children.* Philadelphia, W. B. Saunders Company.

Haas-Becket, B. (1987). Removing the mysteries of parenteral nutrition. *Pediatr. Nurs.* 13:37–41.

Haddock, B., Merrow, D., and Vincent, P. (1988). Comparisons of axillary and rectal temperatures in the preterm infant. *Neonatal Network,* April: 67–71.

Kaufman, J., and Hardy-Ribakow, D. (1988). What parents need to know about trach care. *RN* Oct.:99–103.

Kenney, M. (1987). Hospital to home: Care of the child with a tracheostomy. *Neonatal Network* Aug.:21–24.

Kilijanowicz, A. (1982). *In* Brunner, L., and Suddarth, D. (eds). *The Lippincott Manual of Nursing Practice,* 3rd ed. Philadelphia, J. B. Lippincott Company.

Kubler-Ross, E. (1983). *On Children and Death.* New York, Macmillan Publishing Company.

Long, S., and Henretig, F. (1987). Fever in children. *Pediatr. Consult* 6. Woodbury, N.Y., McNeil Consumer Products Company.

Moen, J., Chapman, S., Sheehan, A., and Carter, P. (1987). Axillary versus rectal temperatures in preterm infants under radiant warmers. *JOGNN* Sept.–Oct.:348–351.

Mott, S., James, S., and Sperhac, A. (1990). *Nursing Care of Children and Families.* Redwood City, CA, Addison-Wesley.

Rimar, Joan (1982). Guidelines for the intravenous administration of medications used in pediatrics. *Am. J. Maternal/Child Nurs.* 7:184–197.

Whaley, L., and Wong, D. (1987). *Nursing Care of Infants and Children.* St. Louis, C. V. Mosby Company.

Wong, D. (1989). From sites to sensors: Taking infants' temperatures. *Am. J. Nurs.* Mar.:321.

Wong, D. (1988). Taking accurate blood pressure in children. *Children's Nurse* 6:1–4.

STUDY QUESTIONS

1. Observe a patient being admitted. How could the nurse have carried out this function more effectively?
2. Describe how and why measurement of blood pressure differs when the patient is a child.
3. Nine year old Chris Jones has just been admitted to the unit with a severe laceration of the leg. You are assigned to take his blood pressure. How would you explain this to Chris?
4. What is the purpose of the playroom?
5. Compile a list of safety measures that would be effective on the children's unit in your hospital. Underline those measures that apply to the nurse.
6. List several ways in which children show their insecurities.
7. Of what value are visiting hours to the child, the parents, and the nurse?
8. Discuss how you would obtain a urine specimen from a 4 month old baby.
9. Mrs. Lang, the head nurse, has just told you to prepare Room 101 for a new admission who is suspected of having meningitis. The patient is 6 years old. How would you do this?
10. What is the role of the nurse in assisting with a lumbar puncture?
11. What special precautions must be taken when giving medications to children? How and where are medications charted in your hospital?
12. Choose a drug that is administered to adults and children. Investigate the use of the drug thoroughly, using the drug circular. What information is given about pediatric dosage and administration? Is this information adequate for your purposes? Present your findings to your classmates.
13. Rhonda, age 3 years, was admitted with acute laryngotracheobronchitis. She is crying anxiously in her croupette. State the rationale for placing Rhonda in oxygen. Devise a nursing care plan suitable to Rhonda's age and condition.

14. Rita, age 5 years, has been in isolation for meningitis for about a week. She is making satisfactory progress. How does her care differ from the care given to children who are not in isolation? List several diversions that appeal to the 5 year old.
15. Discuss how you would assess a 4 year old child for pain.
16. You have just given a 3 month old infant an injection. What would your next nursing action be?
17. Discuss your feelings about caring for a child who is dying.

C H A P T E R 4 _____

Chapter Outline

ADAPTATIONS OF THE NEWBORN INFANT
INITIAL ASSESSMENT OF THE NEWBORN INFANT
PHYSICAL DEVELOPMENT AND NURSING
 ASSESSMENT OF THE NEWBORN INFANT
CHARACTERISTICS OF THE NEONATE
 Nervous System
 Sensory System
 Respiratory System
 Circulatory System
 Musculoskeletal System
 Genitourinary System
 Integumentary System
 Gastrointestinal System
NEONATAL NUTRITION
BREAST FEEDING
BOTTLE FEEDING
INFECTION
PREVENTION OF INFECTION
SIGNS AND SYMPTOMS OF INFECTION
CARE OF THE PATIENT UNIT
ROOMING-IN
BONDING/ATTACHMENT
SIBLINGS
SPIRITUAL CARE
DISCHARGE TEACHING

Objectives

Upon completion and mastery of Chapter 4, the student will be able to
- Define the vocabulary terms listed.
- Identify the range of average head circumference in the newborn infant and the significance of a particular measurement to the nurse.
- Briefly describe three normal reflexes of the neonate (including approximate age of disappearance) and the tests for their appearance.
- Summarize the principles involved in teaching a new mother how to breast-feed her baby, bathe her baby, and protect her baby from infection.
- List four signs of infection in the neonate.
- Using a systems approach, summarize the pertinent nursing interventions in the care of Marcia, a 2 day old neonate (for example, "circulatory system—check color and warmth, explain principles to parents").
- Compare and contrast breast feeding and formula feeding.
- Describe precautions you would take while caring for a newborn baby to prevent infection.
- Discuss behaviors that would indicate that bonding is taking place between the infant and the mother.

THE NEWBORN INFANT

Terms

acrocyanosis (89)
airway (77)
Apgar score (78)
circumcision (91)
fontanel (83)
icterus neonatorum (92)
Moro reflex (85)
NICU (78)

Adaptations of the Newborn Infant

When a baby is born, an orderly process of adaptation from fetal life to extrauterine life takes place. All the body systems undergo some change. Respirations are stimulated by chemical changes within the blood and by chilling. Sensory and physical stimuli also appear to play a role in respiratory function. In the past, the infant was slapped on the buttocks or heels to provide stimulation for breathing. This has been replaced with gentle physical contact. Cold, pain, touch, movement, and light are other stimuli that affect the stimulation of respirations. The first breath initiates the opening of the alveoli. The baby then enters the world of air exchange, beginning an independent existence. In addition, this process begins cardiopulmonary interdependence. Fetal circulation is depicted in Figure 4–1. The ability of the neonate to metabolize food is hampered by immaturity of the digestive system, particularly deficiencies in enzymes from the pancreas and liver. The kidneys are developed structurally, but their ability to concentrate urine and maintain fluid balance is limited because of a decreased rate of glomerular flow and limited renal tubular reabsorption. Most neurological functions are primitive (see also individual body systems later in this chapter).

Initial Assessment of the Newborn Infant

Airway. Regardless of the site of delivery (home, birthing room, taxicab), clearing the neonate's airway is an immediate concern. A rubber bulb syringe or a special trap connected to suction may be used. This produces very low suction, which protects the delicate tissues while removing secretions. Spontaneous breathing should begin within a few seconds. If this does not occur, resuscitative measures are begun. When there are no complications, the baby is placed on a warming table with head down to facilitate drainage of mucus and is dried gently. Mothers who are alert are given their child to hold and inspect.

Umbilical Cord. The umbilical cord, which is attached to the placenta at birth, is cut by the attending physician. Before applying the clamp the cord is inspected to determine that two arteries and one vein are present. A single umbilical artery is often indicative of genitourinary anomalies. The findings are recorded.

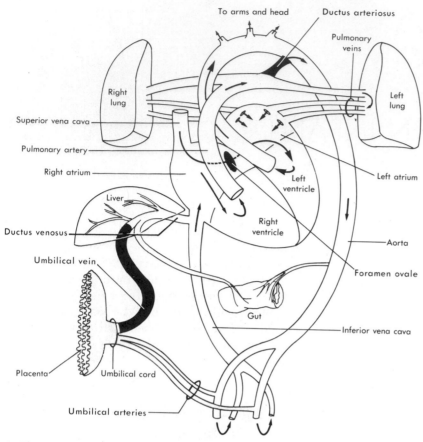

▲ **Figure 4–1**

Diagram of fetal circulation showing the placenta, umbilical vein, and umbilical arteries. The fetal bypasses (ductus venosus, ductus arteriosus, and foramen ovale) are also shown. (From Burroughs, A. [1986]. *Bleier's Maternity Nursing,* 5th ed. Philadelphia, W. B. Saunders Company.)

The cord stump gradually shrinks, discolors, and finally falls off. The blood vessels of the cord and their extension into the abdomen are a potential portal of entry for disease organisms until the umbilical wound is completely healed. Redness, odor, or discharge from this area should be reported to the physician. The nurse observes the cord for bleeding, particularly during the first 24 hours.

Immediate Assessment. A system for recording the condition of the neonate and the need for resuscitation was devised by Dr. Virginia Apgar and is widely used. The first assessment is made 1 minute after delivery. This is generally the lowest score. A second evaluation is made after 5 min-

utes. The *Apgar score* is shown in Table 4–1. An infant with a score of 7 to 10 is in good condition and will need only routine suction and observation. Babies with a score of 3 to 7 will require some form of resuscitation and close observation. An infant with a score of 0 to 2 will need ventilatory support and care in the neonatal intensive care unit (NICU). Apgar scores alone are not evidence of sufficient hypoxia to result in neurological damage (American Academy of Pediatrics, 1986).

Resuscitation. If the neonate has difficulty breathing, resuscitation measures are immediately instigated. The need for resuscitation often can be anticipated by the history of the mother's pregnancy, abnormal progression of labor, size of the

Table 4–1. THE APGAR SCORING SYSTEM

The Apgar scoring system provides a quick and accurate way of evaluating a baby's physical status right at birth, regardless of any combination of weaknesses or debilities. The physician or nurse observes the five vital signs and records the score for each. Each sign is evaluated according to the degree to which it is present; 0 (poor), 1 (fair), or 2 (good). The five scores are then added together; Apgar scores range from 0 to 10. A score of 10 means the baby is in the best possible condition. A score of 9, 8, or 7 indicates good condition; 6, 5, or 4 indicates fair condition. A score of 3, 2, 1 or 0 indicates poor condition and the need for prompt diagnosis and treatment of specific disorders.

Sign	0	1	2	Score
Heart rate: strong and steady?	Not detectable	Slow (less than 100)	Above 100	_____
Respiratory effort: breathing frequently and regularly?	Absent	Slow, irregular	Good; crying	_____
Muscle tone: kicking feet and making fists?	Flaccid	Some flexion of extremities	Active motion	_____
Reflex irritability; lusty cry elicited if catheter is pushed up one nostril or soles of feet are prodded?	No response	Grimace	Cry; cough or sneeze	_____
Color: pink all over, or hands and feet bluish?	Blue, pale	Body pink, extremities bluish	Completely pink	_____
			TOTAL	_____

neonate, and difficulty of delivery. Well-trained personnel and equipment that is properly functioning are imperative. Periodic review of techniques is also required. Resuscitation methods are directed toward clearing the airway, inflating the lungs, and maintaining circulation. The administration of appropriate drugs, such as sodium bicarbonate, epinephrine, dextrose, or calcium gluconate, also may be warranted. Procedures go from the simple to the more complex. Measures such as tactile stimulation (rubbing the neonate's back), assisted ventilation by bag and mask or endotracheal tube, intermittent positive pressure breathing (IPPB), and external cardiac massage may be necessary. The infant is transferred to the nursery in a prewarmed transport Isolette. Assisted ventilation via a mechanical respirator may be required in the nursery.

Meconium Aspiration Syndrome. Aspiration of stained amniotic fluid is sometimes seen in the term or post-term newborn infant. It signals that the fetus had been in distress while in utero.

Aspiration of meconium may occur with the first breath. This results in small airway obstruction manifested by tachypnea, retractions, grunting respirations, and cyanosis. Respiratory distress may be immediate or delayed, and pneumothorax may result. If the course is mild, improvement may occur within 48 hours.

Immediate suctioning of the nasopharynx is indicated. A chest x-ray study may show coarse, patchy intensities. Atelectasis sometimes occurs. Resuscitated neonates are transferred to the intensive care nursery for close observation.

Identifying the Neonate. Proper identification of the newborn baby is insured by tagging both the mother and the baby before they are separated in the delivery room (Fig. 4–2). The American Academy of Pediatrics recommends that two identical identification bands be placed on the infant while in the delivery room. Bracelets are placed on both wrists, both ankles, or one of each. The neonate loses weight after birth, so bracelets must be snug. The Academy also recommends finger-

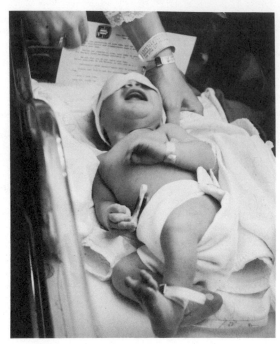

▲ **Figure 4–2**

Identification. Note double identification bands on mother and 2 day old baby. (Eye mask is for phototherapy.)

printing the mother and newborn baby (or footprinting the baby as an alternative). Identification is reaffirmed upon admission to the nursery and before transferring the infant to a regional care center.

Providing Warmth. Radiant warmers are available in most delivery rooms. The baby is thoroughly dried (especially the hair) and placed uncovered under radiant heat. If the baby is placed on the mother's chest, skin to skin contact should be maintained. In an out-of-hospital delivery, the newborn infant and mother can be wrapped together in a sleeping bag. A cap for the baby will prevent heat loss. The nurse remains with the mother and child to ensure their safety and to monitor progress (Table 4–2).

Protection from Infection. *Handwashing by all persons involved in the delivery room and nursery is imperative.* Clean covergowns or scrubs are worn. Clamping of the umbilical cord is carried out using aseptic technique. A 0.5 per cent erythromycin solution is instilled in the neonate's eyes to pre-

vent chlamydial ophthalmia and gonococcal ophthalmia. A 1 per cent tetracycline solution is also effective against these organisms. Silver nitrate, 1 per cent, may be used in some areas but is not effective against chlamydial ophthalmia and can cause a chemical conjunctivitis.

NURSING BRIEF ▶ ▶ ▶ ▶ ▶ ▶ ▶ ▶
Advise parents to limit the neonate's exposure to crowds during the early weeks of life.

Reactivity. Following delivery, the vigorous neonate exhibits a characteristic pattern of activities. These patterns are termed the *first and second periods of reactivity.* During the first period, which lasts for about 30 minutes after birth, the neonate is awake and active. The heart and respiratory rates are rapid, and grimacing, sucking movements, and random motor activity occur. This is followed by a period of rest, which lasts from 2 to 4 hours. At this time the neonate is disinterested in sucking and stimulation. A second period of reactivity occurs on awakening. This lasts from 4 to 6 hours. The neonate's responsiveness returns. Periods of apnea may be seen, and there is an increase in mucus. The color of the newborn infant may vary between mildly mottled and cyanotic. Bowel sounds become audible, and meconium stools are passed. "The sequence of clinical behavior just described is common to all newborns after birth regardless of gestational age or route of delivery. However, the time sequence of changes is altered in infants who are immature or who have demonstrated difficulty in establishing respiration promptly on delivery (low Apgar score infants)" (Levine and colleagues, 1983).

Vitamin K Administration and Screening Tests. Vitamin K (Aqua-Mephyton) is given in many hospitals to promote blood clotting and prevent hemorrhage in the neonate. A mild vitamin K deficiency is not unusual in newborn infants and is common in preterms. The neonate's intestinal flora is sterile at birth; thus, the baby is unable to synthesize vitamin K. Normal intestinal flora is established after birth. Vitamin K is administered intramuscularly, using the lateral aspect of the thigh, and given in the nursery.

Blood work such as a hematocrit and a glucose recording may be indicated. Screening tests for phenylketonuria (PKU), galactosemia, and hypo-

Table 4–2. HEAT LOSS IN NEONATES

TYPE OF HEAT LOSS	MECHANISM	CONDITIONS CONTRIBUTING TO HEAT LOSS	NURSING INTERVENTION
Conduction	Conduction to surfaces that touch skin	Cool temperature of contact surfaces Thermal conductivity of material of contact surfaces	Avoid placing infant on cold surface (e.g., scales, x-ray plates, examining tables); pad with a warm diaper or blanket Warm hands, equipment before touching baby
Evaporation	1. Insensible evaporation from skin	Insensible evaporation accounts for 25 percent of heat loss	Maintain relative humidity of 50 to 80 percent
	2. Evaporation of moisture on skin (e.g., amniotic fluid, bath water)	Increased skin premeability leads to insensible water loss and thus evaporative heat loss	Keep skin dry Do not bathe baby unless the temperature is stable
	3. Evaporation from the mucosa of respiratory tract	Tachypnea increases rate of heat loss from respiratory tract	Bathe and dry only small area at a time Warm any soaks or solutions applied to skin; keep warm Change wet diapers quickly
Convection	1. Air moving over the skin	Exposure to currents of air, including oxygen that has not been warmed and humidified	Avoid currents of air moving across skin
	2. Warm air expired during respiration	Thermal sensors on face and forehead are sensitive to cold even when rest of body is warm	Warm and humidify oxygen When infant must leave nursery (e.g., for surgery), transport in prewarmed incubator
	3. Convection of heat to skin surface		
Radiation	Transfer from infant's skin to surrounding environment	Difference between skin temperature and environment (e.g., walls of single-walled incubator) Total radiating surface of infant—the smaller the infant, the greater the surface area in relation to weight and thus the greater the loss Large surface area of infant's head exacerbates loss	Room temperature should be no more than 7° C. below environmental temperature Raise incubator air temperature to 36° C Clothe infant when possible Keep infant's bed away from outside walls and out of drafts Use a heat shield in incubator Swaddle infant Put cap or bonnet on baby (nearly doubles insulating effect of infant's own tissues)

From Moore, M. L. (1981). *Newborn Family and Nurse*, 2nd ed. Philadelphia, W. B. Saunders Company.

thyroidism may also be administered in approximately 1 week. For the measurement of PKU to be accurate, the infant must have ingested protein for at least 48 hours. False-negative results can occur; retesting is suggested and is usually done in 2 to 4 weeks. With the current trend of early discharge of mothers and babies, it is imperative that follow-up be undertaken.

Physical Development and Nursing Assessment of the Newborn Infant

CHARACTERISTICS OF THE NEONATE

Maturity. There are several differences between the premature infant and a full-term one. Muscle tone is decreased in the infant who is not term. The position of the infant also can indicate low gestational age. The full-term infant lies with the pelvis high and the knees drawn up under the abdomen when in the prone position. The premature infant lies with the pelvis low and the knees at the side of the abdomen, the hips flexed. In the supine position, the infant of 28 to 32 weeks' gestational age lies in a "froglike" position with the lower limbs extended and the hips abducted. The full-term infant lies with the limbs strongly flexed. There are also differences in moving the hand of the infant across the chest to the opposite side of the neck. The 28-week gestational-age infant reaches well past the acromion. The hand of the full-term infant does not go beyond the acromion. If the hand is put behind the neck to the opposite side, the same difference between the ages is noted. This is called the *Scarf sign* (Fig. 4–3).

Head. The newborn infant's head is proportionately large in comparison with the rest of the body, for the brain grows rapidly before birth. The normal limits of head circumference range from 13.2 to 14.8 inches (Fig. 4–4). The head may be out of shape from *molding* (the shaping of the fetal head to conform to the size and shape of the birth

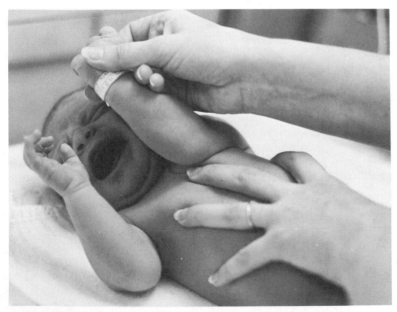

▲ **Figure 4–3**

Examining the newborn baby for maturity. The full-term neonate's elbow resists attempts to be brought farther than the midline of the chest. Little or no resistance is seen in the preterm infant. This is called the Scarf sign.

Table 4–3. AGES OF APPEARANCE AND DISAPPEARANCE OF NEUROLOGICAL SIGNS PECULIAR TO INFANCY

RESPONSE	AGE AT TIME OF APPEARANCE	AGE AT TIME OF DISAPPEARANCE
Reflexes of position and movement		
Moro reflex	Birth	1 to 3 months
Tonic neck reflex (unsustained)*	Birth	5 to 6 months (partial up to 2 to 4 years)
Palmar grasp reflex	Birth	4 months
Babinski response	Birth	Variable†
Reflexes to sound		
Blinking response	Birth	
Turning response	Birth	
Reflexes of vision		
Blinking to threat	6 to 7 months	
Horizontal following	4 to 6 weeks	
Vertical following	2 to 3 months	
Postrotational nystagmus	Birth	
Food reflexes		
Rooting response—awake	Birth	3 to 4 months
—asleep	Birth	7 to 8 months
Sucking response	Birth	12 months
Other signs		
Handedness	2 to 3 years	
Spontaneous stepping	Birth	
Straight line walking	5 to 6 years	

*Arm and leg posturing can be interrupted by child despite continued neck stimulus.
†Usually of no diagnostic significance until after age 2 years.
Adapted from *Children Are Different*, Ross Laboratories, Columbus, Ohio, November 1978; from Smith, D. W., et al (1978). *The Biologic Ages of Man*, 2nd ed. Philadelphia, W. B. Saunders Company.

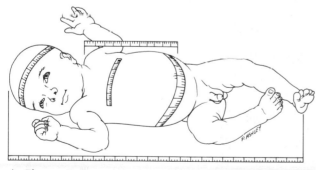

▲ **Figure 4–4**

Measuring head, chest, and abdominal circumference. (From Marlow, D., and Redding, B. [1986]. *Textbook of Pediatric Nursing*. Philadelphia, W. B. Saunders Company.)

canal) (Fig. 4–5). Occasionally, a hematoma (*hemato*, blood + *oma*, tumor) protrudes from beneath the scalp. This condition usually clears up within a few weeks. Some neonates have a large amount of black hair, which eventually is replaced by new hair. The infant's hair is washed daily when the baby is bathed and is brushed into place.

Fontanels are junctures at the cranial bones that can be felt as soft spots on the cranium of the young infant. Two can be palpated on the neonate's head. The fontanels may be smaller immediately after birth than several days later because of molding. The anterior fontanel is diamond-shaped and located at the junction of the two parietal and two frontal bones. It usually closes by 12 to 18 months of age. The posterior fontanel

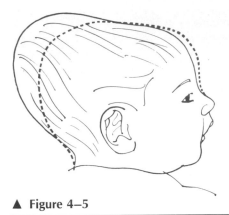

▲ **Figure 4–5**

Molding of the head occurs as a result of overriding of the parietal bones as the head passes through the birth canal. The head appears to be longer than normal. This condition disappears without treatment within a few weeks. The dotted line shows the normal contour of the head as compared with the molded head of the newborn infant. (From Leifer, G. [1982]. *Principles and Techniques of Pediatric Nursing.* Philadelphia, W. B. Saunders Company.)

is triangular and located between the occipital and parietal bones. It is much smaller than the anterior fontanel and is usually ossified by the end of the second month. The pulsating of the anterior fontanel may be seen by the nurse. These areas are covered by a tough membrane, and there is little chance of their being injured with ordinary care.

The features of the newborn baby's face are small. The mouth and lips are well developed, as they are necessary to obtain food. The neonate can both taste and smell. In fact, the mother's scent appears to stimulate the neonate to smell breast milk and search for the nipple.

Nervous System

Reflexes (Table 4–3). The nurse will recall that the nervous system directs most of the body's activity. The neonate can move arms and legs vigorously but cannot control them. The reflexes a full-term baby is born with, such as winking, sneezing, gagging, sucking, and grasping (Fig. 4–6), help keep the child alive. The infant can cry, swallow, and lift the head slightly when lying on the stomach. If the crib is jarred, the baby will extend the extremities and then draw the legs up and fold the arms across the chest in an embrace position. The hands open, but the fingers often

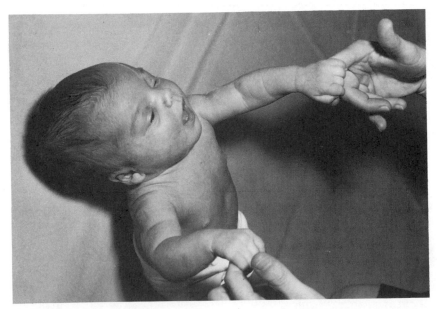

▲ **Figure 4–6**

Grasp reflex and head lag help determine the maturity of the newborn infant. (From Marlow, D. [1977]. *Textbook of Pediatric Nursing*, 5th ed. Philadelphia, W. B. Saunders Company.)

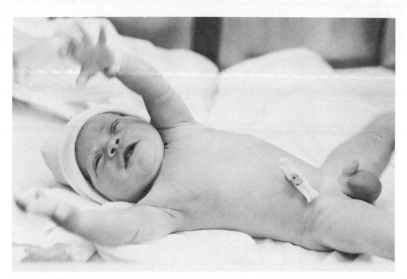

▲ **Figure 4–7**

Moro reflex. Sudden jarring causes extension and abduction of the extremities and spreading of the fingers. This is followed by abduction of the arms in an embrace position.

remain curved. This is normal and is called the *Moro reflex* (Fig. 4–7). Its absence may indicate abnormalities of the nervous system. The *rooting reflex* causes the infant to turn the head in the direction of anything that touches the cheek, in anticipation of food. The nurse should remember this when helping a mother breast-feed her infant.

If the breast touches the infant's cheek, the baby will turn toward it to find the nipple.

The *tonic neck reflex* (TNR) is a postural reflex that is sometimes assumed by babies while asleep. The head is turned to one side and the arm and leg are extended on the same side, while the opposite arm and leg are flexed in a "fencing"

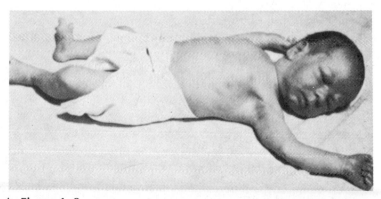

▲ **Figure 4–8**

Spontaneous tonic neck reflex. (From Behrman, R. E., and Vaughan, V. C. [1983]. *Nelson Textbook of Pediatrics*, 12th ed. Philadelphia, W. B. Saunders Company.)

position. This reflex disappears about the 20th week of life (Fig. 4–8). Prancing movements of the legs, seen when a baby is held upright on the examining table, are termed the *dancing reflex*.

Sensory System

Vision. Although vision is the most poorly developed sense, the neonate can see sizes, shapes, colors, and patterns and is able to fixate points of contrast. The infant shows preference for observing a human face and will follow moving objects. Visual stimulation thus becomes an important ingredient in caring for the baby. Auditory toys and contrasted colors attract the neonate. Sensory overload, of course, should be avoided.

Most newborn infants appear cross-eyed because their eye muscle coordination is not fully developed. At first the eyes appear to be blue or gray; however, the permanent coloring becomes fixed between the third and sixth month.

Hearing. Hearing is felt to be keener than was once believed. Increased response to vocal stimulation, particularly higher-pitched female voices, can be documented. The ears and nose need no special attention except for cleansing during the bath with a soft cloth. Occasionally, they may be *externally* cleansed with a cotton wisp moistened slightly with water. Toothpicks or wooden applicator sticks are dangerous to use. They may cause injury if the baby moves suddenly.

Sleep. The baby sleeps approximately 15 to 20 hours a day. There is a gradual change in the quantity and quality of sleep as the neonate matures. Differentiation between active and quiet sleep is based primarily on whether *rapid eye movement* (REM) occurs. The sleep of the newborn infant consists of approximately half REM sleep, as opposed to only 20 per cent in the 5 year old. During REM sleep, respirations are rapid and more irregular, movements of the eye are evident beneath the eyelid, and movements of the limbs and mouth may be seen. Premature infants have an even higher proportion of REM sleep than babies born at term. Investigators theorize that REM sleep may be an internal stimulus to the higher brain centers, at a time when external stimulation is minimal because of only brief periods of arousal. The baby awakes for feedings, and after feedings should be placed on the stomach with the head turned outward or on the right side to reduce the danger of choking from food or vomitus. Occasionally putting the baby's head at the foot of the crib prevents always sleeping on one side of the head and also provides a change of scene. In good weather, the child can sleep outdoors in a carriage or portable carrier or bed.

NURSING BRIEF ▶ ▶ ▶ ▶ ▶ ▶ ▶ ▶
Advise parents that even the youngest of babies can roll off a changing table or bed if left unattended.

Conditioned Responses. A conditioned response or reflex is one that is learned over time. Basically it is an unconscious response to an external stimulus. An example is the hungry baby who stops crying at simply hearing the footsteps of the mother. Emotions are particularly subject to this type of conditioning. As an infant matures, the mere sight of an object that once caused pain can precipitate fear. Learning mechanisms such as these are of particular interest to *behavior theorists,* who hold that the proper study of psychology is that of behavior alone.

The *Neonatal Behavioral Assessment Scale,* developed by Brazelton (1984), has increased our understanding of the neonate's capabilities. Among other things, the scale measures the inherent neurological capacities of the neonate, as well as responses to selected stimuli. Areas tested include alertness, response to visual and auditory stimuli, motor coordination, level of excitement, and organizational processes in response to stress.

Respiratory System

Before birth, a baby is completely dependent on the mother for all vital functions. The fetus needs oxygen and nourishment in order to grow. These are supplied through the blood stream of the pregnant woman by way of the placenta and umbilical cord. The fetus is relieved of the waste products of metabolism through the same route. The lungs are not inflated and are almost completely inactive. The circulatory system is adapted only to life within the uterus. Little blood flows through the pulmonary artery, owing to natural openings within the heart (foramen ovale) and vessels that close at birth or shortly thereafter. When the umbilical cord is clamped and cut, the lungs take on the function of breathing in oxygen and removing carbon dioxide. The first breath taken helps expand the collapsed lungs. The physician assists the first respiration by holding the infant's head down and removing mucus from the passages to the lungs. The baby's cry should be strong and healthy. The most critical period for the neonate is the first hour of life, when the drastic change from life within the uterus to life outside the uterus takes place.

Respirations may be irregular and should be counted for 1 full minute. Normal respirations are 40 to 60 breaths per minute and then will drop to 30 to 50 breaths per minute after the first 24 hours.

The baby is wrapped in a light blanket and carried to the nursery. The nursery nurse removes excess blood from the baby's face and scalp with a soft, moist cloth. The baby is weighed and measured if this has not been done in the delivery room. During this procedure the nurse observes the baby's general condition. The baby is then dressed in a diaper and shirt and placed in a bassinet, either on the abdomen or one side, under a light blanket. The foot of the bassinet is elevated. The newborn remains in this position for the first 24 hours to promote the drainage of mucus from the respiratory passages. A routine blood glucose test to detect hypoglycemia, using capillary blood obtained by heel prick, may be performed at this time. Results are compared with a color chart.

The nurse refers to the patient's chart to review the Apgar score (see page 78) and to determine whether or not there were any particular difficulties during the birth process. The orders left by the doctor are reviewed. The nurse must observe the baby *very closely*. Respiratory distress may be shown by the rate and character of respirations (Fig. 4–9), color (watch for cyanosis), and general behavior. Sternal retractions should be reported immediately (Fig. 4–10). Mucus may be seen draining from the nose or mouth. It is wiped away with a sterile gauze square. Gentle suctioning via a bulb syringe may also be indicated. The bulb is depressed and the tip is inserted into the nose or mouth. The depression is slowly released, creating the necessary suction. When this procedure is done orally, the tip is inserted into the side of the mouth to avoid stimulating the gag reflex. Instruct parents in the use of the bulb syringe and keep one alongside the infant during the early weeks.

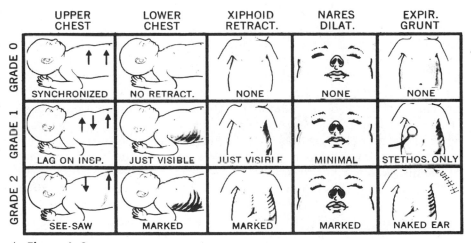

▲ Figure 4–9

Criteria of respiratory distress. Grade 0 for each criterion indicates no respiratory distress; grade 2 for each criterion indicates severe distress. Abbreviations: DILAT., dilation; EXPIR., expiratory; INSP., inspiration; RETRACT, retraction; STETHOS, stethoscope. (Courtesy of Mead Johnson & Company, Evansville, Indiana. Adapted from Silverman, W., and Anderson, D. [1956]. Controlled clinical trial of effects of water mist on obstructive respiratory signs, death rate and necropsy finding among premature babies. *Pediatrics* 17:1.)

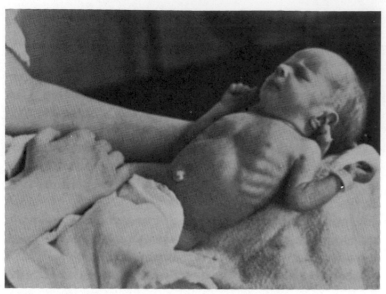

▲ **Figure 4–10**

Sternal retractions. Note the triangular indentation over the sternal area of the chest, which indicates marked retraction during inspiration. Intercostal retractions are also evidenced. The infant is inactive. All of his energy is being used to breathe. (From Kalafatich, A. [1966]. *Pediatric Nursing*. New York, G. P. Putnam's Sons.)

Circulatory System

The mother's blood has brought essential oxygen to each cell of the fetus during life in the uterus. The obstetrician cuts off this supply when he or she severs the umbilical cord. From this time on the newborn infant has not only a systemic circulation but also a pulmonary circulation. (There is some pulmonary circulation prior to birth, although not as great as after the lungs have expanded.) (Normal blood values are given in Appendix D.)

The circulation of the fetus differs from that of the newborn baby in that most of the blood bypasses the lungs (see Fig. 4–1). Some of the blood goes from the right atrium to the left atrium of the heart through an opening (the foramen ovale) in the septum. Some of the blood goes from the pulmonary artery to the thoracic aorta by way of the *ductus arteriosus* (see Fig. 4–1).

"Murmurs" are caused by blood leaking through openings that have not yet closed. Murmurs may be thought of as functional (innocent) or organic (due to improper heart formation). Functional murmurs are due to the sound of blood passing through normal valves. Organic murmurs are due to blood passing through abnormal openings or normal openings that have not yet closed. The majority of heart murmurs are not serious. However, they should be checked periodically to rule out other possibilities.

An apical pulse is auscultated (Fig. 4–11). The pulse rate is between 120 and 140 beats per minute. This rate may be increased if the infant is crying. Blood pressure is low, and use of the correct sized cuff is very important. The average blood pressure at birth is 80/46. If the pulse is elevated to 160 or drops below 120, it should be reported.

Thermoregulation. The neonate has an immature heat regulating system. The baby's temperature falls immediately after birth to about 35.5°C (96°F). Within a few hours it climbs slowly to a range of 36.6 to 37.2°C (98 to 99°F). The body temperature is influenced by the temperature of the room and the number of blankets covering the

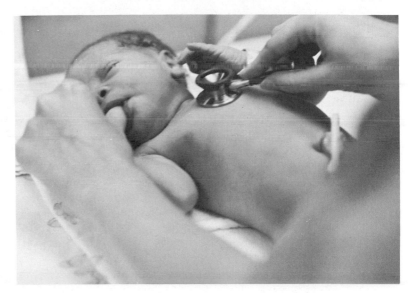

▲ **Figure 4–11**

Apical pulse. An apical pulse is obtained from neonates and infants. The average heart rate for newborn infants is 120 to 140 beats per minute.

baby. The temperature of the nursery, or the mother's room in the case of rooming-in, should be 20 to 23.8° C (68 to 75°F). The humidity should be 45 to 55 per cent. The air in the room needs to be fresh, but there should be no drafts.

Another sign of the neonate's system immaturity is acrocyanosis (*acro,* extremity + *cyanosis,* blue color) or peripheral blueness of the hands and feet, and sometimes the lips. The hands and feet will also be cooler than other parts of the body. The neonate has difficulty adapting to changes in temperature. The baby should be wrapped in a blanket when leaving the nursery. Since heat perception is poor, the nurse must be very careful when applying any form of external heat.

The most accurate way to determine body temperature is measurement with a thermometer. The initial temperature of the neonate is taken in the rectum to determine that the rectum is patent, although stooling is the definitive sign of patency. The nurse must be gentle in order to avoid injuring the rectal mucosa. Daily routine temperatures are taken in the axilla. Refer to Chapter 3 (page 37) for review of the procedures for taking vital signs.

Musculoskeletal System

Movements, Eye Coordination, Tremors. The bones of the newborn infant are soft because they are made up chiefly of cartilage, in which there is only a small amount of calcium. The skeleton is flexible. The joints are elastic to accommodate the passage through the birth canal. Since the bones of the child are easily molded by pressure, the position must be changed frequently. If the baby lies constantly in one position, the bones of the head can become flattened.

The movements of the neonate are random and uncoordinated. The infant lacks the muscular control to hold the head steady. The development of muscular control proceeds from head to foot and from the center of the body to the periphery (see cephalocaudal control, page 16). The baby will therefore hold up the head before sitting erect. In fact, the head and neck muscles will be the first ones under control. The legs are small and short and may appear bowed. There should be no limitation of movement. Fingers clenched in a fist should be separated and observed.

Most neonates appear cross-eyed because their eye muscle coordination is not fully developed. At first the eyes appear to be blue or gray; however, the permanent coloring becomes fixed between the third and sixth month.

Freedom of movement is needed as the baby stretches, sucks, and makes faces. The whole body moves vigorously when the baby cries. Tremors of the lips and extremities during crying are normal. Constant tremors during sleep may be pathological. These are often accompanied by eye movements and are not related to any particular stimuli. The morning bath provides excellent opportunities for the infant to exercise and the nurse to inspect and assess the baby's condition. When handled, the infant should not feel limp. General body proportions are noted. Bathing is also an excellent way to provide stimulation to the neonate.

Length and Weight. The length of the average neonate is 19 to 21.5 inches. The weight varies from 2700 to 4000 g (6 to 9 pounds) (Fig. 4–12). Girls generally weigh a little less than boys. In the first 3 to 4 days after birth the baby loses about 6 to 10 ounces. This may be due to withdrawal from maternal hormones, withholding of water, and the loss of feces and urine. It is expected and natural, and the mother need not be alarmed by it. Some hospitals prefer not to tell the mother the daily weight of the baby in order to avoid upsetting her. The nurse should comply with this rule if it is used in the hospital where she or he is employed.

Neonates are weighed at the same time each day, when morning care is given. Breast-fed babies may sometimes be weighed before and after feedings. (Instructions for measuring and weighing the baby are outlined in Chapter 3.)

Genitourinary System

The kidneys function normally at birth but are not fully developed. The glomeruli are small. Renal blood flow is only about one third that of the adult. The ability to handle a water load is reduced, as is the excretion of drugs. The renal tubules are short and have a limited capacity for reabsorbing important substances such as glucose, amino acids, phosphate, and bicarbonate. There is a decrease in the ability to concentrate urine and to cope with fluid imbalances. The infant should void within the first 24 to 48 hours after birth. The baby may void in the delivery room, and it may not be observed. The nurse must keep an accurate record of the frequency of urination. Anuria, changes in color, and any unusual findings should be brought to the attention of the physician.

Male Genitalia. The genitals are undeveloped at birth. The testes of the male child descend into the scrotum before birth. Occasionally, they remain in the abdomen or inguinal canal. This condition is called cryptorchidism (undescended testes). The prognosis is good with proper surgical treatment.

The penis is covered by a sleeve of skin called the foreskin or prepuce. If possible, the foreskin is gently retracted daily at bath time. It is cleansed to remove *smegma* (a cheeselike substance) and bacteria that might cause irritation. The foreskin should be retracted only to the extent that it will not cause pressure. It must be returned all the

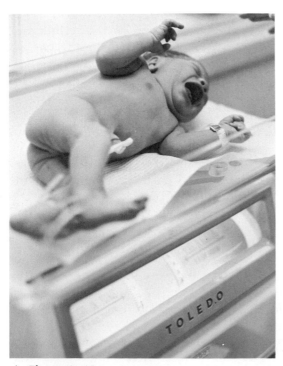

▲ **Figure 4–12**

Weight loss of about 10 per cent occurs within the first 2 days because of fluid shifts.

way to its normal position; otherwise, constriction may cause swelling and impairment of circulation. The foreskin may not be retractable until several weeks after birth, as the prepuce is normally tight during this period. Parents are taught how to retract the foreskin and are encouraged to ask questions concerning this at well visits. Erection of the penis is common and has no significance.

Circumcision is the surgical removal of the foreskin. The procedure has been subject to much controversy. The risks include infection and hemorrhage, among others. Infants with congenital anomalies of the penis, such as hypospadias (the opening of the urethra on the undersurface of the penis), should not be circumcised because the skin may be needed for surgery. Studies linking cancer and the absence of circumcision are considered by some to be incomplete. A discussion of the pro's and con's of this procedure is included as part of prenatal and postpartum education. Regardless of whether the boy is circumcised, he is taught daily hygiene of the genitals when it is age-appropriate. This includes special attention to skin folds, retraction of the foreskin, cleansing of the penis, and examination for lumps or swelling. The nurse must assess the parents' knowledge in this regard and also determines their understanding of circumcision. A surgical consent form must be obtained prior to performing this procedure.

When circumcision is desired, it is performed shortly after birth. This stress should be avoided directly following delivery, when it may also interfere with the bonding process. The baby is restrained on a circumcision board. The foreskin is freed by the use of a scalpel, Gomco clamp, or Hollister Plastibell. A thin layer of Vaseline gauze may be applied to the end of the penis to protect it from moisture and from sticking to the diaper. Postoperatively, the nurse observes for bleeding, irritation, and voiding.

When a Plastibell is used, no incision is made. The foreskin is tied over a fitted plastic ring. The rim usually drops off 5 to 8 days after circumcision. Parents are instructed not to remove it prematurely. No special dressing is required and the baby may be bathed and diapered as usual. A dark brown or black ring encircling the plastic rim is natural. This will disappear when the rim drops off. Instruct parents to consult their physician if there are any questions or if there is increased swelling, if the ring has not fallen off within 8 days, or if the ring has slipped onto the shaft of the penis.

The Jewish religious custom of circumcision, comparable to baptism in the Christian faith, is performed on the eighth day after birth if the baby's condition permits. The baby receives his Hebrew name at this time.

Female Genitalia. The female genitals may be slightly swollen. A blood-tinged mucus may be discharged from the vagina. This is due to hormones transmitted from the mother at birth. The nurse should cleanse the vulva from the *urethra to the anus,* using a clean cotton ball or different sections of a washcloth for each stroke to prevent fecal matter from infecting the urinary tract. The importance of this is stressed to parents.

Integumentary System

Skin. The skin of newborn white babies is red to dark pink in color. The skin of black babies is a reddish brown. Infants of Latin descent may appear to have an olive or yellowish tint to the skin. The body is usually covered with fine hair called *lanugo,* which tends to disappear during the first week of life. This is more evident in premature infants. *Vernix caseosa,* a cheeselike substance that covers the skin of the neonate, is made up of cells and glandular secretions and is thought to protect the skin from infection. White pinpoint pimples caused by obstruction of sebaceous glands may be seen on the nose and chin. These are called *milia* and disappear within a few weeks. *Mongolian spots,* bluish discolorations of the skin, are common in babies of black parents, Native Americans, and those of Mediterranean races. They are usually found over the sacral and gluteal areas. They disappear spontaneously during the first years of life. Pallor or generalized cyanosis is not normal and should be reported.

Many hospitals identify newborn babies by footprints. The skin is so constructed with ridges and grooves that each person has a unique pattern that never changes except to grow larger.

Tissue turgor refers to the condition of the skin in regard to how hydrated or dehydrated the newborn is. To test tissue turgor (elasticity), the nurse gently grasps and releases the skin (Fig. 4–13). It should spring back into place immediately.

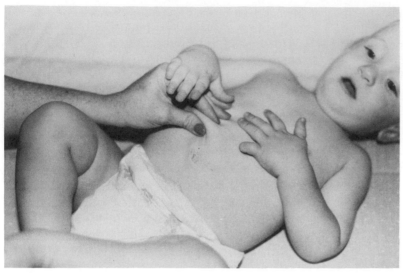

▲ **Figure 4–13**

Testing tissue turgor.

When the skin remains distorted, tissue turgor is termed poor.

Desquamation, or peeling of the skin, occurs during the first weeks of life. Areas such as the nose, knees, elbows, and toes may break down because of friction from rubbing against the sheets. The area involved should be kept dry, and the baby's position should be changed frequently. The buttocks need special attention. A wet diaper should be changed immediately to prevent chafing. The buttocks should be washed and dried well.

Physiological jaundice, also called *icterus neonatorum,* is characterized by a yellow tinge to the skin. It is caused by the rapid destruction of excess red blood cells, which the baby does not need in an atmosphere that contains more oxygen than could be obtained during prenatal life. Plasma levels of bilirubin rise from a normal 1 mg/dl to an average of 5 to 6 mg/dl between the second and fourth day. Physiological jaundice becomes evident between the third and fifth day of life and lasts for about a week. This is a normal process and is not harmful to the baby. However, genetic and ethnic factors may affect its severity, resulting in pathological hyperbilirubinemia. Evidence of jaundice is reported and charted, and the neonate is evaluated frequently to ensure safety.

BATHING THE BABY

The bath is an excellent time to observe the naked newborn infant. Special attention must be given to areas of the skin that come in contact with each other, because chafing may occur. These are found in the neck, behind the ears, in the axillae, and in the groin. They should be dried well. Because powder can be irritating to the respiratory tract, it is not used in the hospital, and parents are discouraged from using it at home. Lotions and the type of soap used will vary with each institution. No bath is necessary after delivery if the blood is wiped from the neonate's face and scalp, because the vernix caseosa is protective. The procedure for bathing the newborn infant is described in the *Home Care* section of this chapter.

Gastrointestinal System

Stools. The normal functions of the gastrointestinal tract begin after birth: food is prepared for absorption into the blood and is absorbed, and waste products are eliminated. *Meconium,* the first stool, is a mixture of amniotic fluid and secretions of the intestinal glands. It is dark green, thick, and sticky, is passed 8 to 24 hours following birth, and continues about 3 days. The stools gradually change during the first week. They become loose and are a greenish-yellow with mucus. These are called *transitional* stools.

The stools of a breast-fed baby are bright yellow, soft, and pasty. There may be three to six stools a day. With age, the number of stools decreases. The bowel movements of a bottle-fed baby are more solid than those of the breast-fed baby. They vary from yellow to brown and are generally fewer in number. There may be one to four a day at first, but gradually this decreases to one or two a day. The stools will be darker when a baby is receiving iron and green when the baby is under the bilirubin lamp. Small, putty-like stools, green watery stools, and bloody stools are abnormal and should be reported. The nursery nurse keeps an accurate record of the number and character of stools each neonate has daily.

Constipation. Constipation refers to the passage of hard, dry stools. Neonates differ in regularity. Some pass a soft stool every other day. This is not constipation. The nurse explains to parents that straining in the newborn period is due to undeveloped abdominal musculature. This is normal and no treatment is required.

Hiccups. Hiccups appear frequently in neonates and are normal. Most disappear spontaneously. Burping the baby and offering warm water may help.

Digestion. Breast-fed babies may be put to breast on the delivery table to help stimulate milk production and for its psychological benefits. Bottle-fed babies usually begin their first feeding by 5 hours of age. A baby's hunger is evidenced by crying, restlessness, sucking the fist, and the rooting reflex. The capacity of the stomach is about 90 ml. Emptying time is 2 to 3 hours, and peristalsis is rapid. Deficiency of pancreatic lipase limits fat absorption. The liver is immature, especially in its ability to conjugate bilirubin, regulate blood sugar, and coagulate blood.

Neonatal Nutrition

BREAST FEEDING

Breast Milk

Breast milk provides immunological, nutritional, and psychosocial advantages. The current trend is toward nursing the newborn infant. Most mothers can nurse their infants (Fig. 4–14). The nurse can play an important role in teaching, supporting, and encouraging the nursing mother.

Compared with cow's milk, breast milk contains more iron, sugar, vitamins A and C, and niacin. Breast milk has less protein and calcium than cow's milk, but the amounts present are better utilized by the baby. Breast milk is more digestible because its fat globules are smaller, and it is pure, i.e., free from bacteria. It provides the baby with greater immunity to certain childhood diseases. Breast-fed babies are less prone to intestinal upsets. In brief, the quality of mother's milk is suited to the needs of the baby.

Practical factors in favor of breast milk are that it saves time and money, it is delivered to the baby in the proper quantity, and it aids the mother physically. As the baby nurses, the mother's

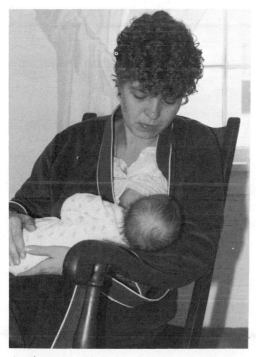

▲ **Figure 4–14**

The mother is seated comfortably with her arm supported when nursing. The baby's entire body is turned toward the breast.

uterus contracts, thus hastening its return to normal size and shape. Mothers receive emotional satisfaction, and bonds of attachment are enhanced during feeding.

Contraindications. Nursing may be contraindicated in mothers with poor physical or mental health. Certainly the mother who has a personal preference not to breast feed should not be forced to do so. Breast feeding may be interrupted for 1 to 2 days in infants with hyperbilirubinemia. Resumption of feeding does not increase bilirubin levels significantly (Behrman and Kleigman, 1990). One disadvantage to the mother of breast feeding is the necessity of being available to the baby, particularly if she works. Breast milk can be expressed manually and given to the baby separately if necessary.

The nurse must keep in mind that even though breast feeding is highly recommended, the choice of the mother should be respected and the decision never criticized. The new mother tends to be especially vulnerable to criticism. She needs rest and a secure environment to prepare her for the busy duties of motherhood. Her stay in the hospital should be a pleasant one, unmarred by thoughtless conversation or personality conflicts.

NURSING BRIEF ▷ ▷ ▷ ▷ ▷ ▷ ▷ ▷ ▷

If a pacifier is used to provide extra sucking, instruct parents to obtain the type that is of one-piece construction to prevent choking. It is not to be tied around the neonate's neck. If the pacifier is continued after 5 to 6 months, it is apt to become a transitional object, which may become more difficult to give up.

Technique of Breast Feeding

In the establishment of lactation, the mother's milk goes through three stages: colostrum, transitional milk, and mature milk. Colostrum secretion is watery and yellowish, begins early in pregnancy, increases, and may last for several days after delivery. Transitional milk replaces colostrum after 2 to 4 days and lasts until about 2 weeks post partum, when mature breast milk is present. The neonate is generally put to breast immediately or shortly after delivery (Fig. 4–15). Current research supports this practice, because it appears to in-

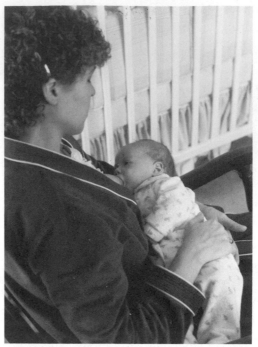

▲ **Figure 4–15**

It is important that the newborn infant grasp a large amount of areola to compress the milk ducts below.

crease early maternal-infant attachment, increase milk production, and decrease the chances of engorgement. The sucking of the neonate stimulates the production of milk; therefore, many doctors suggest that the baby nurse from both breasts at each feeding. The *let-down reflex* by which the milk is squeezed into the large ducts and nipples is stimulated by the infant's sucking or sometimes by the baby's crying. The mother feels a vague tingling sensation in her breasts when this occurs. If she is tense or tired, this feeling can be inhibited. The crying infant does not usually stimulate the let-down reflex until the mother has been conditioned to the infant's crying. Supplemental nursery feedings are to be avoided in favor of more frequent nursing. If the mother has a good fluid intake, an ample diet with extra milk, an adequate vitamin intake, and moderate rest and exercise, most difficulties will be eliminated. Factors to be emphasized are depicted in Table 4–4.

Possible Problems. Although many women nurse successfully with few problems, some fre-

Table 4–4. SUMMARY OF BREAST-FEEDING INSTRUCTIONS FOR THE MOTHER

INFORMATION	RATIONALE
1. Wash hands before proceeding; wash nipples with warm water, no soap	Prevents infection of the newborn and breast

2. Position
  a. Comfortably seated in chair with back and arm support (baby in football position)
  b. Side lying with pillow beneath head, arm above head
  c. Mother will need to experiment initially to find most comfortable positions for her
  d. Entire body of infant turned to mother's breast
	Alternating positions facilitates breast emptying and prevents sore nipples

3. Stroke baby's cheek with nipple	Utilizes rooting reflex; baby will turn toward nipple
4. Baby's mouth should cover entire or large amount of areola	Compresses ducts, lessens tension on nipples
5. Both breasts are used; the first side for about 10 minutes. On the other breast feed for unlimited time.	Allows for letdown on the first breast
6. At next feeding the infant starts to feed on breast used to finish the preceding feeding	Nursing at second breast will increase milk production
7. Retract breast tissue from baby's nose during sucking	Baby will release nipple if unable to breathe
8. Break suction by placing finger in corner of baby's mouth	Removing baby in this way prevents irritation to nipples
9. The neonate is nursed shortly after birth and approximately every 2 to 3 hours thereafter	Initial feedings provide colostrum; establishing a pattern helps baby develop own schedule
10. Burp baby after each breast and after feeding	Rids stomach of air bubbles, reduces regurgitation

quently discussed concerns include the neonate who fiddles, sore and cracked nipples, and breast engorgement. Some babies do not seem to nurse vigorously and fall asleep after 5 minutes, only to wake when they are put in their crib. The mother can first try shifting the baby to the other breast. Babies generally obtain a major portion of what is in the breast after 5 minutes of nursing. Assume that a pacifier may provide for further sucking needs. A baby generally outgrows this behavior in a few weeks as the digestive and nervous systems become more mature.

There are several remedies for sore and cracked nipples. It is important to instruct mothers to be certain that the baby takes a large amount of the areola into the mouth when sucking. To accomplish this, the mother slides all the fingers under the breast to lift and support it for the baby. The thumb is placed above the areola. Move the breast so that the nipple lightly tickles the baby's lower lip. Bring the baby to the breast and not the breast to the baby. Time limits on each breast are no longer thought to prevent nipple soreness. When breaking suction prior to removing the infant from the breast, the mother should insert a finger into the infant's mouth beside the nipple. Frequent nursing will provide continued stimulation of the breast and relieve fullness. The nipples and areola should be washed with water and then allowed to dry thoroughly. Airing the nipples and applying an ointment such as lanolin or Eucerin are also helpful. Avoid using soap or alcohol on the nipples. Keep breast pads dry.

Breast engorgement occurs mainly in the first week of nursing. The breasts become swollen, firm, and tender, and there is less nipple protrusion. Prevention consists of drainage of at least one breast at each feeding. The nurse also instructs the mother to purchase a well-fitting nursing bra and to wear it 24 hours a day. Treatment consists of breast massage and frequent feedings (every 2 to 3 hours). It may be necessary to soften the areola region first by hand expression of milk if the nipple is too hard to get into the baby's mouth. Warm moist compresses or a warm shower provides relief. Ice packs may be applied between feedings.

Since many mothers are being discharged within 48 hours or less after delivery, literature such as *The Womanly Art of Breastfeeding* by the La Leche League is very helpful.

BOTTLE FEEDING

Newborn babies who are not breast-fed are given formula. Modern research has made such feedings safe and nutritionally adequate.

Studies have indicated that babies tolerate cold formula equally as well as formula that has been heated slightly. If cold formula is used, there is no chance of burns from overheated bottles, and time and energy are conserved. There is also a growing concern over burns caused by microwaving bottles. The formula tends to get too hot in the center and give a false reading to the person feeling the bottle on the outside.

The mother or nurse needs to be relaxed and comfortable when feeding the neonate. The head and back are supported in the crook of the arm (Fig. 4–16). The baby should be warm and dry. Propping the bottle on a pad deprives the baby of the pleasure of being held and loved and is dangerous because the baby may choke if the flow of milk is too rapid. The natural tendency for a baby to push the tongue out when the nipple is placed in the mouth (the tongue retrusion reflex) should not be taken as an indication that the infant is not hungry.

Use of Formula

The majority of formulas used today in hospitals and homes are commercially prepared. Brand name formulas, such as Similac, Enfamil, and SMA, are popular. These may be purchased with or without iron, according to the physician's preference and the neonate's needs. Vitamins have been added. Modified formulas such as Special Care or Enfamil Premature are best for preterm infants because of the whey-casein and calcium-phosphorus ratios. Bottles and formula are not routinely sterilized today in homes with a city water supply and available refrigeration.

Always wash hands before handling formula. In homes with dishwashers, the high temperature of the water is excellent for cleansing. Nipples

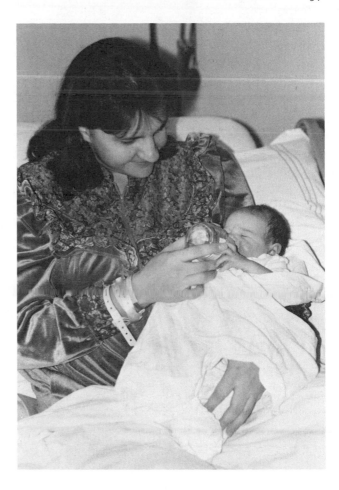

▲ **Figure 4–16**

Position for bottle feeding the newborn infant. (Courtesy of HCA North Hills Medical Center, Fort Worth, Texas.)

should be washed and rinsed by hand, as they may be damaged by the high temperature.

Basically, prepared formulas come in four forms: (1) ready to use in cans; (2) ready to use in disposable bottles; (3) concentrated form in 13-ounce cans, which must be diluted with an equal amount of water; and (4) powdered form in 16-ounce cans—1 level tablespoon of powdered formula for every 2 ounces of water. *When using powdered formula or concentrated liquid, it is important that the nurse determine the mother's understanding of the proportions by reviewing product directions with her.* Some products sold in the United States are packaged with directions in several languages. Tap water may be mixed with powder if the water is from an uncontaminated source. If there is any question, boil the water rapidly for 5 minutes and cool.

Expense governs the choice of formula for many families. In general, the more convenient, the higher the cost. Some nursing bottles utilize sterilized thin plastic nursing containers that come in rolls. These are inserted into the holder and filled according to the manufacturer's directions.

Leftover formula should not be rewarmed for future feedings, as bacteria thrive at room temperature. This can be averted by filling the bottle with the approximate amount the baby generally drinks. Persons who need to sterilize formulas because of travel or personal circumstances are taught the aseptic or terminal heat methods. These are well outlined in government pamphlets and baby books. The services of the public health nurse are invaluable in many instances. Cultural considerations that have a bearing on practices such as feeding a newborn baby can be evaluated at this time.

Regardless of the method used, all bottles, nipples, caps, and other utensils must be thoroughly cleansed. Bottles and nipples are scrubbed with a bottle brush in hot soapy water and rinsed well in hot clear water. Water is squeezed through nipple holes during washing and rinsing. Bottles are placed upside down on a rack to drain. Nipples and caps are put in a clean jar or an area especially designated for them. It is helpful to rinse bottles and nipples immediately after feeding to prevent the milk from forming a film. Nipple covers, made of assorted materials, including paper, are used for the purpose of keeping nipples sterile. If screw cap bottles are utilized, the disc is used to push the shoulder of the nipple through the cap. The disc is then removed and the cap put on the bottle.

Technique of Bottle Feeding

The following points should be observed when feeding the baby by bottle:

1. Wear a covergown.
2. Change diaper as needed. Wash hands following this.
3. Hold the baby unless contraindicated. If a baby cannot be removed from the crib, sit by the child and elevate the head and shoulders.
4. Observe the kind and amount of formula in the bottle.
5. Let a few drops of formula fall on the inner aspect of your wrist to test (only necessary if it was warmed).
   a. Temperature: it should be warm but not hot.
   b. Size of nipple hole: formula should drop but not flow in a steady stream. If the holes are too small, the weak neonate will tire and fail to finish the feeding. If they are too large, the baby may choke or miss the satisfaction received from sucking.
6. Do not contaminate the nipple.
7. Hold the bottle so that the nipple is full of formula. This prevents the baby from swallowing air.
8. Burp the baby halfway through the feeding and at the end by one of the following methods:
   a. Place a diaper or small towel over your shoulder to protect your gown. Place the

baby firmly against your shoulder and pat the back.
   b. Place the baby in a sitting position. Put a towel beneath the chin. Support the chest and head with one hand. Gently rub the back with the other.
9. The feeding should take 15 to 20 minutes. Do not hurry the baby or force the infant to eat too much.
10. Leave the baby clean and dry. Place the baby on the abdomen or right side to promote digestion and prevent aspiration of regurgitated milk or vomitus.
11. Chart the amount of formula offered, the amount taken and retained, regurgitation or vomiting, how the formula was taken, and whether or not the baby appeared satisfied following the feeding. (Note that regurgitation is an overflow of milk that occurs shortly after feeding. Vomiting means bringing up a more substantial amount of partially digested milk.)

In the hospital, newborn babies are fed according to individualized schedules. The majority are fed every 3 or 4 hours. In the home, the baby who is fed when hungry ("demand feedings") will soon adopt a flexible schedule. Prompt fulfillment of the baby's needs assures the infant that the world is a good place in which to live.

Infection

Infections that are relatively harmless to an adult may be fatal to the newborn infant. Symptoms are often subtle in the early stages, the recognition of which can be crucial (Table 4–5). Portals of entry are the respiratory tract, the gastrointestinal tract, the genitourinary tract, and breaks in the skin. The portals of exit are the same as those just mentioned, and the organisms are in the excretions from the various systems: sneezes, sputum, vomitus, feces, saliva, urine, and discharges from the skin and mucous membranes. Nursery standards are developed and enforced by various professional agencies such as the American Academy of Pediatrics, hospital accreditation boards, and local health agencies. Provisions governing space, control of temperature and humidity, light-

Table 4–5. CLINICAL FEATURES OF NEONATAL SEPSIS

GENERAL
Poor feeding
Irritability
Lethargy
Temperature instability

RESPIRATORY
Grunting
Nasal flaring
Intercostal retractions
Tachypnea/apnea

CNS
Hypotonia
Seizures
Poor spontaneous
movement

SKIN
Petechiae
Pustulosis
Sclerema
Hyperemia

GASTROINTESTINAL
Diarrhea
Hematochezia
Abdominal distention

HEMATOPOIETIC
Thrombocytopenia
Leukocytosis,
leukopenia

CARDIOVASCULAR
Bradycardia/
tachycardia
Hypotension
Cyanosis

From Klaus, M., and Fanaroff, A. (1986): *Care of the High-Risk Neonate.* Philadelphia, W. B. Saunders.

ing, and safety from fire and other hazards are considered. Each newborn infant has her or his own crib, bath equipment, and linen supply. Any communal equipment is sterilized following each use.

PREVENTION OF INFECTION

The nurse caring for neonates may wear a covergown over the uniform to prevent cross-infection and to protect the infant. Some nursery personnel wear scrub gowns while in the nursery and put covergowns on if they leave the nursery. Students should investigate the policy of the institution in which they are practicing. A nurse who has a fever, skin infection, or gastrointestinal disease should not work in the nursery. Since many hospitals have open visiting, all visitors should be cautioned not to come if they are sick.

Handwashing Technique

The most effective procedure employed in the prevention of infections is *proper handwashing*. The nurse must conscientiously wash and rinse the hands and forearms before handling each baby and before and after handling equipment. Although most organisms are transmitted by direct contact, some are capable of remaining alive for a time outside the body and may be transferred indirectly by articles. Personnel entering the newborn nursery scrub their hands with an antiseptic. In other areas of the hospital hands are washed with soap under running water. Parents and relatives should be taught the importance of this simple but highly effective procedure.

PROCEDURE ▶ ▶ ▶ ▶ ▶ ▶ ▶ ▶ ▶

Equipment. Running water, soap, paper towels.

Method
1. Keep the hands lowered over the basin throughout the procedure.
2. Wet the hands.
3. Soap hands well, working up a lather.
4. Rinse the bar of soap, leaving it clean for the next use.
5. Use friction. Rub well between the fingers and around the nails. Wash the entire hands, wrists, and forearms; rinse well.
6. Repeat steps 2, 3, 4, and 5 three times.
7. Dry the hands well.
8. If there is no foot pedal, turn faucet off with a paper towel.

SIGNS AND SYMPTOMS OF INFECTION

The following signs and symptoms of infection in newborns and infants should be reported:

1. Temperature elevation (to 37.8°C, 100°F) or depression below 36°C (97°F).
2. Refusal to take nourishment.
3. Rashes or skin lesions.
4. Loose, watery stools.
5. Discharge from eyes, nose, umbilicus.

6. Vomiting.
7. Lethargy, irritability.
8. Others as indicated in Table 4–5.

The sick newborn is removed from the nursery and placed in an isolated room or special isolation nursery if contagious. Persons who care for an infected baby must not enter the regular newborn nursery.

Care of the Patient Unit

A baby in the newborn nursery is usually placed in a small, transparent bassinet equipped with a bath tray that can be pulled out. On the children's unit the baby may be placed in the same type of bassinet or in a crib. When making a crib, the nurse places the baby at the bottom and tucks the clean sheet in at the top of the mattress, and then puts the baby at the top of the crib and tucks the sheet in at the bottom. The nurse must guard the infant when the crib side is down. If the crib is large, it may be easier to place the baby on the far side of it and apply the clean sheet lengthwise. The nurse tucks in the closer side, raises the cribside, and finishes the other side of the mattress.

The newborn infant in the hospital needs to wear only a shirt and a diaper and to be covered with a light blanket. A shirt that ties or snaps on in a double-breasted fashion is easy to put on and gives added warmth to the chest. Most hospitals use disposable diapers, although there is discussion now about returning to cotton diapers for environmental reasons.

Rooming-In

Rooming-in is the term given to the hospital experience in which the mother keeps her newborn baby by her bedside and takes as much care of the infant as her condition permits and she desires. Its advantages are that the baby receives individual attention from and becomes better ac-

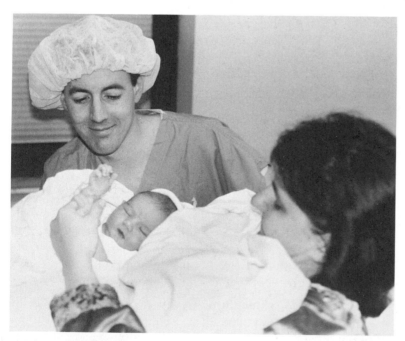

▲ Figure 4–17

The beginning of the bonding process immediately after delivery. (Courtesy of HCA North Hills Medical Center, Fort Worth, Texas.)

quainted with the parents and that the mother need not worry that her baby is being neglected in the busy nursery. It also provides an excellent opportunity for the caregiver to teach parents many aspects of infant care. The nurse who calls the baby by name, encourages holding the baby en face, discusses particular behavior patterns, and points out unique characteristics helps enhance the bonding process (Fig. 4–17). This is especially important if the parents' "fantasy child" differs from the "real" child in terms of sex, physical attributes, or health. Nursing assessment includes observation of specific parenting behavior, such as amount of affection shown to the baby, level or lack of interest in the child, amount of physical contact, stimulation, and eye-to-eye contact, and amount of time spent interacting with the baby. The extent to which the parents encourage involvement of siblings and grandparents with the infant's arrival is also noteworthy in assessing the attachment process. This information provides a basis for nursing intervention that may serve to foster positive family relationships.

BONDING/ATTACHMENT

The terms *bonding* or *attachment* are sometimes used interchangeably although they have different meanings. Bonding is thought to occur soon after birth, and attachment occurs gradually during the first year of the infant's life (Fig. 4–18). Maternal attachment behaviors include gazing at, kissing, touching, holding the infant en face, and talking to the infant in a higher-pitched voice than normal. The father is included in the bonding process, as are other significant others in untraditional families (Fig. 4–19). The nurse can point out various behaviors of the neonate, encourage eye contact, and provide periods of privacy for the couple.

SIBLINGS

Brothers and sisters (or siblings) are less likely to regard their new baby as an intruder or a rival if they are made to feel that the baby is theirs as well as their parents'. If the other children are made to feel wanted, accepted, and cherished,

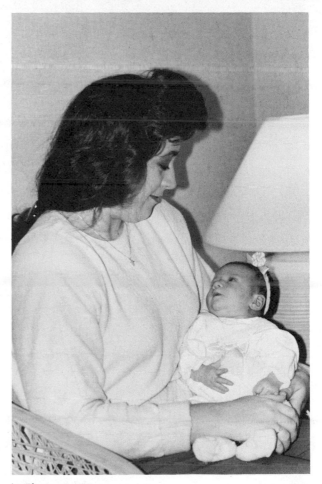

▲ **Figure 4–18**

Parental bonding from the earliest weeks appears to be a major determinant in the quality of attachment. (Courtesy of HCA North Hills Medical Center, Fort Worth, Texas.)

their jealousy of the newborn baby will be kept at a minimum (Fig. 4–20).

Classes to help siblings prepare for the new baby are held in some hospitals. Questions are answered, and a tour of appropriate areas is held. This generally includes the nursery and the "room where Mom will be." The children have their picture taken and these are placed in the mother's file. The pictures remain there until the baby is born and are then taped to the corresponding bassinet. This helps young children to locate "their baby" on the first hospital visit. These classes help

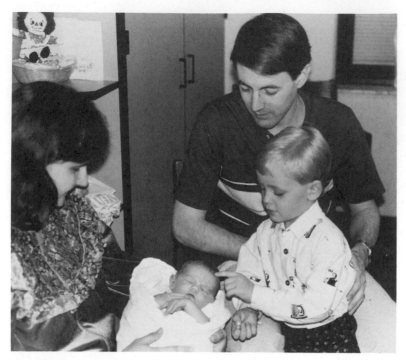

▲ **Figure 4–19**

The bonding room. (Courtesy of HCA North Hills Medical Center, Fort Worth, Texas.)

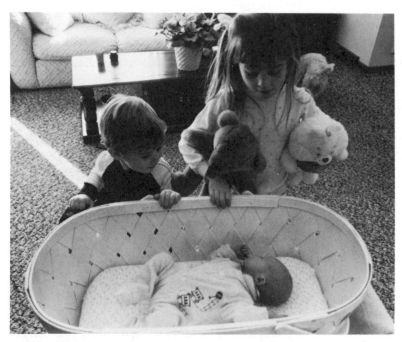

▲ **Figure 4–20**

The arrival of a newborn baby has an impact on the established pattern of the family. The family has changed and a new balance must be found by siblings.

the staff become acquainted with the rest of the family prior to delivery and directly involve the siblings. Two common questions from toddlers are "Why doesn't the baby have any hair?" and "When are you going to take the baby back to the hospital, Mommy?"

NURSING BRIEF ▷ ▷ ▷ ▷ ▷ ▷ ▷ ▷ ▷
Upon return from the hospital, if siblings are waiting it is helpful if father arrives carrying the baby. This leaves mother's arms free for hugs before introductions are made.

Spiritual Care

If the condition of a neonate is poor, parents who are Christians may wish to have the baby baptized. The minister or priest should be notified. In an emergency, the nurse may perform the baptism by pouring water on the baby's forehead while saying "I baptize thee in the name of the Father, and of the Son, and of the Holy Spirit." Should there be any doubt as to whether the baby is alive, the baptism is given conditionally: "If you are capable of receiving baptism, I baptize you in the name of the Father, and of the Son, and of the Holy Spirit."

Occasionally parents will pin small medals to the baby's blankets or clothing. The nurse must be extremely careful not to lose these because they are of great sentimental and religious value to the parents, particularly if the baby dies.

Discharge Teaching

As the number of postpartum hospital days continues to decrease, the importance of discharge teaching increases. Prior to discharge, follow-up appointments for visits with both the pediatrician and obstetrician are made. Many families are cared for by physicians and nurses in hospital clinics and public health clinics. Mothers should be informed of the location of these facilities and appointments made there prior to discharge. The social worker may be involved in the planning and implementation of this care. This insures that the infant will receive care in well-baby clinics in the areas of anticipatory guidance, immunizations, growth and development, physical assessment, nutrition, and emotional health.

Parents should receive instruction in the following areas:

1. Feeding
2. Bathing (bathing time can vary and is not necessary each day)
3. Elimination (skin should be cleansed after each diaper change)
4. Temperature
5. Growth and development
6. Safety
7. Follow-up medical care (well-baby check-ups, immunizations)
8. Skin care (it is not necessary to use lotions, oils, and so on)
9. Detection and removal of "cradle cap"

The following method for giving a sponge bath may be used in the nursery or pediatric unit and in the home until the cord has healed. The nurse will have to adapt it to the patient's condition and the routine of the hospital. Involve the baby's parents in this procedure as much as possible.

PROCEDURE   ▶ ▶ ▶ ▶ ▶ ▶ ▶ ▶ ▶

Equipment. Linen: bath towel, washcloth, shirt, diaper, quilted pad, crib sheet, receiving blanket. Bath tray: cotton balls, mild soap, baby oil or lotion, comb. Paper bag; wash basin; clean covergown for nurse.

Method
1. The bath can be given when it best fits into the schedule of the family. It should not be given immediately after a feeding. Temperature of room should be 23.8 to 26.6°C (75 to 80°F), temperature of water 37.7 to 40.6°C (100 to 105°F) (test with elbow or bath thermometer). Wash hands. Don clean covergown.
2. Wash baby's face with plain water and dry.
3. Clean outer nostrils as needed. Use a separate cotton wisp moistened with water for each side of the nose.

4. Wrap washcloth around one finger and cleanse outer ear.

5. Squeeze cheeks gently to examine mouth. Gums should be pink and clean, breath should be sweet.

6. Wash scalp by making a lather of soap on the hands. Go over the scalp thoroughly. Observe fontanels.

7. Hold head over tub, and rinse soap off with a wet washcloth. (If there is a scaly crust [cradle cap], apply oil at night and the scale will come off more readily with the next morning's shampoo.) Dry gently with a soft towel.

8. Remove diaper and cleanse diaper area with cotton dipped in water. Wash from front to back, using a separate cotton ball for each stroke.

9. Remove shirt, soap hands, and go over the entire body, front and back. Rinse with washcloth. Pay special attention to creases, folds, and genitals.

10. Pat dry and re-dress. Comb hair.

11. Apply clean crib sheet and quilted pad to crib. Cover baby with clean receiving blanket. Tidy unit.

NURSING BRIEF ▷ ▷ ▷ ▷ ▷ ▷ ▷ ▷
Emphasize flexibility in the time of the bath. Stress the need to gather all materials beforehand to avoid leaving the neonate unattended and/or chilled. The nurse attempts to help parents relax by emphasizing that there is nothing baffling about bathing a baby.

Home Phototherapy. In the past the hospital stay of infants was prolonged when they received phototherapy. Currently, many women are leaving the hospital within the first 24 hours of birth. This further complicates the treatment of physiological jaundice and would necessitate the return of the infant to the hospital and separation of the mother and child. Home therapy allows the mother and baby to leave the hospital together, thus maintaining continuous bonding and control of the care of the infant at home (Ludwig, 1990).

Referral for home phototherapy is based on the infant's health, weight, and bilirubin levels and the suitability of the family to comply with the home program. The equipment is usually provided by an outside vendor. A nurse assists the family in the discharge teaching, set-up, and care throughout the treatment. The family keeps records concerning the baby's temperature, feedings, appearance of the eyes (color, drainage, lesions), number of wet diapers, and number and description of stools. Nursing care of the infant receiving phototherapy is further developed in Chapter 5.

References

American Academy of Pediatrics (1986). Use and abuse of the Apgar score. *Pediatrics* 78:1148–1149.

Behrman, R., and Kleigman, V. (1987). *Nelson Essentials of Pediatrics.* Philadelphia, W. B. Saunders Company.

Brazelton, T. B. (1984). *Neonatal Behavioral Assessment Scale,* ed. 2. Philadelphia, J. B. Lippincott Co.

Levine, M., Carey, W., Crocker, A., and Gross, R. (1983). *Developmental-Behavioral Pediatrics.* Philadelphia, W. B. Saunders.

Ludwig, M. (1990). Phototherapy in the home setting. *J. Pediatr. Health* 4:304–308.

Bibliography

Behrman, R., and Vaughan, V. (1987). *Nelson Textbook of Pediatrics,* 13th ed. Philadelphia, W. B. Saunders Company.

Foster, R., Hunsberger, M., and Anderson, J. J. (1989). *Family-Centered Nursing Care of Children.* Philadelphia, W. B. Saunders Company.

Heffern, D. (1990). Reminders for building confidence in breast-feeding Moms. *Maternal-Child Nurs* 15:267.

Marlow, D., and Redding, B. (1988). *Textbook of Pediatric Nursing,* 6th ed. Philadelphia, W. B. Saunders Company.

Mott, S., James, S., and Sperhac, A. (1990). *Nursing Care of Children and Families.* Redwood City, CA, Addison-Wesley.

Olds, S., London, M., and Ladewig, P. (1988). *Maternal-Newborn Nursing,* 3rd ed. Menlo Park, CA, Addison-Wesley.

Shrago, L., and Bocar, D. (1990). The infant's contribution to breastfeeding. *JOGN* 19:209–220.

Whaley, L., and Wong, D. (1987). *Nursing Care of Infants and Children.* St. Louis, C. V. Mosby Company.

STUDY QUESTIONS

1. What is the meaning of an Apgar score of 7?
2. Define the following: meconium; vernix caseosa; fontanels; Moro reflex; rooting reflex; tonic neck reflex.

3. It is feeding time and you have just brought Mrs. Webster and Mrs. Jones their babies. Mrs. Webster is nursing her baby; Mrs. Jones' baby is bottle-fed. They are discussing feedings and ask your opinion. What would your reply be in this situation?

4. What principles will you include when teaching Mrs. Loomis to bottle-feed her newborn baby?

5. What care is given to the umbilicus of the neonate? Why is this care important?

6. Define circumcision. Describe how you would teach Mrs. Zimmerman how to care for newly circumcized Harold.

7. What measures must the nurse take to prevent infection of the newborn infant in the newborn nursery? On the children's unit?

8. Describe how a nurse guides and assists a mother in the process of bonding.

9. Baby Rand is crying loudly in her bassinet. List several discomforts that might be the cause of her unhappiness. What can the nurse do to alleviate them? How can you help Mrs. Rand interpret her baby's crying?

10. Define skin turgor. How does the nurse test for good skin turgor?

11. Discuss three areas concerning care of the newborn baby that you would cover with a parent prior to discharge.

CHAPTER 5 _____

Chapter Outline

THE PRETERM INFANT
CAUSES OF PRETERM BIRTH
RISKS RELATED TO PREMATURITY
SPECIAL NEEDS AND CARE OF THE PRETERM
  INFANT
FAMILY REACTION TO THE PRETERM INFANT
THE POST-TERM INFANT
INFANTS OF DIABETIC MOTHERS (IDMs)
TRANSPORTATION OF THE HIGH-RISK
  NEONATE

Objectives

Upon completion and mastery of Chapter 5, the
student will be able to
- Define the vocabulary terms listed.
- Differentiate between the preterm and the low
  birth weight neonate.
- List three causes of preterm birth.
- Describe the handicaps of preterm birth and the
  nursing goals associated with each handicap. (For
  example, "Poor control of body temperature—
  Keep warm with incubator.")
- Contrast the techniques of feeding the preterm
  and the full-term neonate.
- Discuss two ways to help facilitate the maternal-
  infant bonding process for a preterm neonate.
- List three characteristics of the post-term baby.

THE HIGH-RISK NEONATE

Terms

atelectases (111)
grunting (111)
high-risk (107)
lanugo (111)
macrosomia (118)
previability (111)
respiratory distress syndrome (111)
transport team (119)

The Preterm Infant

The high-risk infant is any infant who is at risk of developing medical, developmental, or psychological problems. The goal is prevention or early detection of these problems. With increased specialization and sophisticated monitoring techniques, many babies who would have died if born a few years earlier are now surviving. The nurse's role has become more and more complex, with greater emphasis on subtle clinical observations. This chapter serves only to acquaint the student with the high-risk infant in order to encourage appreciation of this baby's struggle for survival and the intense responsibility placed on those entrusted with care.

Any neonate whose life or quality of existence is threatened is considered to be in a *high-risk category* and requires close supervision by professionals. Prematurity and low birth weight often occur at the same time, and both factors are associated with increased neonatal morbidity and mortality. The less a baby weighs at birth, the greater the risks to life during delivery and immediately thereafter. According to the National Infant Mortality Surveillance Project, the high infant mortality rate in this country is attributed to the steady increase of low birth weight infants born (Swartz, 1990).

In the past, a newborn infant was classified solely by birth weight. Those infants weighing less than 2500 g are classified as low birth weight (LBW) and those less than 1500 g as very low birth weight (VLBW). Likewise, those infants weighing above the 90th percentile on intrauterine growth curves are referred to as large for gestational age (LGA). Emphasis is now also placed on gestational age and level of maturation (Fig. 5–1). Current data also indicate that intrauterine growth rates are not the same for all babies and that individual factors must be considered.

Gestational age refers to the actual time, from conception to birth, that the fetus remains in the uterus. A full-term infant is born between 38 and 42 weeks. Those infants who are born at less than 38 weeks are called preterm and those born at more than 42 weeks are called post-term. The Dubowitz scoring system is used to determine gestational age. The Dubowitz scoring system consists of evaluation of physical characteristics and neuromuscular tone (Fig. 5–2).

Level of maturation refers to how well developed the baby is at birth and the functional ability of the organs to exist outside the uterus. The physician can determine a great deal about the maturity of the neonate through careful physical examina-

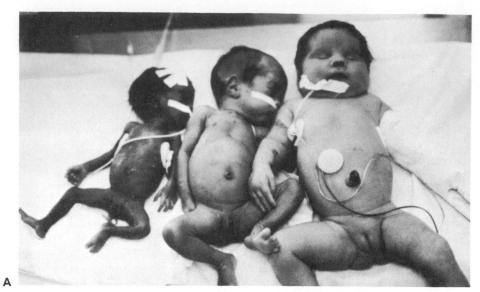

A

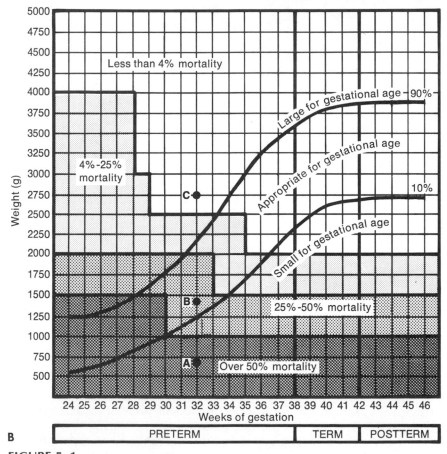

B

▲ **FIGURE 5–1**

See legend on opposite page

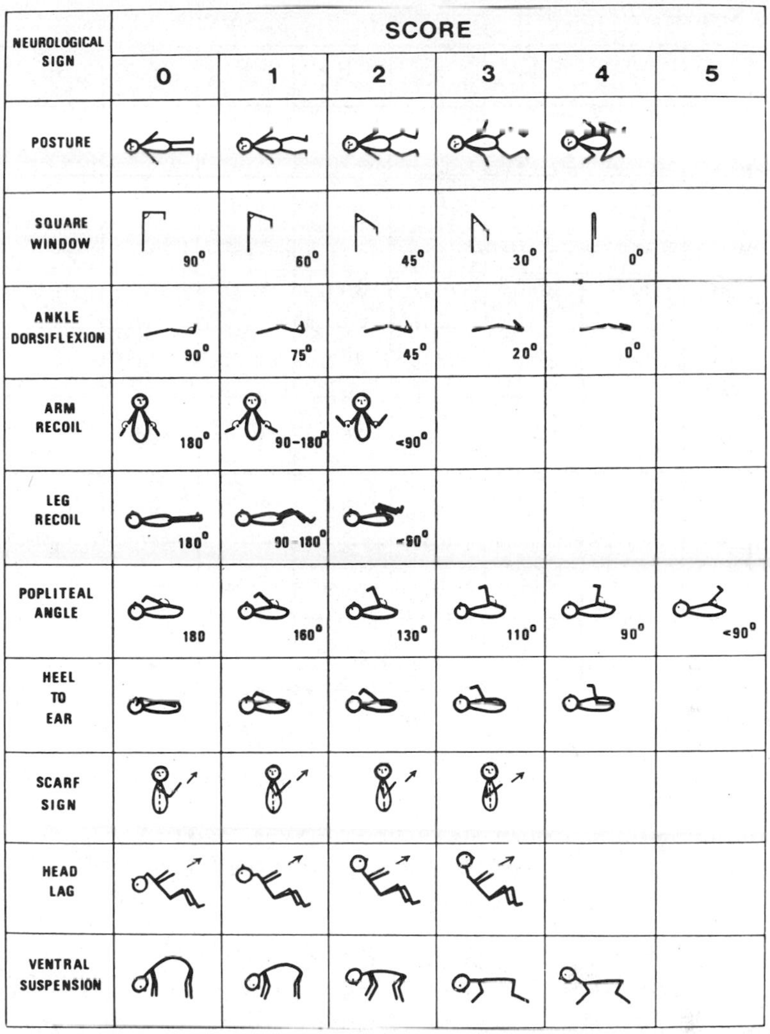

NEUROLOGICAL SIGN	SCORE					
	0	**1**	**2**	**3**	**4**	**5**
POSTURE						
SQUARE WINDOW	90°	60°	45°	30°	0°	
ANKLE DORSIFLEXION	90°	75°	45°	20°	0°	
ARM RECOIL	180°	90-180°	<90°			
LEG RECOIL	180°	90-180°	<90°			
POPLITEAL ANGLE	180	160°	130°	110°	90°	<90°
HEEL TO EAR						
SCARF SIGN						
HEAD LAG						
VENTRAL SUSPENSION						

A

▲ **FIGURE 5–2**

A, Dubowitz scoring system for neuromuscular criteria. Add scores for all signs and apply score to *B.*

Illustration continued on following page

▲ **FIGURE 5–1**

A, Three babies of the same gestational age (32 weeks) weighing 600, 1400, and 2750 g, respectively. (From Korones, S. B. [1986]. *High Risk Newborn Infants. The Basis for Intensive Care,* 4th ed. St. Louis, The C. V. Mosby Company.) *B,* Classification of the newborn infant as indicated by relationship of weight to gestational age. The status of babies of the weights shown in *A* is plotted at 32 weeks (dots A, B, and C). (From Whaley, L. F., and Wong, D. L. [1983]. *Nursing Care of Infants and Children,* 2nd ed. St. Louis, The C. V. Mosby Company; adapted from Battaglia, F. C., and Lubchenco, L. C. [1967] A practical classification of newborn infants by weight and gestational ages. *J. Pediatr.* 71:59.)

Score   **Units**

	0	1	2	3	4	5	6	7	8	9
0						26.0	26.0	26.5	26.5	27.0
10	27.0	27.5	27.5	28.0	28.0	28.5	29.0	29.0	29.5	29.5
20	30.0	30.0	30.5	30.5	31.0	31.0	31.5	31.5	32.0	32.0
30	32.5	33.0	33.0	33.5	33.5	34.0	34.0	34.5	34.5	35.0
40	35.0	35.5	35.5	36.0	36.0	36.5	36.5	37.0	37.5	37.5
50	38.0	38.0	38.5	38.5	39.0	39.0	39.5	39.5	40.0	40.0
60	40.5	40.5	41.0	41.0	41.5	42.0	42.0	42.5	42.5	43.0
70	43.0									

B

▲ **FIGURE 5–2** *Continued*

B, To determine gestational age in weeks, take score from examination, find on chart, and read off value in weeks. For example, for a score of 44, find 40 in the far left column. Then read across to the column headed by 4. The gestational age is 36.0 weeks. (From Dubowitz, L. M., Dubowitz, V., and Goldberg, C. [1970]. *J. Pediatr.* 77:1.)

tion, observation of behavior, and family history. A baby who is born at 34 weeks' gestation, weighs 3.5 pounds at birth, has not been damaged by multifactorial birth defects, and has had a good placenta may be healthier than a full-term small for gestational age baby whose placenta was insufficient for any of a number of reasons. This infant is also probably in better shape than the heavy but immature baby of a diabetic mother. Each child has different, distinct needs.

CAUSES OF PRETERM BIRTH

The causes of prematurity are numerous; in many instances the cause is unknown. Prematurity may be caused by multiple births, illness of the mother (e.g., malnutrition, heart disease, diabetes mellitus, or infectious conditions), or the hazards of pregnancy itself, such as toxemias, placental

abnormalities that may result in premature rupture of the membranes, placenta previa (the placenta lies over the cervix instead of higher in the uterus), and premature separation of the placenta.

Studies also indicate that there are relationships between prematurity and smoking, alcohol consumption, and substance abuse. Third trimester use of cocaine by pregnant women has been reported to induce a sudden onset of uterine contractions and fetal tachycardia (Smith, 1988). Adequate prenatal care to prevent preterm birth is extremely important. There is evidence that inadequate prenatal care correlates with low birth weight infants and premature delivery (Hogue and Ray, 1989). The presence of parents in special care nurseries is commonplace. This encourages bonding and attachment. Many of these premature infants are born into families with numerous problems. The parents may not be prepared to handle the additional strain imposed by a preterm infant.

Parent aides and other types of home support and assistance are vital, particularly because current studies indicate a correlation between high-risk births and child abuse and neglect.

RISKS RELATED TO PREMATURITY

Premature birth deprives the neonate of the complete benefits of intrauterine life. The baby whom the nurse sees in the incubator will resemble pictures of a fetus of 7 months' gestation. The skin is transparent and loose. Superficial veins may be seen beneath the abdomen and scalp. There is a lack of subcutaneous fat, and fine hair called *lanugo* covers the forehead, shoulders, and arms. The cheeselike vernix caseosa seen in more mature infants is conspicuously absent. The extremities appear short, and the abdomen protrudes. The nails are short. The genitals are small. In girls, the labia majora may be open.

Inadequate Respiratory Function

Important structural changes occur in fetal lungs during the second half of pregnancy. The alveoli, or air sacs, enlarge, which brings them closer to the capillaries in the lungs. The failure of this phenomenon leads to many deaths attributed to *previability* (*pre*, before + *vita*, life). In addition, the muscles that move the chest are not fully developed; the abdomen is distended, causing pressure on the diaphragm; the stimulation of the respiratory center in the brain is immature; and the gag and cough reflexes are weak because of inadequate nerve supply.

Respiratory Distress Syndrome

Description. Respiratory distress syndrome (RDS) is a disorder that is most frequent among small neonates. The United States Department of Health and Human Services (1989) reported that of the 250,000 premature infants born in the United States in 1989 with RDS, about 5000 die (Ioli and Richardson, 1990). Because of the immaturity of the lungs, there is decreased gas exchange. This, together with pulmonary structural immaturity, results in absolute or functional deficiency of surfactant. Surfactant prevents collapse of the alveoli during expiration by reducing surface tension in the lung. Without surfactant, the alveoli must be re-expanded with each breath so that adequate gas exchange can occur. The result is an infant who is using all available energy to breathe.

Signs and Symptoms. Signs of RDS may develop at birth, but more mature infants (of at least 34 weeks' gestation) may not show signs until 3 to 4 hours after birth (Behrman and Kleigman, 1990). Manifestations of RDS include cyanosis, tachypnea, nasal flaring, intercostal and sternal retractions, and grunting. Infants with severe RDS develop edema, apnea, and respiratory failure that requires mechanical ventilation.

Treatment. If insufficient amounts of surfactant are detected by means of amniocentesis, it is possible to speed up its production by giving the mother injections of corticosteroids such as betamethasone. Administration 1 or 2 days before delivery may reduce the chances of RDS. Surfactant replacement therapy has recently been approved. Surfactant is administered into the infant's endotracheal tube so that the drug can be instilled directly into the lungs (Ioli and Richardson, 1990). Although this technique is in its infancy, some of the indications at this time are that surfactant will reduce pulmonary complications, improve gas exchange, and require shorter intensive care stays for the infant (Ioli and Richardson, 1990). Other studies have failed to show a reduction in morbidity or mortality (Reynolds and Wallander, 1990). Continued research will be needed to perfect the administration of this drug.

Atelectasis

Description. The lungs are collapsed during fetal life; their failure to expand after birth is known as atelectasis. Some lung expansion must take place with the first breath, although full development may be several days later. *Primary* atelectasis, in which the alveoli fail to expand, may occur in preterm infants, infants of mothers oversedated before delivery, and infants with damage to the respiratory center in the brain. *Secondary* atelectasis occurs when the lungs collapse after they have once inflated. This may be caused by pulmonary disease, aspirated mucus, or a foreign body.

Symptoms. The infant exhibits irregular, rapid respirations. These may be accompanied by a respiratory grunt and flaring of the nostrils. The skin is cyanotic and mottled. Inter-rib and sternal retractions may be noticeable. X-ray studies that reveal increased density, sometimes throughout both lungs, confirm the diagnosis. The prognosis depends on the general condition of the baby and the cause.

Apnea

Apnea in the preterm infant is fairly common. Premature infants have periods of rapid respirations, followed by very slow breathing, and then a period of no apparent respirations. Apnea is defined as the cessation of breathing for 20 or more seconds. This may be accompanied by bradycardia (fewer than 100 heart beats per minute) and cyanosis.

Nursing Care. Apnea monitors, usually set at 15 seconds, help alert nurses to a cessation of respirations. This does not remove the nurse's responsibility to observe the infant for signs of respiratory distress. If the monitor alarm sounds, the nurse should first assess the infant for signs of distress: color and respirations. It is not unusual for the monitor to have false alarms due to loose leads and other mechanical causes. If an apneic spell has occurred, the nurse can gently rub the infant's feet, ankles, and back. If stimulation fails, the nurse should suction the nose and oropharynx and reposition the head by raising the head to a "sniffing" position. If breathing still does not begin, the infant should be ventilated via an Ambu bag.

Sepsis

Sepsis refers to a generalized infection in the bloodstream. All neonates are at risk of developing sepsis, but preterm infants are at even greater risk. The infant has diminished immunity, and usually there is no local inflammatory response at the site of the infection, which makes the signs and symptoms vague.

Signs and Symptoms. Manifestations of sepsis are often vague and are sometimes based on an infant's "not looking right." All the body systems may be affected by sepsis. Some of the more common manifestations include hypothermia, fever, and changes in feeding, color, and activity. Table 4–5 shows the various system responses to sepsis.

Nursing Care. Prevention of sepsis is the goal of the nurse when caring for a preterm infant. Good handwashing is imperative before and after handling the baby or the equipment used in the infant's care. Nurses caring for infants in the neonatal intensive care unit (NICU) wear gowns and gloves when handling the infant or touching any objects in the baby's environment. The infant is handled gently, and a thermoregulated environment is provided to conserve energy. Infants with sepsis are isolated to prevent the spread of infection to other neonates.

Necrotizing Enterocolitis

Premature infants weighing between 1400 and 1500 g and with a mean gestational age of between 30 and 32 weeks are most often affected by necrotizing enterocolitis (NEC) (Rushton, 1990). The cause of NEC is controversial, but there seems to be a relationship among intestinal ischemia, bacteria in the area, and the feeding of formula.

Signs and Symptoms. Early signs, such as temperature instability, apnea, and bradycardia, are difficult to differentiate from those of other diseases. More specific manifestations include a distended abdomen, bilious vomitus, blood in the stool, and diarrhea.

Nursing Care. Early recognition of the signs and symptoms of the disease aids in early treatment. Rectal temperatures should not be taken because of the danger of perforation. Strict handwashing and other infection control measures are implemented. The nurse monitors vital signs and reports any abnormal findings. Orders for resuming feedings are followed closely.

Hypoglycemia and Hypocalcemia

Hypoglycemia. In the preterm infant, this is defined as glucose plasma concentrations of less than 30 mg/dl (Bobak and Jensen, 1991). The preterm infant has not remained in the uterus long enough to have sufficient supplies of fat or glycogen to mobilize glucose.

Signs and Symptoms. Besides the obvious low glucose level, determined by plasma or blood, the nurse should observe for other manifestations of hypoglycemia. They include feeding difficulty, hunger, lethargy, apnea, irregular respiratory effort, cyanosis, weak and high-pitched cry, jitteriness, twitching, eye rolling, and seizures.

Nursing Care. Nursing care is primarily the identification of signs and symptoms that might indicate this disorder. The nurse should also control the thermal environment to prevent increased energy needs for the infant to adjust to a cold environment. Feeding the infant also aids in prevention.

Hypocalcemia. *Hypocalcemia* (*hypo*, below + *calcemia*, calcium in the blood) is also seen in preterm infants and sick neonates. Calcium is transported across the placenta throughout pregnancy but particularly during the third trimester. Early birth can result in babies with lower serum calcium levels. Other stressors, such as perinatal asphyxia, trauma, infants born to diabetic mothers, and so on, may predispose the newborn infant to hypocalcemia. "Early" neonatal hypocalcemia is seen in the first 2 or 3 days of life. It usually is temporary. "Late" hypocalcemia appears about 1 week after birth. It results when babies are fed unmodified cow's milk, which depresses activity of the parathyroid glands. This condition is also referred to as "neonatal tetany." Serum calcium levels are monitored for all high-risk neonates. Normal levels range from 8.0 to 10.5 mg/dl. Hypocalcemia is treated by early feedings and calcium supplements when possible.

Hemorrhagic Disease

Infants are born with a deficiency of vitamin K. The neonate's intestinal tract is also sterile and unable to synthesize the vitamin until feedings are begun.

Signs and Symptoms/Treatment. Manifestations of the disease usually occur on the second or third day. The nurse should observe for oozing from the umbilicus or circumcision site, bloody or black stools, hematuria, bruising, and epistaxis (nose bleed). Vitamin K is given intramuscularly during the first 24 hours to prevent this disorder.

Retinopathy of Prematurity

This disorder is caused by the effect of oxygen toxicity on the developing blood vessels of the premature infant's retina. Retinopathy of prematurity is the leading cause of blindness in infants weighing less than 1500 g. The incidence may be reduced by careful monitoring of arterial blood gases in infants receiving oxygen.

Jaundice

The liver in the neonate is immature and takes 3 to 7 days to start functioning effectively. Physiological jaundice was discussed on page 92 and occurs during the third to fifth postpartum day. Preterm infants may have higher peak levels of bilirubin (15 mg/dl), and the peaks occur later (5th day) (Behrman and Kliegman, 1990). Jaundice on the first day of life is always pathological and should not be confused with physiological jaundice. Phototherapy is the treatment for reducing or preventing rising bilirubin levels when they are related to physiological jaundice. The light waves assist in the breakdown of bilirubin in the skin into excretable byproducts. Nursing Care Plan 5–1 is a nursing care plan for newborns receiving phototherapy in the hospital.

SPECIAL NEEDS AND CARE OF THE PRETERM INFANT

Care of the preterm infant is similar to that of the term infant in that the infant is assessed at birth and resuscitation performed if indicated. When respiratory function is established, the infant is then examined for any other problems that may be present. Routine care may be delayed until the infant is stable. Stabilization of respirations and thermoregulation take priority over all other types of care. The infant may need to be transferred from a community hospital to an NICU.

CARE PLAN 5–1

THE NEONATE RECEIVING PHOTOTHERAPY

Nursing Diagnosis	Goals/Outcome Criteria	Intervention
Potential for injury to eye, related to phototherapy	Infant will not experience eye damage Infant displays no evidence of eye irritation as evidenced by the absence of discharge or corneal irritation	Apply eye patches over infant's closed eyes while under lights Remove patches at least once per shift to assess eyes for conjunctivitis Remove patches to allow eye contact during feeding Remove patches to promote parental bonding
Skin impairment, related to immature structure and function, immobility	Infant will not develop skin breakdown Skin remains intact as evidenced by absence of skin rash, excoriation, or redness	Observe for maculopapular rash Cleanse rectal area gently, as stools are often green and liquid Reposition at least every 2 hours Assess for jaundice or bronzing (*Note*: serum bilirubin may be high even though baby may not appear jaundiced under lights) Observe for pressure areas
Potential for dehydration, related to increased water loss through skin and loose stools	Infant will not become dehydrated Infant displays no signs of dehydration as evidenced by good skin turgor, moist mucous membranes, and maintenance of weight	Monitor IV fluids Check skin turgor Observe for depressed fontanel Anticipate the need for additional water between feedings Daily weights unless contraindicated
Potential for hyperthermia or hypothermia	Infant will maintain normal body temperature Infant's temperature will be maintained between 36.3 and 37.4°C (97.4 and 99.4°F)	Monitor newborn's temperature Adjust incubator to maintain neutral thermal environment Infant is naked except for eye patches and cap
Potential for neurological damage, related to nature of hyperbilirubinemia	Infant will not experience neurological damage Infant will show no signs of neurological involvement (lethargy, twitching)	Anticipate daily bilirubin blood levels Turn phototherapy lights off when blood is being drawn to avoid false readings Observe parameters for neurological deficit (e.g., twitching, lethargy)

CARE PLAN 5–1 *Continued*

THE NEONATE RECEIVING PHOTOTHERAPY

Nursing Diagnosis	Goals/Outcome Criteria	Intervention
Nutrition alterations: less than body requirements	Infant will receive adequate nutrients Infant will show signs of adequate nutrition as indicated by weight gain	Provide feedings as ordered Assist mother to re-establish breast feeding if temporarily halted
Injury potential, related to immobility, electrical apparatus	Infant will be protected from injury Infant will show no signs of burns or other breaks in skin integrity	Ascertain that all electrical outlets are grounded Record number of hours lights have been in use, change prn Use Plexiglas cover or shield to protect infant in case of lamp breakage
Parental anxiety, related to knowledge deficit, crises	Parents will have a decrease in anxiety Parents will verbalize fears concerning infant's disease and treatment	Explain procedures and treatment Provide reassurance Provide follow-up

This may mean immediate separation of the infant from the family unit. Obviously, issues of bonding and attachment need to be addressed.

Thermoregulation. One of the most critical needs of the high-risk infant is the control of body temperature. The preterm infant lacks insulating fat and there is excessive heat loss by radiation from a surface area that is large in proportion to body weight. After birth, all high-risk infants should be dried immediately to eliminate evaporative heat loss. A radiant warmer should also be provided for these infants (Behrman and Kleigman, 1990) (Fig. 5–3).

The infant is placed in an incubator or radiant warmer. The infant's temperature is maintained at a constant level by a heat-sensitive probe that is taped to the abdomen or back. The infant's axillary temperature is also monitored. Overhead radiant warmers have the advantage of providing easier access to the patient while maintaining a neutral environment. The nurse should also

1. Prewarm all surfaces that will come in contact with the infant.
2. Avoid drafts in the room.
3. Use discretion in bathing the infant. Regular assessment has a much higher priority than a routine daily bath because of the danger of loss of heat through evaporation.
4. Provide a plastic heat shield for very low birth weight infants.
5. Use knitted caps and booties if the infant is removed from the radiant warmer (Fig. 5–4).
6. Wrap the infant in a blanket if the infant is removed from the radiant warmer.

Nutrition. The feeding of the preterm infant may be oral, by gavage (feeding by tube), or parenteral. Sick and very premature infants are usually given intravenous fluids. IVs given through a catheter passed into the umbilical vein may be started shortly after delivery. Small amounts are given, sometimes as little as 5 ml per hour. Preterm infants younger than 32 to 34 weeks are usually fed through a nasal or gastric tube because of their immature sucking and swallowing reflexes. As the infant progresses, nipple and gavage feedings may be alternated. The nurse observes the infant's suck and swallow reflexes, weight gain, and lack of respiratory distress to determine whether nipple feeding is being tolerated. Breast milk that has been expressed and

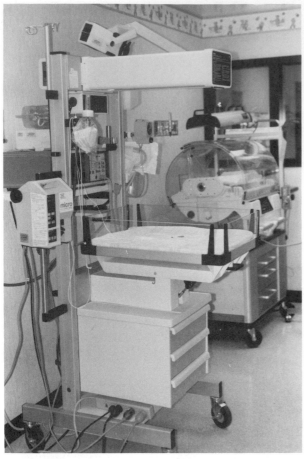

▲ FIGURE 5–3

The radiant warmer is used to conserve and maintain the infant's body heat. (Courtesy of HCA North Hills Medical Center, Fort Worth, Texas.)

stored properly or formula may be fed to the infant when ordered. Special small and soft nipples are available for the small infant.

The feeding should take no longer than 15 to 20 minutes. Feeding for longer periods will use more calories than will be supplied by the feeding. The infant is fed in a semisitting position and burped gently after each half-ounce. After the feeding the infant should be placed on the abdomen or side with the head slightly raised.

Fluid intake is recorded scrupulously. The nurse reports the number of voids and color and specific gravity of the urine, and observes for signs of edema. The hydration needs of the patient are reviewed daily on the basis of intake, output,

weight, blood chemistry studies, and general appearance.

Close Observation. The doctor examines the premature baby when the patient's condition permits and writes specific orders concerning treatment and nursing care. When he or she leaves the nursery, the doctor relies on the nurses for notification of any significant changes in the baby's condition (Fig. 5–5). The experienced nurse in the premature nursery observes and charts care and treatment with great accuracy. For example, a chapter could be spent on observations of the premature infant's behavior during feedings. Table 5–1 lists *general* observations to serve as a guide in premature care. Sudden changes are reported immediately.

Position and Skin Care. The premature infant with a great deal of mucus is placed in the head-down position or turned from side to side at least every 2 hours. Plan feedings and postural drainage times so that both can provide maximum benefits without interference with the other. The premature baby should not be left in one position for long periods, as it is uncomfortable and may be harmful to the lungs. Changing the baby's position will also prevent pressure breakdowns on the

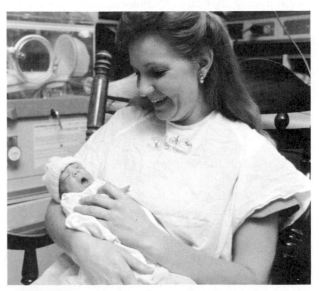

▲ FIGURE 5–4

When the infant is removed from the radiant warmer, a knitted cap and booties should be worn. (Courtesy of Cook–Fort Worth Children's Medical Center, Fort Worth, Texas.)

Parents need to be prepared for comments by relatives on the baby's small size and slower development. In general, base the growth and development of the preterm infant on current age minus the weeks preterm, e.g., if born at 36 weeks' gestation, a 1 month old infant would be at a newborn achievement level. This way, no one has unrealistic expectations for the infant.

Parents need guidance throughout the infant's hospitalization to help prepare them for this new experience. They may be disheartened by the unattractive appearance of the premature baby. They may believe that they are to blame for the baby's condition. They may fear that the baby will die but are unable to express their feelings. They need time to look at and touch the baby, and to begin to see this child as uniquely their own. This touch and immediate human contact are vital for the infant as well. The mother is usually concerned with her ability to care for such a small and helpless creature. When she feels ready, she may

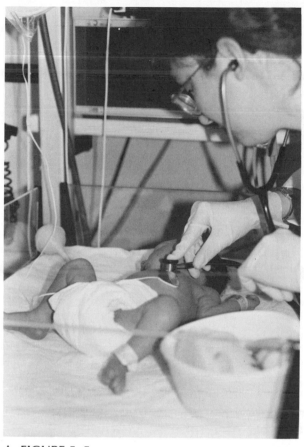

▲ FIGURE 5–5

Physical assessment of the premature infant is an ongoing process. (Courtesy of HCA North Hills Medical Center, Fort Worth, Texas.)

delicate skin. If such a breakdown should occur, the area is exposed to the air and a suitable ointment is applied as prescribed by the physician. (See page 91 for a more extended discussion on the skin of the neonate.)

FAMILY REACTION TO THE PRETERM INFANT

In the absence of severe birth defects and complications, the growth rate of the preterm infant nears that of the term baby by about the second year. Very low birth weight infants may not catch up, especially if there has been chronic illness, insufficient nutritional intake, or inadequate caretaking (Behrman and Vaughan, 1987).

Table 5–1. NURSING OBSERVATIONS IN CARE OF PRETERM INFANTS

CHARACTERISTICS	THINGS TO LOOK FOR
Color	Paleness; cyanosis; jaundice
Respirations	Regularity; apnea; sternal retractions; labored breathing
Pulse	Rate and regularity
Abdomen	Distention
Stools	Frequency; color; consistency
Skin	Rashes; irritations; pustules; edema
Cord	Discharge
Eyes	Discharge
Feeding	Sucking ability; vomiting or regurgitation; degree of satisfaction
Mucous membranes	Dryness of lips and mouth; signs of thrush
Voiding	Initial; frequency
Fontanels	Sunkenness or bulging
General activity	Increase or decrease in movements; lethargy; twitching; frequency and quality of cry; hyperactivity

assist the nurse in diapering, bathing, feeding, and so on. During these times other aspects of baby care are also stressed.

When infants need special care and are separated from their parents, there may be difficulties with bonding and attachment. Nurses need to be aware of this and facilitate the attachment process. Encouragement of visiting, calling, and participating in care, when possible, are all ways of supporting the family through this crisis. Parents can help siblings accept the infant by naming the child and using the name, sharing news of progress, taking pictures of the infant, and encouraging them to send drawings and cards to the infant. Some hospitals have special areas where siblings may visit through a window.

Discharge planning should begin at the baby's birth. Parents may experience anxiety when they take their infant home. They may question their ability to handle an infant who has been receiving specialized care. They need to be confident in routine infant care as well as any special care the infant requires. Instructions in prevention of infection should be a priority teaching goal. Follow-up visits are scheduled, and any home health care needs are identified and met. The nurse stresses the importance of well-baby examinations and immunizations for this infant.

NURSING BRIEF ▷ ▷ ▷ ▷ ▷ ▷ ▷ ▷
Encourage parents to talk about their feelings and fears concerning the preterm infant and how they will care for this child at home.

The Post-Term Infant

The newborn baby is considered post-term if a pregnancy goes beyond 42 weeks. This is a great psychological strain on both the mother and the other members of the family who are eagerly awaiting the birth of the baby. What causes postmaturity is not yet clear; however, it is known that the placenta does not function adequately as it ages, which could result in fetal distress. Very large neonates, such as those of diabetic mothers, are not necessarily postmature but are instead larger than normal because of rapid abnormal growth before delivery. The mortality rate of "late" babies is two to three times higher than that of newborn infants delivered at term, particularly when the lateness exceeds 3 weeks. The fetal death rate is greater than that of the neonate. Once the baby makes it through delivery, the risks are less.

The post-term infant is long and thin and looks as though she or he has lost weight. The skin is loose, especially about the thighs and buttocks. There is little downy hair (lanugo) or vernix caseosa. Loss of this cheeselike protection leaves the skin dry; it cracks and peels and is almost parchment-like in texture. The nails are long and may be stained with meconium. The baby has a good head of hair and looks alert. Many postmature babies suffer few adverse effects from the delay, but they still require careful observation in the nursery.

When it is determined, by testing, that a pregnancy is past 42 weeks, the well-being of the mother and infant determine the course that is taken. Cesarean sections are performed if there is fetal distress or a risk to the mother.

Infants of Diabetic Mothers (IDMs)

The successful regulation of diabetes has led to increasing numbers of diabetic women bearing children. These infants are considered at high risk because they were exposed to high levels of maternal glucose before birth. The pancreas of the fetus responds by producing more insulin, which is an important regulator of fetal growth and metabolism. This is believed to account for the large size of these babies. The mortality rate is high. *Macrosomia* (*macro*, large + *soma*, body) has been considered a classic symptom of diabetic babies. The baby's face is large and puffy, resembling a child on steroids. These infants are also candidates for problems such as perinatal asphyxia, birth trauma, polycythemia, hyperbilirubinemia, hyaline membrane disease, and other complications. It is imperative that these babies be born in centers where there is expert supervision or be transferred to a regional care center shortly after birth.

Transportation of the High-Risk Neonate

Transportation of the high-risk neonate requires organization and the expertise of a special team. Successful transport depends upon anticipating the need for transport, stabilizing the infant prior to transport, and preparing the parents (Gellis and Kagan, 1990). Many hospitals have special transport teams, which may include a nurse, a respiratory therapist, and sometimes a physician. Baseline data, such as vital signs and blood work (blood gases and glucose levels), are ascertained. The neonate is weighed if this is not contraindicated. Copies of all records are made. This includes the baby's record, the mother's prenatal history and delivery, and pertinent admission data. A transport incubator is provided for warmth. Batteries are kept fully charged.

The mother is shown the baby prior to the departure. If she is unable to hold the infant because of the condition, the incubator is wheeled to her bedside so that she may observe and touch the baby. A Polaroid picture is taken and given to the parents. On occasion, a mother is unable to see her baby because of her own unstable condition. Such situations require special empathy from nursing personnel.

Once the baby has safely reached the destination, the parents should be contacted by telephone. It is also thoughtful if the receiving hospital personnel provide feedback to the transport team so that they may enjoy the results of their efforts.

References

Behrman, R., and Kleigman, R. (1990). *Nelson Essentials of Pediatrics*. Philadelphia, W. B. Saunders Company.

Behrman, R., and Vaughan, V. (1987). *Nelson Textbook of Pediatrics*, 13th ed. Philadelphia, W. B. Saunders Company.

Bobak, I., and Jensen, M. (1991). *Essentials of Maternity Nursing*, 3rd ed. St. Louis, C.V. Mosby.

Gellis, S., and Kagan, B. (1990). *Current Pediatric Therapy*. Philadelphia, W. B. Saunders Company.

Hogue, C., and Ray, Y. (1989). Preterm delivery: Can we lower the black infant's first hurdle? *JAMA* 264:548–549.

Ioli, J., and Richardson, M. (1990). Giving surfactant to premature infants. *Am. J. Nurs.* March:59–60.

Reynolds, M., and Wallander, K. (1990). Surfactant for neonatal respiratory distress syndrome. *J. Pediatr. Health Care* 4:209–215.

Rushton, C. (1990). Necrotizing enterocolitis. *Maternal-Child Nurs.* 15:296–313.

Smith, J. (1988). The dangers of prenatal cocaine use. *Maternal-Child Nurs.* 13:174–179.

Swartz, M. (1990). Infant mortality: Agenda for the 1990s. *J. Pediatr. Health* 4:169–174.

Bibliography

Foster, R., Hunsberger, M., and Anderson, J. J. (1989). *Family-Centered Nursing Care of Children*. Philadelphia, W. B. Saunders Company.

George, D., Stephen, S., Fellows, R., and Bremer, D. (1988). The latest on retinopathy of prematurity. *Maternal-Child Nurs.* 13:254–258.

Martin, L., and Reeder, S. (1991). *Essentials of Maternity Nursing*. Philadelphia, J. B. Lippincott Company.

Meier, P., and Anderson, G. (1987). Responses of small preterm infants to bottle- and breast-feeding. *Maternal-Child Nurs.* 12:97–105.

Mott, S., James, S., and Sperhac, A. (1990). *Nursing Care of Children and Families*. Redwood City, CA, Addison-Wesley.

Olds, S., London, M., and Ladewig, P. (1988). *Maternal Newborn Nursing*, 3rd ed. Menlo Park, CA, Addison-Wesley.

Wilks, S., and Meier, P. (1988). Helping mothers express milk suitable for preterm and high-risk infant feeding. *Maternal-Child Nurs.* 13:121–123.

STUDY QUESTIONS

1. List the risks related to prematurity.
2. What is an incubator? A radiant warmer?
3. How does the nursing care of the premature baby differ from that of the full-term neonate?
4. Define the following: preterm; sternal retractions; phototherapy.
5. What is retinopathy of prematurity?
6. Close observation is extremely important in the care of the premature infant. List several significant changes that should be reported to the nurse in charge.
7. What problems confront the parents of the premature infant? In what ways might the nurse facilitate maternal-infant bonding?

C H A P T E R   6 _____

Chapter Outline

**MALFORMATIONS PRESENT AT BIRTH
  (CONGENITAL)**
NERVOUS SYSTEM
    Hydrocephalus
    Myelodysplasia/Spina Bifida
CARDIOVASCULAR SYSTEM
    Congenital Heart Disease (CHD)
GASTROINTESTINAL SYSTEM
    Cleft Lip
    Cleft Palate
MUSCULOSKELETAL SYSTEM
    Clubfoot
    Congenital Hip Dysplasia
DOWN SYNDROME
PERINATAL DAMAGE
HEMOLYTIC DISEASE OF THE NEWBORN:
    ERYTHROBLASTOSIS FETALIS
INTRACRANIAL HEMORRHAGE
INFECTIONS
THRUSH (ORAL CANDIDIASIS)
INFECTIOUS DIARRHEA
THE SKIN
    Impetigo
    Staphylococcus aureus Infection
IMMUNE SYSTEM
    AIDS, AIDS-Related Complex
      (ARC)

Objectives

Upon completion and mastery of Chapter 6, the student will be able to

- Define the vocabulary terms listed.
- List and define the more common disorders of the newborn period.
- Differentiate between communicating and noncommunicating hydrocephalus.
- Outline the preoperative and postoperative nursing care of a neonate with spina bifida cystica.
- Summarize the nursing goals significant to the care of the neonate with a congenital heart defect and discuss what, if any, modifications of these goals are necessary following surgery.
- Describe two feeding techniques used for the patient born with a cleft lip or cleft palate and provide the rationale for such modifications.
- List three ways in which the nurse can help facilitate maternal-infant bonding when a baby is born with a birth defect.
- Discuss the nursing measures for the patient in a body cast and provide the rationale for each.
- Describe the nursing care of the neonate with infectious diarrhea, including the types of precautions that are necessary to prevent the spread of infection throughout the nursery.

DISORDERS OF THE NEWBORN

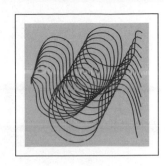

Terms

choroid plexus (122)
congenital malformation (121)
habilitation (125)
hemodynamics (128)
hyperbilirubinemia (144)
multifactorial (127)
shunt (123)
tenesmus (147)
TORCH (122)
transillumination (122)

In the United States, approximately 100,000 infants are born each year with serious congenital anomalies (U.S. Department of Health and Human Services, 1989). Each year, 1.2 million infants, children, and adults are hospitalized for treatment of health problems related to congenital anomalies.

An abnormality of structure, function, or metabolism may result in a physical or mental handicap, may shorten life, or may be fatal (Birth Defects, 1986). Table 6–1 depicts the current system of classification of birth defects. Because these disorders include so many conditions, it has been necessary to limit the number discussed in this chapter and to place others in relevant areas of the text (see index for specific conditions).

Defects present at birth often involve the skeletal system; limbs may be missing, *malformed*, or duplicated. Some abnormalities, such as congenital hip dysplasia, are more subtle and require alertness on the part of nurses to detect. Inborn errors of metabolism include a number of inherited diseases that affect *body chemistry*. There may be an absence or a deficiency of a substance necessary for cell metabolism. This is usually an enzyme. Almost any organ of the body may be damaged. Examples of inborn errors of metabolism include cystic fibrosis and phenylketonuria. In disorders of the blood, there is a reduced or missing blood component or an inability of a component to function adequately. Sickle cell anemia, thalassemia, and hemophilia fall into this category. Chromosomal abnormalities number in the hundreds. Most involve some type of mental retardation, and some are incompatible with life. The newborn infant with Turner syndrome or Klinefelter syndrome may be retarded in physical growth and sexual development. Perinatal damage has many causes and is seen in a variety of forms, most common of which is premature birth. "Few birth defects can be attributed to a single cause. The majority are thought to result from an interplay between environment and heredity, depending on inherited susceptibility, stage of pregnancy, and degree of environmental hazard" (Birth Defects, 1986).

Malformations Present at Birth (Congenital)

NERVOUS SYSTEM

Hydrocephalus

Description. Hydrocephalus (*hydro*, water + *cephalo*, head) is a condition characterized by an increase of cerebrospinal fluid (CSF) in the ventricles of the brain, which causes an increase in the

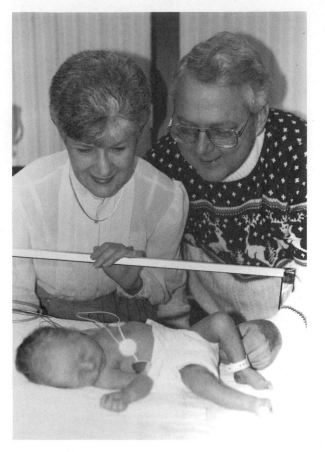

▲ **FIGURE 6–1**

Visits from relatives are encouraged in the neonatal unit when a newborn infant has an extended stay. (Courtesy of HCA North Hills Medical Center, Fort Worth, Texas.)

size of the head and pressure changes in the brain. It occurs as a result of an imbalance between production and absorption of CSF. Hydrocephalus may be congenital or acquired. It may occur in conjunction with a meningomyelocele or as a sequela of infections (including congenital TORCH infections,* encephalitis, or meningitis) or of perinatal hemorrhage. The symptoms depend on the site of obstruction and the age at which it develops. Although there are many causes of hydrocephalus, all result in either an impairment of CSF absorption within the subarachnoid space (communicating hydrocephalus) or an obstruction of CSF flow within the ventricles (noncommunicating

*TORCH stands for *t*oxoplasmosis, *o*ther, *r*ubella, *c*ytomegalovirus, and *h*erpes simplex.

hydrocephalus). Hydrocephalus may proceed slowly or rapidly. Two forms of hydrocephalus are the Arnold-Chiari malformation and the Dandy-Walker syndrome. Because this condition can cause progressive cerebral damage, early recognition and treatment are very important.

The nurse will recall that the brain and spinal cord are surrounded by fluid, membranes, and bone. The three membranes, called *meninges,* are the dura mater, the arachnoid, and the pia mater. The arachnoid, or middle membrane, resembles a cobweb, with its spaces filled with fluid. Cerebrospinal fluid is also found in spaces of the brain called *ventricles.* The primary site of formation is believed to be the *choroid plexus.*

Signs and Symptoms. These depend upon the time of onset and the severity of the imbalance. The classic sign both in congenital hydrocephalus and in hydrocephalus with onset in infancy is an increase in head size. The direction of skull expansion depends on the site of obstruction. Transillumination (*trans,* across + *illuminare,* to enlighten), the inspection of a cavity or organ by passing a light through its walls, is a simple diagnostic procedure useful in visualizing fluid. A flashlight with a sponge rubber collar is held tightly against the infant's head in a dark room. The examiner observes for areas of increased lu-

---

Table 6–1. CLASSIFICATION OF BIRTH DEFECTS

MALFORMATIONS PRESENT AT BIRTH: Structural defects such as hydrocephalus, spina bifida, congenital heart malformations, cleft lip and palate, clubfoot, congenital hip dysplasia, others
INBORN ERRORS OF METABOLISM (body chemistry): Cystic fibrosis, PKU, Tay-Sachs, others
BLOOD DISORDERS: Sickle cell anemia, hemophilia, thalassemia, defects of white blood cells and immune defense, others
CHROMOSOMAL ABNORMALITIES: Down syndrome, Klinefelter syndrome, Turner syndrome, trisomies 13 and 18, many others
PERINATAL DAMAGE: Infections, drugs, maternal disorders, abnormalities unique to pregnancy (Rh disease, difficult labor or delivery, premature birth)

Data from Birth Defects (1985). Tragedy and Hope. White Plains, N.Y., March of Dimes Birth Defects Foundation.

minosity. Another sign is a bulging anterior fontanel and separation of cranial sutures. The scalp is shiny, and the veins are dilated. The infant is helpless and lethargic. The body becomes thin, and the muscle tone of the extremities is often poor. The cry is shrill and high-pitched. Irritability, vomiting, and anorexia are present, and convulsions may occur. In severe infantile hydrocephalus, the eyes may appear deviated downward ("setting sun" sign) (Fig. 6–2). Children with onset of hydrocephalus later in childhood may have minimal enlargement of the head and will present with signs and symptoms of increased intracranial pressure.

Diagnosis and Treatment. The child's head is measured daily. Echoencephalography, a computed tomography (CT) scan, or magnetic resonance imaging (MRI) is most frequently used to show the enlarged ventricles and locate the level of obstruction. A ventricular tap or puncture may be performed in the treatment room, using sterile technique. The equipment needed is the same as

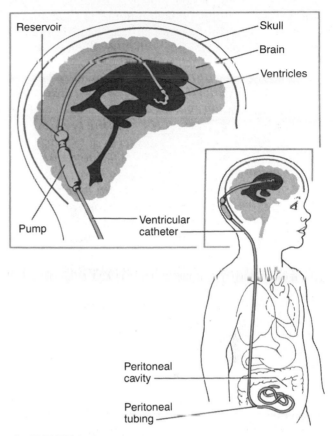

▲ **FIGURE 6–3**

Placement of the ventriculoperitoneal shunt. (From Foster, R., Hunsberger, M., and Anderson, J. J. [1989]. *Family-Centered Nursing Care of Children*. Philadelphia, W. B. Saunders Company.)

that for a lumbar puncture. The specimen is labeled and sent to the laboratory for analysis.

After careful evaluation of these and other preoperative tests, the doctor decides whether or not to operate. The surgeon attempts to bypass or *shunt* the point of obstruction. The cerebrospinal fluid may thus be carried to another area of the body, where it will be absorbed and finally excreted. This is accomplished by inserting special tubing, which is replaced at intervals as the child grows (Fig. 6–3). Two types of shunts are used: the ventriculoperitoneal (VP) shunt and the ventriculoatrial (VA) shunt. The VP shunt is most common (Fig. 6–3). The prognosis for this condition has improved with modern drugs and surgical techniques. If the brain is not seriously damaged before the operation, mental function may be

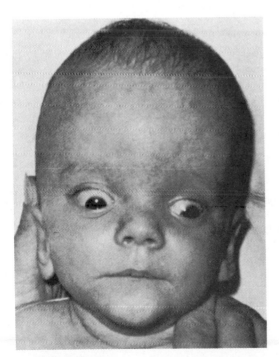

▲ **FIGURE 6–2**

Marked hydrocephalus with "setting sun" sign and divergence of the eyes. (From Youmans, J. R. [1982]. *Neurological Surgery*. 2nd ed. Philadelphia, W. B. Saunders Company, p. 1384.)

preserved. Motor development is sometimes slower if the child cannot lift the head normally. Complications of shunts are usually mechanical flaws (kinking or plugging of tubing) or infection. The shunt acts as a focal spot for infection and may need to be removed if infection persists. The shunt will also have to be replaced as the child grows.

NURSING CARE

The general nursing care of an infant with hydrocephalus who has not undergone surgery presents several problems. The child may be barely able to raise the head. Mental development is delayed. Lack of appetite, a tendency to vomit easily, and poor resistance to infections present challenging problems.

The position of the patient must be changed frequently to prevent hypostatic pneumonia and pressure sores. Hypostatic pneumonia occurs when the circulation of the blood in the lungs is poor and the patient remains in one position too long. It is particularly prevalent in patients who are poorly nourished or weak, or who have a debilitating disease. When the nurse turns the patient with hydrocephalus, the head must always be supported. To turn the patient in bed, the weight of the head should be borne in the palm of one hand and the head and body should be rotated together to prevent a strain on the neck. When the patient is lifted from the crib, the head must be supported by the nurse's arm and chest. The head circumference is measured daily. Because this measurement is so critical, the child's head is marked with a marking pen where the measurement is taken.

Pressure sores may occur if the patient's position is not changed at least every 2 hours. The tissues of the head and ears as well as the bony prominences have a tendency to break down. A pad of lamb's wool or sponge rubber placed under the head may help avoid these lesions. If the skin becomes cracked, it should be given immediate attention to prevent infection. The patient must be kept dry, especially around the creases of the neck, where perspiration may collect.

In most cases the nurse may hold the infant for feeding. The nurse sits with the arm supported, since the baby's head is heavy. A calm, unhurried manner is necessary. The room should be as quiet as possible. Following the feeding, the infant is placed on the side. Do not disturb after he is once settled, since the baby vomits easily. The nurse must organize daily care so that it does not interfere with meals.

Observations to be made include type and amounts of food taken, vomiting, condition of skin, motor abilities, restlessness, irritability, lethargy and changes in vital signs. Fontanels are palpated for size and bulging. Changes in vital signs associated with increased intracranial pressure (ICP) are usually a later sign in infancy. They include an elevated blood pressure and a decrease in pulse and respirations. Signs of a cold or other infection are reported to the nurse in charge immediately and are recorded.

Postoperative nursing care is complex. Often students assist or are coassigned with a graduate. In addition to routine postoperative care and observations, the nurse observes the patient for signs of ICP and of infection at the operative site or along the shunt line.

Bacterial infection is a life-threatening complication that sometimes makes it necessary to remove the shunt. Signs of infection include poor feeding, elevated vital signs, decreased level of consciousness, vomiting, and seizure activity. The nurse also should observe for signs of inflammation at the shunt insertion site. The surgeon will indicate the position desired and the activity level of the child.

If the fontanels are sunken, the infant is kept flat, since too rapid reduction of fluid may lead to seizures or cortical bleeding. If the fontanels are bulging, the patient is usually placed in the semi-Fowler position to assist in drainage of the ventricles through the shunt. The patient is always positioned so as to avoid pressure on the operative site. Head and chest measurements are recorded; in patients with peritoneal shunts the abdomen also should be measured or observed to detect malabsorption of fluid. Skin care continues to remain a priority. As the patient's condition improves, parents are instructed in the care of the shunt.

In the presence of increased intracranial pressure, the shunt can be tested for patency by compressing the antechamber or reservoir. The physician may order the pump to be depressed a certain number of times per day to facilitate drainage.

Myelodysplasia/Spina Bifida

Myelodysplasia refers to a group of central nervous system disorders characterized by malformation of the spinal cord, one of which is spina bifida.

Description. *Spina bifida* (divided spine) is a congenital embryonic neural tube defect in which there is an imperfect closure of the spinal vertebrae. There are two forms, *occulta* (hidden) and *cystica* (sac or cyst). Spina bifida occulta is a relatively minor variation of the disorder in which the opening is small and there is no associated protrusion of structures. It is often undetected and occurs most commonly at L5 and S1 levels. There may be a tuft of hair, a dimple, a lipoma, or a port-wine birthmark at the site. Generally, treatment is not necessary unless neuromuscular symptoms appear. These consist of progressive disturbances of gait, footdrop, or disturbances of bowel and bladder sphincter function.

Spina bifida cystica consists of the development of a cystic mass in the midline of the spine (Fig. 6–4). *Meningocele* and *meningomyelocele* are two types of spina bifida cystica. A meningocele (*meningo*, membrane + *cele*, tumor) contains portions of the membranes and cerebrospinal fluid. The size varies from that of a walnut to that of the head of a newborn infant.

More serious is a protrusion of the *membranes* and *spinal cord* through this opening, or a *meningomyelocele*. Although it resembles a meningocele, there may be associated paralysis of the legs and poor control of bowel and bladder functions. Hydrocephalus is common.

Treatment. The treatment is surgical closure to prevent meningeal infection. The child is observed for the development of hydrocephalus and is shunted if this occurs. Urinary retention is managed by catheterization. The prognosis depends on the extent of the motor deficit, the status of the bladder innervation, and any other anomalies (Behrman and Vaughan, 1987). Care of the child involves a multidisciplinary approach including neurology, neurosurgery, urology, pediatrics, physical therapy, occupational therapy, and nurs-

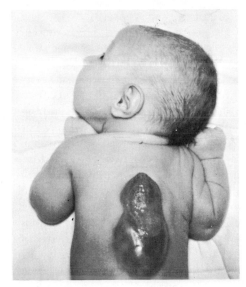

▲ **FIGURE 6–4**

Newborn infant with spina bifida. (From Burroughs, A. [1986]. *Bleier's Maternity Nursing,* 5th ed. Philadelphia, W. B. Saunders Company.)

ing. Depending upon the extent of the defect, the child may have problems with hydrocephalus, orthopedic defects, genitourinary abnormalities, and paralysis. *Habilitation* is necessary after surgery to minimize the child's handicap and put to constructive use the normal parts of the body. Every effort is made to help the child develop a healthy personality so that he or she may live a happy and useful life. Eventually the child may attain some degree of fecal continence and some type of emptying of the bladder (intermittent clean catheterization). Mobility is assisted through bracing, surgery, and the use of a wheelchair.

NURSING CARE

The student nurse will need demonstrations and careful explanations when assisting with the care of these infants in the hospital. The main objectives of the extensive nursing care required include prevention of infection of or injury to the sac; correct position to prevent pressure on the sac and deformities; good skin care, particularly if the baby is incontinent of urine and feces; adequate nutrition; tender, loving care; accurate observations and charting; education of the parents; continued medical supervision; and habilitation.

Immediate care of the sac is essentially the same whether or not the cord is involved. Upon delivery the neonate is placed in an Isolette. Moist sterile dressings of saline or an antibiotic solution may be ordered to prevent drying of the sac. Some method of protecting the mass will be necessary if surgery is to be delayed. Pertinent nursing observations include a description of the newborn infant, the size and area of the sac, and any tears or leakage. The extremities are observed for deformities and for movement. There may be spasticity or paralysis of the limbs or they may be normal, depending on the type and location of the cyst. The head is measured to determine the possibility of associated hydrocephalus. Fontanels are observed in order to provide baseline data. Lack of anal sphincter control and dribbling of urine are significant in the differential diagnosis. In general, the higher the defect is on the spine, the greater the neurological deficit. Data are recorded along with the routine observations made for every newborn infant.

Positioning of the patient is of importance. The goal is to avoid pressure on the sac and to prevent postural deformities. When positioning patients with multiple deformities, the nurse must try to guard against aggravating existing problems. These children may also have hip dysplasia, which can be a factor in positioning the infant. The infant is usually placed prone with a pad between the legs to maintain abduction and counteract hip subluxation, and a small roll is placed under the ankles to maintain a neutral foot position. The position can be maintained through the use of diaper rolls, blankets, or sandbags.

Postoperative nursing care involves neurological assessment and prevention of infection. The status of the fontanels and any signs of increased intracranial pressure, such as irritability or vomiting, are significant. Sometimes a shunt is performed along with the closure of the spine; the nursing care of the patient with a shunt is discussed on page 123. Complications that can be life-threatening include meningitis, pneumonia, and urinary tract infection.

Urological monitoring is essential, since many of these patients are incontinent of urine. Medication to prevent urinary tract infections is given routinely. Prolonged use of the Credé method has been replaced by clean intermittent catheterization. This is a simple procedure that ensures total emptying of the bladder. It can be performed by parents and learned by young children. The use of this method has nearly eliminated the need for surgical urinary diversion (Myers, 1990). It is important that this procedure be performed regularly and in a clean manner. Implanted artificial sphincters are used in some cases.

Skin care is a challenge. Diapering is generally contraindicated. Constant dribbling of feces and urine irritates the perineal area and can infect the sac or the incision. Meticulous cleanliness is necessary. Bedding must be dry and wrinkle-free. Frequent cleansing, application of a prescribed ointment or lotion, and light massage help maintain skin integrity. If range of motion exercises are ordered, they are performed gently.

Feeding of the patient is facilitated by early closure of the defect. In delayed cases gavage may be used. To bottle-feed the patient, one nurse may hold the infant over the shoulder while another administers the formula. Nipple holes should be large enough to prevent exhaustion by making the infant work to get food. A side-lying position in or out of the crib (on the nurse's lap) is effective with some babies.

These patients need cuddling and sensory stimulation. If infants cannot be held, the nurse soothes them by touch. Talk to them and when possible provide face-to-face (en face position) communication. Mobiles are placed appropriately. Moving the incubators or cribs periodically will provide diversity of view. Soft music is also soothing.

Special consideration must be given to the establishment of parent-infant relationships. This problem is complicated if the infant is transferred to a large medical center. Understanding and support are given to the parents, who may be overwhelmed. It is not unusual for them to be overwhelmed by the cyst. Most experience a sense of loss for what was to have been their "perfect baby." Steps of the grieving process may be recognized by the nurse. If the malformation is complex and incompatible with life, a decision must be made about the feasibility of surgical intervention. This is a crisis situation for the most mature of people and an area in which guidelines are not clearly defined. Information and education concerning this disorder can be obtained from the Spina Bifida Association of America.

A crucial factor for nurses is recognition of their

own feelings about these patients, which often include sorrow, anger, frustration, guilt, and fear of incompetence. Group discussions that provide a safe, nonthreatening environment for nurses to externalize their feelings are healthy. Physical outlets such as exercise, active sports, and screaming rooms will prevent illness and displacement of repressed feelings on innocent parties. These resources are a must if emotional "burn out" is to be avoided (see also Facing Death, page 70).

CARDIOVASCULAR SYSTEM

Congenital Heart Disease (CHD)

General Description. A baby born with congenital heart disease has a defect in the structure of the heart and/or in one or more of the large blood vessels that lead to and from the heart. The heart or vessels have failed to develop properly. The incidence of congenital heart disease is approximately 8 per 1000 live births.

You will recall that the heart of the fetus is completely developed during the first 8 weeks of pregnancy. A mother who contracts German measles early in her pregnancy or who is poorly nourished may bear a child with a faulty heart. Other prenatal or maternal factors associated with increased risk include alcoholism, exposure to coxsackievirus, diabetes mellitus, ingestion of lithium salts, and advanced maternal age. Genetic factors such as a history of CHD in other family members, patients with Down syndrome or other chromosomal aberrations, and patients who have other congenital defects often contribute to the incidence of CHD. Research now indicates that most congenital heart lesions are produced by a genetic-environmental interaction, that is, they are *multifactorial*. In other words, congenital heart diseases are not all one disease; there is a hereditary predisposition determined by many genes, and an environmental trigger acts on the predisposed individual to push that fetus over the threshold from normal development to abnormal development (Table 6–2).

Heart defects are the principal cause of death (except for prematurity) among the congenital anomalies during the first year of life. It is important, therefore, that the nurse stress the need for good prenatal care and impress upon the parents the value of regular checkups at baby clinics. Many organic heart murmurs have been detected early in infancy at a periodic checkup. A careful health history is particularly useful. The symptoms, as indicated in Table 6–3, depend upon the location and type of heart defect. Some patients have mild cases and can lead a fairly normal life under medical management. Others are treated medically until the optimal time for surgery. Most

Table 6–2. DIAGNOSTIC PROCEDURES IN CONGENITAL HEART DISEASE

History	Echocardiography
Physical examination	Hemoglobin and
Roentgenographic	hematocrit
examination	determinations
a. Thoracic	Angiocardiography
roentgenogram	Heart catheterization
b. Cardiac fluoroscopy	
Electrocardiography	

Table 6–3. GENERAL SIGNS AND SYMPTOMS OF CONGENITAL HEART ABNORMALITIES

INFANTS	
Dyspnea	Failure to gain weight
Difficulty with feeding	Heart murmurs
Stridor or choking spells	Cyanosis
Pulse rate over 200	Cerebral vascular
Recurrent respiratory	accidents
infections	Anoxic attacks
CHILDREN	
Dyspnea	Cyanosis
Poor physical	Squatting
development	Clubbing of fingers and
Decreased exercise	toes
tolerance	Elevated blood pressure
Recurrent respiratory	
infections	
Heart murmur and thrill	

From Ross Laboratories (1986). *A Study Guide to Congenital Heart Abnormalities.* Reproduced with permission of Ross Laboratories, Columbus, Ohio 43216. © 1986 Ross Laboratories.

cardiac surgery is corrective, although some is palliative. There is no medical cure for congenital heart disease (Nadas, 1990).

Classification. In the past, congenital heart defects were divided into two groups: cyanotic and acyanotic. This has proved inaccurate since children with acyanotic defects may develop cyanosis and those with cyanotic disease may be pink. To present the student with a more accurate picture, defects are classified according to the effect the defect has on the movement of circulating blood.

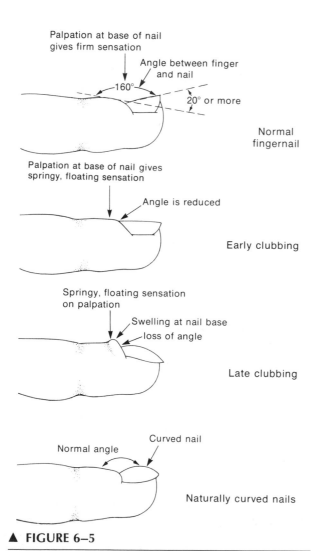

Palpation at base of nail gives firm sensation

Angle between finger and nail

160°

20° or more

Normal fingernail

Palpation at base of nail gives springy, floating sensation

Angle is reduced

Early clubbing

Springy, floating sensation on palpation

Swelling at nail base

loss of angle

Late clubbing

Curved nail

Normal angle

Naturally curved nails

▲ **FIGURE 6–5**

Clubbing in infant's fingers, caused by poor oxygenation. (From Foster, R., Hunsberger, M., and Anderson, J. J. [1989]. *Family-Centered Nursing Care of Children.* Philadelphia, W. B. Saunders Company.)

Table 6–4. NURSING DIAGNOSES ASSOCIATED WITH CONGENITAL HEART DEFECTS

Potential for infection, related to reduced body defenses, debilitated state

Fluid volume, alteration in, excess, related to compromised cardiac function

Nutrition, alteration in, less than body requirements, related to fatigue, chronic hypoxia

Activity intolerance, related to imbalance of oxygen supply and demand

Growth and development, alteration in, related to stress of chronic illness, chronic hypoxia

Knowledge deficit, related to chronic disease

Family process, alteration in, related to child with a long-term disease

Defects can be classified as *defects with increased pulmonary blood flow, obstructive defects, defects with decreased pulmonary blood flow, and mixed defects.* The study of blood circulation is termed *hemodynamics* (*hemo,* blood + *dynamis,* power) (Whaley and Wong, 1991).

Signs and Symptoms. The child with congenital heart disease may be small for age and the condition may be classified as a physiological failure to thrive. This is secondary to the difficulty the child has feeding and breathing at the same time. Exercise intolerance first may be identified when the infant experiences dyspnea when feeding. Or, it may not be evident until the toddler period when the child tends to be more active. The child may assume a *squatting position* to decrease venous return by occluding the femoral veins and thus lessen the workload of the right side of the heart. The infant can gain this same effect by lying in the knee-chest position. Clubbing of the fingers is thought to be caused by anoxia (Fig. 6–5). Finally, the child tends to have frequent respiratory infections because of the pulmonary vascular congestion. Some common nursing diagnoses associated with the child with a congenital heart defect are listed in Table 6–4.

The normal heart is illustrated in Figure 6–6.

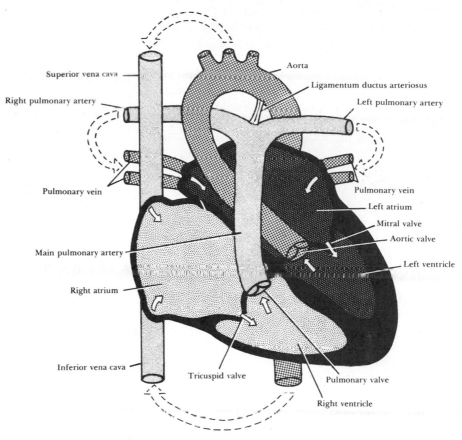

▲ FIGURE 6–6

The normal heart. (From Clinical Education Aid No. 7, reproduced with permission of Ross Laboratories, Columbus, Ohio 43216. © 1986 Ross Laboratories.)

Patent Ductus Arteriosus

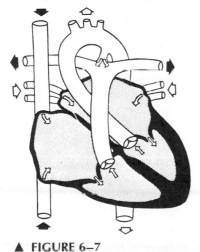

▲ FIGURE 6–7

(From Clinical Education Aid No. 7, reproduced with permission of Ross Laboratories, Columbus, Ohio 43216. © 1986 Ross Laboratories.)

DEFECTS WITH INCREASED PULMONARY BLOOD FLOW

Patent Ductus Arteriosus (PDA) (Fig. 6–7). As was previously mentioned (on page 88), the circulation of the fetus differs from that of the neonate in that most of the fetal blood bypasses the lungs. The *ductus arteriosus* is the passageway by which the blood crosses from the pulmonary artery to the aorta and avoids the deflated lungs. This vessel closes shortly after birth; however, when it does not close, blood continues to pass from the aorta, where the pressure is higher, into the pulmonary artery. This causes oxygenated blood to recycle through the lungs, overburdening the pulmonary circulation and making the heart pump harder. The symptoms of this disorder may go unnoticed during infancy. However, with growth, the child experiences dyspnea, the radial pulse becomes full and bounding on exertion, and there may be growth retardation.

Patent ductus arteriosus is one of the most common cardiac anomalies. The word patent means "open." It occurs twice as frequently in females as in males. Closed heart surgery is performed in all diagnosed patients if there are no other complications. If this condition is left uncorrected, the patient eventually could develop congestive heart failure or endocarditis. The opening is closed by ligation or by division of the ductus. Indomethacin has been used medically to close the ductus in premature babies. The prognosis is excellent.

OBSTRUCTIVE DEFECTS

Atrial Septal Defect (ASD) (Fig. 6–8). This is one of the more common congenital heart anomalies. The incidence is higher in females than in males. There is an abnormal opening between the right and left atria. Blood that contains oxygen is forced from the left atrium to the right atrium. This type of arteriovenous shunt does not produce cyanosis unless the blood flow is reversed by heart failure. Less serious types of this defect can be corrected by open heart surgery. With the use of the heart-lung bypass machine, the condition can be corrected in a dry or bloodless field. The hole is then sutured or patched. The prognosis depends upon the location of the atrial defect in the septum.

Atrial Septal Defect

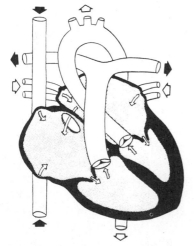

▲ **FIGURE 6–8**

(From Clinical Education Aid No. 7, reproduced with permission of Ross Laboratories, Columbus, Ohio 43216. © 1986 Ross Laboratories.)

Ventricular Septal Defect

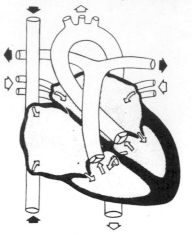

▲ **FIGURE 6–9**

(From Clinical Education Aid No. 7, reproduced with permission of Ross Laboratories, Columbus, Ohio 43216. © 1986 Ross Laboratories.)

Ventricular Septal Defect (VSD) (Fig. 6–9). As the name suggests, there is an opening between the right and left ventricles of the heart. Increased pressure within the left ventricle forces blood into the right ventricle. A loud, harsh murmur combined with a systolic tremor is characteristic of this defect. The condition may be mild or severe. Surgical risk is high during infancy; therefore, postponement of surgery is advised until early childhood. The correction is similar to that of atrial septal defects. A *staged* procedure by way of closed heart surgery is sometimes done on babies to provide relief from symptoms until the optimal time for definitive surgery. A large percentage of small VSDs will close spontaneously by 2 years of age.

Coarctation of the Aorta (Fig. 6–10). The word *coarctation* means a "tightening." In this condition, there is a constriction or narrowing of the aortic arch or of the descending aorta. Hemodynamics consists of increased pressure proximal to the defect with decreased pressure distally. The patient may not develop symptoms until later childhood. Treatment is surgical. The surgeon resects the narrowed portion of the aorta and joins its ends. The joining is called an *anastomosis.* If the section removed is large, an end-to-end graft using tubes of dacron or similar material may be necessary. Since the graft will not grow but the aorta will, the best time for surgery is between the ages of 3 and 6 years. As in patent ductus arteriosus, closed heart surgery is performed because the

Coarctation of the Aorta

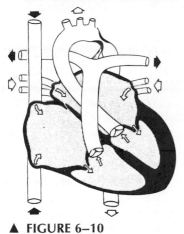

▲ FIGURE 6–10

(From Clinical Education Aid No. 7, reproduced with permission of Ross Laboratories, Columbus, Ohio 43216. © 1986 Ross Laboratories.)

structures are outside the heart. The prognosis is favorable if there are no other defects.

DEFECT WITH DECREASED PULMONARY BLOOD FLOW

Tetralogy of Fallot (Fig. 6–11). *Tetra* means four. In this condition, there are four defects: (1) stenosis or narrowing of the pulmonary artery, which decreases the blood flow to the lungs; (2) hypertrophy of the right ventricle, which enlarges because it has to work harder in order to pump blood through the narrow pulmonary artery; (3)

Tetralogy of Fallot

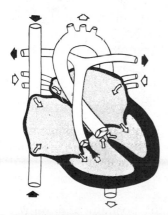

▲ FIGURE 6–11

(From Clinical Education Aid No. 7, reproduced with permission of Ross Laboratories, Columbus, Ohio 43216. © 1986 Ross Laboratories.)

dextroposition (*dextra*, right + position) of the aorta, in which the aorta is displaced to the right and blood from both ventricles enters it; and (4) ventricular septal defect.

When venous blood enters the aorta, severe heart trouble is evident in the infant. Cyanosis increases with age, and clubbing of the fingers and toes is seen. The child rests in a "squatting" position to breathe more easily. Feeding problems, growth retardation, frequent respiratory infections, and severe dyspnea upon exercise are prevalent. The red blood cells of the body increase, causing polycythemia (*poly*, many + *cyt*, cells + *hema*, blood) in an effort to compensate for the lack of oxygen.

All children with cyanotic congenital heart disease are at risk for neurological sequelae such as cerebrovascular accident. Blackouts and convulsions may occur. The child is treated medically until surgery can be endured. Staged surgery may be done to increase the flow of blood to the lungs. Open heart surgery is performed for permanent correction of the defect. The optimal age for elective repair is after age 3 or 4 years but prior to starting school. Sometimes a complete repair is necessary during infancy. This operation is becoming more successful.

MIXED DEFECT

Transposition of the Great Arteries (TGA) (Fig. 6–12). In this defect, the pulmonary artery leaves

Complete Transposition of the Great Vessels

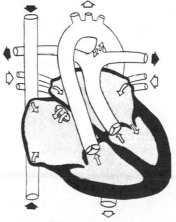

▲ FIGURE 6–12

(From Clinical Education Aid No. 7, reproduced with permission of Ross Laboratories, Columbus, Ohio 43216. © 1986 Ross Laboratories.)

the left side of the ventricle and the aorta leaves the right ventricle. Because the body receives only desaturated blood, there must be other defects in order to maintain life (septal defects, PDA). The condition of the child depends upon how much mixing of systemic and pulmonary venous blood is taking place. Infants with large septal defects or a PDA may not be as cyanotic but will develop symptoms of congestive heart failure. No murmur is associated with TGA. If a murmur is present, it is related to the other defects. Prostaglandin E and a balloon atrial septostomy may be used as palliative measures. Corrective surgery is usually performed between 3 weeks and 1 year, depending upon the procedure. The mortality rate depends upon the severity of the defect, maturity of the infant, type of procedure, and any other complicating factors.

CONGESTIVE HEART FAILURE

An infant with a severe heart defect may develop congestive heart failure. Congestive heart failure is not a disease within itself but rather symptoms caused by an underlying heart defect. The nurse must constantly be on the alert for signs and symptoms of this condition. Some of these are cyanosis, pallor, rapid respiration, rapid pulse, feeding difficulties, fatigue, failure to gain weight, edema, and frequent respiratory infections.

Cyanosis. When observing the baby's color, the nurse notes whether the cyanosis is general or localized. If it is localized, the exact location is recorded in nurse's notes, e.g., hands, feet, lips, or around the mouth. Is the cyanosis deep or light? Is it constant or transient? Sometimes a baby's color improves when crying, sometimes it gets worse; this is significant. If overt cyanosis is not apparent in the black infant, observe the palms of the hands and bottoms of the feet. Clubbing of the fingers and toes as a result of pooling of the blood in the capillaries of the extremities may be evident. The infant may be very pale or may have a mottled appearance.

Rapid Respirations. Over 60 respirations per minute in a newborn infant at rest indicates distress. The amount of dyspnea does vary; in more acute cases, it is accompanied by flaring of the nostrils, mouth breathing, and sternal retractions. The baby has more trouble breathing when flat in bed than when being held upright. Air hunger is indicated if the patient is irritable and restless. The cry is weak and hoarse.

Rapid Pulse. This is *tachycardia*. A pulse rate of over 150 beats per minute is significant. The heart is pumping harder in an effort to get sufficient oxygen to all parts of the body.

Feeding Difficulties. When the nurse tries to feed these infants, they tire easily. They may refuse to suck after a few ounces. When placed in the crib, they cry and appear hungry. They may choke and gag during feedings; the pleasure of sucking is spoiled by their inability to breathe.

Poor Weight Gain. The patients fail to gain weight. A sudden increase in weight may indicate the beginning of heart failure.

Edema. Watch for puffiness about the eyes and, occasionally, in the legs, feet, and abdomen.

Exercise Intolerance. The infant may sleep excessively and fall asleep during feedings. As the children grow, they may not be as active as other children and may be delayed in motor development. Older children may fatigue easily and be intolerant to exercise.

NURSING GOALS AND TREATMENT IN CONGENITAL HEART DISEASE

The nursing goals in the care of the newborn infant can be adapted for all children with heart defects. These are: (1) to reduce the work of the heart, (2) to improve respiration, (3) to maintain proper nutrition, (4) to prevent infection, (5) to reduce the anxiety of the patient, and (6) to support and instruct the parents.

The nurse must organize care so that the baby is not unnecessarily disturbed. The patient needs a great deal of energy. A complete bath and linen change are luxuries that an infant with a serious heart defect cannot afford. The infant should be fed early if crying and late if asleep. The doctor will order the position in which the infant should be placed. In some cases, the knee-chest position facilitates breathing; in other cases, a slanting position with the head elevated may be helpful. Older babies may be placed in infant seats.

Small frequent feedings are scheduled. The infant is fed in an upright position and burped frequently. The nipple should be soft and the hole large enough for easy sucking. Older children generally tolerate a "no added salt" diet with a restriction on high-sodium foods. In some cases, nasogastric tube feedings are advantageous because they are less tiring for the patient. Oxygen is administered to relieve dyspnea. As breathing becomes easier, the baby begins to relax. A soft voice with gentle care will soothe the patient. Whenever possible, the infant is held and loved during feedings.

Digitoxin and digoxin (Lanoxin) are the commonly prescribed oral digitalis preparations. In pediatric patients, Lanoxin is preferred because of its rapid action and shorter half-life. The action of these agents is to slow and strengthen the heart beat. The nurse counts the patient's pulse for one full minute before administering them. A resting apical pulse is most accurate. Because normal pulse ranges vary at different ages, the physician will usually indicate at what pulse rate the drug is to be withheld. If this information is not available, it should be obtained from the physician as soon as possible to prevent confusion and a possible error. When the drug is withheld, the physician is notified. A common guideline is to withhold the medication if an infant's pulse is below 90 to 110 beats per minute and below 70 beats per minute in older children. However, the nurse should also be aware of significant drops from the child's previous reading. Tachycardia and irregularities in the rhythm of the pulse are significant and should be reported. Symptoms of toxicity include nausea, vomiting, anorexia, irregularity in rate and rhythm of the pulse, and a sudden change in pulse.

If the baby is discharged while still receiving medication, the parents are taught how to take the pulse and what signs to be alert for when administering the drug.

Diuretics such as furosemide (Lasix) or chlorothiazide (Diuril) are useful in reducing edema. Careful monitoring of serum electrolyte levels will prevent electrolyte imbalance, particularly potassium depletion. Teach parents of older patients to recognize foods high in potassium, such as bananas, oranges, milk, potatoes, and prune juice. Diapers are weighed to determine urine output. Daily weights of the baby will also help the physician determine the effectiveness of the diuresis.

Complications other than cardiac decompensation (heart failure) may arise before or after surgery. Owing to the increase in numbers of red blood cells circulating within the body (polycythemia), the blood becomes sluggish and prone to clots. When this is accompanied by dehydration, the threat of cerebral thrombosis may become a reality.

An accurate record of intake and output is essential. Signs of dehydration, such as thirst, fever, poor skin turgor, apathy, sunken eyes or fontanel, dry skin, dry tongue, dry mucous membranes, and a decrease in urination, should be brought to the immediate attention of the nurse in charge. Pneumonia can occur rapidly. Fever, irritability, and an increase in respiratory distress may indicate this condition. The patient's position is changed regularly to help prevent this setback.

Chest tubes may be used postoperatively to remove secretions and air from the pleural cavity and to allow re-expansion of the lungs. These are attached to underwater seal drainage bottles or a commercially manufactured disposable system such as Pleur-Evac. Units for infants and older children are available. This system must be *airtight* to prevent collapse of the lung. Drainage bottles are always kept below the level of the chest to prevent backflow of secretions. This is especially important during transportation. Two rubber-shod Kelly clamps are available at all times for emergency clamping of tubes. These are applied to the tubes as close as possible to the child's chest if a break in the system occurs.

The nurse working in a cardiac unit should be alert for emergencies such as cardiac and respiratory arrest and should be competent in cardiopulmonary resuscitation techniques and the necessary modifications required for pediatric patients. *The parents of the child need support and understanding over a long period of time.* A mother's fears and dependencies come to the surface when she gives birth to a baby with a defect. Since the heart is the body's most vital organ, this type of diagnosis causes a great deal of apprehension. The physician has to reassure the parents without minimizing the danger involved. If the condition permits, the infant is sent home under medical supervision until the preferred age for surgery. Every effort must be made by the family to provide a normal environment that is within the infant's limits. It is easy for parents to become overpermissive because they do not wish the child to become unnecessarily excited. The child senses this and soon gains control of the home. This is difficult for everyone but is especially exhausting and confining for the mother. Limit setting, such as 5 minutes of chair time, if done with consistency, is beneficial.

The patterns formed during infancy can build the framework of a healthy personality for the patient. The child with a heart condition who is well integrated into family life has a decided advantage over the child who is made to think she or he is an invalid. Routine naps and early bedtime will provide adequate rest for most patients. As the patients grow, they usually set their own limits on the amount of activity they can handle. Substitutions can be made for strenuous activities, such as bicycle riding, and for rigorous competitive games. The child receives the usual childhood immunizations. Prompt treatment of infections is important. A suitable diet with adequate fluids is necessary. Encourage iron-rich foods. Dental care should be regular. All-day attendance in school may be too tiring for the child; therefore, special provisions in this area may be necessary. The child will need careful evaluation before any type of minor surgery, such as tonsillectomy, is performed.

Some children will need hospitalization occasionally for various tests or problems. Simple explanations must be given to the patients regarding this condition. They should be allowed to handle and to see hospital equipment prior to its use whenever feasible. Cardiac surgery is generally performed at a regional medical center where the necessary costly equipment is available. The American Heart Association has established standards and recommendations for centers that care for children with congenital heart defects. Whenever possible, a continuum of nursing care by an experienced registered nurse who follows the patient throughout hospitalization is desirable for both the physical and the psychological welfare of the patient. The physician may refer the baby to a local crippled children's service for evaluation and follow-up. The financial burden to the parents throughout the years for medical and surgical necessities is phenomenal. All avenues for financial aid should be explored by qualified personnel.

GASTROINTESTINAL SYSTEM

Cleft Lip

Description. A cleft lip is characterized by a fissure or opening in the upper lip and is a result of the failure of the embryonic structures of the face to unite. In many cases it seems to be caused by hereditary predisposition, coupled with a minor deviation of the intrauterine environment. This disorder appears more frequently in boys than in girls and may occur on one or both sides of the lip. The extent of the defect may vary from slight to severe. Sometimes it is accompanied by a *cleft palate,* a fissure in the midline of the roof of the mouth. Cleft lip and palate are common congenital anomalies, occurring in about 1 in 600 to 1250 births.

TREATMENT AND NURSING CARE

The initial treatment is surgical repair. The cleft lip is repaired first, because it interferes with the infant's ability to eat. The baby cannot create a vacuum in the mouth and is unable to suck. Surgery not only improves the infant's sucking but also greatly improves the appearance. Currently the operation is performed any time after birth if the infant's general health is good and there is no infection.

Prior to surgery a complete physical examination is given, and blood tests are ordered. Photographs may also be taken. Any signs of infection such as a cold should be reported to the head nurse. The doctor may order restraints to prevent the patient from scratching the lip and to accustom the patient to them, since they will be necessary postoperatively. An Asepto syringe with a rubber tip is used to feed the baby before and after surgery, since sucking motion must be avoided to decrease tension on the suture line. Sometimes a soft, crosscut nipple can be used prior to surgery.

Feeding Method for Neonates with Cleft Lip, Cleft Palate, or Both. The following feeding method may be used for babies with both cleft lip and cleft palate. The nurse will need to allow more time than the usual 20 minutes required for bottle feedings.

PROCEDURE ▶ ▶ ▶ ▶ ▶ ▶ ▶ ▶ ▶

Equipment. Sterile medicine dropper with rubber tip or Asepto syringe with rubber tip, formula, covergown for nurse, bib.

1. Check to see that the baby is dry and warm. Change the diaper as needed. Wash hands following this. Leave restraints on during feeding.

2. Hold the baby in a sitting position. Draw the formula into an Asepto syringe or medicine dropper.

3. Place the rubber tip of the feeder just inside the lips, on the opposite side of the mouth from the cleft or repaired area.

4. Exert gentle pressure on the bulb of the feeder, allowing a small amount of fluid to drop into the mouth.

5. Allow the baby to swallow before giving more. Prevent sucking motions as much as possible.

6. Bubble frequently. Sit the baby up and gently pat the back with one hand while supporting the chest with the other. Note: The doctor may wish to have the formula followed by a small amount of sterile water to cleanse the mouth.

7. Following the feeding, return the baby to the crib. Place the baby on the right side. Support the back with a rolled blanket or small pillow.

8. Chart: Time of feeding, method, amount offered, amount taken and retained, and untoward results (vomiting).

Postoperative Care. Postoperative nursing goals for this patient include: (1) preventing the baby from sucking and crying, which could cause tension on the suture line; (2) careful positioning (never on the abdomen) to avoid injury to the operative site; (3) cleansing of the suture line to prevent crusts from forming that could cause scarring; (4) applying restraints to prevent injury to the operative site and use of a *Logan bow* (to reduce tension on the suture line); and (5) cuddling and other forms of affection to provide for the infant's emotional needs, which is of particular importance because the baby is unable to obtain the usual satisfactions from sucking.

The wound may be kept moist through the application of a bacterial ointment. When applying the ointment, use a cotton-tipped swab and a gentle rolling motion to avoid injuring the surgical site. The same procedure should be used when cleaning the area with sterile saline.

The infant receives feedings by dropper until the wound is completely healed (from 1 to 2 weeks). The mother who has fed her baby preoperatively and has been allowed to assist with feedings during hospitalization will not find it too difficult to continue after discharge. The immediate improvement as a result of surgery is very encouraging to the parents, particularly if the child must have further surgery for cleft palate repair.

Cleft Palate

Description. A cleft palate is more serious than a cleft lip. It forms a passageway between the nasopharynx and the nose, which not only complicates feeding, but easily leads to infections of the respiratory tract and middle ear and is generally responsible for speech difficulties, which occur in later life. Unlike cleft lip, cleft palate is more common in girls than in boys.

Treatment. The best time for surgery is subject to controversy, although some surgeons prefer to operate before 18 months of age if at all possible, so that speech patterns will not be affected. To facilitate communication, a dental speech appliance may be used if surgery has been deferred or has been contraindicated because of extensive malformation. This appliance must be changed periodically as the child grows.

The management of the child with a cleft lip and palate requires expert teamwork over a long period. The emotional problems that sometimes occur with this condition require more extensive attention than the repair itself. A child born with a facial deformity encounters many problems. It is difficult not to be attractive when society places such importance on good looks. A mother's first reaction to a disfigured newborn infant is one of shock, hurt, disappointment, and guilt. Some parents regard the deformity as a result of their inadequacies. There may be a desire to hide the child from relatives and friends. Feedings are difficult and are not relaxed in the initial period. As the child grows, irregular tooth eruptions, drooling, delayed speech, and the need for intermittent hospitalization and frequent clinic appointments can be frustrating. The developing child senses the feelings of the parents and acquires either a positive or a negative attitude about self. The patient and the family need understanding, concrete basis for hope, and practical advice.

In large cities, special cleft palate clinics are available where several specialists can work together in convenient consultation. The parents should be instructed as to the resources available in the state in which they live. Financial assistance is usually indicated because of the length of treatment required.

POSTOPERATIVE MANAGEMENT AND NURSING CARE

Nutrition. Fluids are best taken by a cup, although an Asepto syringe with a rubber tip (gravity feeder) may be used. The nurse should clarify the preference of the plastic surgeon prior to feeding the child. Hot foods and liquids should be avoided to prevent injury to the surgical site. All objects should be kept out of the mouth. This includes straws, tongue blades, spoons, forks, and pacifiers. A wide-bodied spoon may be used if the food is fed from the side of the spoon and does not come in contact with the roof of the mouth. The diet progresses from a clear to a full liquid diet. The child may go home on a soft diet (nothing harder than mashed potatoes).

Oral Hygiene. The mouth is kept clean at all times. Feedings should be followed by a little water. The doctor may prescribe a mild antiseptic mouthwash.

Restraints. Elbow restraints are generally sufficient. They should be removed one at a time periodically to prevent constriction of circulation and to allow normal movement. In the home they may be made out of rolled cardboard tied with a string. Prevent the child from placing fingers or objects in the mouth. Teach the child to keep the tongue away from the sore part of the mouth.

Speech. Speak slowly and distinctly to the patient and encourage the child to pronounce words correctly. Children who have had extensive repairs or have associated deafness need the help of a speech therapist. Others require a minimum of help from their parents.

Diversion. Crying is to be avoided as much as possible. Play should be quiet, particularly in the immediate postoperative period. Read to the child or help the child color.

Complications. Otitis media and dental problems may accompany this condition. The parent must be instructed to take the child to the physician at the first signs of earache. Visits to the dentist should be regular.

MUSCULOSKELETAL SYSTEM

Clubfoot

Description. Clubfoot, one of the most common deformities of the skeletal system, is a congenital anomaly characterized by a foot that has been twisted inward or outward. The incidence is about 1 in 700 to 1000 live births. Many mild forms are due to improper position in the uterus and clear up with little or no treatment when the extremity is allowed unrestricted activity. In contrast, true clubfoot does not respond to simple exercise. Many believe that this is because of an abnormal degree of compression and molding of the infant's feet in the uterus. Several types are recognized. Talipes (*talus*, heel + *pes*, foot) equinovarus (*equinus*, extension + *varus*, bent inward) is seen in 95 per cent of cases. The feet are turned inward and the child walks on the toes and the outer borders of the feet. It generally involves both feet. Boys are affected twice as often as girls.

TREATMENT AND NURSING CARE

The treatment of clubfoot should be started as early as possible; otherwise the bones and muscles will continue to develop abnormally. During infancy, conservative treatment, consisting of manipulation and casting to hold the foot in the right position, is carried out (Fig. 6–13). Manipulation and casting are repeated every few days for the first 1 to 2 weeks and then at 1- to 2-week intervals. This is done to allow for the rapid growth during this period. If manipulation does not work, surgery is performed.

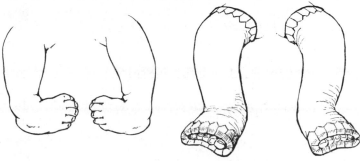

▲ FIGURE 6–13

Bilateral talipes equinovarus (clubfoot) before and after application of plaster casts. Adhesive "petals" have been placed around the ends of the casts to prevent plaster from irritating the skin. (From Marlow, D. [1977]. *Textbook of Pediatric Nursing*, 5th ed. Philadelphia, W. B. Saunders Company.)

Cast Care. Casts are made of either plaster or synthetic materials (fiberglass, polyurethane, or a combination). The plaster cast is placed in warm water before being applied over stockinette and cotton batting. It takes approximately 24 to 48 hours for the cast to dry. The cast should be left uncovered until it dries. The cast dries from the inside out. The child should be turned every 2 hours. When lifting the cast, the palms, not the fingers, should be used, to prevent indentations that could press on the underlying skin and cause damage.

Synthetic casts dry quickly (less than 30 minutes) and are lighter, which allows for greater mobility. However, they are not as strong as plaster and are more expensive.

NURSING BRIEF ▷ ▷ ▷ ▷ ▷ ▷ ▷ ▷

Of importance in the long-term care of orthopedic patients is education of the parents in terms of orthopedic devices, cast care, exercise and hygiene, and treatment goals. The nurse explains the importance of frequent clinic visits, reinforces physician information, and clarifies directions as necessary.

The toes are left exposed for observation. *The nurse checks them for signs of poor circulation—pallor, cyanosis, swelling, coldness, numbness, pain, or burning.* If circulation is impaired, the cast may be slit to relieve the pressure, or it may need to be removed and reapplied. The nurse should also report irritation of the skin around the edges

of the cast and lack of movement of the toes. Adhesive petals may be placed around the edges of the cast to prevent skin irritation.

It is difficult to keep a child's cast free of food particles, which cause skin irritation. The patient needs careful supervision during mealtime to prevent placing bits of food under the edges of the cast. Powder and oil are not used following the bath because they may cause irritation.

If surgery on tendons and bones has been performed, the nurse must also observe the cast for evidence of bleeding. If a discolored area appears on the cast, it is circled and the time is recorded. Further bleeding can then be estimated. If bleeding is noted, the patient's vital signs are also checked and compared with preoperative readings.

Emotional Support. The nurse is an important figure in the care of the long-term patient. Nurses should review the normal growth and development of children in the patient's age range, to anticipate some of the problems and to educate caretakers in parenting.

In general, children from birth to 4 years of age suffer the most from being separated from their parents. They cry loudly when visiting hours end and need the nurse to console them. They may be slow in developing certain motor abilities and in many cases regress to their baby ways. This is particularly true of bowel and bladder control. The nurse should not shame a child if an "accident" occurs.

The parents can give much helpful information

about their child. Be a good listener. Parents should be encouraged to participate in the care of their hospitalized child, for it will bring them emotional relief and will reassure the child.

The financial burdens of hospitalization, surgery, and continued medical supervision pose a real problem. If the nurse suspects that the parents need financial help, a social service referral should be made.

Congenital Hip Dysplasia

Description. Congenital hip dysplasia is a common orthopedic deformity. The incidence is about 1 in 1000 live births. The term *hip dysplasia* is a broad description applied to various degrees of deformity—subluxation or dislocation, either partial or complete. The head of the femur is partly or completely displaced from a shallow hip socket (*acetabulum*). Both hereditary and environmental factors appear to be involved in the cause. Hip malformation, joint laxity, breech position, and race may all contribute. Congenital hip dysplasia is seven times more common in girls than in boys.

Newborn infants seldom have complete dislocation. When the baby begins to walk, the pressure exerted on the hip can cause a complete dislocation. Accordingly, the nurse can understand why early detection and treatment are of particular importance in this condition.

Symptoms. A dislocation of the hip is commonly discovered at the periodic health examination of the baby during the first or second month of life. One of the most reliable signs is a limitation of abduction of the leg on the affected side. When the infant is placed on the back with knees and hips flexed, the doctor can press the femur of the normal hip back until it almost touches the examining table. This can be accomplished only partially on the affected side. The knee on the side of the dislocation is lower and the skin folds of the thigh are deeper and are often asymmetrical. When the infant is prone, one hip is higher than the other (Fig. 6–14). In some infants younger than 4 weeks; the physician can actually feel and hear the femoral head slip into the acetabulum under gentle pressure. This is called Ortolani's sign or Ortolani's click and is considered diagnostic. The child who is walking and has had no

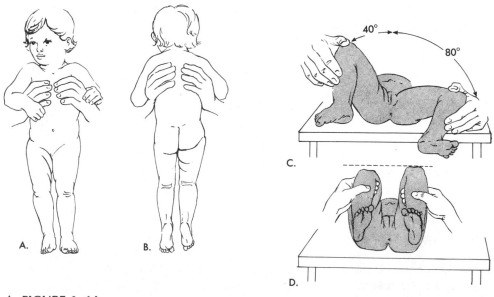

▲ **FIGURE 6–14**

The three "classic" signs of congenital hip dysplasia: *A* and *B*, unequal skin folds, *C*, limitation of abduction, and *D*, unequal knee height. (From Tachdjian, M. [1990]. *Pediatric Orthopedics*, 2nd ed, p. 326. Philadelphia, W. B. Saunders Company.)

treatment displays a characteristic limp. Bilateral dislocation may occur; however, unilateral dislocation is more common. X-ray films will confirm the diagnosis.

Treatment. Treatment is begun immediately upon detection of the dislocation. The physician attempts to form a normal joint by keeping the head of the femur within the hip socket. This constant pressure enlarges and deepens the acetabulum; thus, it corrects the dislocation. The nurse will recall that the bones of small children are fairly pliable because they contain more cartilage than bones of adults.

Treatment of the hip dysplasia depends upon the age of the child. In the neonate, the abduction of the hips is maintained through the use of the Pavlik harness or Frejka pillow. The Pavlik harness is the treatment of choice in most cases. If the dislocation is severe or has not been detected until the child has begun to walk, it may be necessary to use traction. This pulls the head of the femur down to the correct position opposite the acetabulum. After the traction has stretched the tissues to allow the hip to be placed in the acetabulum, the dislocation is reduced under general anesthesia, and a spica cast is applied to hold the abduction. This type of cast is shown in Figure 6–15. The length of time that the patient remains in a cast varies according to progress and growth and the condition of the cast; however, it is usually from 5 to 9 months. During this time, the cast may be changed about every 6 weeks. Sometimes surgery is required. In this case, open reduction of the dislocation or repair of the shelf of the hip bone is done. A cast is applied following surgery to keep the femur in the correct position.

NURSING BRIEF ▷ ▷ ▷ ▷ ▷ ▷ ▷ ▷
Three signs of congenital dislocation of the hip are (1) unequal skin folds on the thighs and buttocks, (2) limited abduction on the affected side, and (3) unequal knee height.

NURSING CARE

The nursery nurse carefully observes each infant during the morning bath to detect signs of a dislocated hip. When the baby is prone, the nurse observes the buttocks for variation in size. The legs of the infant should be equal in length. The

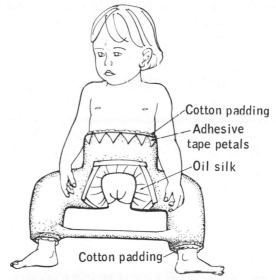

▲ **FIGURE 6–15**

A body (spica) cast. This body cast maintains the legs in a froglike position and is used to treat congenital dislocations of the hip. Note that the child is able to move the toes freely. All edges are padded with cotton and protected by adhesive "petals." (From Leifer, G. [1982]. *Principles and Techniques in Pediatric Nursing,* 4th ed. Philadelphia, W. B. Saunders Company.)

infant should be kicking both legs, not just one leg. There should be no difference in the depth of the skin folds of the baby's upper thighs. In the well-baby clinic, the nurse notes the posture and gait of older children and records observations.

Infants who progress well with the Pavlik or Frejka splint or similar brace remain at home. The parent and baby visit the physician regularly. The parents need assurance that they may hold the baby and sit him or her in a chair. They should be encouraged to ask questions of the clinic nurse and doctor.

The child who is admitted to the hospital with a diagnosis of a congenital dislocated hip should be given as much personal attention as possible. The first admission will set the pattern for future hospitalization; therefore, it is important that the child make a satisfactory adjustment. The nurse should become familiar with the child's Habit and Care sheet. Every effort should be made to provide patients who are hospitalized for many weeks with a homelike environment.

The type of cast that is used is called a *body*

spica. It encircles the waist and extends to the ankles or toes. General cast care, discussed on page 137, should be reviewed at this point. Other aspects pertinent to this particular type of cast are discussed in the following paragraphs.

Firm, plastic-covered pillows are placed beneath the curvatures of the cast for support. Older children may benefit from an overhead bar and trapeze. The room should be adequately ventilated. A fracture pan should be available in the bedside table.

The head of the patient's bed is slightly elevated so that urine or feces will drain away from the body of the cast. Do not elevate the head or shoulders of a child in a body cast by means of pillows, as this thrusts the patient's chest against the cast and will cause discomfort or respiratory difficulty. The child who is not toilet trained may be placed on a Bradford frame to facilitate nursing care. To prevent soiling of the cast from urine and feces, plastic wrap can be tucked around the edges of the cast at the openings between the legs. A disposable diaper can be tucked under the edges around the buttocks for the same purpose. As these coverings become soiled, they must be changed immediately. Frequent change of position is important; bed patients need to be turned often. Infants may be held in the nurse's lap after the cast has dried. A ride on a stretcher to the playroom or around the hospital provides a change of position as well as a change of scene.

Turning a Child in a Body Cast. The following method should be used to change the position of a child in a body cast.

PROCEDURE   ▶ ▶ ▶ ▶ ▶ ▶ ▶ ▶ ▶

Two people, one on each side of the bed, are needed to turn a child in a body cast.

1. Move the child to the edge of the bed as far as possible, so that the nurse who will receive the child is farther away from the child.

2. The nurse nearer the child places one hand under the head and back and one hand under the leg part of the cast and turns the child to the midway point on the side.

3. The nurse farther away then accepts the support of the weight and cast as the child is turned completely onto the abdomen.

The supporting bar between the legs should not be used as a lever when turning the child. All body curvatures should be supported with pillows or sheet rolls. Whenever possible, the older child should be on the abdomen during mealtime to facilitate swallowing and self-feeding. When placing a child in a body cast on a bedpan, support the upper back and legs with pillows so that body alignment is maintained.

Itching is a particular problem with a patient in a body cast. If at all possible, prior to applying the cast a strip of gauze is placed beneath the cast to the opened area required for toilet needs. It is gently moved back and forth beneath the cast to provide relief from itching. When the strip becomes soiled, a clean one is tied to one end of the soiled gauze and pulled through the cast; the soiled portion is removed. Other methods that might cause injury to the skin beneath the cast are discouraged, since any break in the skin under a cast is very difficult to heal.

The child with a long-term disability such as this needs help in meeting the everyday needs of life. This child is growing and developing rapidly. Therefore, frequent adjustments in home and clinic care are necessary. Dressing and clothing are a problem. The child cannot fit into regular furniture or much of the play equipment enjoyed by other children. Transportation is difficult. Children in spica casts can be transported from their rooms by placing them in a wagon that has been built up with pillows. They can also be elevated with pillows when eating. Refer parents to home health care, if appropriate.

Down Syndrome

Description. Down syndrome is a congenital defect of the embryo. In the past, children with the defect were called "mongoloid" because of the oriental appearance of their faces, but this term is now considered inappropriate. The incidence of Down syndrome is approximately 1 in 600 to 800 live births; it is higher in mothers 35 years or older. Sometimes, a baby with Down syndrome is the first child of a young mother; usually, however, her subsequent children are normal. There are three known causes of Down syndrome—all of which involve abnormalities of the chromosomes. In the most common type, *trisomy 21 syndrome,* the total chromosome count is 47 instead of the normal 46 (see Fig. 2–2). This accounts for 95 per cent of cases. It is a result of *nondisjunction,* the failure of a chromosome to follow the normal separation process into daughter cells. The earlier in the embryo's development this occurs, the greater the number of cells affected. The other two types are *translocation,* which is hereditary, and *mosaicism.* In translocation, a piece of chromosome in pair 21 breaks off and attaches itself to another chromosome. In mosaicism, some cells of the body have an extra chromosome 21.

Symptoms. The signs of this condition, which are apparent at birth, are close-set and upward-slanting eyes, small head, round face, flat nose, protruding tongue that interferes with sucking, and mouth breathing. Also, the hands of the baby are short and thick, and the little finger is curved. There is a deep straight line across the palm, which is called the *simian crease.* There is also a wide space between the first and second toes. The undeveloped muscles (hypotonia) and loose joints enable the child to assume unusual positions. Physical growth and development may be slower than normal (see Tables 6–5 and 6–6). Most children are mildly to moderately retarded. However, owing to medical, educational, and social advances, the Down syndrome child today develops much further than in past generations (Miola, 1987). Congenital heart deformities may be associated with this condition. No one child has all the physical characteristics that a child with Down syndrome could exhibit (Fig. 6–16).

These happy-go-lucky children are very lovable. They are restless and somewhat more difficult to train than the normal youngster. Their resistance to infection is poor, but the life spans of children with Down syndrome have been increased with the widespread use of antibiotics. The incidence of acute leukemia is higher in these children than in the normal population, however. These children are also at risk of developing respiratory infections and otitis media. Children with Down syndrome are also prone to have speech and hearing problems. Plastic surgery on the face of Down syndrome children has been performed and results are still being monitored. The surgery facilitates nose breathing, speech, and eating (Miola,

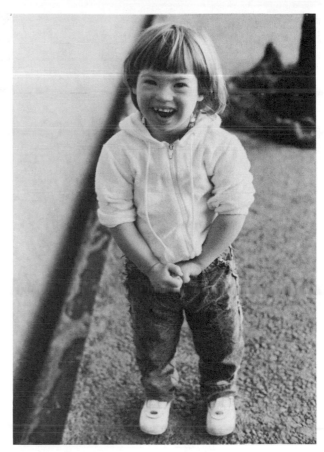

▲ **FIGURE 6–16**

Child with Down syndrome.

1987). It has also been suggested that if the children look "normal," then they will be encouraged and allowed to develop their potential (Tables 6–5 and 6–6).

Attitude of the Nurse. Nurses need to be aware of their own feelings before they can give effective support to the handicapped child and the parents. They must have patience and understanding. The children are encouraged to help themselves within their ability, even though it may take more time. This is especially true when they are ill and hospitalized. Early infant stimulation is emphasized in order to enable the children to reach milestones as rapidly as possible (Fig. 6–17).

The child with Down syndrome is no longer commonly institutionalized. The increased stimulation at home, together with love and encouragement, increases the child's progress (Miola, 1987) (Tables 6–5 and 6–6).

Table 6–5. SELF-HELP SKILLS

	CHILDREN WITH DOWN SYNDROME		"NORMAL" CHILDREN	
	Average (Months)	Range (Months)	Average (Months)	Range (Months)
Eating				
Finger feeding	12	8 to 28	8	6 to 16
Using spoon and fork	20	12 to 40	13	8 to 20
Toilet training				
Bladder	48	20 to 95	32	18 to 60
Bowel	42	28 to 90	29	16 to 48
Dressing				
Undressing	40	29 to 72	32	22 to 42
Putting clothes on	58	38 to 98	47	34 to 58

From Levine, M., et al. (1983). *Developmental-Behavioral Pediatrics*. Philadelphia, W. B. Saunders Company.

As funds are made available, more and more community facilities and programs suited to the short-term and long-term needs of Down syndrome patients, such as group, foster, and boarding homes, are common. The nurse should become familiar with services located in and adjacent to the community. Sometimes parents cannot accept the fact that their baby is retarded and are ashamed to tell anyone of the baby's condition. The parents need to cry. They are grieving the loss of the normal child they do not have. This should not be interpreted as a lack of love for the child they do have. It takes exceptional strength to accept this diagnosis. Empathy from the nurse is of particular importance. Allowing parents to become involved in care and planning for the infant from the start helps facilitate bonding. The warm concern of the staff cannot be overestimated. Pampering the baby by putting a little curl in the hair, for example, shows that others care even though this baby is different. Parents watch for evidence of rejection of their child; they are

Table 6–6. DEVELOPMENTAL MILESTONES

	CHILDREN WITH DOWN SYNDROME		"NORMAL" CHILDREN	
	Average (Months)	Range (Months)	Average (Months)	Range (Months)
Smiling	2	1.5 to 4	1	0.5 to 3
Rolling over	8	4 to 22	5	2 to 10
Sitting alone	10	6 to 28	7	5 to 9
Crawling	12	7 to 21	8	6 to 11
Creeping	15	9 to 27	10	7 to 13
Standing	20	11 to 42	11	8 to 16
Walking	24	12 to 65	13	8 to 18
Talking, words	16	9 to 31	10	6 to 14
Talking, sentences	28	18 to 96	21	14 to 32

From Levine, M., et al. (1983). *Developmental-Behavioral Pediatrics*. Philadelphia, W. B. Saunders Company.

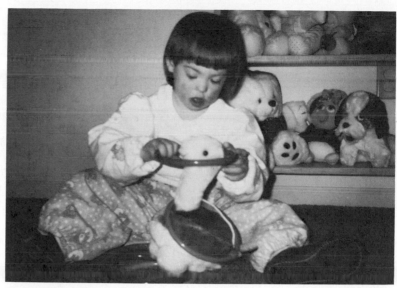

▲ FIGURE 6–17

Stimulation of the child with Down syndrome is critical in the child's development.

sensitive to such things as placement in the nursery.

Several organizations provide support to the child with Down syndrome: National Down Syndrome Congress, National Association for Retarded Citizens, National Association for Down Syndrome.

Perinatal Damage

HEMOLYTIC DISEASE OF THE NEWBORN (HDN): ERYTHROBLASTOSIS FETALIS

Description. Erythroblastosis fetalis (*erythro*, red + *blast*, a formative cell + *osis*, disease condition) is a disorder that becomes apparent late in fetal life or soon after birth. It is one of many congenital hemolytic diseases found in the neonate. There is excessive destruction of the red blood cells of the baby, due to an incompatibility between the red blood cells of the mother and those of the fetus. In other words, a sensitized Rh-negative mother is pregnant with an Rh-positive child. Sensitization refers to the phenomenon in which the

mother, during her first pregnancy or through exposure to Rh-positive blood by transfusion, developed anti–Rh-positive antibodies. The incidence of erythroblastosis fetalis has greatly decreased as a result of the protective administration of Rh antibody (RhoGAM) to women at risk. Incompatibility of ABO factors is now more common and generally less severe than Rh incompatibility. The process of *maternal sensitization* is depicted in Figure 6–18. The mother accumulates antibodies with each pregnancy; therefore, the chance that complications may occur increases with each gestation. Severe reactions can cause kernicterus, severe anemia, brain damage, and death.

Diagnosis and Prevention. Erythroblastosis fetalis should be suspected when the mother is Rh-positive and the father is Rh-negative. An amniocentesis can be done to detect bilirubin levels in the amniotic fluid. This procedure is not without its risks and, in some cases, can sensitize the mother. During the prenatal period, an indirect Coombs test can show previous exposure to Rh-positive antigens. Postnatally, a direct Coombs test is done on umbilical cord blood; a positive result usually indicates Rh incompatibility.

Prevention of erythroblastosis by the use of

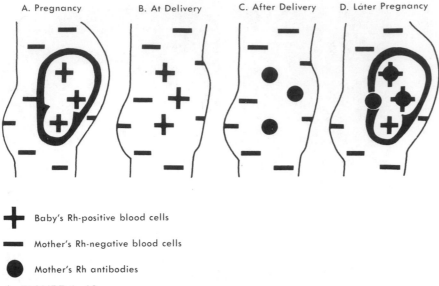

A. Pregnancy B. At Delivery C. After Delivery D. Later Pregnancy

+ Baby's Rh-positive blood cells

— Mother's Rh-negative blood cells

● Mother's Rh antibodies

▲ **FIGURE 6–18**

While an Rh-negative mother is carrying an Rh-positive baby (*A*), some of the baby's Rh-positive blood enters the mother's body (*B*). Her body produces antibodies against this factor (*C*). When she carries a subsequent Rh-positive baby, the antibodies cross the placenta and attack the baby's red blood cells (*D*).

RhoGAM is now routine. An intramuscular injection is given to the mother within 3 days of delivery, provided she has not previously been sensitized (Fig. 6–19). RhoGAM may also be given to the pregnant woman at 27 to 33 weeks' gestation. This is of importance in a primigravida who may unknowingly have miscarried or in a multigravida who may not have received her postpartum RhoGAM. It is also administered, when appropriate, in cases of abortion (Burroughs, 1986). Mothers who deliver at home and are potential candidates for sensitization must not be overlooked.

Symptoms. The symptoms of erythroblastosis fetalis vary with the intensity of the disease. Anemia and jaundice are present. The anemia is due to hemolysis of large numbers of erythrocytes. The jaundice, termed *pathological*, differs from *physiological* jaundice in that it becomes evident within 24 hours following delivery. The liver is unable to handle the massive hemolysis, and bilirubin levels rise rapidly, causing hyperbilirubinemia (*hyper*, excess + *bilis*, bile + *rubor*, red + *emia*, blood). Early jaundice should be reported immediately to the physician.

Enlargement of the liver and spleen and extensive edema may develop. The circulating blood usually contains an excess number of immature nucleated red blood cells (*erythroblasts*), produced by attempts by the baby's body to compensate for the destruction of its cells. The oxygen-carrying power of the blood is diminished, as is the blood volume, so shock or heart failure may result. Severe jaundice may cause *kernicterus*, serious damage to the brain that may leave the neonate mentally retarded and frequently results in death.

Treatment. Treatment includes a combination of phototherapy and exchange transfusion. Phototherapy may reduce the likelihood of the infant's needing a transfusion or may reduce the number of transfusions needed. It should not be regarded as an alternative to an exchange transfusion if the transfusion is required (Nielsen, 1990). These treatments are instituted according to established guidelines based on laboratory findings, weight, and general condition of the infant. Nursing care of the child receiving phototherapy is presented on page 114.

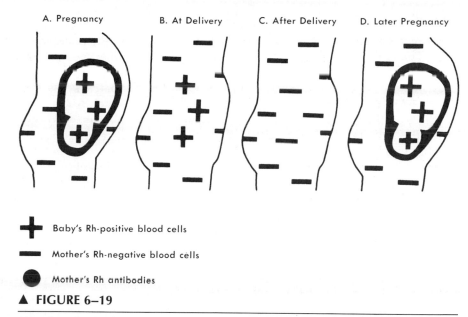

A. Pregnancy   B. At Delivery   C. After Delivery   D. Later Pregnancy

+ Baby's Rh-positive blood cells

— Mother's Rh-negative blood cells

● Mother's Rh antibodies

▲ **FIGURE 6–19**

(*A*) After the birth of a baby, its blood is tested. If the blood is Rh positive, RhoGAM is given to the Rh-negative mother (*B*) within 72 hours after delivery. It prevents formation of Rh antibodies (*C*), and the next Rh-positive fetus (*D*) is protected. The procedure is repeated with each pregnancy or miscarriage.

INTRACRANIAL HEMORRHAGE

Description. Intracranial hemorrhage, the most common type of birth injury, may result from trauma or anoxia. It occurs more frequently in the preterm infant, in whom the blood vessels are fragile. Blood vessels within the skull are broken, and bleeding occurs into the brain. When the diagnosis is made, the specific location of the hemorrhage may be noted, i.e., subdural or subarachnoid, or intraventricular. This injury may also occur during precipitated delivery or prolonged labor or when the newborn's head is large in comparison with the mother's pelvis.

Symptoms. The symptoms of intracranial hemorrhage may occur suddenly or gradually. Some or all are present, depending on the severity. They include inability to move normally, lethargy, poor sucking reflex, irregular respirations, cyanosis, twitching, forceful vomiting, a high-pitched, shrill cry, and convulsions. Opisthotonic posturing may be observed. The fontanel may be tense and under pressure, rather than soft and compressible. One pupil of the eye is apt to be small and the other large. If the symptoms are mild, there is a good

chance of complete recovery in most cases. Death results if there is a massive hemorrhage. The infant who survives an extensive hemorrhage may suffer residual defects such as mental retardation or cerebral palsy. The diagnosis is established by the history of the delivery, CT scan, MRI, evidence of an increase in pressure of the cerebrospinal fluid, and the symptoms and course of the disease.

TREATMENT AND NURSING CARE

The newborn is placed in an incubator, which allows proper temperature control, ease in administering oxygen, and continuous observation. The baby is handled gently and as little as possible. The head is elevated. The doctor may prescribe vitamin K to control bleeding and phenobarbital if twitchings or convulsions are apparent. The baby is fed carefully because the sucking reflex may be affected. The infant vomits easily. The nurse observes the baby for signs of increased intracranial pressure and convulsions and assists the physician with such procedures as lumbar punctures and aspiration of subdural hemorrhage.

If a convulsion occurs, observation of its character by the nurse will aid the doctor in diagnosing the exact location of the bleeding (see also Chapter 12). The following are of particular importance: Were the arms, legs, or face involved? Was the right or left side of the body involved? Was the convulsion mild or severe? How long did it last? What was the condition of the infant before and after the seizure? The nurse records observations in the nurses' notes.

Infections

THRUSH (ORAL CANDIDIASIS)

Description. Thrush is an infection of the mucous membranes of the mouth, caused by the fungus *Candida.* This organism is normally present in the mother's vagina and is nonpathogenic. However, the altered conditions in the vagina produced by pregnancy may lead to the development of *monilial vaginitis.* The mucous membranes of the baby's mouth may become infected by direct contact with this infection during delivery, or by contact with the mother's or nurse's contaminated hands. Cross-infection of other newborn infants may then result.

Symptoms. White patches that resemble milk curds are visible on the tongue, inner lips, gums, and oral mucosa. These are painless but will not wipe away. Anorexia may be present. The systemic symptoms are mild if the infection remains in the mouth; however, it can pass along the mucous membranes into the gastrointestinal tract, causing inflammation of the esophagus and stomach.

TREATMENT AND NURSING CARE

This infection responds well to local application of antibiotic suspensions. Nystatin, for example, may be applied by swab. The mouth is swabbed three or four times a day, between feedings, with a sterile applicator moistened with the prescribed solution. The remainder of the dose is deposited in the infant's mouth to be swallowed to treat any other lesions of the gastrointestinal tract. With treatment, the disease is usually self-limiting in an otherwise healthy infant.

Individual feeding equipment is necessary, and the equipment should be sterile. Disposable bottles or prefilled formula bottles are used. Nipples require scrupulous cleansing because they come in direct contact with the lesions. Disposable nipples, as well as bottles, are preferred. Nurses who care for neonates with thrush should direct their care toward prevention of spread of the infection and correct application of the medication.

The prevention of this infection begins in the prenatal period. Mothers suspected of having *Candida* infection can then be properly treated. Effective handwashing to prevent reinfection from the mother is necessary. This is particularly true if she is breast-feeding her infant. Nurses and other personnel must maintain a high quality of nursing care to prevent cross-infection.

INFECTIOUS DIARRHEA

Description. Despite improved care of the neonate, infectious diarrhea continues to be a serious problem in many areas of the world. It is defined as the excessive loss of water and electrolytes in stools, which usually results from disturbed solute transport in the intestine. Infectious diarrhea is highly contagious and may be fatal. It may be caused by a variety of organisms, and often the offender cannot be identified. Viral gastroenteritis is the most widespread type and is self limiting. Rotavirus is the major agent during the winter months (Behrman and Kleigman, 1990). *Escherichia coli* often affects children under 2 years of age. *Shigella, Salmonella,* and *Staphylococcus* may also cause diarrhea. Diarrhea may accompany antibiotic therapy, which sometimes alters the normal flora of the intestinal tract. Food allergies, emotional strain, fatigue, and the unwise of laxatives can precipitate this disorder in older children. Overfeeding, unbalanced diets containing excessive amounts of sweets, and spoiled foods are additional offenders in the early years.

A carefully obtained medical history yields valuable information. The age of the child is significant with regard to etiology. Travel, personal contacts, and history of food allergy are relevant. Diarrhea may last from a few days to several weeks. *Functional* diarrhea differs from infectious diarrhea in that it is due to an organic disease rather than to infection.

Symptoms. The symptoms of diarrhea may be mild or extremely severe. The stools are watery and are expelled with force. They may be yellowish-green in color. The baby becomes listless, refuses to eat, and loses weight. The temperature may be elevated, and the infant may vomit. Dehydration is evidenced by sunken eyes and fontanel and dry skin, tongue, and mucous membranes. The frequency of urination may decrease. In severe cases, the excessive loss of bicarbonate from the gastrointestinal tract results in *acidosis.*

TREATMENT AND NURSING CARE

Constant observation of each neonate in the nursery is of utmost importance. If diarrhea is suspected, it is reported immediately and the baby is isolated. A warm stool specimen is sent to the laboratory for culture. The nurse must describe the stools accurately in the nurses' notes as to consistency, frequency, color, odor, the presence or absence of blood, mucus, or pus, and the forcefulness with which the stool is expelled. In older patients, cramping and *tenesmus*, or involuntary straining to empty the bowel, may be observed and should be recorded.

The gastrointestinal tract of the newborn infant is especially vulnerable to infection. The nurse must constantly seek to protect babies against exposure to pathogenic organisms and must adhere strictly to nursery routines. The preparation of formula requires undivided attention to prevent microorganisms from being carried to the infant through this medium. Careful feeding techniques are necessary. If a nipple becomes contaminated, a new one must be applied. Proper handwashing is essential. If clothing or blankets touch the floor, they must be relaundered before being used.

The skin of the buttocks must receive special care to prevent excoriation. Removing the diaper and exposing the area to the air may be helpful. Daily *accurate weights* are taken to help ascertain the amount of water loss. Careful observation and charting of intravenous fluids are necessary. The child is on *strict* intake and output recording.

Diarrhea caused by bacteria and parasites may respond to drug therapy. Other cases are viral and treatment is supportive. The focus is electrolyte imbalance and dehydration.

Oral glucose-electrolyte rehydration is the treatment of choice when possible. Certainly this is effective in the infant with mild to moderate dehydration (Table 6–7). Infants with moderate to severe dehydration may require intravenous replacement of fluids and electrolytes. Prolonged "bowel rest" is no longer considered the best approach in this disorder (Ulshen and Shub, 1990). Oral rehydration has been associated with quicker recovery and shorter hospitalization without the complications of parenteral nutrition (Ulshen and Shub, 1990). The mother who is breast-feeding should continue to breast feed.

Table 6–7. CLINICAL SIGNS OF DEHYDRATION IN AN INFANT

MILD DEHYDRATION (<5%)
Watery diarrhea
Increased thirst
Slightly dry mucous membranes/thickened saliva
Oliguria

MODERATE DEHYDRATION (6–9%)
Loss of skin turgor
Oliguria
Sunken eyes
Very dry mucous membranes
Sunken anterior fontanel
Restlessness or apathy

SEVERE DEHYDRATION (≥10%)
Signs of *moderate* dehydration plus one or more of the following:
    Peripheral vasoconstriction
    Hypotension
    Cyanosis
    Coma or marked irritability

Reprinted with permission from Cohen, M. B., and Balistreri, W. F. (1989). Diagnosing and treating diarrhea. *Contemp. Pediatr.* 6:104. © 1989 by Contemporary Pediatrics.

Mild diarrhea in older children may be treated at home under a physician's direction, provided there is a suitable caregiver. Treatment is essentially the same as that for the hospitalized child with the exception of administering intravenous fluids. Oral rehydration may be given. Clear fluids, e.g., flat ginger ale, gelatin, tea, and popsicles, are usually tolerated well. High-sodium broths are avoided to prevent electrolyte imbalance. Fruit juices are diluted because they are high in carbohydrate content. Other foods are added to the diet gradually. A regular intake is usually resumed within 2 to 3 days. Medications such as Lomotil, paregoric, and pectin, which slow intestinal mobility, are avoided in the treatment of children.

New babies must not be admitted to the nursery when infants with acute diarrhea are present. Separate personnel are needed to care for uninfected neonates. When the epidemic has ceased, the nursery must be thoroughly scrubbed, and all equipment must be cleaned and sterilized according to hospital procedure.

THE SKIN

Impetigo

Description. Impetigo is an infectious disease of the skin caused by staphylococci or by group A beta-hemolytic streptococci. The bullous form seen primarily in infants is usually staphylococcal, whereas nonbullous types are more commonly seen in children and young adults. Both organisms usually can be cultivated in the latter. The neonate is susceptible to this infection because resistance to skin bacteria is low. Impetigo tends to spread from one area of skin to another and is quite contagious.

Symptoms. The first symptoms of a bullous lesion are red papules. These eventually became small vesicles or pustules surrounded by a reddened area. When the blister breaks, the surface beneath is raw and weeping. The lesions may occur anywhere but are most often found on the face, neck, and extremities. In older children a crust may form, and scratching may cause further infection.

TREATMENT AND NURSING CARE

The lesions may be cleaned three or four times a day with soap and water to remove crusts. This is followed by the application of topical antibiotic ointment. Parenteral antibiotics may also be given in severe cases. The prognosis with proper treatment is good. The nursing care consists primarily of preventing this disease by proper aseptic methods. Once the diagnosis is made, the baby is isolated to prevent other newborn infants from becoming infected. Nephritis may occur as a complication of beta-hemolytic streptococcal infections.

Staphylococcus aureus Infection

Description. The genus of bacteria called *Staphylococcus* comprises very common bacteria that are found in dust and on the skin. Under normal conditions they do not present a problem to the healthy body defenses. If the number of organisms increases in preterm infants and neonates, whose general resistance is low, skin infections may occur. An abscess may form, and in some cases infection may enter the bloodstream. This condition is called *septicemia*. Pneumonia, osteomyelitis, or meningitis may result. Primary infection of the neonate may develop in the umbilicus or circumcision wound. It generally occurs while the newborn infant is in the hospital but may appear after discharge. This infection spreads readily from one infant to another. Small pustules on the neonate must be reported immediately.

TREATMENT AND NURSING CARE

Antibiotics effective against the particular strain are administered. Ointments may be applied locally.

In past years, the staphylococci that invade the body have developed resistance to the drugs that had been used. Penicillinase-resistant semisynthetic penicillins should be used except when staphylococci are resistant to these drugs. Vancomycin then becomes the drug of choice (Behrman and Vaughan, 1987). In some hospitals, serious epidemics have occurred in the newborn nursery and among surgical patients. It is difficult to control the spread of this infection because personnel act as carriers. The chief reservoir is the nose.

To prevent staphylococcal infections, no one with a skin infection should be allowed to visit mothers or enter the nursery. Mothers or newborn infants who have acquired this infection must be isolated. Strict standards must be upheld in the nursery: adequate space must be provided for each bassinet to avoid overcrowding, and each baby should have individual equipment. The number and quality of personnel and their health status are also important factors. The hands of all personnel must be scrubbed thoroughly with a bactericide before they enter the nursery. Washing the hands before and after touching each patient and before and after handling equipment is *essential*. Medical supervision of all discharged babies must be continued to detect latent cases.

IMMUNE SYSTEM

AIDS, AIDS-Related Complex (ARC)

Description. Acquired immune deficiency syndrome (AIDS) is caused by a retrovirus identified as the human immunodeficiency virus (HIV). This virus attacks T-helper cells that support immune functioning. T-suppressor cells that shut down the immune system are not altered by the virus. This causes an imbalance between these two cells, and the child is at great risk to develop infections.

In 1982 the first case of AIDS in infants was reported. In the early 1990s it is expected that there will be 3000 cases of the disease, with an additional 2000 children manifesting symptomatic HIV infection but not meeting all the criteria of the disease (Cooper et al., 1988). Of this group, approximately 80 per cent are due to perinatal exposure and 13 per cent to blood transfusion; 5 per cent are hemophiliac and received contaminated blood products.

Since the risk of blood product transmission has been diminished significantly, the main concern at this time is perinatal exposure. Perinatal transmission takes place either transplacentally, from secretions during the birth process, or, in a very few cases, from breast milk. Pregnant women at greatest risk to carry this disease are intravenous drug users and those with multiple sexual part-

ners. The disease can be transferred even if the mother is asymptomatic. Many women do not know they are positive for HIV when they become pregnant. About half the children born to HIV-positive mothers will themselves become positive (Rankin, 1989).

Signs and Symptoms. The most common signs and symptoms in infants include failure to thrive, chronic diarrhea, repeated respiratory infections, oral candidiasis, and enlargement of the liver and spleen. Developmental delays also have been noted. Kaposi sarcoma, which is common in adults, is rare in children.

TREATMENT AND NURSING CARE (Nursing Care Plan 6-1)

At the present time there is no cure for AIDS. Several antiviral drugs are being tested in children. The use of intravenous gamma globulin in children is fairly well accepted as a means of providing passive immunity to children who are having recurrent infections (Thurber and Berry, 1990).

The child with AIDS has many needs, both psychological and physiological. The child should be immunized against the common childhood diseases but should not receive live vaccines. Those caring for the child should observe good hand-washing techniques and avoid contact with anyone who is infectious. Parents should be educated in these two areas.

Assessment for signs of infection, including vital signs, and observation of the skin and general condition of the child, should be done routinely. Particular attention should be paid to the respiratory system because of the child's increased risk of developing infections within this system. The mouth, anal area, and skin should be assessed and care of these areas stressed.

The child should receive a high-protein, high-calorie diet. Frequent, small meals should be served. The child is on intake and output check, and daily weights are taken.

Psychological support of the child and family is critical. The effects of isolation, and in some cases of being ostracized, can be devastating to the developing child. Since the prognosis is poor, the nurse anticipates interventions related to the care of the child with a life-threatening disease. Since

NURSING CARE PLAN 6–1

THE CHILD WITH AIDS

Nursing Diagnosis	Goals/Outcome Criteria	Intervention
Potential for infection, related to altered immunity	Child will remain free of infection Child will show no signs of infection, as evidenced by Temperature between 36.5 and 37.6°C (97.6 and 99.6°F) No signs of respiratory distress (coarse breath sounds, tachypnea, restlessness) Redness, drainage, breaks in skin integrity	Anticipate opportunistic infections, as child's immune system is depressed Monitor respiratory status closely; patient subject to pneumonia, particularly *P. carinii*; watch for restlessness, apprehension Provide adequate hydration Examine child regularly for infection (puncture sites, mouth, rectum, pierced ears) Conserve energy Reposition frequently Administer antipyretics and antibiotics as prescribed
Nutritional alterations: less than body requirements, related to anorexia, anemia, thrush	Child will maintain growth Child will show signs of adequate growth as evidenced by weight gain and intake of 50% of diet appropriate for age	Offer small portions of high-caloric bland foods often Provide oral formula to infants as prescribed Administer nasogastric tube feedings if ordered Provide hyperalimentation therapy if ordered Provide for mobility to ensure muscle strength Chart Intake and Output Daily weights
Potential for injury related to changes in CNS and from decreased blood components	Child will not show signs of injury, as evidenced by absence of petechiae and ability to help with self-care	Provide developmentally appropriate and safe toys and activities Involve in self-care Observe skin for petechiae and bruising, explain to parents Monitor lab reports (prothrombin times, hematocrit, etc.)

NURSING CARE PLAN 6–1 *Continued*

THE CHILD WITH AIDS

Nursing Diagnosis	Goals/Outcome Criteria	Intervention
Impaired skin integrity and mucous membranes, related to immunosuppression	Child's skin will remain intact Child will show no signs of break in integrity of skin and will be able to eat without voicing discomfort	Inspect mouth often for lesions (*Candida albicans*) Apply nystatin suspension if ordered Observe frequently for diaper rash, apply prescribed ointment Maintain skin intactness by thorough, gentle cleansing Avoid citrus fruits
Potential for transmission of infection, related to disease organism	Child will not spread infection Potential for spread of infection is prevented as evidenced by the use of universal blood and body fluid precautions	Observe isolation technique Use universal blood and body fluid precautions Handle secretions and excretions with care Utilize good handwashing techniques
Knowledge deficit of family, related to nature, transmission, outcome	Family will verbalize understanding of disease process and transmission Family will use gloves when handling blood and body fluids and demonstrate good handwashing technique	Clarify misconceptions about the disease Help prepare parents for possible poor prognosis Prepare parents adequately for discharge from hospital (both verbal and written information) Encourage parents to stay abreast of current unfolding information Provide ongoing support services
Fear (parents and child), related to diagnosis, disapproval of society, rumor, inaccurate information	Parents will verbalize fears Family will discuss previous coping skills and demonstrate problem-solving abilities	Encourage family to support one another and keep lines of communication open Alert parents to self-help groups Acquire accurate knowledge about the disease Dispel inordinate fears of general public Involve parents in care of child Provide for consistent caregiver

many of these children will come from a family already in crisis, their support system may be weak. These family-centered interventions are recommended for nurses who care for children with AIDS: (a) answer questions, (b) provide accurate information, (c) assist the parents to move beyond guilt and blame, and (d) assist with concrete service needs (Thurber and Berry, 1990).

References

Behrman, R., and Kleigman, R. (1990). *Nelson Essentials of Pediatrics*. Philadelphia, W. B. Saunders Company.

Behrman, R., and Vaughan, V. (1987). *Nelson Textbook of Pediatrics*, 13th ed. Philadelphia, W. B. Saunders Company.

Birth Defects 1986. *Tragedy and Hope*. White Plains, N.Y., March of Dimes Birth Defects Foundation.

Burroughs, A. (1986). *Bleier's Maternity Nursing*, 5th ed. Philadelphia, W. B. Saunders Company.

Cooper, E., Pelton, S., and LeMay, M. (1988). Acquired immunodeficiency syndrome: A new population of children at risk. *Pediatr. Clin. North Am.* 35:1365–1387.

Miola, E. (1987). Down syndrome: Update for practitioners. *Pediatr. Nurs.* 13:233–236.

Myers, G. (1990). Myelodysplasia. *In* Gellis, S., and Kagan, B. (eds.). *Current Pediatric Therapy*. Philadelphia, W. B. Saunders Company, pp. 53–56.

Nadas, A. (1990). Congenital heart disease. *In* Gellis, S., and Kagan, B. (eds.). *Current Pediatric Therapy*. Philadelphia, W. B. Saunders Company, pp. 133–138.

Nielson, H. (1990). Hemolytic disease of the newborn. *In* Gellis, S., and Kagan, B. (eds.). *Current Pediatric Therapy*. Philadelphia, W. B. Saunders Company, pp. 717–720.

Rankin, W. (1989). AIDS, children, and our fear of death. *J. Pediatr. Nurs.* 4:432–434.

Thurber, F., and Berry, B. (1990). Children with AIDS: Issues and future directions. *J. Pediatr. Nurs.* 5:168–177.

Bibliography

Ulshen, M., and Shub, M. (1990). Protracted diarrhea of infancy. *In* Gellis, S., and Kagan, B. (eds.). *Current Pediatric Therapy*. Philadelphia, W. B. Saunders Company, pp. 186–187.

United States Department of Health and Human Services (1989). *Child Health USA '89*. HRS-M-CH8915. Washington, D.C., Office of Maternal and Child Health.

Whaley, L., and Wong, D. (1991). *Nursing Care of Infants and Children*. St. Louis, C. V. Mosby.

Barrett, D. (1988). The clinician's guide to pediatric AIDS. *Contemp. Pediatr.* 5:24–47.

Cohen, M., and Balistreri, W. (1989). Diagnosing and treating diarrhea. *Contemp. Pediatr.* 6:89–114.

Engel, N. (1989). AZT for children with AIDS. *Maternal-Child Nurs.* 14:121.

Finberg, L. (1990). Assessing the clinical clues to dehydration. *Contemp. Pediatr.* 7:45–57.

Foster, R., Hunsberger, M., and Anderson, J. J. (1989). *Family-Centered Nursing Care of Children*. Philadelphia, W. B. Saunders Company.

Mott, S., James, S., and Sperhac, A. (1990). *Nursing Care of Children and Families*. Redwood City, Ca., Addison-Wesley.

Oleske, J., Conner, E., and Boland, M. (1988). A perspective on pediatric AIDS. *Pediatr. Ann.* 15:319–321.

Rogers, M. (1988). Pediatric HIV infection: Epidemiology, etiopathogenesis, and transmission. *Pediatr. Ann.* 15:324–331.

Scott, G. (1988). Clinical manifestations of HIV infection in children. *Pediatr. Ann.* 15:365–370.

United States Department of Health and Human Services (1987). *Report of The Surgeon General's Workshop on Children with HIV Infection and Their Families*. DHHS Publication No. HRS-D-MC 87–1. Rockville, Md., Division of Maternal and Child Health.

Williams, A. (1989). Nursing management of the child with AIDS. *Pediatr. Nurs.* 15:259–261.

STUDY QUESTIONS

1. What is the most obvious symptom of hydrocephalus?
2. What complications may arise from neglecting to turn the patient with hydrocephalus?
3. List the symptoms of increased intracranial pressure.
4. Define habilitation. What is the nurse's role in habilitative nursing?
5. What does the term *maternal-infant bonding* mean to you? How can the nurse facilitate this process?
6. What is the most effective procedure carried out by the nurse in preventing the spread of infection?
7. What care is given to the buttocks of the infant with diarrhea? List five characteristics of the baby's stool that the nurse must record.
8. Describe the method for feeding the patient with a cleft lip and palate.
9. What resources are available in your community for speech training of the child with a cleft palate?
10. Define clubfoot. Why is it necessary to begin treatment early?

11. Billy, who has congenital clubfoot, had his cast changed in the early morning. List several signs of impaired circulation that might occur.
12. Define the following: patent; anastomosis; acyanotic heart defect; polycythemia; cardiac decompensation.
13. What modern methods are being used for the repair of congenital heart defects?
14. Baby Rico has been admitted with the diagnosis of congenital hip dysplasia. List the signs and symptoms of this orthopedic disorder.
15. Describe the nursing care you would give to the child with AIDS.

CHAPTER 7 ──────────────────────────

Chapter Outline

GENERAL CHARACTERISTICS
**PHYSICAL DEVELOPMENT, SOCIAL BEHAVIOR,
  CARE AND GUIDANCE**
HEALTH MAINTENANCE
IMMUNIZATION
NUTRITION COUNSELING OF PARENTS
WEANING
TEETH
DECIDUOUS TEETH
TEETHING DURING INFANCY

Objectives

Upon completion and mastery of Chapter 7, the
student will be able to

- Define or identify the vocabulary terms listed.
- Discuss the nutritional needs of growing infants.
- Identify the approximate age for each of the
  following: posterior fontanel has closed; central
  incisors appear; birth weight has tripled; child
  can sit steadily alone; child shows fear of
  strangers.
- Describe four developmental characteristics of
  infants that predispose them to certain hazards.
  For example, ''Puts everything into mouth—
  danger of aspiration.''
- List the immunizations given during the first year
  using medical terminology, including the
  approximate age for each and discussing ways to
  educate parents to the merits of this type of
  protection.
- Describe the physical and psychosocial
  development of infants from 1 month to 12
  months, listing age-specific events and guidance
  when appropriate.

THE INFANT

Terms

General Characteristics

Children, unlike adult patients, are in the process of growing while they are hospitalized. In order to give total patient care, the nurse must be able to recognize a patient's needs at various stages of growth and development. The nurse must try to meet these effectively, as well as to administer the specialized nursing care required for the particular patient. *The most common cause for concern about a child is a sudden slowing up, not typical for age, in any aspect of development.*

Each baby develops at an individual rate. Although growth is continuous, there are slow and rapid periods. The first year of life is a period of rapid growth and development. Brain growth is the most critical organic achievement of infancy. The infant is completely dependent on adults during the first months, and gives little in return. Behavior is not consistent. Sucking brings comfort and relief from tensions. The nurse, knowing the importance of sucking to the baby, holds the baby during feedings and allows sufficient time to suck.

Infants who are warm and comfortable will associate food with love. The baby who is fed intravenous fluids should be given added attention and a pacifier so that the necessary satisfaction that sucking provides is received. When the teeth appear, the infant learns to bite and enjoys objects that can be chewed. Gradually, the baby begins to put the fingers into the mouth. When babies can use their hands more skillfully, they will not suck their fingers as much but will be able to derive pleasure from other sources. The *grasp reflex* is seen when one touches the palms of the hands of the infant and flexion occurs. This disappears at about 3 months. *Prehension,* the ability to grasp objects between the fingers and the opposing thumb, occurs slightly later (at 5 to 6 months) and follows an orderly sequence of development. By 7 to 9 months, the *parachute reflex* appears. This is a protective arm extension that occurs when an infant is suddenly thrust downward when prone. By 1 year, the *pincer grasp,* coordination of index finger and thumb, is well established.

Love and security are vital needs of infants. They require the continuous affection given by the parents. Infants' needs should be met in a loving, consistent manner. As this happens, infants begin to learn that they can trust those persons they interact with. Parents should be assured that they will not spoil infants when they respond to their needs. Loving adults assure infants that the world is a good place in which to live. The development of a *sense of trust* is vital to the development of a healthy personality. A sense of trust is thought to be a foundation for subsequent tasks throughout the lifespan. The child who is deprived of this will instead learn to mistrust people, which could have a negative effect for the rest of life.

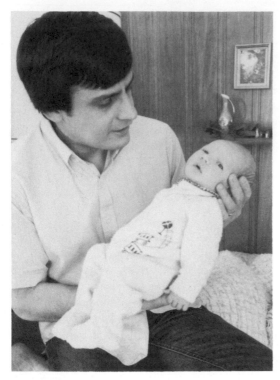

▲ FIGURE 7–1.

The role of father, although neglected in the past, is now seen as an important and integral part of family-centered nursing.

The constant care of an infant is a strain on the most exemplary parents. If the mother is the fulltime caregiver, she needs and deserves the understanding and kind support of her husband or her relatives at home and from the nurses in the hospital. A short break from pressures will give her renewed energy with which to enjoy her baby. A trip to the store, a stroll with the baby in the carriage, or coffee with neighbors affords stimulation and a change of environment for the baby as well as for the mother. The infant who is left constantly in the crib or playpen and who is not introduced to a variety of learning experiences may become shy and withdrawn. *Sensory stimulation is essential for development of the baby's thought processes and perceptual abilities.*

If a mother is unable to room-in with her hospitalized infant, personnel should try to imitate her care by prompt fulfillment of the infant's physical and emotional needs. In the nursery the baby who appears hungry is fed first, rather than adhering to a specific routine. Change wet diapers as soon as possible. Soothe the child who is crying. The exactness of bathing or feeding the infant is not as important as the care with which it is done. Warmth and affection or the lack of it is easily recognized by the baby.

COMMUNICATION ALERT ▶ ▶ ▶ ▶ ▶
The nurse can use the time spent caring for an infant to communicate with the child. While feeding, changing the diaper, and bathing, talk softly, sing, touch, and play simple games with the child.

Physical Development, Social Behavior, Care and Guidance

On the following pages are guides to infant care from the first month to the first year. The material has been arranged under headings and in chronological order so that it may be referred to easily by the student. Though this is convenient, it is merely a summary of data. Some of the aspects of care are important throughout the entire year, e.g., safety measures. The nurse explains to parents that physical patterns cannot be separated from social patterns and that abrupt changes will not take place with each new month. The development of humans cannot be separated into specific areas any more than the body's structure can be separated from its function. **No two infants are just alike at a certain age.** *This is just a guide!* However, individual variations range about central norms that serve as indicators for the evaluation of an infant's or child's progress. The addition of the various solid foods to the diet and the time of immunizations vary slightly depending on the baby's health and the doctor. The types, nevertheless, remain the same.

Health Maintenance

The prevention of disease during infancy is of the utmost importance and includes all measures that improve the physical health and psychosocial adjustment of the child. The concept of periodic health appraisal is not new. In the late 1800s, "milk stations" were established in various localities throughout the United States to provide safe water and milk for babies, in an effort to reduce the number of deaths from infant diarrhea. Skilled health services as we know them today encompass periodic health appraisal, immunizations, assessment of parent-child interaction, counseling in the developmental processes, identification of families at risk (for child abuse, for example), health education and anticipatory guidance, referrals to various agencies, follow-up services, appropriate record keeping, and evaluation and audit by peers. These are provided in a variety of health settings. The kinds and quality of assistance vary. Private group practice, hospital-based clinics, and neighborhood health centers are examples of settings.

Infant health care visits should be regular. A careful health history is obtained. Growth grids during infancy include measures of weight, length, and head circumference (see page 37). The reading and recording of growth charts are described on page 18. There are numerous developmental screening tests. The *Denver Developmental Screening Test,* which is widely used, is discussed in Chapter 9. The *Brazelton Neonatal Behavioral Assessment Scale* is of particular value during the newborn period; it helps describe the emerging personality of the baby and includes evaluation of infant reflexes, general activity, alertness, orientation to spoken voice, and response to visual stimuli.

The physical examination is adapted to the needs of the infant. Routine assessments of hearing and vision are an integral part of the examination. Loud noises in the newborn period should precipitate the *startle* or *Moro reflex.* Localization of sound during infancy can be roughly ascertained by standing behind the child seated on the mother's lap and ringing a bell or repeating voice sounds. The baby's response is compared with the average for the age level. Vision is mainly assessed by light perception. The examiner shines a penlight into the eyes and notes blinking, following to midline, and other responses. Laboratory tests include a hemoglobin or hematocrit determination to detect anemia, and a urinalysis. Screening tests for a variety of asymptomatic diseases are assuming greater importance; examples of these are the test for phenylketonuria (PKU), tuberculin test, and sickle cell test.

IMMUNIZATION

The importance of immunizations must be repeatedly stressed to parents by health personnel. A delay can lead to undue risks of serious illness, with sometimes fatal complications. Measles, pertussis, and other preventable diseases continue to strike children in the 1990s. Health experts warn that unless more young children are immunized epidemics could occur. There has been an increase in the outbreak of measles since 1986. In response to the increase, changes have been made regarding the recommended measles immunization policy (American Academy of Pediatrics, 1989). The nurse can stress to employed parents the fact that an unprotected child may become sick, making it necessary for them to lose valuable working hours. Immunization also prevents numerous doctor and hospital expenses and is required prior to school entry. A delay or interruption in a series does not interfere with final immunity. It is not necessary to restart any series, regardless of the length of delay. Accurate record keeping will prevent confusion. *Contraindications* to routine immunizations include acute febrile conditions, some chronic diseases, recent blood transfusion or injection of immune serum globulin, allergy, severe reaction following previous diphtheria-tetanus-pertussis (DTP) vaccine, malignancy, and steroid therapy. Other stipulations are described in drug circulars. The common cold is not considered sufficient reason for delay. Any questions regarding these or other maladies should be brought to the attention of the physician *prior to immunization.*

Recent changes have been made in the recommendations for giving the measles, mumps, and rubella vaccine (MMR). There is still discussion about when the second dose of this vaccine should

Text continued on page 170

PHYSICAL DEVELOPMENT, SOCIAL BEHAVIOR, CARE AND GUIDANCE FOR FIRST 12 MONTHS

ONE MONTH
Physical Development

Weighs approximately 8 pounds. Has regained weight lost after birth. Gains about 1 inch in length per month for the first 6 months.

Lifts head slightly when placed on stomach. Pushes with toes. Turns head to side when prone. Head wobbles. Head lag when pulled from lying to sitting position. Clenches fists. Stares at surroundings.

Vaginal discharge in girls and breast enlargement in boys and girls from maternal hormones received in utero are not unusual and will disappear without treatment.

Social Behavior

Makes small throaty noises. Cries when hungry or uncomfortable.

Sleeps 20 out of 24 hours. Awakes for 2 A.M. feeding.

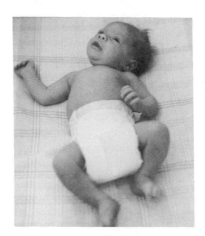

Joel at one month of age.

TWO MONTHS
Physical Development

Posterior fontanel closes. Tears appear. Can hold head erect in midposition. Follows moving light with eyes. Holds a rattle briefly. Legs are active.

Social Behavior

Smiles in response to mother's voice. Knows crying will bring attention. Awakens for 2 A.M. feeding.

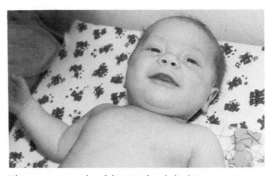

The two month old's smile delights parents.

Care and Guidance

Sleep. On stomach with head turned to side following feedings. If prefers side-lying position, support back with blanket roll. Use a firm, tight-fitting mattress in a crib with bars properly spaced so that the baby's head cannot be caught between them. Raise crib rails. Use no pillow.

Diet. Breast milk every 2 to 3 hours or iron-fortified formula every 4 hours or on demand. Vitamin D (400 IU/day) may be recommended in dark-skinned infants, breast-fed babies, or those infants who are not regularly exposed to sunlight. Plain, cooled water may be given between feedings. Bubble baby well.

Exercise. Allow freedom from the restraints of clothing before bath. Provide fresh air and sunshine whenever possible. Do not leave baby in sun for more than a short while. Provide protection from insects with netting. Avoid exposure to large crowds until immune system becomes more developed.

Support head and shoulders when holding infant. Attend promptly to physical needs. Provide colorful hanging toys for sensory stimulation.

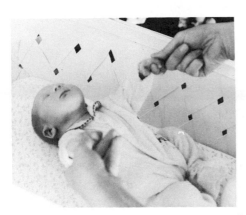

Note head lag of one month old when pulled from lying position.

Care and Guidance

Sleep. Develops own pattern; may sleep from feeding to feeding.

Diet. Breast milk or formula.

Exercise. Provide a safe, flat place for baby to kick and be active. Do not leave baby alone, particularly on any raised surface.

Physical examination by the family doctor, well-baby clinic, or pediatrician.

Immunization. First DTP, an inoculation against diphtheria, tetanus, and pertussis. Oral polio vaccine (TOPV) and *Haemophilus influenzae* type b vaccine (HbOC) may also be started.

Pacifier. If used, select for safety. Choose one-piece construction and loop handle to prevent aspiration.

Hiccups. Are normal and subside without treatment. May offer small amounts of water.

Colic (paroxysmal abdominal pain, irritable crying). Usually disappears after 3 months. Place baby prone over covered hot water bottle. Use pacifier. Relieve caretaker periodically. Avoid overstimulation. Rocking infant swing, music box may help.

Still completely depends on adults for physical care. Needs a flexible routine throughout infancy and childhood.

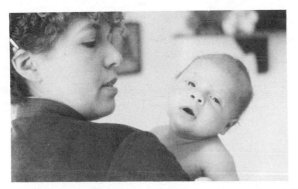

The two month old can hold his head erect in midline for brief periods of time.

PHYSICAL DEVELOPMENT, SOCIAL BEHAVIOR, CARE AND GUIDANCE FOR FIRST 12 MONTHS *Continued*

THREE MONTHS
Physical Development

Weighs 12 to 13 pounds. Stares at hands. Reaches for objects but misses them. Carries hand to mouth.

Can follow an object from right to left and up and down when it is placed in front of face. Supports head steady. Holds rattle.

Social Behavior

Cries less. Can wait a few minutes for attention. Enjoys responding to people talk. Takes impromptu naps.

FOUR MONTHS
Physical Development

Weighs about 13 to 14 pounds.

Drooling indicates appearance of saliva.

Lifts head and shoulders when on abdomen and looks around. Turns from back to side. Sits with support. Begins to reach for objects. Coordination between eye and body movements.

Moves head, arms, and shoulders when excited. Extends legs and partly sustains the weight when held upright. Rooting, Moro, extrusion, and tonic neck reflexes are no longer present. Little head lag.

Social Behavior

Coos, chuckles, and gurgles. Laughs aloud. Responds to others. Likes an audience. Sleeps 8 to 10 hours at night.

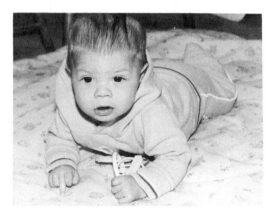

While on his abdomen the four month old can lift his head and shoulders and look around.

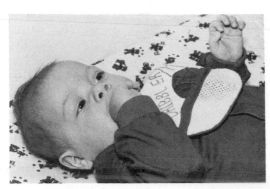

The three month old carries his hand to his mouth.

Care and Guidance

Sleep. Yawns, stretches, naps in mother's arms.

Diet. Breast milk or formula.

Exercise. May have short play period. Enjoys playing with hands.

Care and Guidance

Sleep. Stirs about in crib. Will sleep through ordinary household noises—avoid tiptoeing around.

Diet. Breast milk or formula.

Exercise. Plays with hand rattles and dangling toys. Start acquainting infant with a playpen where rolling safely is possible.

Immunization. Second DTP, polio, and *Haemophilus influenzae* type b vaccine.

Elimination. One or two bowel movements per day. May skip a day.

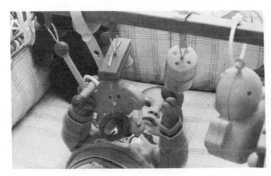

Visual stimulation is important to the growing infant. The four month old reaches for objects. There is increased coordination between eyes and body movement.

PHYSICAL DEVELOPMENT, SOCIAL BEHAVIOR, CARE AND GUIDANCE FOR
FIRST 12 MONTHS *Continued*

FIVE MONTHS
Physical Development

Sits with support. Holds head well. Grasps proffered objects. Puts everything into the mouth. Plays with toes.

Social Behavior

Talks to himself. Seems to know whether persons are familiar or unfamiliar.

May sleep through 10 P.M. feeding. Tries to hold bottle of orange juice at feeding time.

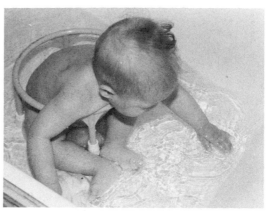

At five months, Joel enjoys water play. Tub safety ring supports child, but *never* leave infant alone in tub. Baby can grasp washcloth and enjoys chewing on it.

Care and Guidance

Sleep. Takes two or three naps daily in crib.

Diet. Breast milk or formula.

Exercise. Provide space to pivot around. Makes jumping motions when held upright in lap.

Safety. Check toys for loose buttons and rough edges before placing them in playpen.

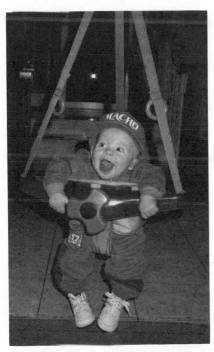

The five month old holds his head well and sits with support

PHYSICAL DEVELOPMENT, SOCIAL BEHAVIOR, CARE AND GUIDANCE FOR FIRST 12 MONTHS *Continued*

SIX MONTHS
Physical Development

Doubles birth weight. Gains about 3 to 5 ounces per week during next six months. Grows about a half inch per month.

Sits alone momentarily. Springs up and down when sitting. Turns completely over. Hitches (moves backward when sitting). Bangs table with rattle. Pulls self to a sitting position. Chewing more mature. Approximates lips to rim of cup.

Social Behavior

Cries loudly when interrupted from play. Increased interest in surrounding world. Babbles and squeals. Sucks food from spoon. Awakes happy.

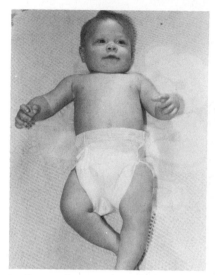

Joel's weight at six months is now 16 pounds, 6 ounces (birth weight: 8 pounds, 4 ounces).

SEVEN MONTHS
Physical Development

Two lower teeth appear. These are the first of the deciduous teeth, the central incisors.

Begins to crawl. Moves forward, using chest, head, and arms; legs drag. Can grasp objects more easily. Transfers objects from one hand to the other. Appears interested in standing. Holds an adult's hands and bounces actively while standing. Struggles when being dressed.

Social Behavior

Shifts moods easily—crying one minute, laughing the next. Shows fear of strangers.

Anticipates spoon feeding. Sleeps 11 to 13 hours at night.

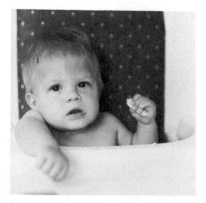

At seven months, Joel enjoys finger foods.

Care and Guidance

Sleep. Needs own room. Should be moved from parents' room if not previously done. Otherwise, with age infant may become unwilling to sleep away from them.

Diet. Introduce first solid foods, usually rice cereal fortified with iron. See Figure 7–3 for progression. Note: The sequence of supplemental foods will vary according to one's physician. This is not as important as offering a wide variety of foods during the first year. Iron is added to breast-fed infants at 6 months. Begin to wean.

Exercise. Grasps feet and pulls toward mouth.

Immunization. DTP, oral polio, and *Haemophilus influenzae* type b vaccine.

Safety. Remove toxic plants from baby's reach. Provide a chewable object such as a teething ring or facecloth for enjoyment.

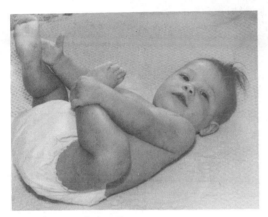

Joel plays with his feet.

Care and Guidance

Sleep. Fretfulness due to teething may appear. This is generally evidenced by lack of appetite and wakefulness during the night. In most cases, merely soothing and offering a cup of water are sufficient.

Diet. Add fruit. Add finger foods, such as toast or zwieback.

Exercise. Rudimentary locomotion.

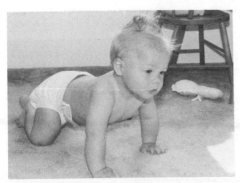

Joel begins to get around.

PHYSICAL DEVELOPMENT, SOCIAL BEHAVIOR, CARE AND GUIDANCE FOR
FIRST 12 MONTHS *Continued*

EIGHT MONTHS
Physical Development

Sits steadily alone. Uses index finger and thumb like pincers. Pokes at objects. Enjoys dropping articles into a cup and emptying it.

Social Behavior

Plays pat-a-cake. Enjoys family life. Amuses himself longer. Reserved with strangers.

Indicates need for sleep by fussing and sucking thumb. Impatient especially when food is being prepared.

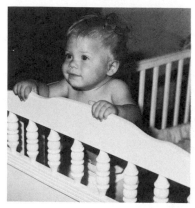

At eight months Joel shows increased interest in standing.

NINE MONTHS
Physical Development

Shows preference for the use of one hand. Can raise self to a sitting position. Holds bottle. Creeps. Carries trunk of body above floor but parallel to it. More advanced than crawling.

Social Behavior

Tries to imitate sounds, e.g., says "ba-ba" for bye-bye. Cries if scolded.

Drops food from high chair at mealtime. May fall asleep after 6 P.M. feeding.

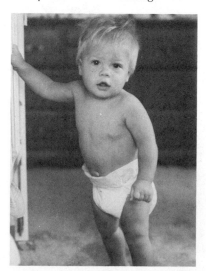

At nine months Joel cruises around holding onto furniture.

Care and Guidance

Sleep. Takes two naps a day.

Diet. Add vegetables. Continue to add new foods slowly.

Exercise. Enjoys jump chair. Rides in stroller. Stuffed toys or those that squeak or rattle are appropriate.

Safety. Remain with baby at all times during bath in tub. Protect from chewing paint from window sills or old furniture. Paint containing lead can be poisonous. Close doors to ovens, dishwashers, washing machines, dryers, and refrigerators. Do not leave standing water in tub, buckets, and so on.

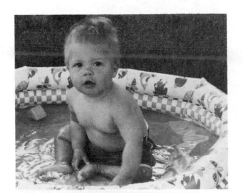

Joel can sit steadily.

Care and Guidance

Sleep. Has generally begun to sleep later in the morning.

Diet. Introduce chopped and mashed foods. Place newspaper beneath feeding table. Use unbreakable dishes. Allow baby to pick up pieces of food by hand and put them into the mouth.

Safety. Keep a supply of syrup of ipecac on hand. Know the phone number of the nearest poison control center. Avoid tablecloths with overhangs baby could reach.

Exercise. Is busy most of the day exploring his surroundings. Provide sufficient room and materials for safe play.

Help baby learn. See that she or he doesn't get into trouble. Distract the curious child from areas of danger.

In this way punishment is limited—avoid excessive spankings and "no's."

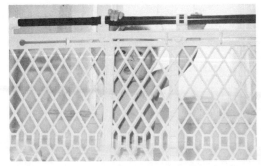

Stairway gates prevent falls for the infant with increased mobility.

**PHYSICAL DEVELOPMENT, SOCIAL BEHAVIOR, CARE AND GUIDANCE FOR
FIRST 12 MONTHS** *Continued*

TEN MONTHS
Physical Development

Pulls self to a standing position in the playpen. Throws toys to floor for mother to pick up. Cries when they are not returned. Walks around furniture while holding onto it.

Social Behavior

Knows own name. Plays simple games such as "peek-a-boo." Feeds self a cookie. May cry out in sleep without waking.

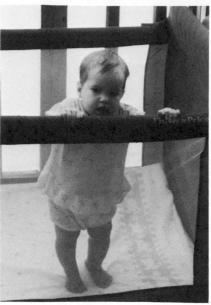

The ten month old child can pull herself to a standing position in a playpen.

ELEVEN MONTHS
Physical Development

Stands upright holding onto adult's hands.

Social Behavior

Understands simple directions. Impatient when held. Enjoys playing with empty dish and spoon following meals.

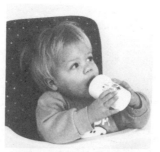

Drinking from a cup is easy for Joel, who is now 11 months old; however, spills still occur.

Care and Guidance

Sleep. Avoid strenuous play before bedtime. A night light is convenient for mother and makes the surroundings more familiar. Pajamas with feet will keep baby warm, as infants become uncovered easily.

Diet. Takes juice and water from cup. Solid foods in general are taken well.

Exercise. Tours around room holding adult's hands. Daytime clothing should be loose so as not to interfere with movement.

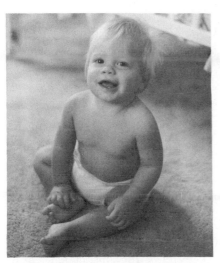

The ten month old. Note lower tooth.

Care and Guidance

Sleep. Greets parents in morning with excited jargon.

Diet. Still spills from cup. Enjoys blowing bubbles.

Exercise. Plays with toys in tub. Enjoys gross motor activity. Kicks, pulls self up.

Safety. Cover electrical outlets with tape. Put household cleaners and medicines out of reach if not previously done. Baby needs to be sat down in playpen at times; tends to stand until becomes exhausted.

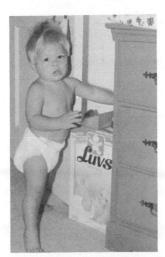

Directions must be simple for the 11 month old.

PHYSICAL DEVELOPMENT, SOCIAL BEHAVIOR, CARE AND GUIDANCE FOR
FIRST 12 MONTHS *Continued*

TWELVE MONTHS
Physical Development

Pulse 100–140. Respirations 20–40 per minute.

Triples birth weight.

Stands alone for short periods. May walk. Puts arm through sleeve, as an aid to being dressed.

Six teeth (four above and two below). Drinks from a cup; eats with a spoon with supervision.

Pincer grasp is well established.

Handedness (the preference for the use of one hand), although not fully established, may be evidenced.

Social Behavior

Friendly. Will repeat acts that elicit a response.

Recognizes "no-no." Verbalization slows owing to concentration on getting about. Enjoys rhythmic music.

Shows emotions such as fear, anger, and jealousy. Will react to these emotions from adults.

Plays with food, removes it from mouth.

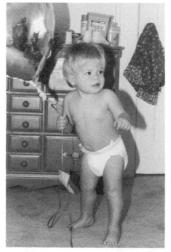

Happy Birthday, Joel! At 12 months Joel weighs 21 pounds, 14 ounces, and is 28¾ inches tall. He can stand alone for brief periods.

be given. Both the Advisory Committee on Immunization Practices (ACIP) and the American Academy of Pediatrics (AAP) recommend the use of MMR as the booster to assure additional protection against mumps and rubella as well as against measles. The ACIP recommendation is for reimmunization prior to school entry (4 to 6 years of age) and the AAP recommendation is for reimmunization prior to junior high school entry (10 to 12 years of age) (Frenkel, 1990). Table 7–1 reflects the recommendation of the AAP. See Table 7–2 for immunization schedules for children after the first year of life.

Side Effects. Parents should be made aware of the possible side effects of the various vaccines. These are usually mild. *The benefits of being protected*

greatly outweigh the risks. The physician may recommend prophylactic use of acetaminophen for fever. Otherwise, no specific treatment is required. Persistent high fever along with other obvious signs of illness is *not* routine and requires further investigation. Possible side effects of DTP vaccine include a mild fever and redness and swelling at the injection site. These last only a day or two. Measles vaccine may produce fever and rash, which occur about 7 to 12 days following vaccination and last only a few days. Encephalitis rarely occurs. Mumps vaccine has essentially no side effects other than occasional mild fever. Rubella vaccine may produce a rash within a few days that may last 1 or 2 days. Joint pain and swelling are sometimes seen about 2 weeks following vac-

Care and Guidance

Sleep. May take one long nap daily.

Diet. Gradually add egg white and fish (baked, steamed, or boiled). Drain oil from tuna or salmon. Add orange juice, if not done earlier. Add well-cooked table foods. Interest in eating dwindles.

Exercise. Plays in own room for an hour in morning. Enjoys putting clothespins in a basket and then removing them. Places objects on head.

Distraction is an effective way to deal with the baby's determination to do what he or she wants regardless of the outcome.

Skin Test. Tuberculin.

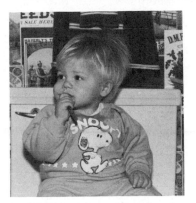

Joel at one year enjoys chewing on his toothbrush.

cine. Be aware of time delay. This is more common in older children. Side effects from polio vaccine are rare.

NUTRITION COUNSELING OF PARENTS

The nutrient needs of infants reflect rates of growth, energy expended in activity, basal metabolic needs, and the interaction of nutrients consumed. The baby is born with a *rooting reflex,* which assists in finding the nipple. The suck is rather immature because of the small mouth. There is a forward and backward movement of the tongue. As the infant grows, neuromaturation of the cheeks and tongue enables advancement to a more mature sucking pattern that utilizes negative pressure to obtain milk. This occurs about the third to fourth month. About this time the *extrusion reflex* (protrusion), which pushes food out of the mouth to prevent intake of inappropriate food, disappears. The digestive system continues to mature. By 6 months it is able to handle more complex nutrients and is less susceptible to food allergens. The stomach capacity expands from 10 to 20 ml at birth to 200 ml by 12 months. This enables the infant to consume more food at less frequent intervals. Most babies dislike spoon feeding at first. They begin by grasping at the spoon. This gradually progresses to the point at which the child scoops a little food but spills most of the contents. As the pincer grasp becomes more de-

Table 7–1. CURRENT AAP IMMUNIZATION SCHEDULE (JANUARY 1991)

2 months	18 months
DTP, TOPV, HbOC*	DTP, TOPV†
4 months	4–6 years
DTP, TOPV, HbOC	DTP, TOPV
6 months	12 years
DTP, HbOC	MMR‡
15 months	every 10 years
MMR, HbCV	dT

Key: DTP = diphtheria-tetanus-pertussis; TOPV = trivalent oral polio vaccine; HbOC = *Haemophilus influenzae* type b conjugate vaccine (diphtheria CRM$_{197}$ protein conjugate; HibTITER); MMR = measles-mumps-rubella; HbCV = Hib conjugate vaccine (ProHIBiT, Pedvax HIB, HibTITER); dT = diphtheria-pertussis

*In October 1990, HbOC (HibTITER) was approved by the FDA for infants starting at 2 months. Makers of other Hib conjugate vaccines have submitted applications.

†Can be given at 15 months.

‡Some states require this dose at 4–6 years.

(From Phillips, C. (1991). Keeping up with the changing immunization schedule. *Contemp. Pediatr.* 8:20–46.)

Note: As of March 1991, two vaccines for *Haemophilus influenzae* have been approved for children under 15 months. See the individual vaccines for exact time of dosage.

veloped, the baby can pick up food with tiny fingers and place it in the mouth. By 2 years, spoon feeding is mastered (Fig. 7–2).

Parents have many concerns about feeding their infant during the first year of life. This is a period when readiness pertaining to nutritional education is usually high; therefore, the nurse looks for opportunities to provide sound information. Assessment of parental knowledge; infant development, behavior, and readiness; parent-child interaction; and cultural and ethnic practices are of importance. Nutritional care plans based on developmental levels will assist parents in recognizing changes in feeding patterns. One means of assessing adequate intake is to determine whether the infant has gained 4 to 7 ounces per week for the first 6 months. The infant should also have at least six wet diapers per day and fall quietly asleep for several hours after feeding (Mott and col-

leagues, 1990). Continued monitoring of weight, height, and skinfold thickness will determine whether the infant's diet is adequate. This can easily be done during the periodic well-baby examinations. Parents should be assured that most children eat enough to grow normally although intake is seldom constant and varies in quantity and quality. Forced feedings are not appropriate.

Infants, in proportion to their weight, require more calories, protein, minerals, and vitamins than do adults. Their fluid requirements are also high. Human milk is the best food for infants under 6 months of age. It contains the ideal balance of nutrients in a readily digestible form. Iron-fortified infant formulas are also available. If an infant cannot tolerate milk-based formulas, soy protein–based formulas are available. These formulas are nutritionally sound and safe alternatives to cow's milk–based formulas. Infants should remain on human milk or iron-fortified formula for the first year of life. Whole cow's milk is not recommended before 1 year of age because (1) cow's milk may create a potential for intolerance of whole milk protein; (2) an increased incidence of iron deficiency anemia is associated with whole cow's milk intake; and (3) from the metabolism of cow's milk, a high level of solute results that stresses renal excretion (Behrman and Kleigman, 1990).

Solid Foods. At about 6 months of age, solids are introduced, based on developmental readiness and the nutrient needs of the infant (Table 7–3). Foods selected may be either commercial or home-prepared. The sequence in which foods are added is shown in Figure 7–3. Rice cereal is recommended as the first solid food, as it is less allergenic than others. Three tablespoons of iron-fortified cereal mixed with breast milk or formula will provide 7 mg of iron (over half the daily requirement). Offer only small amounts at first (1 teaspoonful). Place food on the back of the tongue. The consistency and amounts of solid foods are gradually increased as the infant becomes more familiar with them. A spoon with a small bowl and long straight handle is suggested. Cereal is usually followed by fruits, vegetables, and then meat. New foods should be introduced one at a time, with 4 to 7 days between each food. This makes it easier to determine food allergies if an intolerance is present.

Table 7–2. RECOMMENDED IMMUNIZATION SCHEDULES FOR CHILDREN NOT IMMUNIZED IN FIRST YEAR OF LIFE

RECOMMENDED TIME/AGE	IMMUNIZATIONS*	COMMENTS
Younger Than 7 Years		
First visit	DTP, OPV, MMR	MMR if child ≥ 15 months old; tuberculin testing may also be done at same visit
	HbCV†	For children aged 15–59 months can be given simultaneously with DTP and other vaccines (at separate sites)‡
Interval after first visit		
2 month	DTP, OPV (HbCV)	Second dose of HbCV is indicated only in children whose first dose was received when younger than 15 months
4 months	DTP	Third dose of CPV is not indicated in the U.S. but is desirable in other geographic areas where polio is endemic
10–16 months	DTP, OPV	OPV is not given if third dose was given earlier
4–6 years (at or before school entry)	DTP, OPV	DTP is not necessary if the fourth dose was given after the fourth birthday; OPV is not necessary if third dose was given after the fourth birthday
11–12 years	MMR	At entry to middle school or junior high
10 years later	Td	Repeat every 10 years throughout life
7 Years and Older§, ‖		
First visit	Td, OPV, MMR	
Interval after first visit		
2 months	Td, OPV	
8–14 months	Td, OPV	
11–12 years	MMR	At entry to middle school or junior high
10 years later	Td	Repeat every 10 years throughout life

*Abbreviations are explained in the footnote‡ to Table 7–1

†If child is younger than 15 months, only one HbCV (HbOC), as of October 1990, is approved for use (see *Haemophilus influenzae* infections, page 227 of the Report).

‡The initial three doses of DTP can be given at 1- to 2-month intervals; hence, for the child in whom immunization is initiated at age 15 months or older, one visit could be eliminated by giving DTP, OPV, and MMR at the first visit; DTP and HbCV at the second visit (1 month later); and DTP and OPV at the third visit (2 months after the first visit). Subsequent doses of DTP and OPV 10 to 16 months after the first visit are still indicated. HbCV, MMR, DTP, and OPV can be given simultaneously at separate sites if failure of the patient to return for furture immunizations is a concern.

§If person is ≥ 18 years old, routine poliovirus vaccination is not indicated in the U.S.

‖ Minimal interval between doses of MMR is 1 month.

(Adapted from Report on The Committee on Infectious Diseases, 22nd ed. Elk Grove Village, Ill., American Academy of Pediatrics, 1991.)

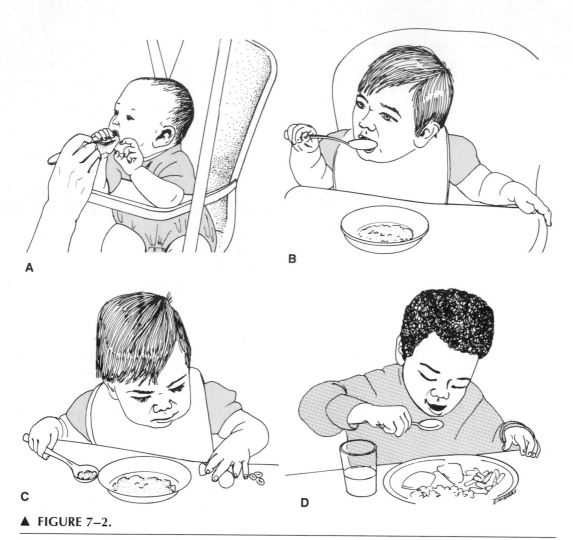

A

B

C

D

▲ **FIGURE 7–2.**

Development of feeding skills in infants and toddlers. *A,* At 7 months the child shows beginning involvement with feeding and reaching for the spoon. *B,* At 9 months the child is beginning to use the spoon independently, although there is difficulty in keeping food on it. *C,* The 9 month old shows a refined pincer grasp to pick up food. *D,* The 2 year old is much more skillful at self-feeding, with the ability to both rotate the wrist and elevate the elbow to keep food on the spoon.

Table 7–3. FEEDING, NUTRITION, AND GROWTH IN INFANCY

AGE	FEEDING BEHAVIORS	PARENTAL CONCERNS	RECOMMENDED NUTRITION	GROWTH RATE

0 to 3 months	Reflexes:
	  Rooting
	  Sucking
	  Extrusion
		Adequacy of intake
		Discomfort with breast feeding
			115 to 130 cal/kg/day
			Breast milk with 400 IU vitamin D and 0.25 mg fluoride or iron-fortified formula
				Weight = 30 g/day (1 oz/day)
				Length = 3.5 cm/mo
				Head circumference = 2 cm/mo

4 to 6 months	Reflexes:
	  Extrusion and rooting gone
	Skills:
	  Sucking
	  Chewing
		Introduction of solids	100 to 110 cal/kg/day
			Breast milk with 400 IU vitamin D and 0.25 mg fluoride or iron-fortified formula
				Weight = 20 g/day (⅔ oz/day)
				Length = 2 cm/mo
				Head circumference = 1 cm/mo

6 to 12 months	Skills:
	  Sucking
	  Chewing
	  Cup drinking (with help)
	  Finger feeding
		Messiness
		Control over feeding
			100 to 110 cal/kg/day
			Solids 50% of total calories
			Limit formula intake to 30 oz/day
				Weight = 15 g/day (0.5 oz/day)
				Length = 1.5 cm/mo
				Head circumference = 0.5 cm/mo

12 to 24 months	Skills:
	  Spoon feeding
	  Cup drinking
	  Fork feeding
		Messiness
		Selective tastes
		Decreased appetite
			90 to 100 cal/kg/day
			Limit milk to 24 oz/day
			No foods that can be aspirated
				Weight = 220 g/mo (7 oz/mo)
				Length = 1 cm/mo
				Head circumference = 0.27 cm/mo (12 to 18 months)
				Head circumference = 0.15 cm/mo (18 to 24 months)

(From Levine, M., et al (1983). *Developmental-Behavioral Pediatrics*. Philadelphia, W. B. Saunders Company.)

If the baby refuses a certain food, omit it temporarily. Keep mealtime pleasant. Let infants try new foods; they may like foods the parent does not care for. Do not introduce new foods when the baby is ill. The amount of food consumed will vary with the individual child. Fruit juices are generally offered at about 5 to 6 months of age, as the infant begins to drink from a cup. An exception to this is the addition of orange juice, which is withheld until the baby is 1 year old, when family members have known allergies. Other highly allergic foods that may be delayed include fish, nuts, strawberries, chocolate, and egg whites.

A spouted plastic cup is helpful at first. Dilute the juice initially. Then gradually increase the quantity to 3 to 4 ounces per day. The directions for preparing baby food at home are listed in Table 7–4. Baby food can be prepared in a food grinder, electric blender, or food mill or by mashing the food to the desired texture.

The infant's height and weight should progress at approximately the same rate. Variations may be due to illness, malabsorption, psychological factors, overfeeding, and underfeeding. It is important to ascertain feeding procedures and practices regularly and to repeat essential information as indicated.

Buying, Storing, and Serving Food. Baby foods stored in jars are vacuum packed. Parents are taught to check safety seals before purchase. (Directions are generally indicated on the jar; e.g.,

Months	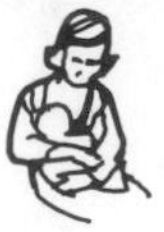 ![breastfeeding icon]	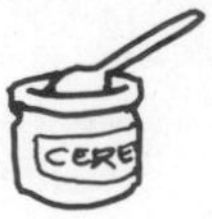 ![cereal icon]	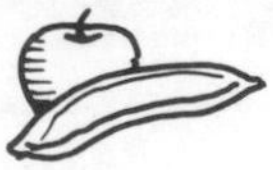 ![fruit icon]	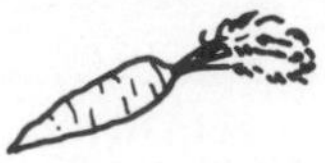 ![vegetable icon]	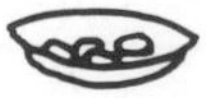 ![meat icon]
0–6	breast milk or formula				
7	breast milk or formula	cereal			
8	breast milk or formula	cereal	fruit		
9	breast milk or formula	cereal	fruit	vegetable	
10	breast milk or formula	cereal	fruit	vegetable	
11	breast milk or formula	cereal	fruit	vegetable	meat

▲ **FIGURE 7–3.**

Order for introducing foods.

reject if safety button is up. Upon opening a jar, a definite "pop" sound is heard as the vacuum seal is broken.) Also check the expiration date of the product. Dates are usually found on the caps of jars and on the sides of cereal and bakery items. Unopened jars of baby food and juices are stored in a dry, cool place. Rotate jars, using those on hand the longest first. Keep baby cereals away from other grain products, which may be insect infested. Transfer food to a serving dish. Do not feed out of the jar or return leftovers to the jar, as saliva may turn certain foods to liquid by digesting them in the jar. Unused portions may be stored in the refrigerator in the original jar. Special precautions should be taken to prevent burning when warming food in the microwave. When food is heated in a microwave, check its temperature, as sometimes food heats unevenly. Test all warmed foods. This can be done by tasting or by dropping a portion of a warmed liquid on the inner wrist.

NURSING BRIEF ▶ ▶ ▶ ▶ ▶ ▶ ▶ ▶
Human milk and properly prepared formula supply adequate water for the infant under normal conditions. During illness or very hot, humid weather, the infant may require additional water.

WEANING

Weaning is usually begun about the sixth month, or when the infant can use a cup. It is done gradually. Extra attention is given to the baby before and after the use of the cup so that pleasure is associated with it. This helps compensate for the loss of satisfaction from sucking. Weaning should not be attempted when the baby is ill. Complementary or relief bottles may be used throughout the period of nursing or only occasionally; the mother should consult her doctor for

Table 7–4. DIRECTIONS FOR HOME PREPARATION OF INFANT FOODS

1. Select fresh, high quality fruits, vegetables, or meats.
2. Be sure all utensils, including cutting boards, grinder, knives, and so on, are thoroughly clean.
3. Wash hands before preparing the food.
4. Clean, wash, and trim the food.
5. Cook the foods until tender in as little water as possible. Avoid overcooking, which may destroy heat-sensitive nutrients.
6. Do not add salt. Add sugar sparingly. Do not add honey to food for infants less than 1 year of age.*
7. Add enough water so that the food has a consistency that is easily puréed.
8. Strain or purée the food using an electric blender, a food mill, a baby food grinder, or a kitchen strainer.
9. Pour purée into ice cube tray and freeze.
10. When food is frozen hard, remove the cubes and store in freezer bags.
11. Unfreeze and heat in serving container the amount of food that will be consumed at a single feeding (in water bath or microwave oven).

*Botulism spores have been reported in honey, and young infants do not have the immune capacity to resist this infection.
(From Krause, M., and Mahan, L. (1991). *Food, Nutrition and Diet Therapy*, 8th ed. Philadelphia, W. B. Saunders Company.)

specific instructions. Decreasing fluid consumption and feedings will assist the mother's milk in drying up.

Teeth

DECIDUOUS TEETH

The development of the 20 *deciduous* or *baby teeth* begins about the fifth month of intrauterine life. The health and diet of the expectant mother affect their soundness. Teeth appear during the first two and a half years of life. It is a normal process and is generally accompanied by little or no discomfort. Wide individual differences occur in tooth eruption in normal, healthy infants. A delay in teething is significant if other forms of immaturity or illness are present. The physician evaluates the process of teething during the baby's regular health checkups. The first tooth generally appears about the seventh month. The 1 year old has about six teeth, four above and two below. The order in which the teeth appear is almost always the same (Fig. 7–4). They are shed in about the same order in which they appear, i.e., lower central incisors first, and so forth.

TEETHING DURING INFANCY

Teething refers to the process in which the crown of the tooth erupts through the periodontal membrane. The gums may be red, swollen, and sensitive. The normal appearance of saliva and drooling at 4 months is frequently attributed, but rarely due, to teething (Graef and Cone, 1985). The first tooth appears about the seventh month. The first (deciduous) teeth act as a guide for the proper positioning of the secondary teeth. Teething does not cause infection. However, at this time the infant's maternal antibody supply is low, making the child more prone to infection. The infant may be fussy and wake during the night. A fever of 38.4°C (101.0° F) should be reported to one's physician. Teething is not responsible for respiratory tract infections, rashes, or diarrhea. Cold appears to soothe inflamed gums. A cool wash cloth, a hard rubber teething ring, or a teething pretzel may bring relief. Acetaminophen is useful when discomfort is clearly related to teeth.

Good oral hygiene at this age consists of offering water following food and gently wiping the teeth with gauze. Calcium, phosphorus, vitamins C and D, and fluoride help ensure healthy teeth. Bottle mouth caries are to be avoided, which can occur when an infant is put to bed with a bottle of milk or sweetened juice. Sugar pools within the oral cavity, causing severe decay. It is seen most often in children between the ages of 18 months and 3 years. Eliminating the bedtime bottle or substituting water is recommended. Nursing bottle caries are also being reported in breast-fed babies, particularly in infants who sleep with their mothers and nurse at will throughout the night. To prevent this, nocturnal nursing should be discouraged, as should frequent intermittent night feedings after the age of 1 year (Brams and Maloney, 1983).

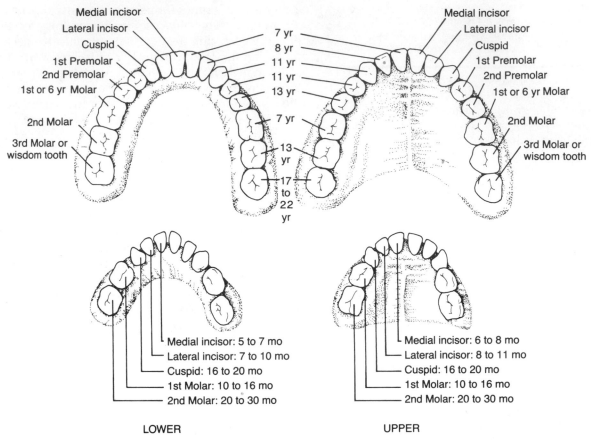

Medial incisor
Lateral incisor
Cuspid
1st Premolar
2nd Premolar
1st or 6 yr Molar
2nd Molar
3rd Molar or wisdom tooth

7 yr
8 yr
11 yr
11 yr
13 yr
7 yr
13 yr
17 to 22 yr

Medial incisor
Lateral incisor
Cuspid
1st Premolar
2nd Premolar
1st or 6 yr Molar
2nd Molar
3rd Molar or wisdom tooth

Medial incisor: 5 to 7 mo
Lateral incisor: 7 to 10 mo
Cuspid: 16 to 20 mo
1st Molar: 10 to 16 mo
2nd Molar: 20 to 30 mo

Medial incisor: 6 to 8 mo
Lateral incisor: 8 to 11 mo
Cuspid: 16 to 20 mo
1st Molar: 10 to 16 mo
2nd Molar: 20 to 30 mo

LOWER

UPPER

▲ **FIGURE 7–4.**

Permanent and deciduous teeth.

An additional cause of erosion of dental enamel is repeated exposure to gastric acids. This is now being recognized in infants with gastroesophageal reflux who are old enough to have teeth and in teenagers with bulimia. When the effects of gastric acid are recognized early, the teeth can be protected with an acrylic sealant (Rosenthal and Rosenthal, 1983). Parents are taught the cariogenic effects of refined sugars, particularly those that are sticky and remain in the mouth for long periods of time.

References

American Academy of Pediatrics (1989). *Measles: Reassessment of the Current Immunization Policy.* Elk Grove Village, Ill.

Behrman, R., and Kleigman, R. (1990). *Nelson Essentials Of Pediatrics.* Philadelphia, W. B. Saunders Company.

Brams, M., and Maloney, J. "Nursing bottle caries" in breast-fed children. *J. Pediatr.* 103:415.

Frenkel, L. (1990). Routine immunizations for American children in the 1990s. *Pediatr. Clin. North Am.* 37:533.

Graef, J., and Cone, T. (1985). *Manual of Pediatric Therapeutics.* Boston, Little, Brown and Company.

Krause, M., and Mahan, L. (1984). *Food, Nutrition, and Diet Therapy,* 7th ed. Philadelphia, W. B. Saunders Company.

Mott, S., James, S., and Sperhac, A. (1990). *Nursing Care of Children and Families.* Redwood City, Cal., Addison-Wesley.

Pipes, P. (1981). *Nutrition in Infancy and Childhood,* 2nd ed. St. Louis, C. V. Mosby.

Rosenthal, P., and Rosenthal, R. (1983). Tooth enamel erosion from vomiting treated with an acrylic sealant. *Clin. Pediatr.* 22:818.

Bibliography

American Academy of Pediatrics (1988). *Report of the Committee on Infectious Diseases,* 21st ed. Elk Grove Village, Ill.

Behrman, R., and Vaughan, V. (1987). *Nelson Textbook of Pediatrics*, 13th ed. Philadelphia, W. B. Saunders Company.

Foster, R., Hunsberger, M., and Anderson, J. J. (1989). *Family-Centered Nursing Care of Children*. Philadelphia, W. B. Saunders Company.

Howard, B. (1990). Growing together: A guide to how babies—and parents—develop. *Contemp. Pediatr.* 7:12–40.

Howard, B. (1990). Growing together: Parents and child from 3 months to 1 year. *Contemp. Pediatr.* 7:81–98.

Marlow, D., and Redding, B. (1988). *Pediatric Nursing*, 6th ed. Philadelphia, W. B. Saunders Company.

Nemethy, M., and Clore, E. (1990). Microwave heating of infant formula and breast milk. *J. Pediatr. Health Care* 4:131–135.

Phillips, C. (1991). Keeping up with the changing immunization schedule. *Contemp. Pediatr.* 8:20–44.

Schmitt, B. (1990). When weaning is delayed. *Contemp. Pediatr.* 7:67–68.

Schmitt, B. (1990). When your baby has colic. *Contemp. Pediatr.* 7:85–86.

Starr, S. (1989). Status of varicella vaccine for healthy children. *Pediatrics* 84:1097–1098.

STUDY QUESTIONS

1. Why must the pediatric nurse be able to recognize the various stages of growth and development in the infant?
2. Of what value is sucking to the baby?
3. Mrs. Jones tells you that she always props baby Sue's bottle, since it saves her so much time. What would you reply?
4. What is the value of attending to the needs of an infant promptly and cheerfully during the first year?
5. Mrs. Piper has been bringing Charlene, who is 4 months old, to the well-child clinic since she was 1 month old. What services are provided by a well-child clinic?
6. How does the infant's environment affect physical growth and development? Mental health?
7. Define *immunity*.
8. List the immunizations given during the first year of life and the diseases they prevent.
9. Tommy is 9 months old. Prepare a day's menu for him.
10. What are deciduous teeth?
11. Prepare diagrams showing the eruption of the deciduous and permanent teeth. Label the teeth and include the approximate month or year that they appear.
12. Joel is 10 months old. You are giving him green beans for the first time. How would you introduce it to him? List four factors to keep in mind in regard to adding solid foods to a baby's diet.
13. Discuss the needs of the newborn infant. How do these needs change during the first year?
14. Observe a 3 month old infant on the children's unit. How do physical growth and development compare with those of the healthy 3 month infant?
15. Jean, 7 months old, shows a fear of strangers. Discuss various ways in which to handle this problem in the home and in the hospital.

CHAPTER 8 _____

Chapter Outline

THE EARS
    Otitis Media
RESPIRATORY SYSTEM
    Nasopharyngitis (The Common Cold)
    Bronchiolitis
THE BLOOD
    Iron Deficiency Anemia
    Sickle Cell Disease
GASTROINTESTINAL SYSTEM
    Inguinal Hernia
    Umbilical Hernia
    Pyloric Stenosis
    Intussusception
    Vomiting
    Fluid Imbalance
        Dehydration
        Overhydration
THE LUNGS
    Cystic Fibrosis
NERVOUS SYSTEM
    Bacterial Meningitis
GENITOURINARY SYSTEM
    Hydrocele
    Undescended Testes (Cryptorchidism)
THE SKIN
    Infantile Eczema (Atopic Dermatitis)
SPECIAL TOPICS
    Sudden Infant Death Syndrome
    Failure to Thrive
    Child Abuse and Neglect

Objectives

Upon completion and mastery of Chapter 8, the student will be able to

- Define the vocabulary terms listed.
- List and define the more common disorders of infancy.
- Illustrate the anatomical difference in the ear canals of adults and children and describe the significance of this difference.
- Explain why infants and young children become more easily dehydrated than adults.
- Recommend four food sources of iron for Robert, age 10 months, who has been found to have iron deficiency anemia.
- Summarize the nursing care for 15 month old Peter, who has infantile eczema, and give the rationale for each nursing measure.
- List four kinds of child abuse and the descriptive behavior often exhibited by parent and child in each case.

Disorders of the Infant

Terms

alkalosis (195)
anastomosis (194)
hypotonia (211)
incarcerated (191)
infarct (187)
opisthotonos (204)
petechia (204)
RSV (184)
SIADH (205)
thrombosis (187)

During infancy, rapid physical and emotional development takes place. Hospitalization during this period is a frustrating experience for infants. They are used to getting what they want when they want it, and they show their displeasure quickly when illness restricts their desires.

Parents are encouraged to stay with the child. This decreases the anxiety the child experiences when hospitalized. Parents should be included in the care of the child and oriented to the routine of the hospital. Mothers who are breast feeding are encouraged to continue. If the mother has other responsibilities and cannot stay, she may use a breast pump in order to continue the child on breast milk. The nurse must be understanding if the parent cannot stay with the child at all times. Parents often have other children as well as financial responsibilities that limit the time they can spend at the hospital. Regression by the child is a normal response to hospitalization. The infant who has been drinking from a cup at home may refuse it entirely when hospitalized.

Nursing personnel must try to meet the needs of infants by protecting them from excess frustration. It is not wise to expect them to develop new habits when they need their energies to cope with their illness and the strange environment. Forcing them to eat or sleep leads only to further difficulties. Gentleness, patience, and ingenuity are not merely qualities attributed to a caring nurse; they are a necessity in caring for children (Fig. 8–1). Every attempt should be made to keep infants on their home schedules. Most hospitals incorporate into their admission record a section devoted to an infant's usual routine. The nurse should use this as a reference and transfer the information to the infant's care plan. Infants also enjoy having their favorite stuffed animal or blanket.

The nurse must also be aware of the parent's needs. The hospital environment may be confusing and stressful for the parent. Parents sometimes feel inadequate because of their lack of knowledge of health care. Prior to hospitalization the parent met all the needs of the child, and suddenly this may not be possible. Every attempt should be made to include the family in all aspects of the infant's care. The family becomes part of the team.

COMMUNICATION ALERT ▶ ▶ ▶ ▶ ▶
Since much of communication with the infant is nonverbal, the nurse uses touch to communicate. The infant is approached slowly, and the nurse uses a calm, soft voice. The infant who is crying loudly can best be soothed by the nurse remaining quiet and calm. Anxiety from the nurse can be transferred to the child.

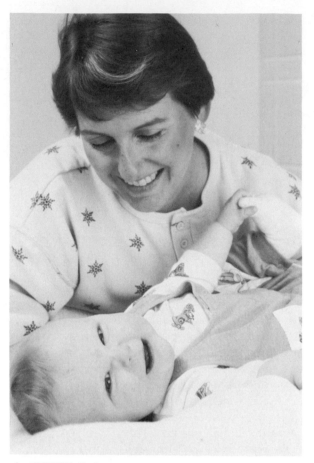

▲ FIGURE 8–1

An integral part of pediatric nursing is the time spent with the child. The nurse uses this time to communicate, nurture, assess, support, and sometimes just play with the child. (Courtesy of Cook–Fort Worth Children's Medical Center, Fort Worth, Texas.)

During convalescence, infants' needs change. One must try to recognize their need for play and social interaction. A warm, continuous relationship with the nurse is important.

The Ears

OTITIS MEDIA

Description. Otitis media (*ot*, ear + *itis*, inflammation of + *media*, middle) is an inflammation of the middle ear. The middle ear is a tiny cavity in the temporal bone. Its entrance is guarded by the sensitive tympanic membrane, or "eardrum," which transmits sound waves through the oval window to the inner ear, which contains the organs of hearing and balance. The middle ear opens into air spaces, or *sinuses*, in the mastoid process of the temporal bone. It is also connected to the throat by a channel called the eustachian tube. These structures—the mastoid sinuses, the middle ear, and the eustachian tube—are lined by mucous membranes. As a result, an infection of the throat can easily spread to the middle ear and mastoid. The eustachian tube also protects the middle ear from nasopharyngeal secretions, provides drainage of middle ear secretions into the nasopharynx, and equalizes air pressure between the middle ear and the outside atmosphere. These protective functions are diminished when the tubes are blocked. Unequalized air within the ear creates a negative pressure that allows organisms to be swept up into the tube if it opens.

Otitis media may be secondary to an upper respiratory tract infection. It is caused by a variety of organisms. The bacteria involved are usually those that cause a sore throat or tonsillitis (hemolytic streptococci or pneumococci), although *Haemophilus influenzae* accounts for about a third of the cases seen in infancy. Infants are more prone to ear infections, for the eustachian tube is shorter, wider, and straighter than that of older children and adults. Since babies lie flat for long periods, microorganisms have easy access from the eustachian tube to the middle ear. This is thought by some to be a contributing factor.

There are two types of otitis media. The acute disease is referred to as suppurative or purulent otitis media. It is most commonly caused by *Streptococcus pneumoniae* and *H. influenzae*. The second type is referred to as serous or nonsuppurative otitis media. The cause is unknown but it often occurs after an acute episode. Serous otitis media may lead to hearing loss.

Symptoms. The symptoms of otitis media are pain in the ear, which is often very severe, irritability, and interference with hearing. Sucking or chewing tends to increase the pain. Fever, which may run as high as 40°C (104°F), headache, and vomiting may also accompany it, as well as diarrhea. The nurse may suspect an earache in the infant who rubs the ear frequently or pulls at it. The infant may also roll the head from side to side and cry piercingly. The older child can point to the place that is tender. Children with serous otitis media may be asymptomatic.

If an abscess forms, a rupture of the eardrum may result and pus may drain from the ear. When this happens, the pressure is relieved and the patient is more comfortable.

Complications of an ear infection include hearing loss, mastoiditis, chronic otitis media, and meningitis. These are rare with modern treatment. Prevention lies in prompt treatment of respiratory infections or infected tonsils and adenoids.

Treatment and Nursing Care

The professional examining the ears first observes their appearance and general hygiene. The lymph nodes about the ear are observed for swelling or tenderness. The patient's head is adequately stabilized to prevent injury to the ear canal from sudden, unexpected movement. Excess cerumen or wax in the ear, which may obstruct visibility, is carefully removed. The examiner ensures that there are no foreign bodies lodged in the outer canal before inserting the otoscope. To straighten the canal and improve viewing, the ear is pulled *down* and *back* in infants and small children and *up* and *back* in older children and adults. The doctor can also incise the tympanic membrane to prevent a tear by spontaneous rupture. This is called a *myringotomy* (*myringo*, eardrum + *otomy*, incision of). This procedure is not performed as routinely today as it once was because of the availability of more effective antibiotics. Alternatively, the doctor may insert a tiny tube into the eardrum to act as a drain. It is called a *tympanic (TM) button* or *tympanostomy ventilating tube*. Eventually this tube will fall out spontaneously.

When an infection is evident, treatment is directed toward finding the causative organism and relieving the symptoms. A throat culture may be taken. Antibiotics are given initially until the specific organism is determined. Amoxicillin and ampicillin are two of the most common drugs used. If these are not effective, sulfamethoxazole/trimethoprim (Bactrim, Septra) may be given. Most physicians give the antibiotic for 10 days. Analgesics and antipyretic drugs may be given to relieve pain and fever. Antihistamines and decongestants are sometimes prescribed but are contro-

versial (Woolbert, 1990). Ear drops are usually not used as they may obscure visualization of the tympanic membrane. All children should be seen at the end of antibiotic therapy to ensure adequate treatment. Parents are taught to give the entire dose of the antibiotic even though the child may appear well.

Heat or cold may be applied to the ear. The child can be placed on the affected side with the ear on top of the hot water bottle (temperature of water: 46°C, or 115°F). If the ear is draining, the outer canal can be cleaned with sterile water or hydrogen peroxide. Parents should be instructed not to use Q-tips in the ears.

NURSING BRIEF ▷ ▷ ▷ ▷ ▷ ▷ ▷ ▷
Children should be fed in an upright position and should not be put to bed with a bottle.

Respiratory System

NASOPHARYNGITIS (THE COMMON COLD)

Description. A cold, the most common infection of the respiratory tract, is caused by one or a number of viruses, principally the *rhinoviruses*, which are spread from one child to another by sneezing, coughing, and direct contact. Group A beta-hemolytic streptococci are the prominent bacterial offenders. Droplets remain suspended in the air and on dust particles for short periods of time. The infection is transferred mainly during the initial stage. In the second phase of a cold, nasal drainage becomes thicker and purulent. Factors that contribute to the individual's susceptibility include age, state of nutrition, general health, fatigue, and emotional upsets.

As the child becomes exposed to more children, the number of colds contracted increases. Parents may notice this particularly during the child's first few years of daycare or school, since the child has had little opportunity to build up resistance. The older the child, the better she or he is able to resist infection. In temperate climates the incidence of rhinoviral infection peaks in September and again in April or May.

To prevent a cold, avoid exposing children to

those with this virus as much as possible. Infants less than 6 months of age can acquire this infection, so they too must be protected from infected persons. Be sure to provide nourishing foods and see that the child or infant gets sufficient rest.

Symptoms. The symptoms of a cold in an infant or small child are different from those in an adult. Children's air passages are smaller and more easily obstructed. Fever as high as 40°C (104°F) is not uncommon in children less than 3 years of age. Nasal discharge, irritability, sore throat, cough, and general discomfort are present, and there may be vomiting and diarrhea. The diagnosis is complicated by the fact that many infectious diseases resemble the common cold during their onset. Complications of a cold include bronchitis, pneumonitis, ear infections, and sinusitis.

Treatment and Nursing Care

There is no cure for the common cold. When a cold is suspected, treatment should be started early. The treatment is designed to relieve the symptoms. Rest, fluids, and proper diet are important. Parents are taught to watch the child for signs of dehydration. If anorexia is present, food should not be forced. The appetite will gradually improve as the condition does. When high fever accompanies a cold, the doctor must be consulted. Acetaminophen (Tylenol) will reduce the temperature, but the correct dosage should be prescribed, particularly in patients less than 1 year of age. Aqueous nose drops will relieve nasal congestion. The older child can help squeeze the bulb of the dropper when drops are instilled. The infant needs nose drops mainly before feedings and at bedtime. When drops are instilled 10 to 15 minutes before nursing, the nasal passages are cleared and the baby can suck easily. Each child needs an individual bottle of nose drops to prevent cross-infection.

Moist air soothes the inflamed nose and throat. An electric cold air humidifier is safe and convenient. It should be cleaned and disinfected regularly. If a great deal of moisture is indicated, as for croup, the infant may be taken to a small room, such as the bathroom, and all the hot water faucets can be turned on to create sufficient steam.

The older child is taught the proper way to remove nasal secretions from the nose. The mouth is opened slightly and secretions are blown gently through both nostrils at the same time. This method prevents infection from being forced into the eustachian tubes. When there is a large amount of nasal discharge, the nurse protects the upper lip by the application of petroleum jelly.

In the hospital, the child is isolated. During the initial stage of the fever the child is kept in bed. Frequent change of position is necessary. In the home it is difficult to keep children with a cold away from other members of the family. They must be taught to cover their mouth and nose when sneezing, and to wash their hands afterwards. Tissues must be properly discarded. The child should stay at home without visitors. Rest, fluids, and adequate nutrition will support recovery.

BRONCHIOLITIS

Bronchiolitis is an inflammation of the small airways. It occurs most often during the spring and winter months and in children under 2 years of age. Bronchiolitis is usually caused by a viral infection. The most common causative organism is the respiratory syncytial virus (RSV). Children are usually exposed through other family members who have symptoms of an upper respiratory infection.

Inflammation of the bronchioles is associated with obstruction due to edema and accumulation of mucus. There may be partial or complete obstruction. The alveoli are usually not affected. Normal gas exchange in the lung is affected. This leads to hypoxemia.

Signs and Symptoms. The infant first shows signs of a mild upper respiratory infection with rhinorrhea, sneezing, cough, and a low-grade fever. The infant's appetite may be affected. Respiratory distress increases, and the child develops rapid breathing and wheezing. Bottle feeding may be difficult because of the rapid respiratory rate interfering with sucking and swallowing. As the disease progresses, nasal flaring, retractions, tachypnea (60 to 80 per minute), and cyanosis may occur. Breath sounds may be diminished if the bronchioles are severely obstructed.

Treatment

Mild cases of bronchiolitis can be managed at home. Increased fluids are ordered, and parents are advised of signs of increased respiratory distress. Indications for hospitalization include a patient less than 6 months of age, sleeping respiratory rates of 50 to 60 per minute or higher, hypoxemia, apnea, and inability to tolerate oral feeding (Behrman and Kliegman, 1990).

Intravenous fluids are started to hydrate the child and thin the secretions. The child is placed in an atmosphere of humidified oxygen (mist tent or Croupette). Antipyretics are given to reduce fever.

When the causative organism is RSV, the infant may be given ribavirin (Virazole). Ribavirin is given to high-risk patients or to those with chronic underlying conditions, such as cardiac disease, pulmonary disease, or a history of prematurity (Nederhand and associates, 1989). Because there is a possibility that the drug could be a teratogen, it is recommended that nurses of childbearing age be cautioned about caring for children receiving this drug.

Nursing Care

NURSING DIAGNOSES

1. Ineffective airway clearance, related to thick mucus.
2. Impaired gas exchange, related to edema and mucus of the bronchioles.
3. Fluid volume deficit, related to insensible fluid loss secondary to tachypnea and decreased intake.
4. Anxiety, related to unfamiliar environment, respiratory distress, and placement in Croupette.
5. Knowledge deficit, related to disease process and treatment.

The child with bronchiolitis is monitored closely for signs and symptoms of increasing respiratory distress. Breath sounds, skin color, depth and rate of respirations, and vital signs are assessed. Changes in alertness and increased anxiety can be signs of impending distress.

Intravenous fluids are monitored in the acutely ill child. As the child improves, oral fluids are increased and frequent small meals are offered. The child is on intake and output recording, and daily weights are taken. The fontanels and the child's skin turgor are also assessed.

The child in a mist tent should have gown and linens changed if they become damp. Also, moisture buildup should be removed from the tubing and sides of the tent. (See Chapter 3 for detailed care of the child in a mist tent.)

As always, parents are encouraged to stay with the child. This may be even more important because the child already may be anxious because of respiratory distress. Parents should understand the importance of the child staying in the tent. They should be included in care and diversional activities for the child.

The Blood

IRON DEFICIENCY ANEMIA

The most common nutritional deficiency of children in the United States today is anemia due to insufficient amounts of iron in the body. The incidence is highest during infancy and adolescence, two rapid growth periods. Anemia (an, without + emia, blood) is a condition in which there is a reduction in the amount and size of the red blood cells or in the amount of hemoglobin, or both. The clinical features are related to the decrease in the oxygen-carrying capacity of the blood. Iron is needed for the manufacture of red blood cells. Iron deficiency anemia may be caused by severe hemorrhage, the child's inability to absorb the iron received, excessive growth requirements, or an inadequate diet. Researchers have also found that whole cow's milk can precipitate gastrointestinal bleeding in some babies.

The prevention of iron deficiency anemias begins with good prenatal care to ensure that the mother has a suitable intake of iron during pregnancy. The newborn infant relies on iron that is stored in the system during fetal life for the first few months following birth. Iron is obtained late in the prenatal period, which has an effect on the infant's iron stores. Premature infants can deplete their iron stores as early as 2 months. The normal term infant who receives unfortified formula will deplete storage of iron by about 4 or 5 months. Breast-fed infants rarely deplete their iron stores until after 6 months (Behrman and Kliegman, 1990).

The highest incidence of this type of anemia occurs from the 9th to the 24th month. During this rapid growth period, the baby outgrows the limited iron reserve that was in the body; in addition, iron-fortified formula and infant cereals may have been eliminated from the diet. Poorly planned meals or feeding problems also contribute to this deficiency. The mother sometimes may rely too much on bottle feedings to avoid conflict at meals. Unfortunately, milk contains very little iron. Instead, the amounts of solid food should be increased and the milk decreased. Boiled egg yolk, liver, green leafy vegetables, iron-fortified cereal, dried fruits (apricots, peaches, prunes, raisins), cooked dry beans, crushed nuts, and whole-grain bread are good sources of iron. Iron-fortified cereals eaten out of the box provide a nutritious snack.

The child's hemoglobin is usually below 10 gm/dl. Children may have much lower hemoglobin levels before they show signs and symptoms. Typically, blood tests are done for hemoglobin, hematocrit, morphologic changes in red blood cells, and iron concentration. A dietary history is also important in the diagnosis.

Symptoms. The symptoms of iron deficiency anemia are pallor, irritability, anorexia, and a decrease in activity. Many babies are overweight owing to excess consumption of milk (so-called milk babies). These infants may look flabby and pale. Sometimes a slight heart murmur is heard. The spleen may be enlarged. Untreated iron deficiency anemias progress slowly, and in severe cases the heart muscle becomes too weak to function. If this happens, heart failure follows. Screening procedures are suggested at 9 to 24 months for full-term infants and earlier, at 6 to 9 months, for low birth weight babies.

Treatment

This disease responds well to treatment. The doctor must first differentiate it from other types of anemia. Iron, usually ferrous sulfate, is given orally two or three times a day between meals.

Vitamin C aids in the absorption of iron; therefore, juice is suggested upon administration. Treatment is recommended for 5 months (Behrman and Kliegman, 1990). Liquid preparations are taken through a straw to prevent temporary discoloration of the teeth. (Recently available iron preparations do not have this disadvantage.) Intramuscular iron is given in cases of malabsorption and when noncompliance with the oral route is a problem. Most children can tolerate the oral drug, and parents should be educated about it so they will comply and the painful injections can be avoided. The injectable drug is an iron-dextran mixture (Imferon), which must be injected deep in a large muscle, using Z tract technique to minimize staining and irritation.

NURSING BRIEF ▷ ▷ ▷ ▷ ▷ ▷ ▷ ▷
Avoid iron poisoning in children by keeping preparations well out of reach. Educate parents about this hazard.

Parent Education. Parents need explicit instructions regarding the proper foods for the infant. The nurse stresses the importance of using iron-fortified formula throughout the first year of life (the absorption of iron from human milk is much better than that from cow's milk). The amount of milk consumed during the night as well as during the day is determined. Infants over 6 months of age receiving formula should not take more than 32 ounces per day. If they are receiving fresh cow's milk, the amount should be less—about 24 ounces per day. Dispel the myth that milk is a perfect food. Infants should be started on solid foods at 6 months. Review solid food intake and suggest specific iron-enriched nutrients. Consider financial, ethnic, and family preferences in discussions. Behavior concerns at mealtime may also need to be addressed.

The stools of babies placed on iron will be a tarry green color. Absence of this finding may indicate poor compliance with therapy by the parents. Oral iron preparations are not to be given with milk, which interferes with absorption. These preparations also should not be given with meals. *It is important to emphasize that both dietary changes and supplemental iron therapy are necessary to eradicate iron deficiency anemia.* Dietary changes must be lifelong to maintain good health and to prevent recurrence. Iron supplements are given until the prescription expires. Parents are encouraged to return for periodic evaluation of the child's blood status. They are also advised to remind new physicians of the condition, even though it may currently be rectified. During discussions, nurses should attempt to support parents, who usually experience guilt feelings or believe they are not successful parents. It may be comforting for the nurse to reiterate that most babies are in the process of "catching up on iron supplies" and that the condition is not uncommon.

SICKLE CELL DISEASE

Description. Sickle cell disease is an inherited defect in the formation of hemoglobin. It occurs mainly in black populations but is also carried by some people of Arabian, Greek, Maltese, Sicilian, and other Mediterranean groups. Many researchers believe that the gene for sickle cell anemia arose in these populations as protection against malaria. Sickling due to decreases in blood oxygen may be triggered by dehydration, infection, phys-

ical or emotional stress, or exposure to cold. Laboratory examination of the affected child's blood shows that the red blood cell has changed its shape to resemble that of a sickle blade, from which the name of the disorder is derived (Fig. 8–2). These cells contain an abnormal form of hemoglobin termed *hemoglobin S* (the sickling type). The membranes of these cells are fragile and easily destroyed. Their crescent shape makes it difficult for them to pass through the capillaries, causing a pile-up of cells in the small vessels. This clumping together may lead to a *thrombosis* (clot) and cause an obstruction. *Infarcts*, or areas of dead tissue, may result when the tissue is denied proper blood supply. These generally develop in the spleen but may also be seen in other areas of the body, such as the brain, heart, lungs, gastrointestinal tract, kidneys, and bones. The patient feels pain in the affected area.

There are two types of sickle cell disorders: an *asymptomatic* (*a,* without + *symptoma,* symptom) version, referred to as *sickle cell trait,* and a much more severe form requiring intermittent hospitalization, termed *sickle cell disease.*

Sickle Cell Trait. This form of the disease occurs

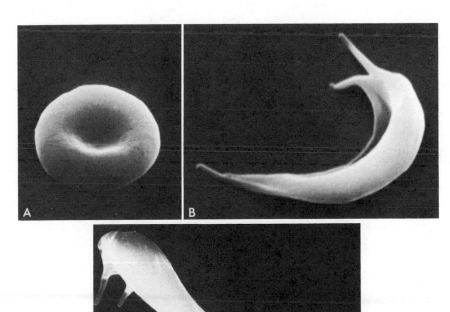

▲ **FIGURE 8–2**

Scanning electron micrograph of erythrocytes. Comparison of a normal cell (*A*) and deoxygenated sickled cells (*B* and *C*). (Courtesy of Dr. James White, from Bunn, H. F., et al.: (1977). *Human Hemoglobins.* Philadelphia, W. B. Saunders Company.)

in about 10 per cent of the African-American population in the United States. The blood of the patient contains a mixture of normal (hemoglobin A) and sickle (hemoglobin S) hemoglobins. The proportions of hemoglobin S are low, since the disease is inherited from only one parent. The doctor can distinguish sickle cell trait from the more severe form by studying the patient's red blood cells and hemoglobin. Sickling is more rapid and extreme in the disease form. In sickle cell trait, the hemoglobin and red blood cell counts are normal. Although there is no need for treatment of the mild form, the patient *is* a carrier, and genetic counseling is important. Advice might be sought from a family physician, pediatrician, or genetic specialist. The nurse encourages and sup-

ports such efforts made by parents. The importance of regular visits to a well-child clinic or family-centered clinic is stressed. The nurse also can suggest organizations that can help with transportation and babysitting problems that so often prevent parents from making maximal use of community facilities.

Sickle Cell Disease. This severe form results when the abnormality is inherited from both parents (Fig. 8–3). *Each offspring* has one chance in four of inheriting the disease (not one of four children). The incidence is about 1:625 black Americans. The symptoms generally do not appear until the last part of the first year of life, although they may occur as early as 1 month. There may be an unusual swelling of the fingers and toes. Damage

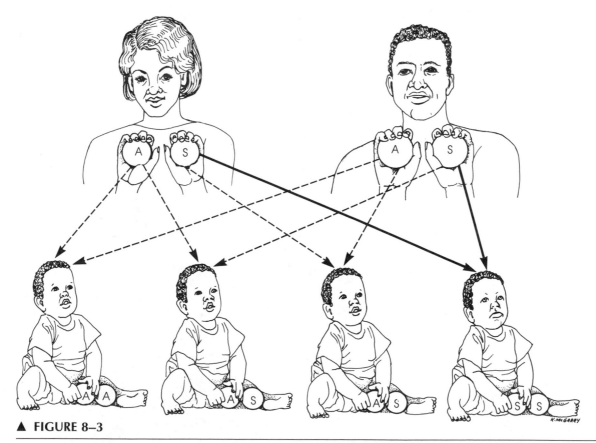

▲ **FIGURE 8–3**

How sickle cell disease is transmitted from parents to children. Parents who are carriers of the sickle cell trait do not show symptoms of the disease because hemoglobin A (the normal form of hemoglobin) in their red blood cells protects them from hemoglobin S (the sickling form). But when two carriers become parents, the possibilities are: One child in four will inherit all normal hemoglobin (AA) and thus be free of the disease. Two children in four will inherit both hemoglobin A and hemoglobin S and thus become carriers (AS) of the trait like their parents. One child in four will inherit all sickling hemoglobin (SS) and thus become a victim of sickle cell anemia.

Table 8–1. SUMMARY OF TYPES OF SICKLE CELL CRISES

TYPE	COMMENT
Vaso-occlusive (painful crises)	Most common type, obstruction of blood flow by cells, infarctions, some degree of vasospasm
	Dactylitis, painful joints and extremities, abdominal pain (infarction or bleeding within liver, spleen, abdominal lymph nodes), CNS strokes, pulmonary disease, priapism
Splenic sequestration	Pooling of large amounts of blood in liver and spleen
	Spleen becomes massive
	Circulatory collapse, shock
	Children between 8 months and 5 years particularly susceptible
	Death may occur within hours of symptoms
	Minor episodes may resolve spontaneously
	Splenectomy may be indicated for children who have one or more severe crises
Aplastic crises	Bone marrow ceases production of RBCs; a number of infections may precipitate this (usually viral)
	Severe anemia
	Child may be transfused with fresh packed red cells
Hyperhemolytic	Rapid rate of hemolysis superimposed on already severe process, rare
Functional hyposplenism and overwhelming infection	Progressive fibrosis of spleen reduces its function; patient becomes more susceptible to infection

(Data from Dickerman, J., and Lucey, J. (1985). *Smith's The Critically Ill Child*, 3rd ed. Philadelphia, W. B. Saunders Company.)

to the kidney's ability to concentrate urine leads to increased urination. Small children are difficult to toilet train and may wet the bed for several years. When this is explained to parents as a side effect of the disease, they may be more able to accept the problem. Teenagers and adults with sickle cell disease may develop painful, slow-healing ulcers on the lower legs, particularly at the ankles.

Chronic anemia is present. The hemoglobin level ranges from 6 to 9 g/dl or lower. The child is pale, tires easily, and loses appetite. These manifestations of anemia are complicated by what is termed the *sickle cell crisis,* which can be fatal. Today, a number of types of crises have been defined. They differ in pathology and may require somewhat different treatment (Table 8–1). Unfor-

tunately, in some cases the sickle cell crisis is the first evidence of the condition. The patient appears acutely ill, with severe abdominal pain. Muscle spasms, leg pains, or painful swollen joints may be seen. Fever, vomiting, hematuria, convulsions, stiff neck, coma, or paralysis can result, depending on the organs involved. The patient may be jaundiced. Cardiac enlargement and murmurs are not uncommon. The sickle cell crises recur periodically throughout childhood; however, they tend to decrease with age. Between episodes patients should be kept in good health. They should refrain from becoming overly tired. They also should avoid situations such as flying in an unpressurized airplane or exercising at high altitude, since oxygen concentrations are already reduced in the blood. Added stress and exposure to cold may lower their resistance, causing additional problems. Overheating, which can lead to dehydration, is also to be avoided.

Treatment and Nursing Care

When the infant or child is hospitalized during a crisis, the treatment is supportive and symptomatic. The patient is confined to bed. Blood transfusions may be given, but they must be given conservatively to avoid iron overload. Antibiotics are given to all children with fever. Prophylactic penicillin significantly reduces both morbidity and mortality from pneumococcal infections (Kinney and Ware, 1988). Fluid intake is increased above the maintenance for the child's age. Analgesics are given for the relief of pain. Children in a severe pain crisis should receive a continuous intravenous narcotic infusion. For continuous infusion, morphine or meperidine (Demerol) are the drugs of choice (Morrison and Vedro, 1989).

The nurse observes the overall appearance of the patient and assesses the developmental stage, body proportions, and the relation of height and weight to age. Facial expressions, degree of restlessness, and areas of pain are noted and recorded. Elevated temperature; rapid, weak pulse; a sunken fontanel in infants younger than 18 months; weight loss; poor tissue turgor; dry skin, lips, and mucous membranes; and a decrease in urination signal dehydration. If vomiting occurs, appropriate oral hygiene is given. The nurse observes and records infusions according to unit policy. An accurate record of intake and output is kept. Careful attention is given to the skin. Jaundice (icterus) can be detected by observing whether the skin (palms and soles) and whites of the eyes have taken on a yellowish tinge. The patient's body position is changed gently.

Because sickle cell disease can affect muscle tone, any rigidity of muscles should be reported. Observe eye movements, swallowing, or sucking. Note whether the child is uncomfortable when the neck is flexed to have the gown changed. Watch for twitching about the face or elsewhere. Sickle cell disease may take a wide variety of courses. Nurses, as always, follow the individual patient's progress. (Pocket-sized index cards containing nursing care plans may be helpful.) They discuss and evaluate the child's progress with their team leader and instructor. They utilize the unit library to increase their knowledge and effectiveness so that they can anticipate problems that might occur with this disease. The prognosis is guarded. Death may result from severe anemia or secondary infection. Pregnancy may increase mortality. There is also an increased likelihood of miscarriage, premature births, and stillborns in women with sickle cell disease. Ideally, all black women should be screened for the disease prior to pregnancy. The sickling test (Sickledex) is commonly used for screening purposes.

Surgery. The approach to splenectomy in children with sickle cell disease has been conservative. Recurrence of acute splenic sequestration becomes less likely after 5 years of age. Routine splenectomy is not recommended, as the spleen generally atrophies on its own because of fibrotic changes that take place in patients with sickle cell disease. However, splenectomy is indicated in selected patients. When possible, the spleen should not be removed until after the age of 2 years (Oski and Stockman, 1985). Since no form of prophylaxis is foolproof and since the duration of treatment is controversial, the child should continue to be carefully supervised for signs of infection. A sickle screening test should be performed on all black patients prior to elective surgery, as general anesthesia places these persons at greater risk for hypoxia. Gallstones can occur in sickle cell patients and have been seen in children as young as 3 years of age (Behrman and Vaughan, 1987). It is sometimes difficult to distinguish abdominal crises from appendicitis or peritonitis.

Gastrointestinal System

INGUINAL HERNIA

Description. An inguinal hernia is a protrusion of part of the abdominal contents through the inguinal canal in the groin. It is more common in boys than in girls. It is also seen frequently in premature infants. Hernias may be present at birth (congenital) or may be acquired and can vary in size. A hernia is termed *reducible* if it can be put back into place by gentle pressure; if this cannot be done, it is called an *irreducible* or an *incarcerated* (constricted) hernia.

Symptoms. The infant with a hernia may be relatively free of symptoms. Irritability, fretfulness, and constipation are sometimes evident. The diagnosis is made when physical examination shows a mass in the inguinal area that reappears from time to time, particularly when the child cries or strains. A *strangulated* hernia occurs when the intestine becomes caught in the passage and the blood supply is diminished. This happens more frequently during the first 6 months of life. Vomiting and severe abdominal pain are present. Emergency surgery is necessary if strangulation occurs, and in some cases a bowel resection is performed.

Treatment and Nursing Care

Inguinal hernias are repaired successfully by the surgical operation called a *herniorrhaphy*. This is a relatively simple procedure that is tolerated well by the child. Most patients are scheduled for same-day surgery units. The benefits of this method are both economical and psychological. Parents remain with the child during the entire time except for the actual procedure. They are encouraged to assist in routine postoperative care if they choose. Often no dressing is applied to the wound. Sometimes a waterproof collodion dressing may be utilized. Postoperative care is directed toward keeping the wound clean. Diapers are left open for this purpose. Wet diapers are changed frequently. The child is discharged in about 2 to 3 hours, when fluids are tolerated. Activity is not limited. Parents are provided with written instructions about home management. Follow-up telephone calls may be made by nursing personnel, and return appointments are scheduled.

Patients who experience incarcerated hernias are hospitalized. Following surgery, vital signs are carefully monitored. Nasogastric suctioning and intravenous fluids are maintained until bowel function returns. The nurse measures and records the patient's intake and output. The child is turned frequently to avoid respiratory complications. The nurse observes the child carefully for signs of peritonitis or bowel obstruction.

UMBILICAL HERNIA

Description. An umbilical hernia is a protrusion of a portion of intestine through the umbilical ring (an opening in the muscular area of the abdomen where the umbilical vessels passed through) (Fig. 8–4). This type of hernia appears as a soft swelling

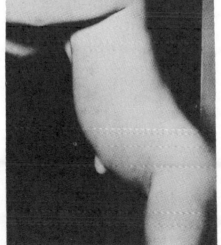

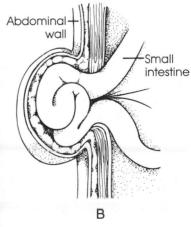

▲ **FIGURE 8–4**

A, Side view of infant with an umbilical hernia. *B,* Diagram of an umbilical hernia. (From Marlow, D. R. (1987). *Textbook of Pediatric Nursing,* 6th ed. Philadelphia, W. B. Saunders Company.)

Abdominal wall

Small intestine

A

B

covered by skin, which protrudes when the infant cries or strains. Most of the small umbilical hernias disappear spontaneously during the first year of life. This type of hernia is not known to become strangulated or to cause other complications.

Treatment

The treatment of this condition is controversial. In general, surgery is not advised unless the hernia causes symptoms, becomes enlarged, or persists until the child is 3 to 5 years of age. Adhesive strapping is no longer recommended to keep the hernia from protruding.

PYLORIC STENOSIS

Description. Pyloric *stenosis* (narrowing) is a disorder of the digestive tract. The pylorus, the lower end of the stomach, becomes partially blocked so that food does not empty properly into the duodenum (Fig. 8–5). Pyloric stenosis is caused by an overgrowth of the circular muscles of the pylorus. The stomach muscles above the obstructed area also enlarge in their attempt to force material through the narrowed passage. An abnormal increase in the size of an organ or part, such as this, is called *hypertrophy*. This condition is commonly classified as a congenital anomaly; however, its symptoms do not appear until the baby is 2 or 3 weeks old. Pyloric stenosis is the most common surgical condition of the digestive tract in infancy. Its incidence is higher in boys than in girls, with a tendency for it to be inherited.

Symptoms. Vomiting is the outstanding symptom of this disorder. The force progresses until most of the food is ejected a considerable distance from the mouth. This is termed *projectile* vomiting and occurs before and after feedings. The vomitus contains mucus and may be blood streaked. The baby is constantly hungry and will eat again immediately after vomiting has occurred. Dehydration—as evidenced by a sunken fontanel, poor turgor, and decreased urination—may occur. In severe cases, the fat pads of the cheeks disappear, giving the patient a "withered old man" look. An olive-shaped mass may be felt in the right upper quadrant of the abdomen. X-ray films confirm an

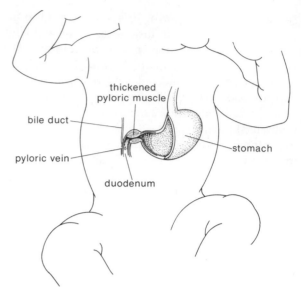

▲ **FIGURE 8–5**

Pyloric stenosis. Hypertrophy or thickening of the pyloric sphincter blocks the stomach contents, causing the infant to regurgitate forcefully. Serious electrolyte imbalances ultimately occur and surgery is necessary to correct the condition. (From Foster, R., Hunsberger, M., and Anderson, J. J. (1989). *Family-Centered Nursing Care of Children.* Philadelphia, W. B. Saunders Company.)

enlarged stomach. It is difficult for the barium to pass into the duodenum. Ultrasonography is commonly used today for diagnostic purposes, as it is noninvasive and accurate. In severe cases, the outline of the distended stomach and peristaltic waves are visible during feedings. The urine and blood are alkaline, since the fluid being lost from the body is mostly hydrochloric acid from the stomach juices. Bowel movements gradually diminish, since little or no food passes into the intestine.

Treatment

Two methods are used to treat pyloric stenosis— one medical and the other surgical. Medical treatment today is rare, since the results from surgery are excellent. The operation performed for pyloric stenosis is called a *pyloromyotomy* (*pyloro* + *myo*, muscle + *tomy*, incision of). The surgeon incises the pyloric muscle in such a way that the opening is enlarged and food may again pass easily through it.

Nursing Care

If the infant is not dehydrated, surgery is usually performed as soon as possible. The dehydrated infant is given intravenous fluids preoperatively to restore fluid and electrolyte balance. If this is not done, shock may occur during surgery. Thickened feedings may be given until the time of operation in hopes that some nourishment will be retained. The doctor prescribes the degree of thickness of the formula, which is given by teaspoon or through a nipple with a large hole. The infant is bubbled *before* as well as during feedings, to remove any accumulated gas in the stomach. The feeding is done slowly, and the baby is handled gently and as little as possible. The infant is placed on the right side following feedings. The pylorus is on the right side of the abdomen; thus, drainage into the intestine is facilitated. If vomiting occurs, the nurse may be instructed to refeed the infant. Charting of the feeding includes time, type, and amount offered; amount taken and retained; and type and amount of vomiting. The nurse also notes whether the baby appeared hungry following the feeding.

The nurse weighs the patient at about the same time each morning and records the weight. Other factors to be charted include the type and number of stools and the color of urine and frequency of voiding. Position is changed frequently, since the infant may be weak and vulnerable to pneumonia. All procedures designed to protect from infection must be strictly carried out.

The care of the patient following surgery includes such procedures as careful observation of vital signs and administration of intravenous fluids. The wound site is inspected frequently for bleeding. Signs of shock are an increase in the rate of pulse and respiration; pale, cool skin; and restlessness. Most infants have a nasogastric tube in place, which is removed soon after surgery in order to begin oral feedings. After the tube is removed, the baby is observed for vomiting. Place the baby on the stomach or right side to prevent the aspiration of vomitus and change the position

gently. When indicated, the doctor prescribes oral feedings of small amounts of sugar and water that gradually increase in amount until a regular formula can be taken and retained. As soon as intravenous feedings are discontinued and oral fluids are tolerated, the baby is fed from a bottle or breast. The nurse must avoid overfeeding the patient. Vomiting is seen following surgery; however, it is not as severe as before the operation and gradually diminishes. The diaper is placed low over the abdomen to prevent infection of the wound.

INTUSSUSCEPTION

Description. Intussusception (*intus*, within and *suscipere*, to receive) is a slipping of one part of the intestine into another part just below it (Fig. 8–6). It is frequently seen at the ileocecal valve, where the small intestine opens into the ascending colon. The *mesentery*, a double fan-shaped fold of peritoneum that covers most of the intestine and is filled with blood vessels and nerves, is also pulled along. Edema occurs. At first this telescoping of the bowel causes intestinal obstruction, but as peristalsis forces the structures more tightly, strangulation takes place. This portion may burst, causing peritonitis.

Intussusception generally occurs in male infants who are otherwise healthy. It occurs before age 5 years, with the highest incidence between 6 and 18 months. The exact cause is still in question. Occasionally the condition corrects itself without treatment. This is termed a *spontaneous reduction*. However, since the patient's life is in danger, the doctor does not waste time waiting for this to occur. The prognosis is good when the condition is treated within 24 hours.

Symptoms. In typical cases the onset is sudden. The infant feels severe pain in the abdomen, evidenced by loud cries, straining efforts, and the kicking and drawing of the legs toward the abdomen. At first the child is comfortable between pains, but the intervals shorten and the condition becomes worse. The child vomits. The stomach contents are green or greenish yellow in color; this is due to bile stain, and the contents are described as *bilious*. If the condition is left untreated, fecal vomiting ensues. Bowel movements diminish and

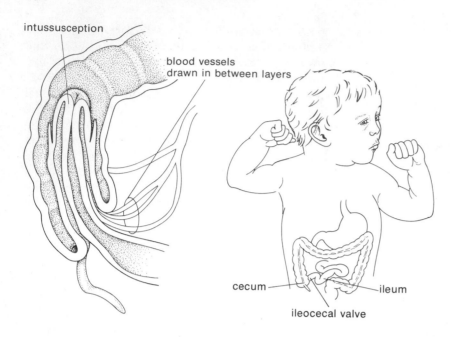

intussusception

blood vessels
drawn in between layers

cecum

ileum

ileocecal valve

▲ **FIGURE 8–6**

Intussusception. The most common type begins at or near the ileocecal valve, pushing into the cecum and onto the colon. At first the obstruction is partial, but as the bowel becomes inflamed and edematous, complete obstruction occurs. (From Foster, R., Hunsberger, M., and Anderson, J., (1989). *Family-Centered Nursing Care of Children.* Philadelphia, W. B. Saunders Company.)

little flatus is passed. Stools of blood and mucus that contain no feces are common about 12 hours after the onset of the obstruction; these are termed *currant jelly stools.* The child's fever may run as high as 41.1°C (106°F) and signs of shock such as sweating, weak pulse, and shallow, grunting respirations appear. The abdomen is rigid.

Treatment

Intussusception is an emergency situation, and because of the severity of the symptoms most parents contact a doctor promptly. The diagnosis is determined by the history and physical findings. The doctor may feel a sausage-shaped mass in the right upper portion of the abdomen during bimanual rectal and abdominal palpation. Abdominal films also may indicate the mass. A *barium enema* is the treatment of choice, with surgery scheduled if reduction is not achieved. Intussusception may recur after reduction by barium enema. For this reason the child is kept for observation after this procedure.

During the operation a small incision is made into the abdomen and the wayward intestine is "milked" back into position. The intestine is inspected for gangrene, and if all is well the abdomen is sutured. Barring complications, recovery is straightforward. If the intestine cannot be reduced or if gangrene has set in, a resection is done and the affected bowel is removed. The cut end of the ileum is joined to the cut end of the colon; this is called an *anastomosis.*

Nursing Care

Preoperative. The patient is admitted to the hospital for procedures that will prepare for surgery and that will prevent postoperative complications. Treatment is aimed at combating shock and restoring blood, fluids, and electrolytes. The doctor or charge nurse obtains a written consent for surgery from the parents or guardians of the child. It is wise for the admitting nurse to confirm this by checking the appropriate sheet in the patient's chart. This procedure takes on even greater importance in emergency situations.

Gastric suction is necessary to prevent stomach distention. This may be continued for some time following surgery, particularly if a resection is done. The nurse applies elbow restraints to the patient to prevent dislodgement of the nasal tube, if this has not already been done for intravenous therapy. The child's identification band is checked to see that it is secure, and voiding prior to surgery is recorded. Preoperative medication is given to relax the patient and to prevent the aspiration of secretions. Once the child has been medicated, the surrounding activity should be kept at a minimum. En route to the operating room, the patient is covered with a light cotton blanket. The medical record accompanies the child. Proper safety precautions are taken during transit.

Postoperative. Following surgery, care is mainly symptomatic. Vital signs are checked frequently, the child's position is changed often, and careful attention is given to the skin. Mouth care is essential, as the patient will be receiving little or nothing by mouth for a while. The nostrils require cleaning and lubricating, as the nasal tube can be irritating. If a urinary catheter has been inserted in the operating room, it is observed for kinks that could hamper flow of urine. The drainage from the catheter is measured and described in the nurse's notes. The operative site is kept clean and dry. Promptly report any odor from the incision. Be on the alert for abdominal distention. Clear fluids are given when bowel sounds are heard. The passage of gas, liquids, or solids through the rectum is of particular significance, as it indicates peristalsis.

Gastric suction will keep the stomach and upper intestine empty. The gastric tube is attached to suction and is run on low to avoid damage to the lining of the stomach. Small saline irrigations are usually ordered to prevent clogging of the tube. The amount used is recorded on the patient's fluid balance sheet. The drainage in the bottle is measured and recorded every 8 hours, or more frequently if necessary. Accurate recording of fluid drainage is essential, because this type of drainage removes salts and hydrochloric acid from the stomach, which must be replaced by intravenous fluids.

As in all of nursing, the patient and the family are given supportive help throughout this ordeal. A pacifier may soothe the young child who is deprived of feeding by mouth. Some of these patients are at an age when fear of strangers is prevalent; thus, their need for the security of the parents is paramount. Parents need assurance that their child is in good hands and that their presence is not a hindrance to the hospital staff.

VOMITING

Description. Vomiting, a common symptom during infancy and childhood, is the result of

sudden contractions of the diaphragm and the muscles of the stomach. It must be evaluated in relation to the child's total health status. Occasional vomiting is to be expected. Persistent vomiting requires investigation, since it results in dehydration and electrolyte imbalance. The continuous loss of hydrochloric acid and sodium chloride from the stomach can cause *alkalosis*. In this condition the acid-base balance of the body becomes disturbed because of a loss of chlorides and potassium. This can result in death if left untreated.

The well child vomits from various causes. Some of them stem from improper feeding techniques. The nurse should ask the following questions when an infant vomits: Was the baby fed too fast? Too much? Was the infant bubbled frequently and properly positioned following the feeding? Has there been a recent formula increase or change? Were any previous feedings vomited? Sometimes the difficulty lies with the formula. If the fat content is too high, it can slow down the emptying process of the stomach. The introduction of foods of a different consistency may also precipitate this symptom. Infants sometimes instigate vomiting by gagging themselves with the fingers or objects of play.

Other factors that cause vomiting are ear, nose, and throat infections. Vomiting is seen in the primary stages of many communicable diseases. Specific disorders such as Reye's syndrome, peptic ulcer disease, increased intracranial pressure, strangulated hernia, and various bowel obstructions are also responsible. In these conditions, the vomiting is not necessarily associated with feedings. When the cause of the illness is discovered and properly treated, the symptom disappears. Aspiration and aspiration pneumonia are serious complications of vomiting. Vomitus becomes drawn into the air passages upon inspiration and causes immediate death in extreme cases.

Treatment and Nursing Care

To prevent vomiting, the nurse must carefully feed and bubble the baby, especially an ill child. The nurse must be relaxed and the surroundings should be peaceful. Treatments are avoided immediately following feedings. The baby should be handled as little as possible at this time. To prevent aspiration of vomitus, the nurse places the infant on the stomach or right side following feedings. When a child begins to vomit, the head is turned to one side, and an emesis basin and tissues are provided. The nurse can relieve some of the strain involved by supporting the patient's head firmly. When the vomiting has ceased, the basin is removed from sight. The infants' hands and face are bathed with warm water. Particular attention is given to the creases of the neck and behind the ears. To change the position, the nurse turns the patient slowly and gently, because motion tends to increase nausea. A clean gown is applied, and the bed linen is changed if necessary.

The nurse may estimate the amount of material vomited by filling a similar basin with water to about the same level as the vomitus and measuring the water. Factors to be charted include time, amount, color (bloody, bile-stained), consistency, force, frequency, and whether or not vomiting was preceded by nausea. The diet following vomiting is prescribed by the doctor. In the hospital, intravenous fluids may be given (see page 54). Oral fluids are withheld for a short time to allow the stomach to rest. Gradually, sips of water are given according to the infant's tolerance and condition. The patient's intake and output are carefully recorded so that the doctor is able to compare the kidney output with the total fluid intake.

When vomiting is persistent, drugs such as trimethobenzamide (Tigan) or promethazine (Phenergan) may be prescribed. They are available in rectal suppository form. The nurse lubricates the suppository and inserts it well into the rectum, where it dissolves. Slight pressure is exerted over the anus for a short time to ensure that the suppository is not expelled. Charting includes the time, name of suppository, and whether or not relief from vomiting was obtained.

FLUID IMBALANCE

Dehydration

When a person is in good health, the intake and output of fluids balance, and *homeostasis* (a uniform state) exists. This is accomplished by appropriate shifts of fluids and electrolytes across cellular membranes and by elimination of those products of metabolism that are no longer needed or that

are in excess. The volume of blood plasma and interstitial and intracellular fluids remains relatively constant. Dehydration occurs whenever fluid output exceeds fluid intake, regardless of the cause.

Disorders of fluids and electrolytes—sodium (Na), potassium (K), calcium (Ca), and magnesium (Mg)—are more complex in children who are growing. A newborn infant's total weight is approximately 77 per cent water, compared with 60 per cent in adults. This varies with the amount of fat. Also, the daily turnover of water in an infant is equal to almost 24 per cent of total body water, compared with about 6 per cent in adults. A baby's body surface in comparison to weight is three times that of the older child; therefore, the baby is subject to greater evaporation of water from the skin. The younger the patient, the higher the metabolic rate and the more unstable the heat-regulating mechanisms. (Elevations in temperature are also higher, increasing the rate of water loss.) Rapid respirations speed up this process, and, when diarrhea is present, additional fluid is lost in the stools. Immaturity of the kidneys impairs the infant's ability to conserve water. Preterm and newborn infants are also more susceptible to dehydration from variations in room temperature and humidity. Cessation of intake alone can result in significant depletion. When this is coupled with higher fluid losses, life-threatening deficits can exist in a few hours.

Problems of fluid and electrolyte disturbance require evaluation of the type and severity of dehydration, clinical observation of the patient, and chemical analysis of the blood. The types of dehydration are classified according to the amount of *serum sodium*, which depends on the relative losses of water and electrolytes. These types are usually termed *isotonic* (the patient has lost equal amounts of fluids and electrolytes), *hypotonic,* and *hypertonic,* because plasma osmolality (pertaining to osmosis) in large part reflects sodium concentrations (Table 8–2); however, in certain instances these interchanged terms may be technically inaccurate.

These classifications are important, since each form of dehydration is associated with different relative losses from intracellular fluid (ICF) and extracellular fluid (ECF) compartments, and each requires certain modifications in treatment. *Main-*

Table 8–2. SIGNS OF ISOTONIC, HYPERTONIC, AND HYPOTONIC DEHYDRATION

AREA OF ASSESSMENT	SIGNS OF DEHYDRATION		
	Isotonic	Hypertonic	Hypotonic
Loss of body weight	Mild dehydration—up to 5% loss of body weight Moderate dehydration—5% to 10% loss of body weight Severe dehydration—over 10% loss of body weight		
Behavior	Irritable and lethargic	Irritable when disturbed; lethargic	Lethargic to delirious; coma
Skin turgor	Dead elasticity	Good turgor; "foam rubber" feel	Very poor turgor; clammy
Mucous membranes	Dry	Parched	Clammy
Eyeballs and fontanel	Sunken and soft	Sunken	Sunken and soft
Tearing and salivation	Absent or decreased	Absent or decreased	Absent or decreased
Thirst	Present	Marked	Present
Urine	Decreased output; SG elevated	Normal to decreased output; SG elevated or decreased	Decreased output; SG elevated
Body temperature	Subnormal to elevated	Elevated	Subnormal
Respiration	Rapid	Rapid	Rapid
Blood pressure	Normal to low	Normal to low	Very low
Pulse	Rapid	Rapid	Rapid
Blood chemistry	BUN increased Na decreased K normal or increased Cl decreased pH usually decreased	BUN increased Na increased K decreased Cl low during correction Ca decreased	BUN increased Na decreased K varied or increased Cl decreased

(From Chinn, P. (1979). *Child Health Maintenance*, 2nd ed. St. Louis, The C. V. Mosby Company.)

tenance therapy replaces normal water and electrolyte losses, and *deficit therapy* restores pre-existing body fluid and electrolyte deficiencies. The replacement of a deficit may take several days, and the deficit will continue unless adequate maintenance therapy is also provided. The physician calculates the volume of fluids to be administered through the use of various formulas based on caloric expenditures, because daily physiological water losses are directly proportionate to caloric expenditure. The patient's temperature and activity (coma, restlessness) must also be considered. Basal calories are determined by the weight of the child. Volume is calculated on a 24-hour basis. Isotonic dehydration is the most common form in children.

Adjustments in fluid therapy are made constantly according to the condition of the patient.

The higher daily exchange of water that occurs in infants leaves them less volume reserve when they are dehydrated. Shock (hypovolemia) is the greatest threat to life in isotonic dehydration. The electrolyte content of oral fluids is particularly significant in the care of infants and small children suffering from disorders of fluid balance and receiving infusions. Commercially prepared electrolyte solutions are available by bottle; however, the nurse should ascertain if they are to be given freely or by doctor's order only. Patients with hypotonic dehydration, i.e., excess water with sodium electrolyte depletion, are at risk for water intoxication. This can also occur if tap water enemas are given to small children. Loss of potassium occurs in almost all states of dehydration. Replacement potassium is administered only after normal urinary excretion is established.

Overhydration

Overhydration results when the body receives more fluid than it can excrete. This can occur in patients with normal kidneys who receive IV fluids too rapidly. It also can occur in a patient receiving acceptable rates of fluid, especially when the patient's illness is related to disorders of fluid mechanism. These would include kidney disease, burns, cardiovascular disease, protein deficiencies, and certain allergies. Hormonal therapy also may disrupt fluid mechanisms.

Edema is the presence of excess fluid in the interstitial spaces. Trauma to or infections of the head can cause cerebral edema, which can be life-threatening. Constrictive dressing may obstruct venous return, causing swelling, particularly in dependent areas. Early detection and management of edema are essential. Taking accurate daily weights is indispensable, as is close attention to body weight changes. Vital signs, physical appearance, and changes in urine character or output are noted. Edema in infants may first be seen about the eyes and in the presacral, occipital, or genital areas. In *pitting edema,* after exerting gentle pressure with the finger, the nurse will notice an impression in the skin that lasts for several seconds.

The Lungs

CYSTIC FIBROSIS

DESCRIPTION

Cystic fibrosis is a generalized disorder of the outward secreting or exocrine glands, in particular the mucous and sweat glands. This disease affects many parts of the body but particularly the lungs and pancreas. It occurs in about 1:1000 to 1:2000 live births. Cystic fibrosis is an inherited congenital disorder, the exact cause of which is unknown. The condition is believed to be inherited as a *mendelian recessive trait* from both parents. The parents, who are *carriers* of this disease, do not show any symptoms. When two *genes* for the disease combine in their child at the time of conception, cystic fibrosis results. The gene associated with cystic fibrosis has been identified, and

it is now possible to identify healthy individuals who carry the cystic fibrosis trait. Cystic fibrosis affects both sexes equally. The survival rate of the children has increased, and many are living into adulthood. Better antibiotic control of pulmonary infection both at home and during hospitalization and increased numbers of cystic fibrosis centers have contributed to this success.

SYMPTOMS

Lung Involvement. Cystic fibrosis is considered the most serious lung problem in children in the United States. The air passages of the lungs become clogged with mucus. There is widespread obstruction of the bronchioles. It is hard for the patient to breathe; expiration is especially difficult. More and more air becomes trapped in the lungs (obstructive emphysema), and small areas of collapse (atelectasis) may occur. Eventually, the chest assumes a barrel shape, with increased diameter across the front and back. The right ventricle of the heart, which supplies the lungs, may become strained and enlarged. Clubbing of fingers and toes, indicating a chronic lack of oxygen, may be present. *Staphylococcus* and *Pseudomonas* infections can easily occur in the lungs, which provide a suitable medium for these organisms to grow. This causes more thickening of the abnormal secretions, irritates and damages lung tissues, and further increases lung obstruction.

The time of onset of this disease varies. Symptoms may appear weeks, months, or years after birth. In general, the earlier the onset, the more severe the disease. The symptoms range from mild to severe. Any or all symptoms may be present in varying degrees of severity in one individual. The patient develops a chronic cough that may produce vomiting. Dyspnea, wheezing, and cyanosis may occur. The patient is irritable and tires easily. Gradually, there is a change in physical appearance. X-ray films of the chest reveal widespread infection. Evidence of obstructive emphysema, atelectasis, and *fibrosis* of lung tissue may also be present. The prognosis for survival depends on the extent of lung damage. However, this is only part of the picture, since cystic fibrosis also affects the pancreas and sweat glands.

Pancreatic Involvement. The pancreas lies behind the stomach. Some of its cells secrete *pan-*

creatic juice. This key digestive juice drains from the pancreatic duct into the duodenum at the same area in which bile enters. Changes occurring in the pancreas are due to obstruction by thickened secretions that block the flow of pancreatic digestive enzymes. As a result, foodstuffs, particularly fats and proteins, are not properly utilized by the body. In infants the stools may be loose. Gradually, because of impaired digestion and food absorption, the feces of the patient become large, fatty, and foul-smelling. They are usually light in color. The baby does not gain weight in spite of a good appetite and may look undernourished. The abdomen becomes distended, and the buttocks and thighs *atrophy* as fat disappears from the main deposit sites. Laboratory tests show a deficiency of pancreatic enzymes (trypsin, lipase, amylase).

An oral pancreatic extract such as Pancrease is given to the child with each meal and snack to replace the pancreatic enzymes the child's body cannot produce. This medication is considered specific for the disease because it aids in the digestion and absorption of food, thus improving the condition of the stools. If the child is ill and not eating, the medication is withheld.

A condition known as *meconium ileus* exists when the intestine of the newborn baby becomes obstructed with abnormally thick meconium while in utero. This is due to the absence of pancreatic enzymes that normally digest proteins in the meconium. The abnormal, putty-like stool sticks to the walls of the intestine, causing blockage. Rupture with signs of shock may occur. The presenting symptoms develop within hours after birth. Absence of stools, vomiting, and abdominal distention lead one to suspect intestinal obstruction. X ray films confirm the diagnosis. The condition is treated surgically. The death rate is high, but the prognosis is more favorable when the obstruction is detected early. Most infants who survive will manifest cystic fibrosis. Fortunately, the incidence of meconium ileus is rare, because the pancreatic enzyme deficiency is seldom complete. Nevertheless, the nurse assigned to the nursery must constantly be on guard for suspicious symptoms.

Sweat Glands. The sweat, tears, and saliva of the patient with cystic fibrosis become abnormally "salty" owing to an increase in the sodium and chloride levels. There is also an increase in the potassium level of sweat glands. The normal amount of chloride in sweat is 1 to 60 mEq/liter. Higher concentrations are considered specific for the disease. The analysis of sweat is a major aid in the diagnosis of the condition. The *sweat test,* using pilocarpine iontophoresis, is the best diagnostic study. A dilute solution of pilocarpine is applied to the arm, and a weak electrical current is used to stimulate sweating. A positive test should be repeated for confirmation. Since the patient loses large amounts of salt through perspiration, he or she must be observed for heat prostration. Liberal amounts of salt should be given with food, and extra fluids and salt should be provided during hot weather.

COMPLICATIONS

Cystic fibrosis is often responsible for rectal prolapse in infants and children. This is partly due to poor muscle tone in the rectal area and excessive leanness of the buttocks of the patient. However, surgery is almost never required, as the patient obtains relief by taking pancreatic medication.

As the disease progresses, the liver may become hard, nodular, and enlarged. There may be edema of the extremities. The retina of the eye may hemorrhage; there may be damage to the eye from swelling, and inflammation in part of the optic nerve may occur. *Cor pulmonale* (*cor,* heart + *pulmon,* lung), heart strain due to improper lung function, is frequently a cause of death. *Osteoporosis* (*osteo,* bone + pore + *osis,* disease) may occur. When it is caused by cystic fibrosis, the bones become porous owing to poor utilization of fat-soluble vitamin D, which is necessary for proper calcium metabolism. There is a deficiency of vitamin A, because the child is unable to absorb fats from which this vitamin is obtained.

Treatment and Nursing Care

A nursing care plan is provided in Nursing Care Plan 8–1.

Respiratory Relief. Antibiotics may be given as a preventive measure against respiratory infection; however, this treatment is subject to controversy. Full dosages of antibiotics are given in an acute infection. The doctor determines the particular antibiotic to be used by the results of throat and

CARE PLAN 8–1

THE CHILD WITH CYSTIC FIBROSIS

Nursing Diagnosis	Goals/Outcome Criteria	Intervention
Ineffective airway clearance related to accumulation of mucus	Respiratory status will stabilize Child will improve aeration as evidenced by absence of dyspnea and tachypnea and will be able to expectorate mucus	Provide adequate hydration Assist patient with aerosol therapy Assist patient with postural drainage Explain importance of breathing exercises Administer medications and explain their use Prevent infection by maintaining a high level of suspicion and proper handwashing; review immunization schedule
Nutritional alterations, related to enzyme deficiencies, anorexia, poor absorption of vitamins, excess sodium loss	Adequate nutrition will be maintained Child will maintain nutrition status as evidenced by weight gain	Administer pancreatic replacement enzymes Administer water-soluble vitamins Monitor salt intake (will need to be increased during hot weather and during increased exercise) Record daily weights and Intake and Output
Infant		Encourage breast feeding, or if bottle-fed, use prescribed formula (Pregestimil, Portagen, Nutramigen) Use enzyme replacement
Child		Provide normal diet for age with supplemental protein, vitamins, minerals; modify fat intake if normal diet is not tolerated
Adolescent		Anticipate anorexia and developmental issues Evaluate nutritional status frequently, provide supplements
Self-care deficit, related to age, developmental level	Child will assist in caring for self Child will maintain self-care as evidenced by ability to participate in daily bath and oral hygiene	Provide good skin care, change position frequently, as child may be malnourished
Infant		Cleanse diaper area, which becomes irritated by stool, observe for breakdown of skin

CARE PLAN 8–1 *Continued*

THE CHILD WITH CYSTIC FIBROSIS

Nursing Diagnosis	Goals/Outcome Criteria	Intervention
Child		Encourage good oral hygiene; patient raises sputum from postural drainage, exercises, etc.
Adolescent		Anticipate problems concerning acne, body size, sexual maturity
Knowledge deficit (parents), related to diagnosis and proper parenting	Child will be maintained at home Parents will verbalize understanding of disease and care of child	Assess level of understanding concerning diet, medication, respiratory therapy regimen, need for frequent follow-up care Assess home environment Encourage parents' participation and acceptance of the child's condition Help parents understand and support the child through various "ages and stages" Initiate referrals, e.g., school and community nurse, National Cystic Fibrosis Research Foundation, local chapter, social worker
Self-concept; disturbance in, related to chronic disease, unrealistic expectations of self	Child will be as self-sufficient as age appropriate Child will verbalize concerns related to self-image	Promote self-care as appropriate Explain new procedures Assist child in understanding the disease Encourage appropriate physical activities Teach child to recognize and report signs of fatigue and infection Educate peers Promote involvement in self-help group Listen empathetically to child Encourage verbalization of feelings

sputum cultures. The route may be oral or IV. Intravenous medication may be given via *heparin lock* or in some cases a *Broviac catheter* (see page 53). This can be employed successfully in both inpatients and outpatients.

Intermittent aerosol therapy is administered to provide medication and water to the lower respiratory tract and to promote evacuation of secretions. Expectorants, especially the iodides, are also employed in an effort to thin secretions. Bronchodilators are used to increase the width of the bronchi, allowing free passage of air into the lungs.

Postural drainage, chest clapping, and breathing exercises are also of importance. These are performed by the respiratory therapist during hospitalization. When postural drainage and chest clapping are done properly, the secretions in the chest are moved up and out. During latent periods or in mild cases, the patient may not raise sputum. This should be explained to the parents so that they will not discontinue this valuable procedure when the child comes home. Instructions may need to be repeated frequently to encourage full cooperation of the parents and child. These procedures should be done following nebulization and at least one hour after eating. General exercise is good for the patient because it stimulates coughing. Somersaults, headstands, and wheelbarrow play within the child's endurance are therapeutic.

Prevention of respiratory infections is very important. The child is isolated from patients and personnel who may harbor infections. The period of hospitalization is kept brief, if possible, to avoid cross-infection. The patient must be given the necessary immunizations against childhood diseases (see page 157). Appropriate boosters should be given so that the immunity obtained is kept up to date.

Diet. The maintenance of adequate nutrition is essential. The diet is high in calories, as much as 50 per cent above normal. There should be increased protein and moderate amounts of fat in conjunction with pancreatic extracts. Simple sugars are easy to digest, and banana products are particularly good. Fruits, cottage cheese, vegetables, and lean meats, which are high in protein and low in fat and starches, are recommended. Restrictions on ice cream, peanut butter, butter, French fries, and mayonnaise are advised. Extra salt may be provided by pretzels and salted bread sticks and crackers. Discrepancies in the diet may be allowed by the doctor to keep meals from becoming drab and to provide a more normal atmosphere. At such times the child is allowed to eat what is desired and is given extra digestive enzymes. Supplements of vitamins A, D, and E in a water-miscible base are given each day in double the recommended dose. Vitamin K also may be given when indicated. Salt tablets may be given to the older child during hot weather. Forcing fluids may be ordered because larger amounts of fluid are lost in the stools. The nurse may be asked to weigh the child daily.

The nurse feeding the infant with cystic fibrosis must be calm and unhurried. The baby may cough, have difficulty breathing, and vomit. Careful bubbling is necessary to avoid abdominal distention. In general, the appetite is good. Older children need small amounts of food served attractively and frequently. Food piled high on a child's tray is discouraging. The child may have eaten a perfectly good meal for the size, but the nurse who carries the remainder of the tray to the kitchen charts "poor appetite." Since mealtime is a social time, the nurse should remain with the child if the parents are not present. It is not necessary to hover over the child to see that every morsel is eaten with the proper utensil. Instead, try to make the meal more satisfying by giving good companionship mixed with a little encouragement. The nurse records the fluid intake at the end of the meal. The child's reaction to new foods and any variations in stools resulting from the food are noted. The food refused and the type, character, and amount of vomiting, if any, are also noted.

General Hygiene. The nurse must pay special attention to the skin of the child with cystic fibrosis. The diaper area is cleansed following each bowel movement. An ointment to protect the skin is advisable, because the character of the stool subjects the diaper area to irritation. The buttocks are exposed to air when a rash occurs. Careful attention to bony areas is necessary to prevent decubitus ulcers. Because the patient has very little fat and muscle, it is important that the position be changed frequently, especially if the child is weak and cannot get out of bed. This will also prevent pneumonia. Be sure that when you change the patient's position the patient is not left staring at a blank wall. This can easily be remedied by turning the crib around. Soiled diapers are immediately removed from the room to prevent offensive odors. The patient wears light clothing to avoid becoming overheated; it should be loose to allow freedom of movement. Good oral hygiene is necessary, since the teeth may be in poor condition owing to dietary deficiencies. Mouth care is given after postural drainage, as foul mucus may be raised, leaving an unpleasant taste in the patient's mouth.

Long-Term Care. Today the child with a lengthy illness spends the majority of time at home and is hospitalized mainly for diagnosis, relapses, and complications. This burden, which the family willingly assumes, is extremely taxing financially, physically, and emotionally. Somehow, the mother must distribute her time and energy within the family yet give careful attention to her sick child or, in the case of cystic fibrosis, sometimes children. How does she keep from spoiling the child? Does she limit the normal activities of the remaining children to spare her sick one? What about birthday parties, camping, Cub Scouts, pets, epidemics at school? What does a trip to the shore or mountains entail? When do the husband and wife find time for themselves? These seemingly overwhelming problems are being faced daily by many people in every community. Parent groups are helpful in promoting exchange of ideas and in providing support. The National Cystic Fibrosis Research Foundation disseminates useful information. The nurse should become familiar with the local chapter to guide parents to reliable sources of information.

Parents of these patients need encouragement and reassurance. When the nurse meets them in the clinic or hospital, he or she should be kind and attentive. If a child looks obviously well cared for, mention this to the parents. If you are asked direct questions about the illness you might say, "Doctor Parker is a fine pediatrician. What did he tell you about Bobby's illness?" This encourages the parents to express themselves and will give you an idea of what the patient has been told. Do not overwhelm parents with information that is difficult to absorb.

Parents need explicit instructions regarding diet, medication, postural drainage, prevention of infection, rest, and continued medical supervision.

Many families require the assistance of a social worker to secure funds for equipment and drugs. Parents should be told that help will be available as the need arises. The mother, who is usually more directly involved, may benefit from these added hints: (1) She needs rest herself; the family must take over some of the responsibilities of the household. Relatives may care for the child periodically so that she can "get away from it all." Respite care is another alternative; it is helpful if she can develop at least one outside interest of her own. (2) An alarm clock set for medication time will remind her of this task. (3) A downstairs bedroom for the child is preferable. (4) Extra spoons and a pitcher of water on the bedside stand save steps.

Emotional Support. The child who is chronically ill finds it hard to accept restricted activity. The amount and kinds of diversion required vary in cystic fibrosis, because the disease affects children of all ages, with variations in severity (see page 298 for a list of suitable toys).

It is felt that children benefit from simple, straightforward answers about the illness. An uncomplicated diagram might be helpful. Children who understand why they are being restricted from certain activities will be more cooperative. They should know why they must take medications with each meal, use the nebulizer, have postural drainage, and so on. They should see and handle the unfamiliar equipment necessary for their care.

The young child finds it difficult to be separated from parents during hospitalization. Even when the prognosis is grave, a child's courage is sustained if the parents are there. Parents are encouraged to stay with the child when possible. Close contact by mail with school, church, and clubs is important for children of school age. It is helpful for patients to develop an activity at which they are good, e.g., piano or art. This will increase their feelings of worth and provide outlets for emotions. Consideration must be given to ways of fostering love, acceptance, trust, fair play, security, freedom of choice, creativity, and maintenance of self-identity.

Nurses learn the patients' likes, dislikes, fears, and interests. They observe them with their families and note the types of relationships that exist. They form their own impressions about the patients and must not be misled by "labels" given them by those with less understanding. Patients have to be allowed to communicate in a manner that is meaningful to them. Sometimes children can express feelings; sometimes they cannot. Drawing with children may stimulate conversation. It is important that nurses be aware of children's facial expressions, posture, eyes, and how they play. What are they saying to their toys, their playmates? Nurses' observations of children's behavior are incorporated into nursing care plans.

Nurses and parents must not show undue concern for a patient's illness. Do not overindulge the children; this makes them demanding. They may then exaggerate small problems. The children's impressions of themselves and their illness are determined a good deal by how they feel physically, how the family feels about their condition, and how others behave toward them. The actions of nurses and their interest or lack of it speak for themselves.

Nervous System

BACTERIAL MENINGITIS

Meningitis is an inflammation of the *meninges,* the covering of the brain and spinal cord. Different organisms cause bacterial meningitis in different age groups (Table 8–3). Organisms may invade

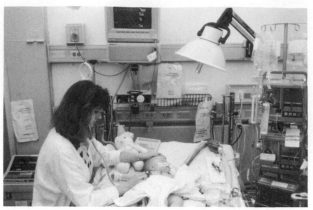

▲ **FIGURE 8–7**

Early identification and treatment of meningitis are key factors in the recovery of the infant. Most children can be cared for on the pediatric floor. The child with severe disease may be placed in the pediatric intensive care unit. (Courtesy of Cook–Fort Worth Children's Medical Center, Fort Worth, Texas.)

the meninges indirectly by way of the blood stream from such centers of infection as the teeth, sinuses, tonsils, and lungs or directly through the ear (otitis media), from neurological procedures, and from a fracture of the skull. Bacterial meningitis is often referred to as *purulent,* i.e., pus-forming, because a thick exudate surrounds the meninges and adjacent structures. This can lead to certain sequelae such as subdural effusion and, less frequently, hydrocephalus. The peak incidence for bacterial meningitis is between 6 and 12 months of age. It is less frequently seen in children older than 4 years. The nursing care for all types is similar.

Symptoms. The symptoms of purulent meningitis result mainly from intracranial irritation. They may be preceded by a cold. There is severe headache, drowsiness, delirium, irritability, restlessness, fever, and vomiting. Stiffness of the neck and spine is yet another symptom. In infants, a characteristic high-pitched cry is noted. Convulsions are common. Coma may occur fairly early in the older child. In severe cases, involuntary arching of the back due to muscle contractions is seen. This condition is called *opisthotonos* (*opistho,* backward + *tonos,* tension). The presence of *petechiae*—small hemorrhages beneath the skin—is suggestive of meningococcal infection.

Table 8–3. ORGANISMS CAUSING BACTERIAL MENINGITIS IN VARIOUS AGE GROUPS	
AGE	**ORGANISM**
Birth to 2 months	Enteric bacilli Group 8 streptococci *Haemophilus influenzae B*
2 months to 12 years	*Haemophilus influenzae .B* *Streptococcus pneumoniae* *Neisseria meningitidis* (meningococci)
Over 12 years	*Neisseria meningitidis* *Streptococcus pneumoniae*

Treatment

At the first indication of meningitis, the physician will perform a spinal tap (lumbar puncture) (see page 44). In the early stages of the illness, the fluid may be clear, but it rapidly becomes full of pus. The pressure is increased, and further laboratory analysis indicates many white cells, sometimes too numerous to count. There is an increase in protein and a decrease in glucose.

The patient is placed in isolation for 24 hours after antibiotic therapy. An IV line is established. The fluid will serve as a vehicle for the administration of antibiotics, which need to be quickly assimilated, and will also aid in the restoration of fluids and electrolytes. Antibiotics are given in combination and are adjusted on the basis of culture and sensitivity reporting. The initial choice is dictated by the CSF Gram-stained smear and the patient's age. They are given according to the patient's progress but are always administered for a minimum of 10 days. Chloramphenicol in combination with ampicillin has proved effective in babies over 2 months of age. More recent drugs with broad-spectrum coverage, such as the third-generation cephalosporins, are widely used. Neonates may be treated with ampicillin, gentamicin, and other combinations. A sedative such as phenobarbital may make the patient less restless. An anticonvulsant such as Dilantin may also be required if the child is having seizures.

Prospective studies have shown that almost 60 per cent of children with bacterial meningitis develop the syndrome of inappropriate secretion of antidiuretic hormone (SIADH). In order to determine the presence of SIADH, body weight, serum electrolytes, and serum and urine osmolarities should be measured at the time of hospital admission. If detected, the syndrome is best treated by fluid restriction.

Initially the patient is given nothing by mouth. An accurate record is kept of fluid intake and output, and vital signs and pupils are checked hourly. Strict isolation is maintained for 24 hours after the start of medications. (It is uncommon for others in the family to contract the disease, but the doctor will order preventive medicines if necessary.) New or persistent fever requires re-evaluation. A computed tomography (CT) scan may be helpful in pinpointing secondary sites of infection.

Prevention. The recent approval by the Food and Drug Administration of two *H. influenzae* type B vaccines to be given in infancy is expected to decrease the number of cases of meningitis.

Nursing Care

The nursing care of the child with meningitis is extensive. The isolation room is prepared in accordance with hospital procedure. Disposable equipment is utilized whenever possible. The room is kept cool and as clean and orderly as time permits.

Since the patient is overly sensitive to stimuli, indirect lighting should be used. Shades are drawn on a bright day. The nurse carefully raises and lowers cribsides to avoid jarring the bed. Padded siderails ensure that the patient will not be injured in the event of a convulsion. The nurse avoids startling the patient by using a gentle touch when waking the child and by speaking in a low voice. This need is also explained to the parents.

The patient is placed on the side to avoid aspiration of vomitus. Since a minimum of handling is necessary during the acute stage, it is important that the nurse organize care so that the patient is disturbed as little as possible yet still receives the treatment necessary for survival and recovery. Frequent change of position is required to prevent pneumonia and to avoid breakdown of the skin. However, careful planning and consolidation of nursing procedures can minimize activity about the patient. As the child's condition improves, nursing care should include range of motion exercises (easily done during bath time) to prevent the development of painful contractures. In long-term patients, splinting of the extremities may also be necessary to avoid this complication.

Frequent monitoring of the patient's vital signs is necessary. Fever may be controlled by antipyretics, sponge baths, and the use of a hypothermia blanket. The nurse observes the child for signs of increased intracranial pressure, especially a change in alertness, or muscle twitchings. The joints are also observed for swelling, pain, and immobility. Oxygen is given as needed.

The patient's intake and output are carefully observed and recorded. *Careful attention is given to maintaining the IV line.* If SIADH occurs, there may be fluid restriction. Good oral hygiene is essential during this stage, when the patient is receiving nothing by mouth. As the patient's condition improves, the diet will progress from clear fluids to regular diet. A special formula may be given when nasogastric feedings are necessary. The nurse promptly reports a decrease in output of urine, which could signal *urinary retention.* Bowel movements are recorded each day to detect constipation and avoid fecal impaction (an accumulation of feces in the rectum). Watch for signs of residual effects from the disease, such as weakness of limbs, speech difficulties, mental confusion, behavior problems, and hearing problems.

The nurse's approach to the patient and the patient's reaction to isolation are discussed on page 63. The diagnosis of meningitis is very frightening to parents, as is the prospect of the child's having to undergo a spinal tap. There is also concern for the health of other members of the family. The nurse should direct attention to the parents. Find a quiet corner for them. Indicate where rest rooms and telephones are located. Parents are encouraged to stay.

Genitourinary System

HYDROCELE

A hydrocele (*hydro,* water + *cele,* tumor), an excessive amount of fluid in the sac that surrounds the testicle, causes the scrotum to swell. Its appearance in the neonate is not uncommon, and in many cases the condition corrects itself as the baby grows.

If a chronic hydrocele persists in the older child, it is corrected by surgery. Routine postoperative nursing care is given. This is outlined on page 65. Same-day surgery may be arranged.

UNDESCENDED TESTES (CRYPTORCHIDISM)

Description. The *testes* are the male sex glands. These two oval bodies begin their development in the abdominal cavity below the kidneys of the embryo. Their function is to produce spermatozoa (male sex cells) and male hormones, particularly testosterone. Toward the end of the fetal period

they begin to descend along a pathway into the scrotum. If, for reasons that are as yet unclear, this descent does not take place normally, the testes may remain in the abdomen or inguinal canal. This condition is common in about 30 per cent of low birth weight infants. When one or both testes fail to lower into the scrotum, the condition is termed *cryptorchidism* (*kryptos,* hidden + *orchi,* testis). The unilateral form is seen more frequently. As the testes are warmer in the abdomen than in the scrotum, the sperm cells begin to deteriorate. If both testes are affected, sterility results. Other complications include increased exposure to injury, an increase in tumor formation, and emotional problems, particularly in the school-age boy, who may be ridiculed by his peers. *Inguinal hernia* often accompanies this condition. Secondary sex characteristics such as voice change, growth of facial hair, and so on are not affected, since the testes continue to secrete hormones directly into the blood stream.

Treatment and Nursing Care

Occasionally, spontaneous descent of the testis or testes occurs during the first year of life. If this does not happen, the patient may first be treated medically. Hormonal management before surgery consists of the administration of human chorionic gonadotropin (hCG). This hormone is useful as a diagnostic aid, and it may also precipitate descent of the testes. If this does not occur, an operation called an *orchiopexy* (*orchio,* testicle + *pexy,* fixation) is performed. The optimal time, at present (although controversial), is about 2 to 3 years of age. Although it is not known whether surgery at this age improves testicular function, it is thought that early scrotal placement and the use of a prosthesis for congenital absence are psychologically important for the growing boy. Although orchiopexy improves the condition, the fertility rate among these patients, even when only one testis is undescended, may be reduced. In addition, although testicular tumors are rare, their incidence is increased in these patients during adulthood. Parents are told to teach the growing child the importance of self-examination of the testes.

The psychological approach of the nurse to the patient and his family is of importance because of the embarrassment felt in many cases of this nature. People may ask the child why he is being operated on when there is no visible evidence of trauma. This problem is frequently compounded by the fact that the older child has been told not to discuss his condition; in addition, his understanding of his problem and just what is going to happen in surgery really may be vague. Therefore, it is important that the nurse caring for the child knows just what he has been told and how he feels about his operation if she or he is to give emotional support during his care. Terminology is clarified. The nurse assures the child that his penis will not be involved in the surgery.

The parents too may have anxieties that they cannot verbalize. It is difficult for many of them to communicate with their child in matters such as these. They may also fear that the child will become homosexual or less virile. A thoughtful, sensitive nurse who tries to anticipate these and other related feelings and fears will be a definite asset to the patient's adjustment.

The Skin

INFANTILE ECZEMA (ATOPIC DERMATITIS)

Description. Infantile eczema, or atopic dermatitis, is an inflammation of a genetically hypersensitive skin. The pathophysiology is characterized by local vasodilation in affected areas. This progresses to *spongiosis*, or the breakdown of dermal cells and the formation of intradermal vesicles. Chronic scratching produces weeping and results in *lichenification*, or coarsening of the skin folds. The exact cause of this condition is difficult to pinpoint, as it is believed to be due mainly to allergy. Infantile eczema is rarely seen in breast-fed babies until they begin to get additional food. It seems to have a definite familial tendency; emotional factors are often involved. Eczema actually is a symptom rather than a disorder. It indicates that the infant is oversensitive to certain substances called *allergens*, which enter the body via the digestive tract (food), by inhalation (dust, pollen), by direct contact (wool, soap, strong sunlight), and by injections (insect bites, vaccines). In most cases, the skin heals by the age of 2 or 3 years, and the eczema does not occur again. Some children develop the triad of atopic dermatitis, asthma, and hay fever.

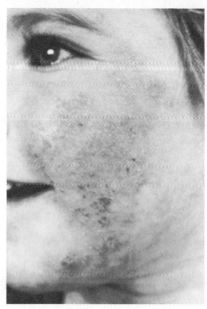

▲ FIGURE 8–8

Atopic dermatitis, showing eczematous lesions on cheeks. (From Krafchik, B. R.: *Pediatr. Clin. North Am.*, 30:673, 1983.)

Symptoms. Although this type of eczema can occur at any age, it is more common during the first 2 years. The lesions form vesicles that weep and develop a dry crust. They are more severe on the face (Fig. 8–8). but may occur on the entire body, particularly in the skin folds. Eczema is worse in the winter than in the summer and has periods of temporary remission. Foods to which these infants are sensitive include egg white, wheat cereal, cow's milk, and citrus fruits.

The baby scratches because the itching is constant and becomes irritable and unable to sleep. The lesions become infected easily by bacterial or viral agents. Herpes simplex is the viral agent of particular concern. Infants and children with eczema should not be exposed to adults with "cold sores." Eczema may flare up following immunization. Laboratory studies may show an increase in IgE and eosinophil rates.

Treatment

The treatment is aimed at making the patient more comfortable by relieving his symptoms. Dermatologists disagree as to the types of ointments and solutions they consider to be most effective. The patient's reaction to an ointment or solution is the best guide. Frequently, the doctor will apply an ointment to a small area of the skin on a trial basis to determine sensitivity to it. If redness and itching occur within a short time, the doctor is notified and the medication is removed. Different types of medications may be used on various parts of the body at the same time. For example, lesion on the face may be of the type that require ointment, while those of the extremities may require wet soaks.

An emollient bath is sometimes ordered for its soothing effect on the skin. Oatmeal or a mixture of cornstarch and baking soda are examples of substances prescribed. The baby's hair is washed with a soap substitute rather than a shampoo. Some dermatologists believe that bathing should be kept to a minimum. Whenever possible, patients are treated at home because of the danger of infection in the hospital.

Corticosteroids may be administered systemically or locally. Antibiotics are needed if infection is present. Medication to help relieve itching is ordered for the patient. A child who is uncomfortable and unable to sleep should receive sedation.

Nursing Care

The nurse plays a vital role in the treatment of patients with skin problems. The doctor's prescribed therapy is of little value if ointments and wet soaks are not applied. It is a rewarding experience for the nurse, who can see the direct results of these efforts more vividly than in other types of nursing.

Infants with eczema are sometimes isolated for their own protection when hospitalized and must therefore receive as much attention as possible. They are unhappy and irritable. They can tolerate the frustration of restraint more easily when they are cuddled frequently in the nurse's lap and their attention diverted from their discomfort. This also shows the parents that the nurse is not repulsed by the baby's appearance and will increase their confidence in the type of care their child will receive.

Children may need to be restrained if they are scratching the area. The kind of restraint used varies with the size and condition of the infant. Combinations of the elbow cuff, abdominal jacket, and ankle restraint are sometimes necessary. The least amount of restraint that accomplishes its purpose is devised. The fingernails must be kept short. Cotton socks or mittens may be placed over the hands and feet to prevent scratching. The restraints are observed frequently to make sure that they are not interfering with proper circulation. They are removed periodically, one at a time, to enable the baby to move about. The child's position must also be changed at short intervals to prevent pneumonia.

Medicated baths may be part of the treatment. Obtain towels and needed clothing in advance. Fill the tub and then run cold water through the faucets before closing them so that they are cool in the event that the baby grasps them. The bath should be 35°C (95°F). Place the infant in the tub for 15 to 20 minutes. Floating toys amuse the infant. *Remain with the baby at all times while it is in the tub.* Children with eczema should not be overdressed, since undue warmth adds to their discomfort. One-piece clothing to prevent binding and irritation should be worn. Wool should be avoided.

Wet dressings are applied to cool the body and in some cases to remove crusts. A gauze bandage is dipped into the prescribed solution, squeezed gently to remove excess fluid, and applied to the involved area. The bandage must cover the entire rash. Soaks are usually ordered to be done continuously, and their effectiveness is measured only in terms of their being *wet*. When they are left on too long and become dried out, itching increases. This type of bandage is *not* covered with towels or rubber sheeting in an effort to protect the bed linens, because the itching is relieved by the cooling effect of the medication, and covering the bandage would prevent evaporation.

Wet compresses may also be applied to the face by means of a mask, which consists of a square piece of gauze material in which places for the eyes, nose, and mouth have been cut out. It is held in place by strings attached to the four corners. When it is necessary to change wet bandages, they are completely removed, soaked in the solution, and reapplied. Observations for the nurse to chart regarding the application of wet soaks include time of application, name of solution, strength of solution, area to which it was applied, length of time, general condition of the involved area (changes in the appearance or area of the rash), and comfort and tolerance of the patient during and following the procedure.

Ointment is usually applied to the skin by hand rather than by a tongue depressor. It is applied evenly and must be kept constantly on the skin to be effective. Since some of these ointments are expensive, the nurse must not be wasteful in using them. Most hospitals provide special linen for their dermatology patients, because many ointments leave a permanent stain on the sheets. Mattresses with special waterproof covering are preferred; rubber sheets would make the patient perspire.

The doctor may prescribe an elimination diet. A basic diet consisting of only hypoallergenic foods is given to the child initially. One new food at a time is added to determine the infant's reaction to it. When the baby is allergic to cow's milk, a substitute such as soybean milk can be used. Vitamin supplements are needed, particularly if the infant is not taking enough of the prescribed fruits and vegetables. The nurse charts the kind and amount of food taken at each meal and any allergic reactions that may have occurred. Plan the time so that treatments do not interfere with mealtime. Elbow restraints are removed from the toddler who is able to eat alone. The nurse assists with the patient's meals and prevents the scratching of irritated skin. Infants are held and loved during feedings, as an emotional climate that discourages tension is very important to the recovery of these patients.

The nurse tries to establish a good working relationship with the parents. They need encouragement, as the course of eczema is unstable and much of the care is given by them to the infant in the home. The nurse should listen to make sure that they understand the doctor's instructions and should clarify matters with the proper authorities as needed.

A nursing care plan is provided in Nursing Care Plan 8–2.

Special Topics

SUDDEN INFANT DEATH SYNDROME

Sudden infant death syndrome (SIDS) is defined clinically as the sudden, unexpected death of an apparently healthy infant for which a routine autopsy fails to identify the cause. It is also referred to as *crib death* or *cot death*. Although precise data are not available, it is estimated that in the United States, SIDS kills about 7,000 infants per year, or about 1 of every 500 babies born. In industrialized countries it is one of the leading causes of death in early infancy; the peak incidence is between 2 and 4 months of age. It is more common in low birth weight babies, in boys, in families with crowded living conditions, and during the winter months. Autopsy may reveal slight respiratory infection or otitis media, petechiae over the pleura, and pulmonary edema. Two clinical features of the disease remain constant: (1) death occurs during sleep, and (2) the infant does not cry or make other sounds of distress. In some cases the baby is found in one corner of the crib with blood-tinged froth coming from the nose.

Theories concerning the cause of crib death are numerous. Although there appears to be an increased incidence among siblings, no genetic pattern has been determined. The risk of SIDS is increased in twins.

Many theories concerning cause, such as suffocation, aspiration allergy, and hormone deficiency, have been disproved. The exact cause is not known. Some researchers propose that crib death results from an interruption of some basic function in the central or autonomic nervous system that causes apnea. Carotid bodies located in the neck and involved in the control of breathing have been found to be abnormal in victims of SIDS. Current opinion holds that SIDS has more than one cause.

Babies with *infantile apnea* (also called near-miss infants) and subsequent siblings of SIDS babies are often monitored at home until they are past the age of danger. Monitors can be leased. Parents are provided with ongoing education and support during this period. Parents are taught CPR prior to having their child monitored.

In dealing with grieving parents after the death of their infant, the nurse must convey some important facts (see also page 70): that the baby died of a disease entity called *sudden infant death syndrome*, that this disease currently cannot be predicted or prevented, and that they are *not* responsible for the child's death. Grieving parents need time to say goodbye to their child. They are encouraged to hold and rock their infant, shed tears, and assist in burial preparations. This proc-

CARE PLAN 8–2

THE CHILD WITH ECZEMA

Nursing Diagnosis	Goals/Outcome Criteria	Intervention
Skin impairment: actual Potential for skin infection, related to scratching and irritation of skin	Skin will remain intact Child's skin will show no signs of break of skin integrity or infection	Describe types of lesions, configuration, and location Provide elbow restraints Hold and comfort child as alternative to restraints Keep fingernails short and cover hands with sock "mittens" Administer medicated baths such as Aveeno Apply wet dressings and teach parents how to do this Administer oral antibiotics and sedatives as prescribed Apply steroid ointments as prescribed
Nutritional alterations: less than body requirements related to irritability, sensitivity to certain foods, increased metabolic needs	Child will maintain adequate nutrition Child will eat 60% of diet and maintain body weight	Administer hypoallergenic diet if prescribed Determine specific food sensitivities from parents if child not on diet Observe child for food sensitivities Administer vitamins and mineral supplements as prescribed Provide adequate fluids
Potential knowledge deficit in parents related to nature of disorder	Parents will verbalize understanding of disease Parents will describe care of the skin of a child with eczema	Advise parents to remove articles that irritate skin, e.g., wool, and to provide loose cotton clothing Encourage parents to use mild detergents, rinse clothes thoroughly Expose infant to sunlight but monitor carefully Help parents identify products in which wheat, milk, eggs may not be readily apparent Advise parents to expect exacerbations and remissions

ess, not common in the past, is conducive to the resolution of grief. One mother who was denied this experience stated that *5 years later,* while visiting a florist shop, she noticed a heart shaped wreath intended for an infant. She unexpectedly burst into tears and wept. Parents experience a great deal of guilt and are catapulted into a totally unexpected bereavement requiring numerous explanations to relatives and friends. Often, needless blame has been placed on one parent by the other or by relatives. The family babysitter and physician may also be targets of attack. Emergency room personnel need to be especially sensitive and supportive during this crisis. There have been occurrences of crib death for which parents have been charged with child abuse and have even been jailed owing to lack of public knowledge about the disease. SIDS can occur in the hospital, and many nurses and physicians have personal experience of the suffering that losing a child to SIDS can cause. Group therapy with other parents of SIDS victims is recommended. Two nationally supported organizations are The Compassionate Friends Inc. and The National Sudden Infant Death Syndrome Foundation. These groups have local chapters in most states.

FAILURE TO THRIVE

Failure to thrive is now used to describe infants and children who, without superficially evident cause, fail to gain and often lose weight. Although this condition can be caused by organic abnormalities as well, this discussion is limited to environmental etiologies. Infants who fail to thrive are frequently admitted to the hospital for evaluation with presenting symptoms of weight loss or failure to gain, irritability, and disturbances of food intake such as anorexia, pica, or abnormal consumption of food. Vomiting, diarrhea, and general neuromuscular spasticity sometimes accompany the condition. Patients fall below the fifth percentile in growth. Their development as ascertained by the Denver Developmental Screening Test and other means is delayed. These children seem apathetic, some have a "rag doll limpness" about them (hypotonia), and often they appear wary of their caretakers. Others appear stiff and unresponsive to cuddling. The "personality" of the baby

may be one that does not foster maternal attachment.

Although causality is sometimes obscured, there appears to be a disturbance in the mother-child or caretaker-child relationship. The situation is complex and is often associated with marital discord, economic pressures, parental immaturity and low stress tolerance, and single parenthood. Alcohol and drug abuse are often present. Many mothers feel deprived and unloved and have conflicting needs. The infant suffers from the inability to establish a "sense of trust" in caretakers. Coping abilities are affected by a lack of nurturing. Outward neglect and physical abuse are not uncommon.

Prevention of environmental failure to thrive consists chiefly of social measures such as parenting classes, family planning, and early recognition and support of families at risk. Treatment involves a multidisciplinary approach in accordance with the circumstance, i.e., physician, nurse, social worker, family agency, and counselor may all participate. If no progress can be made, temporary or permanent placement of the child or children in a foster home may be required.

Treatment of the child who fails to thrive requires maturity on the part of the nurse. It is vital to support rather than reject the mother. Maternal attachment can be facilitated by listening to her and helping her get in touch with her feelings and frustrations and explore her choices. Encourage her to assist with the daily care of her child. Stress the baby's uniqueness and responses to the mother. Point out developmental patterns and provide anticipatory guidance in this area. Avoid lecturing. Try to understand her situation and needs. Take the initiative. Frequently the mother's "lack of interest during visiting hours" stems from her own insecurities and feelings of rejection by hospital staff who seem critical to her. Provide parents with a 24-hour telephone number and encourage them to use it when stress mounts. Parents Anonymous and parent aides are other resources.

The child's meals should be unhurried and pleasant. Frequent snacks and small meals should be offered. The environment should be quiet, and the child should not be distracted. Intake and output is recorded, and the child is weighed daily.

A consistent caregiver should be provided in

order for the child to develop trust in the individual. The caregiver should model appropriate parenting behaviors. The parent should be praised for positive parenting.

Interaction between the parent and child should be observed and documented. Nurses must be diligent about charting only objective observations. Behaviors observed and statements made by the parents meet this criteria. Nurses cannot chart their feelings or instincts about the parent-child relationship.

When the child is hospitalized, nursing measures are similar to those cited for child abuse and neglect (to be discussed next). Hospitalization often leads to dramatic improvement in the form of weight gain and social response. The nurse should feel free to discuss ambivalent feelings toward the parents during staff conferences. Feeling angry is natural. However, expressing anger to parents is damaging and will limit their cooperation. If a nurse is having particular difficulties, reassignment should be considered because body language could be detrimental to the parents' progress.

The prognosis of this condition is uncertain. Emotional abuse, particularly in the early years, can be psychologically traumatic. Inadequacies in intelligence, language, and social behavior have been documented in children who fail to thrive.

CHILD ABUSE AND NEGLECT

The term "battered child syndrome" was coined by C. Kempe in his landmark paper published in 1962 by the JAMA (Journal of the American Medical Association). The term refers to "a clinical condition in young children who have received serious physical abuse, generally from a parent or foster parent." The impact of Kempe's research was considerable and focused the attention of physicians on unexplained fractures and signs of physical abuse (Fig. 8–9). Today, most authorities consider this definition rather narrow and have broadened it to include neglect and maltreatment. Because of the scope of the problem, no one definition seems entirely satisfactory, but efforts are being made to reduce ambiguity. Differences of opinion as to what constitutes child abuse exist from state to state as well as in the criteria of

various agencies concerned with this problem. Nurses must become aware of the mandates of the states and institutions in which they practice.

Approximately 2.4 million cases of child abuse occur each year. The exact number is unknown, as many cases go unreported. There has, however, been an increase in incidence as well as an increase in reporting of cases (Jurgrau, 1990).

The victims are most often between the ages of 3 months and 3 years. The younger the child, the greater the risk of death. Preterm babies have a greater risk of abuse. Adolescent abuse and neglect are also common.

Current thinking recognizes that the temperament of the child as well as the parent can be causal. Children who are different in any way become particular risks. This includes preterm infants; sick, retarded, or disabled children; or merely "unattractive" children. Unwanted or illegitimate babies and stepchildren are particularly vulnerable. Often one child in the family is singled out to be the target of abuse. Ordinal position (e.g., oldest child, youngest child) may also have a bearing.

There are many myths concerning families who maltreat children. Research indicates that only a small percentage of child abusers suffer from psychosis. Not a phenomenon peculiar to the poor, child abuse crosses economic and social boundaries and can exist in any neighborhood. It has been noted that people are often reluctant to report occurrences in middle and upper income families or when the incident involves friends or relatives. Many children suffer from the unrealistic expectations of their caretakers and the lack of knowledge concerning the developmental process in children. Studies indicate that abusers are more likely to be female.

Federal Laws and Agencies. By 1963, the Children's Bureau had drafted a model mandatory state reporting law, which has been adopted in some form in all 50 states. This law aids in establishing statistics and is based on the need to provide therapeutic help to both the child and the family. Immunity from liability is provided for persons reporting suspected cases. Most states have penalties for failure to report child abuse. Originally, only physicians were held responsible for reporting suspected cases; however, many states now include all professionals who are in

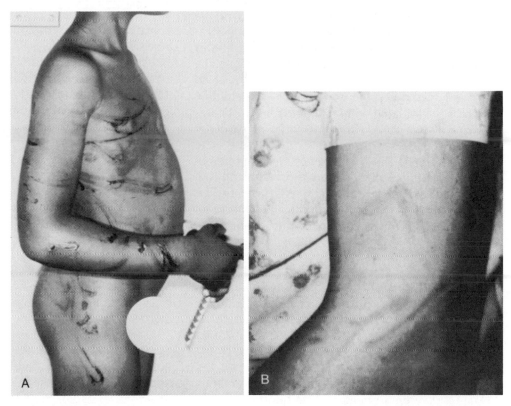

▲ **FIGURE 8–9**

A, Lash marks from an electric cord. Electric cords cause distinct marks. The deep lacerations, which are looped if the cord is looped, result in deep tissue damage and have a potential for keloid formation on healing. *B,* Mark from belt buckle. Manmade geometric articles that have an impact on the skin leave their distinctive imprints. Hospital personnel should become familiar with common instruments with which children are abused. (From Johnson, C. [1990]. *Pediatr. Clin. North Am.,* Aug.:801.)

contact with children, e.g., nurses, social workers, teachers, and clergy. Other laws state specifically that anyone may report an offense. Referrals usually go to Child Protective Services, where a caseworker is assigned to the case.

NURSING BRIEF ▷ ▷ ▷ ▷ ▷ ▷ ▷ ▷

Reporting—A citizen can report suspected child abuse or neglect by contacting the Children's Protective Services (CPS) in the yellow pages of the telephone directory under social service organizations. This can be done with or without the use of the caller's name. After obtaining the facts, the agency will inform the parents that a report is being filed and will check the condition of the child. A visit must be initiated within 72 hours. In most cases this is accomplished within 48 hours or earlier if the situation is life threatening. All persons who report suspected abuse or neglect are given immunity from criminal prosecution and civil liability if the report is made in good faith. As stated earlier, many professionals, such as physicians, nurses, social workers, and so on, are mandatory reporters of child abuse.

Identification and Types. The kinds of child abuse and means of identification are listed in Table 8–4. In the past much of the treatment of child abuse has been after the fact. Current literature stresses the necessity for prevention and early intervention.

Child abuse can be physical, sexual, or emotional. It may entail neglect. It is often difficult to determine whether an injury or situation reflects abuse. Jurgrau (1990) suggests that injuries can happen by accident, but rarely more than once. The nurse should be suspicious when there is a severe injury without evidence of a traumatic event, a pattern of "accidents," or an injury that does not match the history given.

Child abuse is not limited to abuse by parents. Abuse can occur from babysitters, boyfriends, relatives, or casual acquaintances. Drug or alcohol abuse increases the risk of child abuse. Abuse occurs at every socioeconomic level and is often precipitated by a stressful situation within the family (unemployment, marital problems, chronic illness, poverty).

Nursing Care

The prevention of child abuse is of utmost importance. One approach currently being taken is identification of high-risk infants and parents during the prenatal and perinatal periods. Predictive questionnaires are being used as screening tools in some clinics. Many hospitals also provide closer follow-up of mothers and neonates. The process of *maternal-infant bonding* and its significance to later parent-child relationships recently have been explored.

Nurses in obstetrical clinics have the opportunity to casually observe parents and their abilities to cope. The history of the patient, the desirability of the pregnancy, the number of children already in the family, the financial and personal stability of the family, the types of support systems they have, and other factors may have a bearing on how the parents accept the new offspring. Pertinent observations include a description of parent–newborn infant interaction. Both verbal and nonverbal communications are important, as well as the level of body and eye contact. Lack of interest, indifference, or negative comments about the sex, looks, or temperament of the baby could be significant.

In other areas a cooperative team approach is necessary. This includes providing a wide range of services such as family planning, protective services, day care centers, homemakers, education for parenthood classes, "hot lines," self-help groups, family counseling, emergency shelters for children, child advocates, and a massive effort to reduce the incidence of preterm birth. Other related areas include financial assistance, employment services, transportation, emotional support and encouragement, and long-term follow-up. More research and data services are required, as well as an evaluation and reduction of violence generally occurring in our society.

Individual nurses can help detect child abuse by maintaining a high level of suspicion in their work settings. Record-keeping should be factual and objective. Pediatric nurses should make a point of reviewing old records on their patients, which may reveal repeated hospitalizations, x-ray films of multiple fractures, persistent feeding problems, history of failure to thrive, and chronic absentee-

Table 8–4. HOW TO RECOGNIZE CHILD ABUSE AND NEGLECT

TYPE	CHILD'S APPEARANCE	CHILD'S BEHAVIOR	PARENT'S OR CARETAKER'S BEHAVIOR
Physical abuse	Unusual bruises, welts, burns, or fractures Bite marks Frequent injuries, always explained as "accidents"	Reports injury by parents Is unpleasant, hard to get along with, and demanding; often doesn't obey; frequently causes trouble or interferes with others; often breaks or damages things. . . OR Is unusually shy; avoids other people, including children; seems too anxious to please; seems too ready to let other people say and do things to self without protesting Is frequently late for or absent from school; often comes to school much too early; hangs around after school is dismissed Avoids physical contact with adults Wears long sleeves or other concealing clothing to hide injuries The story of how a physical injury occurred is not believable or doesn't seem to fit the type or seriousness of the injury Shows little or no distress at being separated from parents Seems frightened of parents Is apt to seek affection from any adult	Has a history of abuse as a child Uses harsh discipline that doesn't seem right for the age, condition, or offense of the child being punished Offers an explanation of child's injury that doesn't seem to make sense or to fit the type and seriousness of the injury, or offers no explanation at all Seems unconcerned about the child Sees the child as "bad," "a monster," etc. Misuses alcohol or other drugs Attempts to conceal the child's injury or to protect the identity of the person responsible
Neglect (physical, emotional)	Often is not clean, is tired, and has no energy Comes to school without breakfast; often does not have lunch or lunch money	Is frequently absent from school Begs or steals food Causes trouble in school; often has not done homework	Misuses alcohol or other drugs Has a disorganized, upset home life Seems not to care much about what happens;

Table continued on following page

Table 8–4. HOW TO RECOGNIZE CHILD ABUSE AND NEGLECT *Continued*

TYPE	CHILD'S APPEARANCE	CHILD'S BEHAVIOR	PARENT'S OR CARETAKER'S BEHAVIOR
Neglect (physical, emotional) *Continued*	Clothes dirty or wrong for the weather Seems to be alone often, for long periods of time Needs glasses, dental care, or other medical attention	Uses alcohol or drugs Engages in vandalism and/or sexual misconduct	gives the impression that he or she feels nothing is going to make much difference anyway Lives very much isolated from friends, relatives, neighbors Does not seem to know how to get along well with others Has a long-term or chronic illness Has a history of neglect as a child
Emotional abuse (often verbal)	Signs are less obvious than in other forms of mistreatment Behavior is best indication	Is unpleasant, hard to get along with, and demanding; frequently causes trouble; won't let others alone. . . OR Is unusually shy; avoids others; is too anxious to please; puts up with unpleasant acts or words from others without protesting Is either unusually adult in actions or overly young for age (for example, sucks thumb, rocks constantly) Is "behind" for age in physical, emotional, or intellectual development	Blames or belittles the child Is cold and rejecting Withholds love from the child Treats children in the family unequally Does not seem to care much about the child's problems
Sexual abuse	Has torn, stained, or bloody underclothing Experiences pain or itching in the genital area Has venereal disease	Appears withdrawn or engages in fantasy or baby-like behavior Has poor relationships with other children Is unwilling to participate in physical activities Is engaging in delinquent acts or runs away States that he or she has been sexually assaulted by parent or caretaker	Is very protective or jealous of the child Encourages the child to engage in prostitution or sexual acts in his or her presence Misuses alcohol or other drugs Is frequently absent from home

(Data from *New Light on an Old Problem: 9 Questions and Answers About Child Abuse and Neglect* (1978.) DHEW Publication No. (OHDS) 79–31108. Washington, D.C., Head Start and National Center on Child Abuse and Neglect, pp. 6–11.)

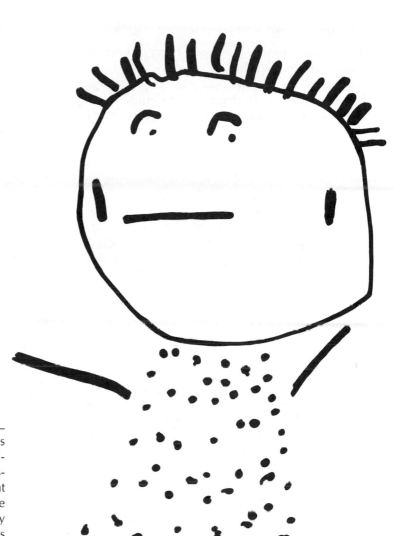

▲ FIGURE 8–10

Five year old girl's self-portrait. The child was sexually abused, and the portrait shows feelings of fear (hair standing on end), helplessness (no hands, legs, or feet), shame (bright red cheeks), and reluctance to talk of the experience (tightly closed mouth). (Courtesy of Iowa Children's and Family Services, Des Moines, Iowa.)

ism in school. Delay or neglect in seeking medical attention for a child or failure to obtain immunization and well-child care is sometimes significant. Children who seem overly upset about being discharged need to be brought to the attention of the physician.

NURSING BRIEF ▷ ▷ ▷ ▷ ▷ ▷ ▷ ▷

Bruises heal in various stages according to color (0 to 2 days, swollen, tender; 0 to 5 days, red; 5 to 7 days, green; 7 to 10 days, yellow; 10 to 14 days, brown; 14 to 28 days, clear). Does this bruise match the caretaker's explanation of what happened?

The abused child is approached quietly, and preparation for treatments is carefully explained in advance. The number of caretakers should be kept to a minimum. The child may be able to express some hostility and fear through play (Fig. 8–10). It is not unusual for these patients to be either unresponsive or openly hostile or to show affection indiscriminately. Keep direct questioning to a minimum. Use praise when appropriate. Encourage activities that promote physical and sensory development. Avoid speaking to the child about the parents in a negative manner. Consult with other professionals about setting limits for poor behavior.

The nurse must acknowledge that in cases of child abuse there are always two victims, the child *and* the abuser. Because of personal problems, the abuser often leads an isolated life. Some have themselves been "battered" or "neglected" children. Many have unrealistic expectations regarding the child's intelligence and capabilities. There may be a role reversal, in which the child becomes the comforter. Although removing the child from the home is one answer, many authorities feel that this can be more detrimental in the long run. Being open to parents in this type of crisis is difficult but essential if the nurse wishes to be part of the solution rather than part of the problem. When placement in a foster home is necessary, parents experience feelings of grief, loss, and remorse. The child will also mourn the loss of the family even if there has been abuse. The nurse should be aware of the child's needs and facilitate expression of feelings of loss. The nurse who recognizes the potential for violence that lies in all persons is better able to deal with this complex problem.

References

Behrman, R., and Kliegman, R. (1990). *Essentials of Pediatrics.* Philadelphia, W. B. Saunders Company.

Behrman, R., and Vaughan, V. (1987). *Nelson Textbook of Pediatrics.* Philadelphia, W. B. Saunders Company.

Jurgrau, A. (1990). How to spot child abuse. *RN,* Oct. 1990, pp. 26–32.

Kinney, T., and Ware, R. (1988). Advances in the management of sickle cell disease. *Pediatr. Consult* 7:1–8.

Morrison, R., and Vedro, D. (1989). Pain management in the child with sickle cell disease. *Pediatr. Nurs.* 15:595–599.

Nederhand, K., Solon, J., Sweet, J., and Conner, S. (1989). Respiratory syncytial virus: A nursing perspective. *Pediatr. Nurs.* 15:342–345.

Oski, F., and Stockman, J. (1985). *1985 Year Book of Pediatrics.* Chicago, Year Book Medical Publishers.

Woolbert, L. (1990). Do antihistamines and decongestants prevent otitis media? *Pediatr. Nurs.* 16:265–267.

Bibliography

Chinh, L. (1988). Otitis revisited: Are ear tubes the answer? *Contemp. Pediatr.* 5:24–45.

Chonmaitree, T. (1990). Viral otitis media. *Pediatr. Ann.* 19:522–532.

Clarke, P., and Deeds, N. (1988). The child in a mist tent. *Pediatr. Nurs.* 14:446–450.

Cunningham, J., and Taussig, L. (1988). *A Guide to Cystic Fibrosis for Parents and Children.* Tucson, The University of Arizona Health Sciences Center.

Cupoli, J. (1987). Piecing together the pattern of abuse. *Contemp. Pediatr.* 4:12–30.

Davis, N., and Sweeney, L. (1989). Infantile apnea monitoring and SIDS. *J. Pediatr. Health Care* 3:67–75.

Marchant, C. (1990). Otitis media today. *Pediatr. Consult* 8:1–8.

Miles, A. (1990). Caring for families when a child dies. *Pediatr. Nurs.* S16:346–347.

Prows, C. (1989). Ribavirin's risks in reproduction—How great are they? *Am. J. Maternal-Child Nurs.* 14:400–404.

Soditus, C. and Mock, D. (1988). Interrupting the cycle of child abuse. *Am. J. Maternal-Child Nurs.* 13:196–199.

Tammelleo, A. (1988). If you suspect child abuse. *RN,* July 1988, pp 57–58.

STUDY QUESTIONS

1. What measures can the nurse take to prevent the spread of the common cold in the home? In the hospital?
2. Four year old Jimmy has a head cold. How would you teach him to blow his nose?
3. How does the nurse recognize an earache in the infant?
4. Peggy, age 11 months, is admitted to the hospital with the diagnosis of meningitis. List the symptoms of meningeal irritation.
5. How do allergens enter the body?
6. Discuss the nursing care of the infant with eczema. Include the rationale for each measure. What factors must the nurse chart in regard to this condition?
7. You are working the evening shift with Mrs. Green, a registered nurse, who is assisting the doctor in the treatment room. Lee, who is 1 year old, has an intravenous infusion running. What would you observe about the baby and the intravenous infusion set as you made your rounds in the ward?
8. List the symptoms of pyloric stenosis. Why must infants with pyloric stenosis be fed so carefully?
9. Discuss the pathophysiological process of cystic fibrosis as it relates to the following structures: respiratory system, sweat glands, pancreas.
10. Prepare a day's menu for an 11 month old baby with anemia.
11. Describe how bruises heal.
12. Identify the symptoms of physical abuse in terms of the parent's behavior. In terms of the child's behavior.
13. Develop a nursing care plan for Jeffrey, an 8 month old baby with "failure to thrive." Suggest positive approaches you might take in dealing with the patient's mother.

CHAPTER 9 _____

Chapter Outline

GENERAL CHARACTERISTICS
GUIDING THE TODDLER
SPEECH DEVELOPMENT
DAILY CARE
NUTRITION COUNSELING
DENTAL HEALTH
TOILET INDEPENDENCE
PLAY
DAY CARE
ACCIDENT PREVENTION
    Parent Education
    Injury Prevention
    Epidemiological Framework

Objectives

Upon completion and mastery of Chapter 9, the student will be able to

- Define the vocabulary terms listed.
- List two developmental tasks of the toddler period.
- Identify four potential safety hazards peculiar to the toddler, as well as anticipatory guidance for caretakers to prevent such accidents.
- Discuss how adults can assist small children to combat their fears.
- Identify the principles of toilet training (bowel and bladder) that will assist you in guiding parents' efforts to provide toilet independence.
- Describe the physical and psychosocial development of children from 1 to 3 years of age, listing age-specific events and guidance when appropriate.

THE TODDLER

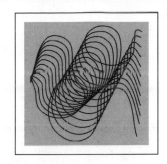

General Characteristics

Children between the ages of 1 and 3 years are referred to as *toddlers*. They are able to get about under their own powers and are no longer completely dependent persons. By this time they have generally tripled their birth weights and gained control of head, hands, and feet. The remarkably rapid growth and development that took place during infancy begin to slow down. The toddler period presents different challenges for the parents and the children. This chapter deals with what they are like as persons and with ways in which adults can help them overcome some of the obstacles they must face.

Toddlers are curious explorers who get into everything. They gain more control of their bodies as each month passes. Soon they are walking, running, jumping, and climbing. They enjoy repeating these new skills, and with practice they become less clumsy and awkward. Their desires to touch, taste, smell, and smear lead them into

difficulties. They quickly discover that much of their conduct is alarming to their parents. Parents no longer accept their actions willingly and without question, as they did when toddlers were infants. Since toddlers cannot understand the need for restrictions, they revolt. Temper tantrums are common, and behavior is not consistent. They are negative and unreasonable and say "no" frequently. *Ritualism* is a characteristic of toddlers. By making rituals of simple tasks, they increase their sense of security and mastery of themselves. *Dawdling* serves essentially the same purpose. *Egocentric* thinking predominates.

The developmental tasks seen during this period are based on a continuum of trust established during infancy. Toddlers are now ready to give up total dependence. They begin to differentiate self from others, particularly from mother. They can tolerate brief periods of separation. They learn to delay gratification and to incorporate rudiments of socially acceptable behavior as determined by the limits of their family's culture. Important self-regulatory functions include toilet independence, eating, sleeping, and perfection of new-found physical skills (Fig. 9–1). The gradual control of these activities provides toddlers with a sense of mastery and contributes to their positive self-concept.

Certain physical changes foster this process (Fig. 9–2). Toddlers' bodies change proportions. Legs and arms lengthen owing to ossification and growth in the epiphyseal areas of the long bones. The trunk and head grow more slowly. The growth of the brain decelerates. The increase in head circumference during infancy is 10 cm (4 inches). During the second year it is only 2.5 cm (1 inch). Chest circumference continues to in-

221

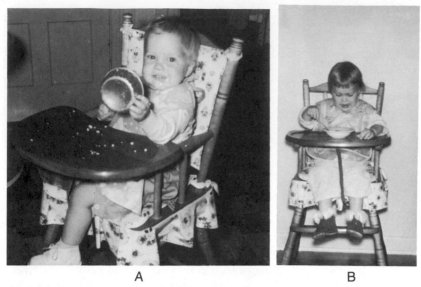

▲ **FIGURE 9–1**

A, One cannot expect much in table manners from the 15 month old toddler. Note plastic bib and unbreakable dish. *B,* At age 2 years, Tina feeds herself well.

crease. The size and strength of muscle fibers increase. Myelination of the spinal cord is practically complete by 2 years, allowing for control of anal and urethral sphincters. Respirations are still mainly abdominal but shift to thoracic as the child approaches school age. The toddler is more capable of maintaining a stable body temperature than the infant. The shivering process in which the

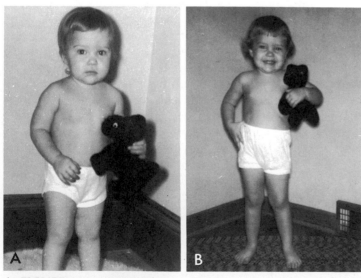

▲ **FIGURE 9–2**

Compare the growth and development of the child of 1 and a half years *(A)* and the child of 2 and a half years *(B).*

capillaries constrict or dilate in response to body temperature has matured. The skin becomes tough as the epidermis and dermis bond more tightly, protecting the child from fluid loss, infection, and irritation. The defense mechanisms of the skin and blood, particularly *phagocytosis*, are working more effectively than in infancy. The lymphatic tissues of the adenoids and tonsils enlarge during this period. Eruption of deciduous teeth continues.

The senses of toddlers do not function independently of one another or of their motor abilities. Two year old toddlers reach, grasp, inspect, smell, taste, and study objects with their eyes. Their attention becomes centered on those characteristics of their surroundings that capture their interest. They can correlate sight with sound, as in the ringing of a bell. Binocular vision is well established by the age of 15 months. By 2 years, visual acuity is about 20/40. Memory strengthens; toddlers can compare present events with stored knowledge. They assimilate information through trial and error plus repetition. They try alternative methods of accomplishing a goal. Thought processes advance, preparing the way for more complex mental operations. Language development parallels cognitive growth. The increase in the level of comprehension is particularly striking and exceeds their verbalization. By 3 years, toddlers have a rather extensive vocabulary of about 900 words. Speech is more than 90 per cent intelligible.

Developmental norms in the use of language have been established. One widely used tool is the *Denver II* (Appendix G). This test is a revision of the *Denver Developmental Screening Test (DDST)*. The Denver II differs from the DDST in selected items, test form, and interpretation. The number of items has been increased, some items have been modified or eliminated, and the age scale is based on the American Academy of Pediatrics' suggested schedule for health maintenance. Each item in the new test was evaluated to determine whether significant differences existed between subpopulations. These subpopulations included gender, ethnic group (black, white, Hispanic), maternal education, and place of residence (rural, semirural, urban).

The test assesses the developmental status of children during the first 6 years in four categories: personal-social, fine motor-adaptive, language, and gross motor. It is neither an intelligence nor a neurological test. Failure merely indicates a need for further evaluation. It is designed for use by both professionals and paraprofessionals. Because it is a standardized test, proper administration and interpretation are paramount. Specific instructions for administering the test, scoring of the results, as well as further description of the test, are included in a manual that may be purchased from the publisher.

Guiding the Toddler

Toddlers' emotions fluctuate greatly. They show ambivalence. They love mother one minute and hate her the next. They will cry, kick, and slap when they have decided to play outdoors longer than mother wants and then turn around and kiss mother for giving them a drink of water. It may be difficult for parents to understand these mood swings. Toddlers are usually trying to assert their independence. It may be best to ignore this behavior as long as the children are not hurting themselves or someone else. After the tantrum, parents should divert toddlers to some pleasant activity.

One of the objectives in the management of toddlers is to help them establish controls for themselves and find socially acceptable outlets for their behavior (Fig. 9–3). Parents who direct all their child's activities cannot expect that toddler to develop self-confidence.

Rituals play an important part in toddlers' ability to achieve independence. They provide them with known routines and people and places to come back to for security. Children's rituals (as at bedtime) should be incorporated into the hospital routine.

COMMUNICATION ALERT ▶ ▶ ▶ ▶ ▶
Children should be given choices when possible. "Would you like to take your medication from a medicine cup or the syringe?" "Would you like Mommy to put the medicine in your mouth"? Never say, "Do you want to take your medicine?" If the child replies "No," the nurse will have created a communication block.

1½ YEARS

Physical Development
Abdomen protrudes
Climbs stairs and on furniture
Anterior fontanel closes
Trunk long, legs short and bowed
Builds a tower of three blocks
Takes off shoes and socks
Runs clumsily
Has sphincter control
Turns pages of books

Social Behavior
Gets into everything
Speaks about 10 words
Rapid shifts of attention
Temper tantrums may occur
Egocentric behavior
Awareness of ownership
Points to common objects when named by adult

2 YEARS

Physical Development
Weight 26 to 28 pounds
Height about 33 inches
Pulse 90 to 120 per minute
Respirations 20 to 35 per minute
16 baby teeth
Head circumference 49 to 50 cm (19.6 to 20 inches)
Builds a tower of six cubes
Runs with a steady gait
Visual acuity 20/40

Social Behavior
Talks in short sentences
Dawdles
Enjoys stories and music
Imitative play
Has trouble sharing
Attention span is increased

2½ YEARS

Physical Development
Has all deciduous teeth
Throws a ball
Builds a tower of eight cubes
Jumps and prances about
May be toilet trained
Walks on tip toes
Walks up and down stairs, one step at a time
Can jump in place

Social Behavior
Balky—cannot make decisions
More fearful than before
Stuttering is common
Speech resembles a monologue
Knows first and last name

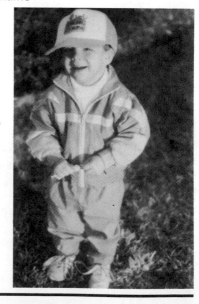

▲ **FIGURE 9–A**

The toddler likes to wear Dad's hat.

AND CARE AND GUIDANCE FOR THE TODDLER

Care and Guidance

Sleep: May stay awake in crib after being put to bed
Eating Habits: Drinks well from cup. Holds and fills spoon; spills contents. Likes to play with food
Immunization: DPT booster. Oral polio vaccine (trivalent OPV)
General: May begin to signal for potty
If temper tantrum occurs, remove child from focus of attention. Keep comments brief. Divert child's attention
Avoid punishment and giving too much attention
Incorporate repetition into routines
Identify and repeat names of items and encourage speech

Care and Guidance

Sleep: Has a nighttime ritual. Tries to postpone bedtime. May climb out of crib
Eating Habits: Feeds self quite well. Appetite fluctuates
Exercise: Enjoys outdoor play. Needs fenced-in area or constant supervision
General: Setting limits on behavior increases sense of security. Praise obedience
Encourage self-help in dressing

Care and Guidance

Sleep: May awaken during night. Needs reassurance
Eating Habits: Dawdles at table. Easily distracted
Exercise: Plays actively
Becomes overtired if left to own impulses

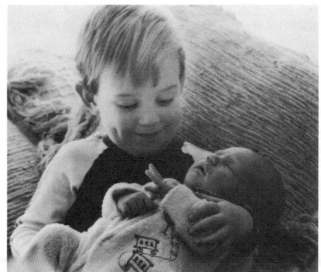

▲ FIGURE 9–B

The toddler needs to be prepared for the changes precipitated by the arrival of a new brother or sister.

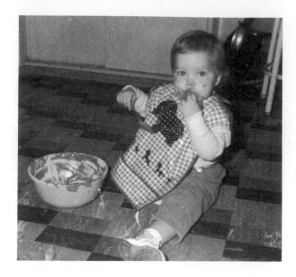

▲ **FIGURE 9–3**

The toddler needs adults to assist in finding socially acceptable outlets for behavior.

Toddlers need a certain amount of discipline. They get into many situations over their head. When adults make a firm decision for them, the problem is resolved, at least for the time being. Children feel secure because parents have helped them escape from their own primitive natures. There is controversy concerning spanking children. A 5-minute time-out period is effective. Do not start timing until the child has settled down.

Children, like adults, seek approval. It is effective and helps increase their self-confidence. Take the positive approach as much as you can. Assume that the toddler is going to be good rather than bad. "Thank you, Johnny, for giving me the matches" will make them arrive in your hand more quickly than "Give me those matches right now" said in a threatening tone.

Separation continues to be a major issue with this age group. They are beginning to separate somewhat from their parents but remain very interested in where their parents are. They have developed the concept that, although their parents might leave, they will return. The younger toddler might exhibit night waking as a response to fear of separation. This same child might have a transitional object (blanket, toy) for consolation when separated from the parent. By 2 years of age the child can separate from the parents and still function (Howard, 1990). The nurse should be reminded that separation fears are increased when a child is under stress.

NURSING BRIEF ▷ ▷ ▷ ▷ ▷ ▷ ▷ ▷ ▷
Caregivers need to provide safe areas for the toddler to explore. They need to watch carefully before saying "no."

Speech Development

At about the end of the first year the baby begins to make noises that sound like "bye-bye," "ma-ma," and "da-da." When toddlers see the happy response to these sounds, they repeat them. This is true throughout the toddler period. For small children to want to learn to talk, they must have an appreciative audience.

At first, children refer to animals by the sounds the animals make. For example, before saying "dog," toddlers repeat "bow-bow." Soon they can say short phrases, such as "daddy gone car." Toddlers respond also to tone of voice and facial expression. If an adult sounds threatening, toddlers may answer "no" and then "no" again in a louder voice. It is well to remember that toddlers who talk remarkably well and understand more than they say still cannot comprehend much of adult conversation. Sometimes when adults forget this, they scold children merely for being too young to understand what is requested of them. Imagine yourself being punished in a foreign country because you could not speak or comprehend the language well enough to defend yourself. Adults who show empathy to small children can help minimize their frustrations.

Toddlers who have just learned to walk may practically give up repeating words because they are so overjoyed at being able to get about independently. As soon as their initial fascination becomes less pronounced, they take up speech again. Delayed speech does not necessarily indicate that a child is mentally slow. The temperament and personality of the child and the family play an important role. No two toddlers have the same vocabulary at the same age. If a mother is concerned about her child's delayed speech, she can discuss it with her doctor during one of the child's routine physical examinations so that it can be evaluated in the light of total physical growth and development. Many late talkers are perfectly normal children who prefer listening to active participation.

Daily Care

Adults must keep their everyday conversation with small children simple. Offering them too many choices will confuse them. When talking to a toddler, adults should position themselves so that they are at eye level with the child. In this way, they will seem less overwhelming. This is of particular importance when the child is in a fear-provoking environment such as the hospital.

By the time a child becomes a toddler, the mother usually has found it easier to give the bath every evening rather than at midmorning. A flexible schedule organized about the needs of the entire household is best. The toddler needs a consistent routine, but it can differ during the summer months, when outdoor water play may make a tub bath optional.

The clothing of toddlers should be simple and easy for them to put on and take off. Slacks with elastic waists are convenient for them to pull down when they go to the toilet. All clothing must be fairly loose to provide freedom of movement for jumping and other strenuous activities. In the summer months, light-skinned children may sunburn quickly and should be protected by clothing and sunscreen to prevent future skin damage. In the winter months, children need outdoor clothing that will protect them from stormy weather. Outdoor garments must be changed when they become wet with snow (Fig. 9–4).

Toddlers wear shoes with firm soles. They should fit the shape of the foot and be one half inch longer and one fourth inch wider than the foot. The heels must fit securely. Children should wear their usual shoes at their periodic checkups because these show how the shoes have been worn, which indicates to the doctor how the children are using their bodies.

Whenever possible toddlers may go barefoot, since this strengthens the foot muscles. Socks must be large enough so that they do not flex the toes. Children are taught to pull socks free from the toes before putting on shoes.

Good posture is the result of proper nutrition, plenty of fresh air and exercise, and sufficient rest. The toddler's mattress must be firm. The chair and play table are adapted to size. In some cases this can be accomplished easily by placing a few magazines in the seat of the chair. A sturdy, small stool placed in the bathroom will bring a toddler to the proper height for brushing the teeth. As in all areas of learning, the child's posture is greatly influenced by that of other members of the family. The toddler who is happy and is allowed gradually

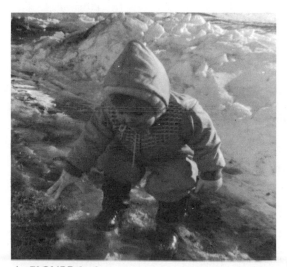

▲ **FIGURE 9–4**

Tina needs security, but she also needs opportunities to explore her world. She must be dressed suitably for the weather.

increasing independence will develop a sense of security, which will be reflected in the posture. Slouching is sometimes seen in children who are insecure and lack self-confidence.

Nutrition Counseling

Toddlers' needs for food are not as great as those of infants because they are not growing as rapidly although their activity level increases. Caloric requirements per unit of body weight decline from 120 kcal/kg during infancy to 100 kcal/kg. Children need an adequate protein intake to cover maintenance needs and to provide for optimal growth. These are mainly provided by milk and other dairy products, meat, and eggs. Milk should be limited to 24 ounces per day. Too few solid foods can lead to dietary deficiencies of iron. Children between the ages of 1 and 3 years are high-risk candidates for anemia. "This risk is due to the rapid growth period of infancy with its increase in hemoglobin mass and the continued need to maintain hemoglobin concentration as well as increase total iron mass during growth" (Krause and Mahan, 1984).

The toddler who is well nourished shows steady proportional gains on height and weight charts and has good bone and tooth development. The diet history is adequate. Laboratory values, such as blood urea nitrogen, albumin, hemoglobin, hematocrit, lymphocyte count, red and white blood cell counts, cholesterol, sodium, potassium, and glucose, are within normal range. Excessive calories and large numbers of vitamins should be avoided.

The toddler is noted for having a fluctuating appetite with strong food preferences. Remind parents that any nutritious food can be eaten at any meal—for example, soup for breakfast, eggs for supper. Serving size is important. Too large servings are discouraging because they can overwhelm the child and can lead to later overeating problems. One suggested way to determine serving size is 1 tablespoon of solid food per year of age. A quiet time before meals provides an opportunity for the child to wind down. The toddlers' refusal to eat may be due to fatigue or to the fact that they are not particularly hungry. They will eat one food with vigor one week and refuse it completely the next. A flexible schedule designed to meet the needs of the toddler and those of the rest of the family must be worked out by the individual family. Forcing toddlers to eat only creates further difficulties. They are quick to sense parental frustration and may then use mealtime as a tool to obtain attention by behaving poorly and refusing to eat. Discipline and arguments during mealtime only upset everyone's digestion.

Toddlers are fond of ritual. This is frequently seen at mealtime. They want a particular dish, glass, and bib. It is best to go along with these wishes, as long as they do not become too pronounced. It gives them a sense of security and in the long run saves time and energy for the adult.

Toddlers have a brief span of attention. They may try to stand in the highchair or wander away from the table. If they have eaten a fair amount of the meal, excuse them; otherwise distraction of some type is necessary. Toddlers who feed themselves regularly may enjoy being helped by mommy. Some restaurants that cater to families provide a pencil and special placemat to keep the small child occupied until adults finish their dinners. In the hospital, the toddler who is fed in a highchair wears a jacket restraint, and the nurse remains with the patient when in the chair.

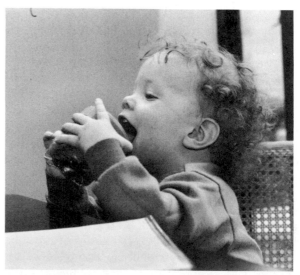

▲ **FIGURE 9–5**

The 18 month old toddler can drink well from a cup. (Photo by Vickie Ashwill.)

The toddler's food is chopped into fine pieces. The portion should be small and separated. Offer a variety of foods and try to plan contrast in colors and textures. A 2 year old likes finger foods such as carrot sticks or a lettuce wedge. Foods are served at moderate temperatures. Candy, cake, and soda between meals are to be avoided. The basic four food groups and the amounts needed are shown in Table 9–1.

Children like colorful dishes, which must be made of an unbreakable substance. Washable plastic bibs and placemats are convenient. Protect the floor around the highchair with newspapers. Silverware should be small enough so that it can be handled easily. Adjust seating equipment so that the child is comfortable and maintains good posture.

Schmitt (1989) suggests the following strategies in aiding toddlers to eat the amount and type of food needed for growth.

1. Teach children to feed themselves as early as possible.
2. Put children in charge of how much they eat.

Table 9–1. RECOMMENDED FOOD INTAKE FOR AGES 1 THROUGH 3 YEARS

Food Group	Servings/Day	Average Serving Size	
		12–23 Months	24–47 Months
FRUITS AND VEGETABLES	At least 4 including:		
Vitamin C source (citrus fruits, berries, tomato, cabbage, cantaloupe)	1 or more (twice as much tomato as citrus)	¼ C juice	¼ C juice
Green vegetables	1	1 to 2 tbsp	3 to 4 tbsp
Other vegetables (potato and other green or yellow vegetables)	2	1 to 2 tbsp	3 to 4 tbsp
Other fruits (apple, banana, etc.)		⅛ C	¼ C
MEAT AND ALTERNATES	4 or more		
Eggs	⎫	½ egg	¾ egg
Lean meat, fish, poultry (liver once a week)	⎬2	1 oz	1½ oz
Peanut butter	⎫	2 tbsp	3 tbsp
Legumes	⎬2*	¼ C	⅜ C
Nuts	⎭	—	¾ to 1 oz
BREADS AND CEREALS (WHOLE-GRAIN)	At least 4		
Bread		½ slice	¾ slice
Ready-to-eat cereals, whole-grain		½ oz	¾ oz
Cooked cereal (including macaroni, spaghetti, rice, etc.; use whole-grain if possible)		¼ C	⅓ C
Infant cereal†		4 to 6 tbsp	—
MILK AND MILK PRODUCTS (1.5 oz cheese = 1 C milk) (C = 8 oz or 240 g)	At least 4	¾ C	¾ C
FATS AND OILS	3		
Butter, margarine, mayonnaise, oils (1 tbsp = 100 calories)		1 tsp	1 tsp

*Use additional servings of meat and eggs when legumes are omitted.
†Iron-fortified infant cereal recommended until 18 months.
(From Endres, J., Rockwell, R. (1986). *Food, Nutrition, and the Young Child.* Columbus, C.E. Merrill.)

3. Never feed children who are capable of feeding themselves.

4. Limit milk to 16 ounces each day. (Some sources say 24 ounces.)

5. Serve small portions of food: less than you think the child will eat.

6. Make mealtimes pleasant.

7. Avoid conversation about eating.

8. Do not extend mealtime or coax the child to eat.

9. Avoid irrational feeding practices (awaken to feed, offer foods every 15 to 20 minutes, and so on).

Dental Health

Good dental health is essential to the growing child. Attractive, healthy teeth promote self-esteem and contribute to physical well-being. Today, techniques are available to prevent dental problems in the majority of children. Unfortunately, many poor children seldom visit the dentist's office. More children are uninsured for health services than in prior years. There has been a decrease in services offered by the public health system (Vanderpool and Richmond, 1990). Both these factors have an impact on preventive as well as acute health care. Nurses must realize that although most middle class children see their dentist regularly, tooth decay is still rampant among the poor. They can play important roles in detection, nutrition education, and teaching oral hygiene. They also can direct parents to dental clinics serving low-income clientele.

Prevention of dental problems consists of good nutrition (a diet high in calcium, phosphorus, and appropriate vitamins), proper brushing and flossing of the teeth, fluoridation of drinking water or fluoride supplements (not both), and regular dental care. In the past, dental care has been advocated at about the age of 2 years. Recent trends in the field of oral health suggest caring for the teeth as soon as they start to develop.

The office visit includes an examination of teeth, gum tissue, and bone structure. It also includes educating parents about proper nutrition, feeding patterns, tooth cleaning procedures, and fluoride treatments. Above all, parents are taught to avoid

using the bottle as a daytime or nighttime pacifier. Constant access to a bottle of milk or juice exposes the tiny teeth to hours of sugary acids that can cause severe damage. Low *cariogenic* snack foods are also important. Sucking on lollipops and chewing sugary gum are to be discouraged, as the sugar remains longer in the mouth. Parents are instructed to read cereal and other product labels for sugar content. Watch in particular for the "–ose" ending of a word, which generally refers to sugar, e.g., sucrose, glucose, fructose, lactose.

When brushing is not practical, teach the child to rinse the mouth several times. The 2 year old enjoys putting toothpaste on a brush. To avoid frustration, allow plenty of time. Technique will improve with practice. Parents may need to assist the child to assure effectiveness.

Toilet Independence

Toilet training has many approaches. Much depends on the temperament of both the individual child and the person guiding her or him. Readiness is important. Voluntary control of anal and urethral sphincters occurs at about 18 to 24 months. If the child wakes up dry in the morning or from naptime, this is an indication of maturity. Children must also be able to communicate in some fashion that they are wet or need to urinate or defecate. They must be willing to sit on the potty for at least 5 to 10 minutes. Toddlers seek approval and like to imitate the actions of their parents. They wander into the bathroom and are curious about what is taking place there. If a mother feels that her child will respond to training at this time, she might first put the toddler in training pants. These can be removed quickly and easily and the child becomes more aware of being wet.

The use of a child's pot chair or a device that attaches to an adult seat is a matter of personal preference. A pot chair may make a toddler feel more secure because it is small sized (Fig. 9–6). It should support the back and arms of the child. The feet should touch the floor. The toilet seat–type must have a belt to strap the toddler in as a safety measure. The child needs time to become

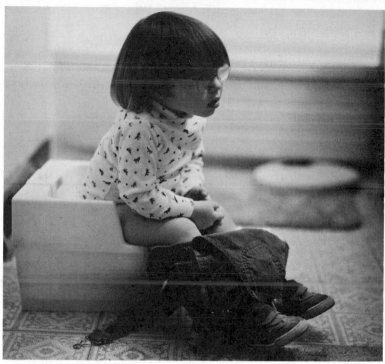

▲ FIGURE 9–6

Toilet training should be a nonstressful experience for the toddler. The nurse assesses the parents' expectations, family and cultural pressures, and the developmental readiness of the child before instruction is begun.

accustomed to this new piece of equipment. Toddlers may want to climb in and out of it and drag it about before they actually try to use it. If a potty seat is not available, a child can sit on a regular toilet facing the toilet tank back. This sitting in reverse gives the child a greater feeling of security.

Bowel training is generally attempted first: however, some toddlers become bladder trained during the day because they enjoy listening to the "tinkle" in the potty. If toddlers have bowel movements at the same time each day, they may progress fairly rapidly. Do not leave them on the pot chair for more than 5 minutes at a time.

If a child's bowel movements are not regular, it might be well to delay training for a while, since the toddler will resent being constantly interrupted from play and taken to the bathroom. Toddlers generally enjoy having their mothers remain with them during the procedure. Most mothers find some phase of toilet training discouraging. Perhaps it is because they work at it too hard, thinking it an obstacle that they must hurdle rather than a normal process that the toddler will easily master when ready. Spankings and threats do more damage than good. Life is smoother for all if the mother remains patient and keeps this new adventure pleasant. Training should not be undertaken when the family or child is under stress, e.g., illness, move to a new city.

Bladder training is begun when the toddler stays dry for about 2 hours at a time. One morning a mother may discover that her toddler has gone the entire night without wetting. It is then logical to put the child on the pot chair and praise success. Bladder training varies widely, particularly during the night. Restricting fluids before bedtime may help. Getting the child up half asleep and putting him or her on the pot chair accomplishes little.

Most children continue to have occasional accidents until the age of 4 or 5 years. If the toddler has a mishap, parents should accept it matter of factly and merely change the clothes. When adults show continuous affection to their children and accept the bad as well as the good days, they surely benefit from it.

NURSING BRIEF ▷ ▷ ▷ ▷ ▷ ▷ ▷ ▷ ▷
Nurses can help parents identify readiness for toilet independence.

The word that toddlers use to signal defecation or urination should be one that is recognized by others besides the immediate family. Sometimes, a parent may forget to inform the babysitter or nursery school teacher of the word that the child uses. This causes children unnecessary frustration because those about them cannot understand what they are trying to tell them.

Toddlers who are toilet trained at home should continue to use the potty in the hospital setting. They literally may be embarrassed at wetting the crib. Nurses regularly consult children's habits and care sheets to make the patients feel more at home. Attentive nurses respond quickly to toddlers' pleas and ask themselves, "Do they need to urinate?" Although regression of bowel and bladder training is common during hospitalization, personnel often contribute to this regression by not taking the time to investigate children's needs.

Play

Toddlers spend much of the day playing. In this way they develop coordination, which contributes to physical well-being. Play also contributes to mental health by bringing relief from emotional tension. Toddlers enjoy *parallel play* at first, i.e., playing near other children but not with them. This is the beginning of socialization. Gradually, as they learn to communicate more easily and become more skilled in handling toys, cooperative play takes place (Fig. 9–7). They learn to give and take and begin to sense moral values of right and wrong. Play is also of educational value. Learning is continuous as they explore and delight in many new play experiences.

It takes time for small children to learn to share. They clutch their toys, shouting "Mine!" Once in a while they will voluntarily offer a toy to a playmate. Parents should not force toddlers to share their possessions. This comes at a later stage of development. If they are constantly corrected for hoarding, they may eventually give up their toys when they are supervised, but they seldom share when left to their own designs.

Toddlers need adult supervision during play, especially when other children are involved. The

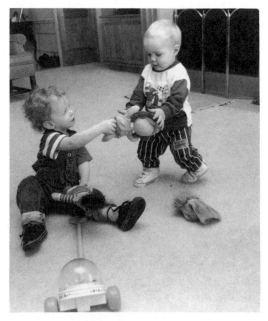

▲ FIGURE 9–7

Occasionally a toddler will offer another child a toy. It takes time to learn to share. (Photo by Vickie Ashwill.)

oldest in the group must be distracted from pushing and hugging and from directing the play of others. The youngest child needs protection from being bullied. Toddlers feel secure when they know they will be rescued from alarming experiences. It is unfair to expect them to rise to situations beyond their capabilities.

The type of toy the toddler selects for play depends on age. The 15 month old is content with pots and pans from mother's kitchen and enjoys repeating acts such as removing clothespins from a bucket and replacing them. The toddler likes certain books and looks at the same pictures over and over again (Fig. 9–8). Some children become very attached to a certain stuffed toy or blanket. Two year olds like to unlace their shoes and remove them frequently. They are fond of water play and may resent being removed from the tub. They enjoy playing in a sandbox, scribbling with a crayon and paper, and prancing to rhythmic music. It is not long before toddlers discover the stairs. Most small children start up them on all fours (Fig. 9–9). As children become more accomplished in walking upright, they shift to the method of placing one foot on the stairs and drawing the other foot up to it, supporting themselves by the handrail. Eventually, they can climb the stairs by using their feet alternately, as in walking.

Toys that can be pedaled, such as a tricycle, are adapted to the size of the child. Wind-up toys as a rule cannot be fully enjoyed by toddlers, since they cannot manipulate them alone. Objects that can be pushed or pulled delight the small child. Toys with small, removable parts are dangerous because of the danger of aspiration.

Table 9–2 summarizes behavior problems that may occur in toddlers, normal expectations for toddlers, and contributing factors to problem behavior.

Day Care

The 1990s will be the first decade to begin with a majority of mothers of children under age 6 years in the labor force (Vanderpool and Rich-

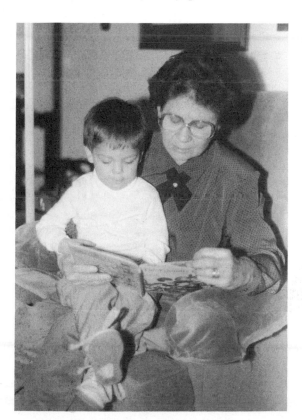

▲ FIGURE 9–8

The toddler loves to have the same story repeated several times. The involvement of grandparents benefits both the child and the parent.

Table 9–2. SUMMARY OF BEHAVIOR PROBLEMS DURING EARLY CHILDHOOD, NORMAL EXPECTATIONS, AND FACTORS THAT CONTRIBUTE TO PROBLEM BEHAVIOR

BEHAVIOR	NORMAL EXPECTATIONS	FACTORS THAT CONTRIBUTE TO PROBLEM BEHAVIOR	
		Child Factors	Parent/Home Environment Factors
Sleep disorders	Occasional nightmares beginning at about 36 months Ritual bedtime routine; attempt to delay sleep peaks between 2 and 3 years Head banging and rocking between 1 and 4 years providing release of tension Waking between 1 and 5 AM occurs infrequently after 6 months of age (less than once a week) Fearful of darkness between 2 and 5 years; will settle down with use of rituals, such as having a favorite toy or a night-light	Excessive napping during the day Insufficient adult interaction during the day, leading to use of bedtime as opportunity to gain adult attention Unusual fears related to darkness, being left alone; rituals and nightlight do not suffice Illness Development of nighttime bowel and bladder control	Anxiety for child's safety results in frequent checking on child, disturbing sleep Inability to set and maintain limits on delaying tactics Unrealistic expectations; cannot tolerate bedtime rituals Environment noisy, not conducive to sleep Excessive stimulation before bedtime Frightening TV shows before bedtime Environmental stress such as new sibling, move, and so on
Temper tantrums	Tantrums peak at 2 years of age, decreasing in frequency and intensity until they rarely occur by about 4 years of age Usually occur in response to frustrated desires of a child, such as wanting a toy that cannot be purchased	Used as a manipulative device to gain control of parental behavior Insufficient positive interaction with adults, leading to use of tantrums to gain attention	Inability to set and maintain limits; parents allow themselves to be manipulated Insufficient positive approaches to child in response to desired behavior Unrealistic expectations; cannot tolerate any tantrum behavior
Toilet training and bedwetting	Child has full physiological capacity for day control by 3 years, night control by 4 years Daytime and nightime "accidents" occur throughout early childhood, decreasing in frequency by 4–5 years	Fears and anxiety in response to negative means of toilet training inhibit ability to gain control Used as an attention-getting device if positive means of gaining attention are lacking Excessive fluid intake before bedtime	Punishment and other negative approaches to toilet training Unrealistic expectations for control; expect normal control before physiological ability is present or expect the child to be accident-free

Table 9–2. SUMMARY OF BEHAVIOR PROBLEMS DURING EARLY CHILDHOOD, NORMAL EXPECTATIONS, AND FACTORS THAT CONTRIBUTE TO PROBLEM BEHAVIOR *Continued*

BEHAVIOR	NORMAL EXPECTATIONS	FACTORS THAT CONTRIBUTE TO PROBLEM BEHAVIOR	
		Child Factors	Parent/Home Environment Factors
	Regression occurs with environmental or social changes, such as arrival of sibling, moving, divorce	Inconsistent recognition of child's signals of needing to use the toilet Inadequate provisions for child's toileting needs, such as small commode Clothing is too difficult for child to maneuver independently Irregular eating patterns	
Aggressive or quarrelsome behavior; sibling rivalry	Ability to play cooperatively begins to emerge at 4–5 years Before this age, child is seldom able to share toys; often wants toys that another child has Predominant use of physical hitting, shoving to express displeasure; verbal abilities begin to emerge during fifth year	Insufficient positive adult attention leads to deliberate use of aggression to gain adult attention Aggression may arise from actual or perceived adult preference for sibling or playmate	Insufficient positive interaction in response to desired behavior Unrealistic expectations for cooperative and sharing behavior Actual preferential attention given to sibling or playmate
Inability to separate; excessive shyness	Child can separate easily by 3 years if the surroundings are consistent, predictable, positive Continues to protest separation if the environment changes or if confronted by total strangers Shy in new and strange surroundings, relaxed and spontaneous in familiar surroundings	Inadequate establishment of self-concept, leading to lack of confidence even in familiar surroundings Uses protest of separation as a manipulative control device Fear of being abandoned	Parental anxiety and guilt over separation Inability to set limits, to leave child after brief, direct explanation Lack of preparation for an anticipated separation, leading to an unpredicted, fearful experience for the child Inconsistent messages and actions, such as telling the child the parent will stay and then sneaking out, or not returning at a predicted time

(From Chinn, P., and Leitch, C. (1979). *Child Health Maintenance*, 2nd ed. St. Louis, The C. V. Mosby Company, pp. 46–47.)

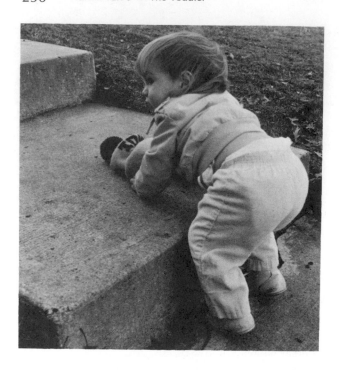

▲ FIGURE 9–9

The toddler usually begins climbing stairs on all fours.

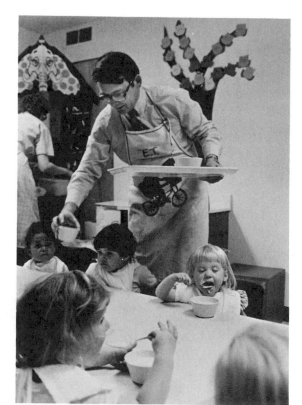

▲ FIGURE 9–10

Parents must take an active role in assuring high-quality day care. An indication of a good program is the child's degree of happiness while attending the day care center. (Courtesy of Blank Memorial Hospital for Children, Des Moines, Iowa.)

mond, 1990). Not only are more mothers working, but they are returning to the work force sooner after the child is born. It is clear that alternative methods of child care are necessary. These arrangements must meet families' personal preferences, cultural perspectives, and financial and special needs. Parents must take an active role in ensuring high quality care (Fig. 9–10). Nurses need to be resource persons and family advocates, as finding adequate day care can be stressful.

There are basically two types of child care: home-based and center-based. In home-based care, caregivers either give care in their own homes or come to the home of the child. These caregivers may be relatives, neighbors, friends, or those who have advertised their services. However, there is very little research on these types of arrangements and few standards of quality control. Center-based care provides care for six or more children, and these are usually private businesses run for profit. They are subject to state regulations regarding physical makeup, number of children per caretaker, education of personnel, and so on. Child care centers run by businesses for their employees are becoming common. Sick child care centers are also available in some areas for children who have minor illnesses that would prevent them from attending conventional types of day care.

For low income families (and increasingly for middle income families) the cost of child care is difficult, if not impossible, to maintain. As the number of working mothers increases, so will the need for quality child care centers. In 1989, Congress passed a bill to support family efforts to obtain child care (Vanderpool and Richmond, 1990). This is only the beginning. Inspection and monitoring of child care facilities in terms of health (physical and mental) and safety standards are paramount. Ideally, all day care programs might include comprehensive health services and health education programs. Primary and episodic health care is being provided in a few school-based clinics located in preschools (Honig, 1991). This concept would increase the access of small children to health care tremendously. Criteria for selecting a day care center are similar to those discussed for nursery schools (see page 291).

Accident Prevention

Accidents kill and cripple more children than any human disease and are the *leading* cause of death in childhood. Unfortunately, we do not have a preventive for this, but we do have a defensive weapon. This weapon is knowledge. If parents understand their child's activities at certain ages, they can prevent many serious injuries by taking necessary precautions. Likewise, when statistics indicate that poisonings or burns are particularly prevalent at a specific age, parents can guard against them (Table 9–3).

The majority of accidents occur in or near the home (Fig. 9–11). Toddlers are especially vulnerable because they have a natural curiosity for investigating their environment. Parents must allow them some natural experiences, which teach them to look out for their own safety. They should also strive to teach toddlers what is safe and what is not.

Nurses demonstrate safety measures to their patients and families. This is done most effectively by good example. Measures pertinent to the pediatric unit are discussed on pages 28 and 29. Nurses in the community often can contribute indirectly to the welfare of others by the example they set and by being aware of emergency medical facilities available in the community.

PARENT EDUCATION

The federal government and concerned private agencies have attempted to regulate some of the variables surrounding certain accidents. A few examples are the use of nonflammable material for children's sleepwear, childproof caps on medicine bottles and certain household products, and the establishment of maximum temperatures for home hot-water heaters. The U.S. Consumer Product Safety Commission has established regulations for crib slats, locks and latches, and mattress size and thickness. Safety warnings on the crib's carton advise buyers to use a snug mattress only.

Laws have been passed in all states that require infants and small children to be restrained while

Table 9–3. ACCIDENT PREVENTION—TODDLER

Behavioral Characteristic	Hazard
	AUTOMOBILE
Impulsive, unable to delay gratification, increased mobility, egocentric	Use car seat, restraints
	Caution children not to run from behind parked cars or snowbanks
	Hold toddler's hand when crossing the street
	Supervise tricycle riding
	Do not allow children to play in a car or leave them alone in it
	Do not allow children to ride in the back of open trucks
	Drivers must look carefully in front and behind vehicles before accelerating
	Teach children what areas are safe for sliding, etc.
	Watch child under 3 years at all times or fence in yard
	BURNS
Children are fascinated by fire	Teach the child the meaning of ''hot''
The toddler can reach articles inaccessible to the infant	Install smoke detectors
	Put matches and cigarettes out of reach and sight
	Turn handles of cooking utensils toward the back of the stove
	Avoid scaldings; do not leave the bathroom when hot water is being drawn or after the tub is filled
	Beware of hot coffee; avoid tablecloths with overhang
	Keep appliances such as coffee pots, electric frying pans, and food processors out of reach
	Test food and fluids heated in microwave ovens to assure that portions are not too hot
	Beware of hot charcoal grills
	Use snug fireplace screens
	Mark children's rooms to alert firemen in emergency
	Keep a pressure-type fire extinguisher available and teach all family members who are old enough how to use it
	Practice what to do in case of fire in your home
	FALLS
Toddlers like to explore different parts of the house. They can open doors and lean out open windows. Their depth perception is immature. *Their capabilities change quickly.* Although they may seem quite grown up at times, they still require constant supervision at home and on the playground	Teach children how to go up and come down stairs when they show a readiness for this task
	Fasten cribsides securely and leave them up when child is in the crib
	Use side rails on a large bed when child graduates from crib
	Lock basement doors or use gates at top and bottom of stairs
	Mop spilled water from floor immediately
	Do not wax floors heavily
	Use car seat restraints
	Keep scissors and other pointed objects away from the toddler's reach
	SUFFOCATION AND CHOKING
Explores with senses, likes to bite on and taste things	Do not allow small children to play with deflated balloons, as they can be sucked into windpipe

Table 9–3. ACCIDENT PREVENTION—TODDLER *Continued*

Behavioral Characteristic	Hazard
Eats on the run	Do not allow small children to play with deflated balloons, as they can be sucked into windpipe Inspect toys for loose parts Remove from reach small objects such as coins, buttons, pins Avoid popcorn, nuts, small hard candies, chewing gum Debone fish, chicken Learn Heimlich maneuver Inspect width of crib and playpen slats Keep plastic bags away from small children; do not use as mattress cover Do not lift child from crib if vomiting, turn on side Avoid nightclothes with drawstring necks Discard old refrigerators

POISONING

Behavioral Characteristic	Hazard
Ingenuity increases, can open most containers Increased mobility provides child access to cupboards, medicine cabinets, bedside stands, interior of closets Looks at and touches everything Learns by trial and error	Store household detergents and cleaning supplies out of reach Lock cabinet if toddler is particularly fascinated by items Do not put chemicals or other potentially harmful substances into food or beverage containers; store in separate cabinets Keep medicines in a locked cabinet; put them away immediately after using them Use child-resistant caps and packaging Flush old medicine down toilet Follow physician's directions when administering medication Do not allow one child to give another medicine Do not refer to pills as candy Keep mouthwash away from small children to avoid potential alcohol poisoning Educate parents as to when and how to use ipecac Explain poison symbols to child (Mr. Yuk stickers, etc.) and to parents not fluent in English Keep telephone number of poison control center available When painting, use paint marked "for indoor use" or one that conforms to standards for use on surfaces that may be chewed by children Wash fruits and vegetables before eating Obtain name of any new plant purchased and record Alert family of location of poisonous plants on or around property

DROWNING

Behavioral Characteristic	Hazard
Lacks depth perception Does not realize danger Loves water play	Watch child continuously while at beach or near a pool Empty wading pools when child has finished playing Cover wells securely Wear recommended life jackets in boats Begin teaching water safety early Lock fences surrounding swimming pools Supervise tub baths; be aware that a young child can drown in a very small amount of water (one 17 month old toddler drowned in a cleaning pail of bleach water)

Table continued on following page

Table 9–3. ACCIDENT PREVENTION—TODDLER *Continued*

Behavioral Characteristic	Hazard
	ELECTRIC SHOCK
Pokes and probes with fingers	Cover electrical outlets
	Cap unused sockets with safety plugs
	Water conducts electricity; teach child not to touch electrical appliances when wet, keep appliances out of reach
	ANIMAL BITES
immature judgment	Teach child to avoid stray animals
	Do not allow toddler to abuse household pets
	Supervise closely

Keep first aid chart and emergency numbers handy
Know location and how to get to nearest emergency facility

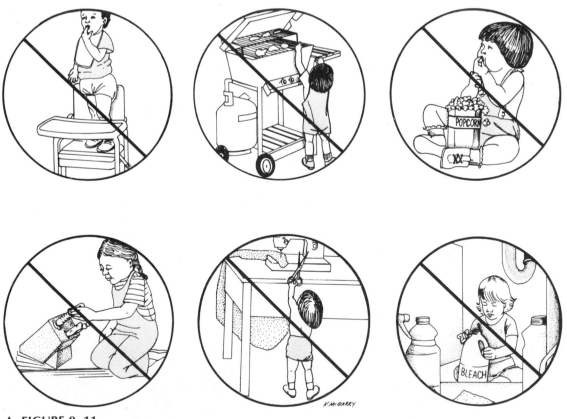

▲ **FIGURE 9–11**

Safety measures should be taken to protect toddlers from these household hazards.

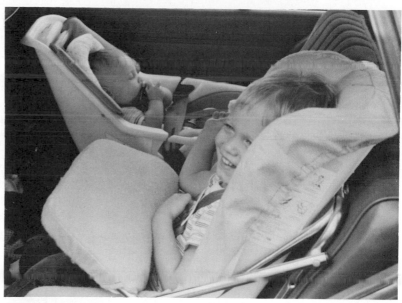

▲ FIGURE 9–12

Automobile seat restraints are mandatory in all states.

riding in automobiles (Fig. 9–12). These restraints must follow standards established by the Federal Motor Vehicle Safety Department. Rental cars also loan child seat restraints. Many parents still do not understand the importance of safety seats and neglect to use them. This is an essential area of patient teaching, beginning with the first ride home from the hospital.

New homes are required to have smoke detectors. Consumers who live in older homes and

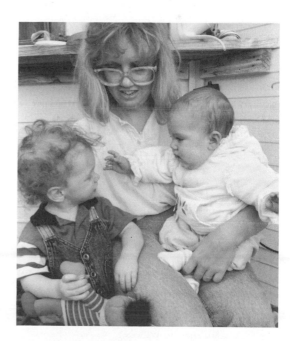

▲ FIGURE 9–13

Family assessment is an integral part of the nursing process.

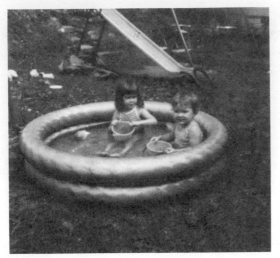

▲ **FIGURE 9–14**

Pam and Tina enjoy water play. Two year olds need continuous supervision for this type of activity.

apartment complexes are also encouraged to install them. Various other safety codes are mandatory for public buildings, with additional measures required for buildings specifically for the handicapped. The problems of surveillance and upkeep nevertheless are considerable. Many children live in substandard housing with little supervision. The education of parents is of monumental importance in decreasing death and disability (Fig. 9–13).

INJURY PREVENTION

Toddlers are at highest risk for accidents involving drowning, motor vehicle injuries, burns, falls, and poisoning (Christoffel, 1990). Many of these accidents are directly related to toddlers' ability to be mobile. Their need for independence, their lack of knowledge of danger, and their curiosity (Table 9–4).

An awareness of the danger of any standing body of water should be instilled in anyone who cares for children. This includes bathtubs, toilets, swimming pools, hot tubs, and even small containers holding water (Fig. 9–14). Parents should be instructed never to turn their back on a child, whether in a tub or standing near a body of water (Fig. 9–15).

Scald burns are the most common type of burn injury in children. Toddlers can pull liquids down upon themselves by tugging at tableclothes, cords, and handles. Knobs, handles, and cords should be placed out of the reach of children. The temperature of the water coming out of the hot-water faucet should be monitored. Small children can turn on the hot water while playing in the bathtub or while playing with the knobs. Matches can cause one of the most devastating types of accidents. Matches should be stored out of the reach of children, and the dangers of playing with matches should be taught. Electrical outlets should

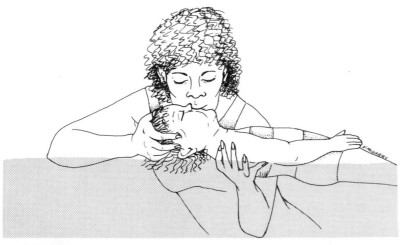

▲ **FIGURE 9–15**

Drowning. Begin mouth-to-mouth resuscitation immediately while the victim is still in the water.

Table 9–4. AGE-APPROPRIATE ADVICE FOR INJURY PREVENTION

The following guide is designed to help you tailor anticipatory guidance about injury prevention to the age of each patient. The left-hand column lists prevention strategies for various injuries. Appropriate ages at which to discuss each strategy with the parents are indicated by Xs in the "Child's Age at Visit" columns, which are based on the standard schedule of well-child visits.

Prevention Strategies*	2 Wk	2 Mo	4 Mo	6 Mo	9 Mo	12 Mo	15 Mo	18 Mo	24 Mo	3 Yr	4 Yr	5 Yr
CHOKING/ASPIRATION/SUFFOCATION												
Learn what to do when a child chokes	X	X	X	X	X	X	X	X	X	X	X	X
Use a crib with slat spacing of not more than 2⅜ inch and a snug-fitting mattress	X	X	X	X								
Remove hanging mobiles or toys before baby can reach them	X	X	X	X								
Allow no cords near crib or around neck	X	X	X	X	X	X	X	X	X			
Keep plastic bags, balloons, and baby powders out of reach	X	X	X	X	X	X	X	X	X			
Keep all small, hard objects out of reach	X	X	X	X	X	X	X	X	X			
Keep sides of mesh playpens up		X	X	X								
Use only unbreakable toys without sharp edges or small parts that can come loose		X	X	X	X	X	X	X				
Avoid foods on which child chokes easily (hot dogs, peanuts, popcorn, chewing gum, and hard fruits and vegetables)				X	X	X	X	X	X	X		
Cut foods into *small* pieces					X	X	X	X	X			
Store toys in a chest *without* a dropping lid						X	X	X	X	X	X	
FIRES AND BURNS												
Never eat, drink, or carry anything hot near or while holding a baby or child	X	X	X	X	X	X	X	X	X			
Turn down water heater so water from the hot water tap is no more than 48.8°C (120°F)	X	X	X	X	X	X	X	X	X	X	X	X
Develop and practice a fire escape plan	X	X	X	X	X	X	X	X	X	X	X	X
Install and maintain smoke detectors	X	X	X	X	X	X	X	X	X	X	X	X
Keep a fire extinguisher in or near the kitchen	X	X	X	X	X	X	X	X	X	X	X	X
Treat a burn immediately with cold water, then call your doctor	X	X	X	X	X	X	X	X	X	X	X	X
Check formula, food, and drink temperatures carefully	X	X	X	X	X	X	X	X	X	X	X	X
Don't smoke near baby	X	X	X	XX	X	X	X	X	X			
Keep hot foods and liquids out of reach		X	X	X	X	X	X	X	X			

Table continued on following page

Table 9–4. AGE-APPROPRIATE ADVICE FOR INJURY PREVENTION *Continued*

Prevention Strategies*	2 Wk	2 Mo	4 Mo	6 Mo	9 Mo	12 Mo	15 Mo	18 Mo	24 Mo	3 Yr	4 Yr	5 Yr
Put shock stops in unused electrical outlets; put cords out of reach			X	X	X	X	X	X	X	X		
Keep hot appliances and cords out of reach			X	X	X	X	X	X	X	X		
Keep all electrical appliances out of the bathroom			X	X	X	X	X	X	X	X	X	
Don't cook with child at feet; use playpen, highchair, or crib as safety area for small child				X	X	X	X	X	X			
Provide nonflammable barriers around hot home heating surfaces and fireplaces				X	X	X	X	X	X	X		
Insulate junction of extension cords with electrical tape				X	X	X	X	X	X			
Use back burners on stove with pan handles out of reach					X	X	X	X	X	X		
Keep matches and lighters out of reach						X	X	X	X			
Do not store items above the stove that attract a child						X	X	X	X	X	X	X
Do not allow child to use stove, microwave, hot curlers, or iron									X	X	X	X
Teach child to drop and roll until fire is extinguished										X	X	X
Teach child emergency phone number and to leave house if fire breaks out											X	X
MOTOR VEHICLE ACCIDENTS												
Never leave child unattended in car	X	X	X	X	X	X	X	X	X	X	X	X
Parents should wear their seat belts	X	X	X	X	X	X	X	X	X	X	X	X
Correctly use an approved car safety seat in the infant position	X	X	X	X								
Be prepared to switch to toddler car seat and position					X	X						
Use approved toddler car seat correctly						X	X	X	X	X	X	
Don't carry child on tractor or riding mower						X	X	X	X	X	X	X
Be prepared to switch to a booster seat and/or seat belt										X	X	
Use child's seat belt consistently										X	X	X
Do not buy motorized vehicles for child											X	X

Table 9–4. AGE-APPROPRIATE ADVICE FOR INJURY PREVENTION *Continued*

Prevention Strategies*	Child's Age at Visit											
	2 Wk	2 Mo	4 Mo	6 Mo	9 Mo	12 Mo	15 Mo	18 Mo	24 Mo	3 Yr	4 Yr	5 Yr
PEDESTRIAN/PEDAL CYCLE INJURIES												
Avoid carrying child as passenger on adult's bike except in special seat, helmeted, and off street					X	X	X	X	X	X	X	X
Hold onto walking child around traffic						X	X	X	X	X		
Fence and/or supervise outside play area						X	X	X	X	X	X	X
Provide play area that prevents balls and riding toys from rolling into street								X	X	X	X	X
Prohibit riding of trikes, bikes, and Big Wheels in or near traffic or on driveways									X	X	X	X
Continue to supervise street crossing										X	X	X
Buy and use bicycle helmet with first two-wheeler											X	X
DROWNING												
Make sure that an adult bathes the baby	X	X	X	X	X	X	X					
Remain in the room during every second of a bath				X	X	X	X	X	X	X	X	X
Provide unbreachable barrier around pool or spa				X	X	X	X	X	X	X	X	X
Continuously supervise child around *any* water				X	X	X	X	X	X	X	X	X
INJURIES FROM FIREARMS												
Unload and lock away all firearms				X	X	X	X	X	X	X	X	X
Don't buy nonpowder firearms (or any toy guns that shoot) for children										X	X	X
FALLS												
Never step away when the baby is on a high surface	X	X	X	X	X	X	X	X	X			
Keep crib sides up	X	X	X	X	X	X	X	X	X			
If infant seat is used out of car, place it on the floor		X	X	X								
Use playpen *with sides locked in up position* as an "island of safety"		X	X	X	X	X						
Avoid using walkers		X	X	X	X	X						
Install safety gates (*NOT* accordion-style) to guard stairways				X	X	X	X	X	X			
Lock doors to dangerous areas like the basement and garage			X	X	X	X	X	X	X	X	X	
Check stability of drawers, tall furniture, and lamps before child cruises; remove tablecloths				X	X	X	X	X	X			

Table continued on following page

Table 9–4. AGE-APPROPRIATE ADVICE FOR INJURY PREVENTION *Continued*

Prevention Strategies*	Child's Age at Visit 2 Wk	2 Mo	4 Mo	6 Mo	9 Mo	12 Mo	15 Mo	18 Mo	24 Mo	3 Yr	4 Yr	5 Yr
Make sure windows above first floor are closed or have screens or guards that *cannot* be pushed out					X	X	X	X	X	X	X	
Don't underestimate climbing ability						X	X	X	X			
Prepare to transfer child out of crib to low bed							X	X	X	X		
Provide soft surface under play equipment							X	X	X	X	X	X
POISONING												
Keep all medicines, vitamins, and cleaning, plumbing, gardening, painting, refinishing, and agricultural chemicals and supplies out of reach, preferably locked away, or dispose of after use				X	X	X	X	X	X	X	X	X
Remove all poisonous plants from the home				X	X	X	X	X	X	X		
Install safety latches to delay access to cabinets				X	X	X	X	X	X	X		
Put poison center number on all phones; call if child puts something in the mouth that *may* be poisonous					X	X	X	X	X	X	X	
Buy syrup of ipecac; use only if directed to do so					X	X	X	X	X	X	X	
Purchase all medicines in containers with safety caps					X	X	X	X	X	X		
Do not transfer toxic substances to drink bottles, glasses, or jars					X	X	X	X	X	X	X	X
ANIMAL BITES												
Don't leave a child alone with pets	X	X	X	X	X	X	X	X	X			
Teach child not to approach pets not well known									X	X	X	X
Teach child not to handle wild animals										X	X	X
CUTS												
Remove (or pad) low furniture with sharp corners from child's living area					X	X	X	X	X	X	X	
Keep sharp objects out of reach (safety latches or locks help delay access)						X	X	X	X	X		
Prohibit use of and proximity to knives, power tools, and mowers									X	X	X	X

*Strategies include, but are not limited to, those recommended in The Injury Prevention Program safety sheets and *Guidelines for Health Supervision* of the American Academy of Pediatrics and the Injury Prevention Counseling Schedule of the Statewide Comprehensive Injury Program of the Massachusetts Department of Public Health.

(From Wilson, M. (1988). Injury Prevention: Protecting the under-6 set. *Contemp. Pediatr.* 5:27.)

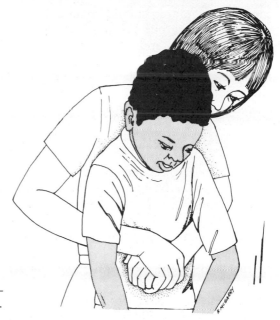

▲ **FIGURE 9–16**

Choking. For a larger child the Heimlich technique can be applied.

have safety guards placed on them to prevent harm.

Legislation mandating car seats has reduced the risk of injury while toddlers are in cars. However, toddlers remain at risk to be hit by a car while playing in their own driveways. Drivers must be alert to the location of a child before they start the car.

With their natural curiosity and new-found mobility, the toddler finds and swallows plant leaves, cleaning materials, medication, and anything else that catches attention. All potentially dangerous substances should be placed out of the child's reach, with a lock attached. Although most medications now have a safety cap, many children have been able to remove these caps. Parents should keep two doses of ipecac syrup at home and have the nearest poison control center number readily available. Specific treatment and care of the poisoning victim is covered in Chapter 10.

Aspiration is one of the leading causes of death in the small child. Hard foods, small objects (e.g., coins, pins, removable toy parts), and balloons are examples of common items that can be aspirated. The Heimlich maneuver is the treatment of choice for the choking child older than 1 year of age (Fig. 9–16). In infants younger than 1 year of age, a combination of back blows and chest thrusts is used (Fig. 9–17).

Over 50,000 emergency room visits a year by toddlers are attributed to playground injuries (Christoffel, 1990). The toddler loves to run and climb and often disregards the danger that this

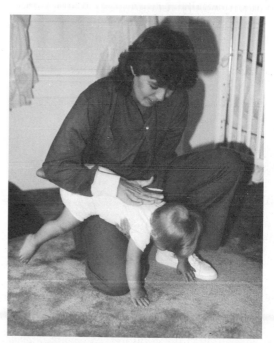

▲ **FIGURE 9–17**

Infants up to 1 year of age who are choking are positioned with the head lower than the trunk. Back blows (adjusted to the size of the child) are instigated.

can cause. Children should be taught safety when playing on playground equipment and riding toys. Doors, windows, and gates should be kept closed or guarded with a screen. When the child begins to climb out of the crib, the parents should consider moving the child to a bed.

EPIDEMIOLOGICAL FRAMEWORK

An *epidemiological* framework for accident prevention is a means of providing a systemic method of evaluation. It consists of three parts, i.e., the characteristics of the host (the child), the agent (the direct cause, for example, poisonous plants), and the environment.

Host and Agent. The individual characteristics of the child must be assessed by the nurse. Particular attention is paid to the parents' description of the child. Some children are much more active, independent, and inquisitive than others. Evaluate carefully children who are aggressive and stubborn and show low frustration tolerance. Children who appear accident prone may be calling attention to themselves in an attempt to reconcile parents (parents usually communicate when an accident happens to a child) and for many other reasons. Children are less receptive to parental advice when they are tired and hungry. The child's age and developmental stage influence the types of accidents that occur. Providing anticipatory guidance is important. Nurses must closely assess children with special needs in terms of safety considerations. Children with handicaps such as visual, motor, or intellectual impairments, convulsive disorders, or diabetes require extended instruction according to the child's particular needs. Immobile children need to be protected from sunburn and inclement weather. Adults must also guard these children from mosquitoes and other vectors. Control of the *agent* refers to some of the methods mentioned under the section on parent education. These include child-proof caps on medication containers, regulations concerning children's furniture, and so on.

Environment. The physical, economic, and social environments of the child are also important in accident prevention. Families may be poor, overcrowded, fatigued, and dysfunctional. Children reared in households burdened by significant stress appear to be more at risk for accidents. A new parent (or babysitter) may underestimate the developmental capabilities of the child. The reverse may occur when a new baby arrives and an older child is given tasks beyond her or his abilities. Some suggest that the time of day has a bearing on accidents. Morning rush hour, after school (particularly for latchkey children), and evening have been cited. Family nationality and lifestyle are also considerations. Vacations and relocations, which place small children in strange environments, are potentially dangerous. The nurse is often the person in close contact with families and can be helpful in determining specific environmental hazards. A room-by-room survey of the home with the parents can be very informative (Surveyer et al., 1985). A discussion of the neighborhood environment, e.g., playgrounds, schoolyard, street lighting, may also be relevant. Explain the necessity for proper "modeling" of safety precautions, as children absorb parental attitudes and behaviors. Utilize community resources such as the library, fire department, police, and so on. Give priority to problem solving, repeat your information, and evaluate its effectiveness.

STUDY QUESTIONS

1. How can adults meet the emotional needs of the toddler during the "negative" stage?
2. Prepare a day's menu for the toddler. Include between-meal snacks.
3. List several situations that frighten you. What can you do to keep from transmitting these fears to others?
4. Define "parallel play." Of what value is play to the child?
5. What is the role of the adult in regard to the development of speech in the child?
6. Stevie, age 3, has recently had his appendix removed. The doctor has written on his chart that Stevie has had a regression in bowel and bladder control. What does this mean?
7. Mrs. Jones, your neighbor, is discouraged because 2 year old Billy signals that he needs to go to the toilet *after* he has soiled his pants. Discuss various ways to cope with this common problem.

8. What factors must be considered when selecting shoes and socks for toddlers?
9. List several factors that contribute to good posture in children.
10. Review your newspaper for one week. Bring to class accounts of various accidents that have occurred to children during that week. Be prepared to discuss how they might have been prevented.
11. Make a list of household substances that are potentially poisonous to small children. In what cases would you want to induce vomiting? When would you not want to make a child vomit?
12. Describe mouth-to-mouth respiration.

References

Christoffel, K. (1990). Prevention of injuries. *In* Green, M., and Haggerty, R. (eds.). *Ambulatory Pediatrics.* Philadelphia, W. B. Saunders Company, pp. 144–156.

Honig, J. (1991). A school-based clinic in a preschool. *J. Pediatr. Health Care* 5:34–39.

Howard, B. (1990). Growing together: The toddler years need not be turbulent. *Contemp. Pediatr.* 7:21–39.

Krause, M., and Mahan, L. (1984). *Food, Nutrition, and Diet Therapy,* 7th ed. Philadelphia, W. B. Saunders Company.

Schmitt, B. (1989). When your toddler or preschooler won't eat. *Contemp. Pediatr.* 6:127–128.

Surveyer, J., et. al. (1985). Prevention of injury. *In* Mott, S., et al. (eds.) *Nursing Care of Children and Families.* Menlo Park, Cal., Addison-Wesley.

Vanderpool, N., and Richmond, J. (1990). Child health in the United States: Prospects for the 1990s. *Public Health* 11:185–205.

Bibliography

Endres, J., and Rockwell, R. (1986). *Food, Nutrition, and the Young Child.* Columbus, C. E. Merrill.

Foster, R., Hunsberger, M., and Anderson, J. (1989). *Family-Centered Nursing Care of Children.* Philadelphia, W. B. Saunders Company.

Levine, M., Carey, W., Crocker, A., and Gross, R. (1983). *Developmental-Behavioral Pediatrics.* Philadelphia, W. B. Saunders Company.

Pipes, P. (1989). *Nutrition in Infancy and Childhood.* St. Louis, The C. V. Mosby Company.

Schmitt, B. (1987). Toilet training refusal: Avoid the battle and win the war. *Contemp. Pediatr.* 4:32–50.

Vaughan, V., and Litt, I. (1990). *Child and Adolescent Development.* Philadelphia, W. B. Saunders Company.

Whaley, L., and Wong, D. (1987). *Nursing Care of Infants and Children,* 3rd ed. St. Louis, The C. V. Mosby Company.

Wilson, M. (1988). Injury prevention: Protecting the under-6 set. *Contemp. Pediatr.* 5:19–34.

CHAPTER 10 _____

Chapter Outline

Objectives

Upon completion and mastery of Chapter 10, the student will be able to

- Define the vocabulary terms listed.
- Describe the three phases of separation anxiety.
- List and define the more common disorders of the toddler period.
- Identify two ways in which the bones of the toddler differ from those of adults.
- Describe the signs of increased intracranial pressure in a child suffering from a head injury; including nursing observations necessary to establish a baseline of information.
- Discuss the nursing care of the child with nephrosis.
- Outline the nursing observation and care necessary for a 2 year old child with croup who requires the use of a mist tent.
- List two measures being taken to reduce acetaminophen poisoning in children.

DISORDERS OF THE TODDLER

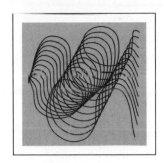

Terms

Separation Anxiety

The world of toddlers revolves around their parents, particularly the mother (or significant other). Hospitalization is a painful experience for them. They cannot understand why they are separated from mother and become very distressed. Toddlers who have a continuous, secure relationship with mother react more violently to separation because they have more to lose.

Three stages of separation anxiety exist: *protest, despair,* and *denial.* Unless toddlers are extremely ill, their grief and sense of abandonment are obvious. They protest loudly. They watch and listen for mother. Their cry is pitiful and continuous until they fall asleep in sheer exhaustion. They call "Mommy, Mommy," and wonder why she does not answer.

The second stage occurs as anger turns to despair. The children look sad and lonely and may refuse to eat. They are depressed and move about less. In the third stage, denial, children may try to deny the need for mother by appearing detached and uninterested in her visits. On the surface it may seem that they have settled in, but this is only a disguise to prevent further emotional pain. The nurse who comprehends the various separation stages will see parental visits as essential, even though the process of separation and reunion is painful. Education of the parents helps promote their continued visits and decrease feelings of inadequacy.

NURSING INTERVENTION

The goals of nursing in care of the hospitalized toddler are presented in Table 10–1.

Table 10–1. NURSING GOALS: CARE OF HOSPITALIZED TODDLER

Reassure parents, particularly the patient's mother
Maintain the toddler's sense of trust
Incorporate home habits of the patient into nursing care plans, e.g., transitional objects
Allow child to work through or master threatening experiences through play and fantasy
Provide individualized flexible nursing care plans in accordance with patient's development and diagnosis

The child and the parent should be oriented to the routine of the hospital (meals, equipment, call bell, visiting rules). The nurse should involve the parent in the care of the child whenever possible. This gives the parent a sense of control and decreases the anxiety of the child.

Pictures of the family and tape recordings of favorite stories are measures that help children remain connected with the family. When the mother leaves, she explains when she will return in terms of the toddler's experience, e.g., after naptime or lunch, and then returns promptly at that time. Nurses do this too. If clinging and protest continue, try to distract the child in some way. A loving hug, goodbye, and prompt exit are then necessary. Repetitive games that deal with disappearance and return are helpful. Peekaboo and hide and seek serve such a purpose. The use of a *transitional* object such as a blanket or favorite toy promotes security.

Parents should not wait until a child falls asleep to depart. This avoids confrontations but disturbs the child's sense of trust. Nurses assure the parents that they will remain with the child and give comfort. The continued reappearance of the parents as promised will be of value in reducing the child's anxiety and re-establishing a sense of trust.

Rooming-in is highly desirable. When rooming-in is impossible, one nurse should be assigned to care for the child and to work with the mother. Nurses should indicate by their approach that they consider the mother's contributions extremely important to the patient's well-being. They interpret the stages of separation anxiety to her. Nurses must also realize that the mother is under stress and should not be asked to assume responsibilities beyond her capabilities. They observe parents for signs of fatigue and suggest appropriate interventions.

The home habits of the toddler are recorded and utilized. Toddlers need routines and rituals, and these are interrupted in the hospital setting. Too often, this information is obtained upon admission but never referred to. The nurse should be aware of the child's time of napping, food preferences, bath time, and favorite toy or object (Fig. 10–1). Children often have special bedtime rituals that become even more important during the anxiety of hospitalization. Provide a pot chair when the child is trained. Expect some regression in behavior. If the toddler still prefers bottles to cups, do not attempt to change this in the hospital. Familiar toys and books are important.

Children should be forewarned about any unpleasant or new experience that they may have to undergo while in the hospital. This is done in keeping with their level of understanding. Be truthful about things that may hurt. This will prevent a child from feeling betrayed. Preparation and explanation should be done immediately before a procedure so that the child will not worry needlessly for an extended period of time. Crying and protest at the time the patient is told about certain procedures that must be performed are healthy expressions of feelings and provide relief of tension.

COMMUNICATION ALERT ▶ ▶ ▶ ▶ ▶
Using a stuffed animal, doll, or puppet to communicate may not be as frightening to a toddler. The nurse can use the inanimate object to assist in gaining the child's cooperation. "Let's see if your doll will take the medicine. She did! Now you try it."

Toddlers are encouraged to play with safe equipment used in their care—tongue blades, stethoscopes, and so on. Whenever possible, they should be allowed out of the crib, as confinement is frustrating for little ones who have just begun to enjoy walking (Fig. 10–2). Supervised playroom activity contributes to intellectual, social, and motor development. Treatments should be done in the treatment room when possible. The child's room should remain a "safe place," and the playroom should never be used for anything but play.

There are indications that the restraint of the child's mobility by surgical and medical procedures involving splints, intravenous therapy, burn dressings, and so on may contribute to the development of subsequent emotional or personality problems or to speech and learning difficulties (Berhman and Vaughan, 1987). Therefore, when restraint is required, it must be accompanied by increased emotional support such as rooming-in, additional attention from nurses, and suitable diversion.

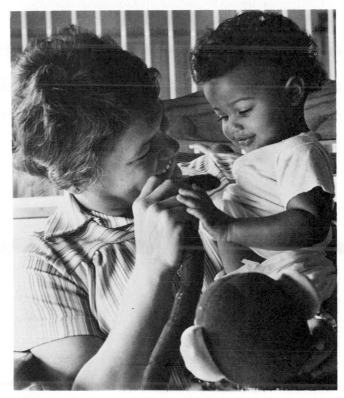

▲ **FIGURE 10–1**

Establishing rapport with the hospitalized toddler. (Courtesy of Blank Memorial Hospital for Children, Des Moines, Iowa.)

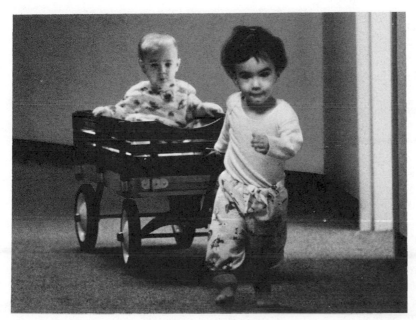

▲ **FIGURE 10–2**

Although supervising toddlers when out of their cribs is at times harrowing, confinement is frustrating for children who have just learned to walk. (Courtesy of Blank Memorial Hospital for Children, Des Moines, Iowa.)

It is common for children to experience changes in behavior upon returning home. They may be demanding and may cling to the mother every minute. "He just won't let me out of his sight" is a common description. The mother should give the toddler extra attention and reassurance until the child's anxiety decreases.

NURSING BRIEF ▷ ▷ ▷ ▷ ▷ ▷ ▷ ▷
Any time the toddler is left by the mother or primary caretaker, some degree of separation anxiety will be experienced, e.g., when left with day care personnel, sitters, or relatives.

Nervous System

CEREBRAL PALSY

Description. Cerebral palsy is a term used to refer to a group of nonprogressive disorders that affect the motor centers of the brain. It is one of the most common crippling conditions seen in children; there are at least 300,000 affected children in the United States. This disease is caused by many factors, some of which are birth injuries, neonatal anoxia, subdural hemorrhage, and infections such as meningitis and encephalitis. Studies indicate that more than one third of children with cerebral palsy weighed less than 2500 g at birth. Head injuries and febrile illness are sometimes responsible during the toddler period. In some cases no single cause can be found.

Symptoms. The symptoms of cerebral palsy vary with each child and may range from mild to severe. Mental retardation sometimes accompanies this disorder; however, many victims have normal intelligence. The disease is suspected during infancy if there are feeding problems, convulsions not associated with high fever, and physical retardation. (The child cannot sit, crawl, creep, stand, and so forth at the approximate age level expected.) *Ataxia* or lack of muscle coordination may be seen. Diagnostic tests may include spinal tap, electroencephalography, pneumoencephalography, computed tomography, and screening for metabolic disorders. Brain tumors must also be ruled out. Early recognition is important.

There are many types of cerebral palsy (Table 10–2). Two of the more common are those marked by *spasticity* and *athetosis* (Fig. 10–3). These conditions occur in about 75 per cent of the cases. *Spasticity* is characterized by tension in certain muscle groups. The stretch reflex is present in the involved muscles. When the child tries to move the voluntary muscles, jerky motions result, and eating, walking, and other coordinated movements are difficult to accomplish. The lower extremities are usually involved. The legs cross and the toes point inward. The arms and trunk may also be affected. In *athetosis,* the patient has involuntary, purposeless movements that interfere with normal motion. Speech, sight, and hearing defects and convulsions may be complications. Emotional problems sometimes present more difficulties than the physical disability.

Treatment and Nursing Care

The objective of treatment is to assist children in making the most of their assets and to guide them into becoming happy, well-adjusted adults performing at their maximal ability. Both short-term and long-term goals must be realistic. Chil-

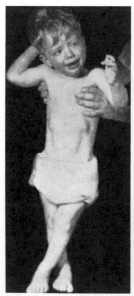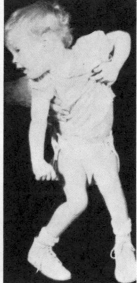

▲ **FIGURE 10–3**

Cerebral palsy. *A,* Spasticity. *B,* Athetosis.

Table 10–2. CLASSIFICATION OF CEREBRAL PALSY

Type	Comment
Spastic Also classified by distribution of muscles involved:	Most common, approximately 65% of cases
Hemiplegia	Limited to one side of the body
Paraplegia	Involves legs only
Quadriplegia	Involves all four extremities (upper and lower limbs equally affected)
Athetosis	Second most frequent type
Ataxia	Least common form, approximately 1–10% of cases; characterized by imbalance, nystagmus, lurching
Mixed types	Most often athetosis and spasticity
Degree of severity Mild	Affects fine precision
Moderate	Affects gross and fine movements and speech; patient is able to perform usual activities of daily living
Severe	Patient is unable to perform usual activities of daily living

dren with cerebral palsy are usually treated at home unless they have surgery. Parents need help in accepting the child and should not be deceived into expecting miraculous cures from the treatment. The sooner the case is diagnosed, the fewer the physical and emotional problems. Parents must be informed of community resources available to them. The patient's religious affiliation should not be overlooked in this respect, as it can become a source of support and help during times of stress. The long course of this disability is a financial burden. Caretakers need respite care from time to time, so that they can refresh their outlook on life. The specific treatment is highly individualistic, depending on the severity of the disease.

It is not uncommon for the parents of children with cerebral palsy to become the "experts" in caring for their child, and therefore it behooves medical personnel to listen and incorporate parents' suggestions when developing nursing care plans.

Many of these children will wear braces, and assessment of the skin is essential. The nurse should observe for areas of redness or pallor. The child might find it helpful to wear a light shirt under the brace. The bedclothes are kept clean, dry, and free of wrinkles.

All precautions are taken to prevent the formation of *contractures* (degeneration or shortening of the muscles due to lack of use). The damage may be permanent, resulting in a loss of function of the part involved, e.g., leg, arm, or finger. A common expression in relation to this is, "What you don't use, you lose." Knowing this, the nurse represses a natural desire to help patients and encourages them to do as much as they can for themselves. When patients take their own baths in the morning, they put muscles and joints through their normal range of motion. When nurses give the bath, they put *their* muscles through the necessary movements, not the patient's. Of course nurses must use their judgment in assessing the patient's capabilities.

Other measures necessary to prevent deformities include frequent change of position, the use of splints, and the carrying out of passive, range of motion, and stretching exercises. The nurse must also assure that the patient maintains good posture while in bed. This is done through the use of footboards and the proper positioning of pillows and other comfort devices. The principles involved in preventing contractures can be applied to the nursing care of all long-term patients. The physical therapist spends many hours with the patient. His or her instructions must be carried out by unit personnel to ensure continuity of care. At some point, the child may need surgery to improve mobility.

Feeding problems may occur due to swallowing and sucking difficulties. During infancy, the child should be fed slowly to prevent aspiration. As children grow older, they should be fitted with a chair with good foot support. The child should be taught as soon as possible to manage special feeding equipment. High-caloric diets are necessary to replace calories used by the constant muscle tension.

The handicapped child needs opportunities to play alone and with other children. Games suited to abilities, such as finger painting, are fun and allow freedom of expression. Activities that require the use of fine muscular movements of the hand cause frustration in the child whose arms and hands are affected by the disease. The nurse can learn a great deal from the parents in regard to types of play enjoyed by the child.

Children with cerebral palsy tire easily but find it difficult to relax. They are under a constant strain to accomplish the simplest of tasks. The nurse must see that they take frequent naps in a quiet room. They should not become overexcited before bedtime.

Public law 94–142 mandates that public schools provide education for handicapped children. When possible, the child should attend regular school. Children with cerebral palsy may need speech and physical therapy, and this can often be provided within the school setting. Mental ability is difficult to evaluate because the type of brain injury associated with cerebral palsy interferes with both verbal and motor expression. The family should be referred to the United Cerebral Palsy Agency.

Mental Health Needs of the Handicapped Child. The requirements for good mental health

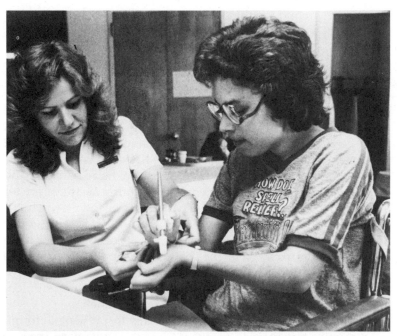

▲ **FIGURE 10–4**

New challenges await the handicapped child as adolescence is reached. Positive encouragement and reinforcement from an early age help the youngster develop a healthy self-concept. (Courtesy of Blank Memorial Hospital for Children, Des Moines, Iowa.)

in handicapped children do not differ greatly from those for all persons. They need to have their basic human drives satisfied and people who are genuinely interested in them. As children grow, they need social experience with both sexes to help them adjust to adolescence. The disabled child needs to participate to the fullest extent in family, school, and community activities (Fig. 10–4). Friendships with other handicapped and nonhandicapped peers are encouraged. Extended family and the community may be important resources or sources of stress. Frequently, families are isolated or stigmatized owing to fear and lack of knowledge on the part of the public. Educational programs are attempting to integrate the handicapped more fully into the community. Barrier-free buildings and modifications that improve accessibility contribute positively to these efforts.

Attitude of the Nurse. Inexperienced nurses may find that they are not immediately attracted to children who are handicapped and may be physically unattractive. Nurses may feel inadequate and may not know how to approach or assist them. Fear of the unknown is natural. The nurse's first problem may be to think of what to say to the child. The best advice is the easiest: be natural and treat the child in a natural manner. Listen to what is being said. Do not be overly kind and solicitous, for this increases dependence. Let the child do as much for the self as possible. Be there to assist if necessary but do not wait on the child hand and foot. The child is happier without pity. Limit setting is essential and provides security. Even patients with the most serious defects can grow up to be happy and self-reliant if they are accepted for what they are and encouraged to perform the tasks they are capable of doing. Expect them to be polite and considerate within reason. They will find security in your firmness. Handicapped children want to be treated like other children of their age and to be loved and accepted as individuals.

Skeletal System

FRACTURES

A *fracture* is a break in a bone and is caused mainly by accidents. It is characterized by pain, tenderness on movement, and swelling. Discoloration, limited movement, and numbness may

also occur. In a *simple fracture* the bone is broken, but the skin over the area is not. In a *compound fracture* a wound in the skin leads to the broken bone, and there is the added danger of infection. A *greenstick fracture* is an incomplete fracture in which one side of the bone is broken and the other is bent. This type of fracture is common in children because their bones are soft, flexible, and more apt to splinter. In a *complete fracture* the bone is entirely broken across.

Healing of a fracture in a child is more rapid than in an adult. The child's periosteum is stronger and thicker, and there is less stiffness upon mobilization. Injury to the cartilaginous *epiphyseal plate*, found at the ends of long bones, is serious if it happens during childhood because it may interfere with longitudinal growth.

If a fracture is suspected, do not allow the child to use the limb or part, and do not move it yourself. If the child is in a safe place, do not move the child, keep the child warm, and prepare for transport via Emergency Medical Services (EMS) to the hospital. An ice pack, covered with a cloth to prevent skin burns, applied to the fracture may minimize swelling. When the fracture is compound, cover the injury lightly with a sterile dressing. If it is necessary to move the child, apply a splint. The joints above and below the break are immobilized by a rolled newspaper or bath towels and tied beyond the injury. Commercially made splints are available, for example, a padded board that is bandaged to the extremity or air splints that can be inflated. If the arm is injured, keep it elevated by a sling to reduce swelling and hemorrhage (Fig. 10–5). If a back or neck injury is evident, do not move the child unless it is life-threatening. Activate the EMS in the area.

Fractures of the Femur

The femur, the thigh bone, is the largest and strongest bone of the body. Children may fracture this bone through a severe fall or an automobile accident. It is one of the most common serious breaks that occur during early childhood. The child complains of pain and tenderness when the leg is moved and cannot bear weight on it. Clothes are gently removed, starting at the uninjured side and proceeding to the injured side. It may be necessary to cut the clothes. X-ray films confirm the diagnosis. Skin traction is used to reduce the

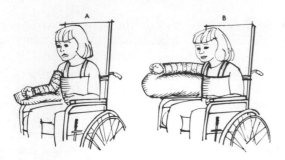

▲ **FIGURE 10–5**

Correct and incorrect positions for a child in a wheelchair. In the incorrect position (*A*), the support is too low to relieve local edema. Correctly positioned (*B*), the arm is elevated, the wrist is higher than the elbow, and the elbow is higher than the shoulder. (From Leifer, G. [1982]. *Principles and Techniques in Pediatric Nursing*, 4th ed. Philadelphia, W. B. Saunders Company.)

fracture, to keep the bones in proper place and to immobilize both legs.

Bryant traction is used for treating fractures of the femur in children under 2 years of age or under 20 to 30 pounds (Fig. 10–6). Weights and pulleys are used to extend the legs vertically. The buttocks should be slightly elevated above the bed. Ninety-ninety skeletal traction with a boot cast on the lower leg and skeletal Steinmann pin or Kirschner wire through the distal femur is used for children over 2 years. Other types of traction that may be used in lower extremity fractures are Russell traction and balanced suspension traction with Thomas splint and Pearson attachment.

The nurse observes the traction ropes to be sure that they are intact and in the wheel grooves of the pulleys and that the child's body is in good position. Elastic bandages should be neither too loose nor too tight. A restraint jacket may be used to keep the child from turning from side to side. Do not remove the weights once they have been applied. Continuous traction is necessary. The weights must hang free, and the pull of the weights must not be obstructed by bedroom furnishings such as a chair. The weights are *not* supported when the bed is moved. The nurse checks the child's toes frequently to see that they are warm and that their color is good. Cyanosis, numbness or irritation from attachments, tight bandages, severe pain, or absence of pulse in the extremities is reported immediately to the nurse

in charge. A specific and serious complication of Bryant traction is *Volkmann's ischemia* (from the Greek *ischein*, to hold back + *haima*, blood), which occurs when the circulation is obstructed. Since the legs are elevated overhead, there is gravitational vascular drainage. Arterial occlusion can cause anoxia of the muscles and reflex vasospasm, which when unnoticed could result in contractures and paralysis. The child is bathed daily, and the back is rubbed frequently to prevent ulceration. The nurse reaches under the patient's body to rub the back and buttocks. A sheepskin or eggcrate padding may also be utilized. The sheets are pulled taut and kept free of crumbs. The jacket restraint is changed when it is soiled.

The child is encouraged to drink lots of fluids and to eat foods that are high in roughage content to prevent constipation due to lack of exercise. Stool softeners may be necessary. A fracture pan is used for bowel movements, and a careful record is kept of eliminations. Deep breathing is encouraged through the use of breathing exercises, blowing bubbles, moving a windmill toy, and so on.

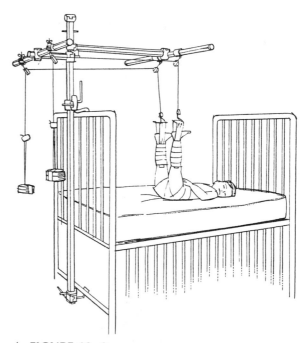

▲ **FIGURE 10–6**

Bryant traction is used for the young child who has a fractured femur. (From Leifer, G. [1982]. *Principles and Techniques in Pediatric Nursing*, 4th ed. Philadelphia, W. B. Saunders Company.)

Diversional therapy is important, as hospitalization lasts for a month or longer. Toys may be suspended over the child's head within reach. Watch for the possibility of strangling from the suspension device. The crib is taken to the playroom when possible, so that the child may take part in the excitement of the activities there. Records, stories, and other forms of entertainment are essential to the total nursing care plan. Parents are encouraged to stay with the child when possible. The prognosis in this condition is good with proper treatment.

Head Injuries

The toddler is famous for the number of blows received to the head. Fortunately, most are not serious, but they are alarming to parents. A *concussion* is a temporary disturbance of the brain that is immediately followed by a period of unconsciousness. It jars the brain stem and is often accompanied by loss of memory with regard to events that occurred immediately prior to (*retrograde amnesia*), during, and after the accident. It is caused by a severe blow to the head and hemorrhage is possible. A *skull fracture* can result from a severe head injury. However, the child's skull is fairly flexible and is able to withstand a great deal of force before the skull is fractured.

After a concussion the child should be observed for signs of intracranial hemorrhage. The child should be checked for pupillary size and reaction to light. Reflexes also should be checked. If the child is alert and the parents are reliable, the child may be sent home with written instructions for observing the child (Table 10–3). The parents are instructed to check the child every 2 hours for any changes in responsiveness. The sleeping child should be awakened to see if he or she can be roused normally.

Complications. The major complications of head injury are hemorrhage, infection, cerebral edema (swelling of the brain), and compression of the brain stem. The brain and its interrelated compartments are tightly confined by the skull. Enlargement of any intracranial component (brain or subarachnoid, venous, or arterial space) may produce *increased intracranial pressure* (ICP), which can lead to permanent brain damage or death. Ag-

Table 10–3. HOME CARE OF A CHILD WITH A MINOR HEAD INJURY

Clean abrasions with soap and water and apply a sterile dressing.
Apply a covered ice pack for 1 hour to decrease swelling.
Give only clear liquids until no vomiting for 6 hours.
Do not give analgesics or anything to sedate the child.
Check reaction of pupils every 4 hours around the clock for 48 hours.
Sleep in room with child during period of observation.
Parents should call their physician if the child
a. vomits more than three times.
b. becomes confused and is acting unusual.
c. has blurred vision or sees double.
d. has difficulty speaking or cannot be roused from sleep.
e. has changes in gait.
f. has pupil changes that include pupils that are dilated or fixed.
g. has headache that increases and interrupts sleep.

gressive medical management, computed tomography (CT) scanning, and intensive therapy to counter intracranial pressure have dramatically altered morbidity and mortality in pediatric head injury (Wisoff and Epstein, 1985).

Frequently, a child who has suffered a blow to the head is brought to the hospital for overnight observation to rule out or confirm the diagnosis. The patient may experience all or some of the following symptoms: headache (manifested by fussiness in the toddler), drowsiness, blurred vision, vomiting, and dyspnea. In severe cases the patient may be completely unconscious. Decerebrate (de + *cerebra*, cerebral cortex) or decorticate posturing may be evident.

A careful history is obtained to determine any pre-existing conditions, and to ascertain the exact circumstances of the accident. Of particular importance is the patient's state of consciousness immediately following the occurrence.

The patients are handled gently and are inspected for injuries to other areas. They are placed in a crib or bed in accordance with size (Fig. 10–7). Siderails are raised as a safety precaution, and seizure precautions are instituted. The room should be quiet and, if the child is restless, the

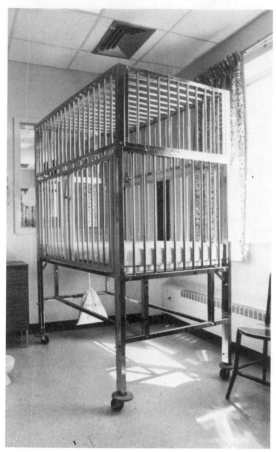

▲ **FIGURE 10–7**

One type of crib used in the hospital to protect toddlers and small children from falls. (Courtesy of St. Joseph's Hospital, School of Practical Nursing, Nashua, New Hampshire.)

siderails should be padded. The head rest is slightly elevated to decrease cerebral edema.

The nurse observes the patient for signs of increasing intracranial pressure. Four components of a cranial or neurological check are (1) *level of consciousness,* (2) *pupil and eye movement,* (3) *vital signs,* and (4) *motor activity.*

Level of Consciousness. Changes in level of consciousness are particularly meaningful and require immediate medical attention. The child's alertness upon admission is recorded for use in baseline data. Response should be correlated with the developmental age of the patient. Parents can be helpful in providing information about the child's usual capabilities. In general, patients should be oriented to person, time, and place (may not be accessible in the toddler). Ask "What is your name?" and "Where are you?" Older children may know the day of the week. The patient should recognize the parents. Point to the mother and ask "Who is this?" The child should be able to follow simple commands such as "turn over." When the patient does not respond to verbal stimuli, pinch the upper arm gently and observe the response. Note the presence or absence of crying or speech. It is not unusual for the child to fall asleep but should be easily aroused. Record changes in sleeping, posture, movements of extremities, and any signs of tremors or restlessness. Observe the bladder for distention, which can contribute to irritability. Incontinence in the child who is toilet trained is significant. Describe behavior in the nurse's notes.

The *Glasgow Coma Scale* (Table 10–4) is valuable in determining various levels of consciousness. It consists of three parts: eye opening, motor response, and verbal response. A numerical value of 1 to 5 is assigned to each part. The lower the score, the deeper the coma. Table 10–5 shows a verbal scale modified for infants.

Pupil and Eye Movement. When observing the patient's eyes, note size, shape, and equality of pupils and their reaction to light and extraocular movements. (Have the patient follow your finger from side to side and up and down to detect movement.) Strabismus, nystagmus, "sunset" eyes, and inability to move eyes in all four quadrants indicate abnormality. The patient should be able to blink the eyes. If intracranial pressure is increasing, pupils will become sluggish to light stimulus, dilated, and eventually fixed.

Vital Signs. Advanced ICP causes an increase in blood pressure, a decrease in pulse, and altered respiratory pattern. This is referred to as the Cushing triad. Temperature is taken rectally because vomiting upon movement is frequently seen. Elevations may be due to inflammation, systemic infection, or damage to the hypothalamus, which regulates body temperature. Body temperature may be reduced by administering antipyretics, giving a sponge bath, or using hypothermia blankets. Mild elevations due to trauma are not uncommon during the first 2 days.

Motor Activity. Because nerves energize the muscle tissue, any damage to the nervous system

Table 10–4. GLASGOW COMA SCALE

	SCORE	
Eyes Opening		**Over 1 Year**
	4	Spontaneously
	3	To verbal command
	2	To pain
	1	No response
Best Motor Response		**Over 1 Year**
	6	Obeys
	5	Localizes pain
	4	Flexion withdrawal
	3	Flexion—abnormal (decorticate rigidity)
	2	Extension (decerebrate rigidity)
	1	No response
Best Verbal Response		**Over 5 Years**
	5	Oriented and converses
	4	Disoriented and converses
	3	Inappropriate words
	2	Incomprehensible sounds
	1	No response
TOTAL	3–15	

will affect body movement. The quality and strength of muscle tone are observed in all four extremities. The patient should be able to squeeze the nurse's hands. The grip should be equal in both hands. The patient should be able to move the legs and push against the examiner's hands with both feet. The face should be symmetrical and the patient can smile and frown. Drooping of the eyes, ptosis, inability to close the eyes tightly, and drooping of the corner of the mouth are considered adverse signs. The patient should be able to raise the arms and extend the palms up and palms down. Abnormal posturing is described and recorded.

Other Nursing Observations. Other factors include examination of wound swelling if a laceration of the head is present. Record the type and amount of drainage from the ears and nose. Check for *nuchal* (Latin *nucha*, back of neck) rigidity, which might indicate infection. Occipital frontal circumference (OFC) should be monitored in infants, as should tension of the fontanels and the presence of a high-pitched cry. Fluids are carefully monitored to control cerebral edema. Overhydration will increase the amount of cerebral fluid.

Feeding difficulties should be noted as the child's diet is increased. Patients are observed for signs of shock, which can also occur. Patients whose condition has remained stable are discharged. Parents are instructed about any additional observations and follow-up care. Post-traumatic epilepsy occurs in about 10 per cent of children with severe head injuries. It usually occurs within 1 year of the injury (Behrman and Vaughan, 1987). More common changes include minor changes in behavior and learning, dizziness, and headache.

Digestive System

PINWORMS

Description. Of the several varieties of worms that affect humans, the most common is the pinworm—*Enterobius vermicularis* (*enteron*, intestine + *bios*, life; *vermis*, wormlike). Pinworms can affect individuals of all ages but are more common in children. Crowded living conditions, institutions (schools and day care centers), and families with

Table 10–5. GLASGOW COMA SCALE (VERBAL RESPONSE, INFANTS)

ONE MONTH
1. None
2. Crying to stimuli
3. Crying spontaneously
4. Blinks when eyelashes touched
5. Throaty noises

TWO MONTHS
1. None
2. Crying to stimuli
3. Shuts eyes to light
4. Smiles when caressed
5. Babbles—single vowel sounds

THREE MONTHS
1. None
2. Crying to stimuli (moans)
3. Stares to response and looks at environment
4. Smiles to sound stimulation
5. Coos, chuckles, *vowels* in a prolonged way

FOUR MONTHS
1. None
2. Crying to stimuli (moans)
3. Turns head to sound
4. Smiles spontaneously or when stimulated, laughs when socially stimulated
5. Modulating voice and perfect vocalization of vowels

FIVE AND SIX MONTHS
1. None
2. Crying to stimuli (moans)
3. Localizes general direction of sound
4. Discriminates family members
5. Babbles to people, toys

SEVEN AND EIGHT MONTHS
1. None
2. Crying to stimuli (moans)
3. ——
4. Recognizes familiar voices and family
4. Babbles
5. "Ba," "Ma," "Da"

NINE AND TEN MONTHS
1. None
2. Crying to stimuli (moans)
3. Recognizes (smiles or laughs)
4. Babbles
5. "MaMa," "DaDa"

ELEVEN AND TWELVE MONTHS
1. None
2. Crying to stimuli (moans)
3. Recognizes—smiles
4. Babbles
5. Words (specifically "Mama" and "Dada")

Courtesy Dr. Kenneth Shapiro, Department of Neurosurgery, Albert Einstein College of Medicine, New York, New York. From Zimmermann, S. S., and Gildea, J. H. (1985). *Critical Care Pediatrics*. Philadelphia, W. B. Saunders Company.

pinworms are factors of high risk. The pinworm looks like a white thread about a third of an inch long. It lives in the lower intestine but comes out of the anus to lay its eggs, generally during the night. These eggs become infective a few hours after they have been deposited. This type of parasite spreads from one person to another, particularly where large groups of children are in close contact. The child infects the self by handling contaminated toys or soiled linen. The route of entry is the mouth. Reinfection takes place by way of the rectum to the fingers to the mouth or by way of the rectum to the clothing to the fingers to the mouth.

Symptoms. The nurse or mother may notice that the child scratches the bottom, may complain of itchiness, and may become irritable and restless. Weight loss, poor appetite, and fretfulness during the night may develop. The rectal area may become irritated from scratching. Worms may be seen on the surface of stools or around the anus. A special pinworm diagnostic tape or paddle or a tongue blade covered with cellophane tape, sticky side out, may be placed against the anal region in an attempt to obtain pinworm eggs. This is done early in the morning or after a period of inactivity. The tape is then put on a glass slide and examined under a microscope. The microscopic eggs are typical.

Treatment and Nursing Care

Several effective anthelmintics are available. Vermox is a single-dose chewable tablet. Antepar, a pleasant-tasting, fruit-colored syrup, is currently popular. Povan suspension, a one-dose treatment, is also effective; nurses should advise parents that Povan stains and will turn the stools red.

If it is determined that a hospitalized child has pinworms, linen and stool precautions are taken. The child must be taught to wash the hands well following bowel movements. The child's fingernails are kept short. A soothing ointment is applied to the rectal area. The patient wears clean underwear that fits snugly. It is changed daily.

All other members of the family are treated for this condition to prevent reinfection. In the home, the toilet seat is scrubbed daily. Underwear and bed linens are washed in hot water. Bed linens are handled carefully to avoid spreading the infec-

tion. The parents are taught the danger of anthelmintic overdosage.

Respiratory System

CROUP

Description. Croup is a nonspecific term applied to a number of conditions, the chief symptom of which is a brassy (croupy) cough and varying degrees of inspiratory stridor. When the larynx is involved, the picture becomes more intense because of possible alterations in respiratory status, e.g., airway obstruction, acute respiratory failure, hypoxia. Acute spasmodic laryngitis is the milder form of the syndrome. Acute laryngotracheobronchitis (LTB) is the most common. It is also referred to as *subglottic croup*, as edema occurs below the vocal cords.

Respiratory infections are common in pediatric patients, especially in children under 5 years of age. Children have smaller air passages than adults do and experience more narrowing with inflammation. Acute infections of the larynx are common in the toddler. Involvement of other parts of the respiratory tract is frequent. A wide variety of organisms cause croup, but most often the infectious agent is a virus. The patient's history is valuable in diagnosis, as there appears to be a familial tendency. Although it can occur at any age, it is most common in children between the ages of 3 months and 3 years.

Signs and Symptoms. Croup usually begins with an upper respiratory infection with or without fever. The child begins to develop hoarseness and a harsh, barking, "croupy" cough. As the subglottic area becomes obstructed due to edema and exudate, the child develops *stridor*, a harsh, high-pitched sound. Cough and stridor are usually worse at night. Although croup is alarming to the child and parents because the child is distressed, most cases are mild and it is not communicable.

Treatment and Nursing Care

Most children can be managed at home. Use of steam from a shower or hot bath in a closed bathroom can often stop the acute respiratory distress and laryngeal spasm. Parents should be instructed to use a cool mist humidifier in the child's room. The vaporizer must be disinfected regularly. Steam vaporizers are usually avoided because of the danger of scalding. Exposure to cold air also relieves stridor. Many a parent has carried a child out into the cold night on the way to the emergency room only to have the child appear quite comfortable when they arrive at the hospital. This may be caused by the cold air being warmed to body temperature and humidified to virtually 100 per cent (Mauro and Poole, 1988). Fluid intake should also be increased.

Children with croup and temperatures over 39°C (102.2°F) should be hospitalized if there is progressive stridor, respiratory distress, or suspected epiglottitis (Behrman and Vaughan, 1987) (Fig. 10–8).

The toddler admitted to the hospital with respiratory distress is anxious and fatigued. The nurse remains calm while preparing the croup tent. Children enjoy special hideaways, and using this tent may appeal to the patient. The nurse also directs attention to the parents, who need reassurance. As the parents become more relaxed, the patient also becomes less apprehensive. Constant attendance is desirable in such cases. Restraining a child who has respiratory distress keeps the patient in one position too long, and complications can develop more easily.

Medications used in the treatment of croup include corticosteroids and racemic epinephrine (Vaponefrin). Although controversy remains about the use of corticosteroids, they have proved helpful in avoiding intubation in seriously ill children. Vaponefrin is inhaled via a face mask. It decreases edema by vasoconstriction and provides immediate relief, although this may be temporary. Vaponefrin may be repeated in several hours if necessary. A single inhaled dose peaks in 10 to 30 minutes, with an overall duration of 2 hours. *Close observation is necessary because some patients may experience a rebound effect and become more obstructed.*

The nurse observes and records temperature, pulse, respirations and blood pressure if ordered. Particular attention is given to the type and rate of respirations. The child's color and degree of restlessness and anxiety are also observed. Respiratory distress should begin to diminish as the child remains in the tent. An increase in respiratory distress is reported immediately, because

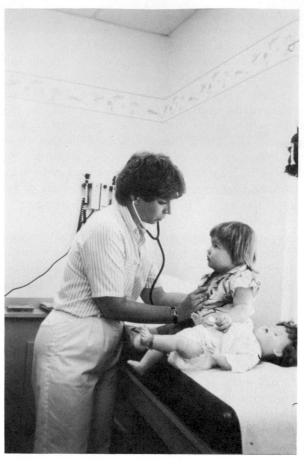

▲ **FIGURE 10–8**

The nurse assesses the child's lung sounds for signs of respiratory distress. (Courtesy of Cook–Fort Worth Children's Hospital, Fort Worth, Texas.)

complications may arise that necessitate endotracheal intubation or *tracheotomy* (trachea + *tomy*, incision of). Specific nursing care is indicated in such cases (see page 57). Intravenous fluids may be started to provide intake and conserve energy. Care should be planned so as to allow time for uninterrupted rest.

EPIGLOTTITIS

Epiglottitis is a swelling of the tissues *above* the vocal cords, i.e., supraglottic. This results in narrowing of the *airway inlet* with the possibility of total obstruction. It is caused by *Haemophilus influenzae* type B (HIB) and occurs most often in the

Table 10–6. ROLE OF THE INTENSIVE CARE UNIT IN A MULTIDISCIPLINARY PROTOCOL FOR EPIGLOTTITIS

Emergency Service

Diagnosis is made clinically and/or radiographically

Child is kept calm, in a comfortable sitting position, with nebulized O_2, if tolerated

Anesthesiology and otolaryngology consultants are assembled in the emergency service, with airway equipment

Child is transported, with consultants, to the operating room

Operating Room

Child is anesthetized with halothane and O_2, and an IV cannula is inserted

The airway is visualized, and an artificial airway is established

The airway is securely taped in place

Blood specimens are drawn, and IV antibiotic therapy is begun

Intensive Care Unit

Self-extubation is prevented by sedating child and splinting both elbows with armboards

After at least 36–48 hours of appropriate antibiotic therapy, the airway is revisualized, preferably in the operating room, and if found to be satisfactorily improved, extubation (or decannulation) is performed. This step can be performed in the ICU, provided that all neccessary personnel and equipment for artificial airway reinsertion, in case that is necessary, are present.

Child is observed in the ICU for 24 hours for development of post-airway edema

When child can take oral antibiotics, therapy is switched to oral for a total of 7–10 days

From Zimmerman, S., and Gildea, J. (eds.) (1985). *Critical Care Pediatrics.* Philadelphia, W. B. Saunders Company.

child from 3 to 6 years of age. It can occur in any season. The course is rapid and progressive. Epiglottitis is a life-threatening medical emergency. Blood gases fluctuate and there is leukocytosis. Bacteremia is often present. *If epiglottitis is suspected, do not examine the pharynx (back of the throat), as laryngospasm may occur followed by respiratory arrest.* The diagnosis can be confirmed by lateral radiograph of the neck. Prophylactic placement of an artificial airway is the treatment of choice, and a skilled endoscopist is required. Nasotracheal intubation is generally selected. Nursing care is given to the critically ill child (Table 10–6).

The HbOC vaccine is a vaccine against *H. influenzae* and can be given at 2 months of age. This should further reduce the incidence of this disease.

PNEUMONIA

Description. Pneumonia or pneumonitis is an inflammation of the lungs in which the *alveoli* (air sacs) become filled with exudate. The affected portion of the lung does not receive enough air. Breathing is shallow. As a result, the blood stream is denied sufficient oxygen.

There are many types of pneumonia (Table 10–7). A text may classify them according to the causative organism, i.e., bacterial and viral; or by the part of the respiratory system involved, i.e., lobar and bronchial; or by various other methods. Respiratory viruses cause a number of cases of pneumonia, particularly in children under 5 years of age. *Staphylococcal pneumonia* is particularly dangerous, since strong strains of this organism do not respond to antibiotic therapy. It may begin as a skin infection in the newborn nursery, pediatric unit, or home. The patient may then carry the germs in the nasal passages until a later date, when the child or a close associate contracts the disease. *Immunocompromised* children frequently develop pneumonia caused by gram-negative organisms, such as *Pneumocystis carinii* and fungi.

Toddlers frequently aspirate small objects such as peanuts or popcorn and develop pneumonia as a result; therefore, such foods are to be discouraged for this age group. The toddler who drinks kerosene may also develop a type of pneumonia. *Hypostatic pneumonia* occurs in older patients who have poor circulation in their lungs and remain in one position too long. The child recovering from anesthesia also needs to be turned frequently to

Table 10–7. SUMMARY OF TYPES OF PNEUMONIA IN CHILDREN

Organism	Age	Comment
BACTERIAL		
Pneumococcal	First 4 years (peak), occurs also in older children and adolescents	Most common bacterial pathogen, occurs late winter to early spring *Pneumococcal vaccine* now licensed for high-risk children over 2 years
Group A streptococcal	3–5 years	Less frequent
Group B streptococcal	Neonates	Leading cause of septicemia and meningitis in newborn infants
Staphylococcal	Neonates, infants	Transmitted primarily by direct contact; pay strict *attention to handwashing*; most serious, rapid progression
Haemophilus influenzae (type B)	Infants, young children under 5 years	Occurs more often in boys Complications frequent (bacteremia, pericarditis, meningitis, others) Vaccine now available for children at 2 months
Mycobacterium tuberculosis	More severe in younger child	Continues to be important owing to immigrant flux, poverty
VIRAL		
Respiratory syncytial virus (RSV)	More serious in infants	Responsible for the largest percentage of cases
Other		
Influenza virus		Less common
Adenovirus		
MISCELLANEOUS		
Pneumocystis carinii	Infants 3–5 weeks Immunocompromised children	Being seen as more children with malignancies are surviving; immunodeficiency diseases (especially under 1 year)
Mycoplasma pneumoniae	School age children Adolescents Young adults	More common in fall and winter Crowded conditions
Aspiration	Infants Toddlers	Avoid feedings that overdistend the stomach, particularly in gavage-fed infants Gastroesophageal reflux (GER) occurs in some babies Inhaled foreign bodies occlude airways Many chemicals (kerosene, gasoline, etc.) cause edema, inflammation
Hypostatic	Immobile child of any age	Prevention is highly important (turn, cough, deep breathe)

stimulate the circulation through the lungs. Early ambulation will also accomplish this.

Pneumonia may occur as the initial or *primary* disease, or it may complicate another illness, in which case it is termed *secondary* pneumonia. Secondary pneumonia may accompany various communicable diseases or may follow surgery. It is more serious than primary pneumonia since the patient is already weak.

Symptoms. The symptoms of pneumonia vary with the age of the patient and the causative organism. They may develop suddenly or be preceded by an upper respiratory tract infection. The cough is dry at first, but gradually becomes productive. Fever rises as high as 39.5 to 40°C (103 to 104°F) and may fluctuate widely during a 24-hour period. The respiration rate may increase to 40 to 80 times per minute in infants, and in older children to 30 to 50 times per minute. Respirations are shallow in an attempt to reduce the amount of chest pain. Sternal retractions may be seen as the assisting muscles of respiration are brought into use. Flaring of the nostrils may appear. The child is listless and has a poor appetite. The patient tends to lie on the affected side.

Treatment

The patient is given a complete physical examination. A tuberculosis skin test is administered as indicated. The doctor pays particular attention to the examination of the child's chest. Radiographs will confirm the diagnosis and determine whether there are complications. A differential white blood cell count is routinely done. Blood specimens show a marked increase in the number of white blood cells (16,000 to 40,000 per cu mm). The number of red blood cells and the amount of hemoglobin may be slightly reduced. The urine is dark amber in color, and there is a decrease in the amount voided. The specific gravity is high. Cultures may be taken from the nose and throat. Tracheal cultures may also be indicated (Fig. 10–9).

Treatment depends upon the severity of the disease and the causative organism. Bacterial pneumonia is treated with antibiotics. Treatment for viral pneumonia is supportive, except in cases of severe RSV infection, at which time ribavirin is given. Antipyretics are given to reduce fever.

Oxygen is administered for dyspnea or cyanosis. When this treatment is begun early, the child is less restless and does not require as many sedatives or drugs to relieve pain. Since drug therapy has become so effective, many uncomplicated cases can be treated at home. Increased fluids are important, particularly clear fluids and "flattened" soft drinks.

Nursing Care

Nursing care in all types of pneumonia is basically the same. The age of the patient determines the nurse's approach and the type of equipment used. (The newborn infant receives oxygen in the Isolette, whereas the older child requires a Croupette or a larger tent.) The child's clothing and bedclothes should be changed if they become damp from the moisture in the tent.

Rest is an important part of the treatment of this disease. The nurse must organize work so the child is not disturbed unnecessarily.

The nurse checks the vital signs at regular intervals. During the acute stages, the temperature may rise as high as 39.5 to 40°C (103 to 104°F). When a child is flushed with fever, *remove heavy clothing and blankets*. The nurse may be asked to give the child tepid sponge baths to help reduce this fever (this procedure is presented on page 39). Smaller children are bathed in a tub or basin. The nurse offers the older patient the bedpan before the procedure is begun.

Intravenous fluids may be given during the acute stage. When oral fluids are begun, small amounts are given slowly. Besides water, the child may be offered Gatorade, juices, or popsicles. The appetite of the child improves as the condition does.

The patient is repositioned frequently. Although this is painful, it is paramount to total recovery. The child will probably prefer the affected side (if pneumonia is unilateral) because it splints the chest on that side and therefore decreases the discomfort. The doctor will prescribe an analgesic to increase the patient's comfort. The nurse assists and encourages the patient to walk about the room and in the hallways when such activity is prescribed. Small children can exercise their lungs by blowing bubbles through a straw. The respiratory

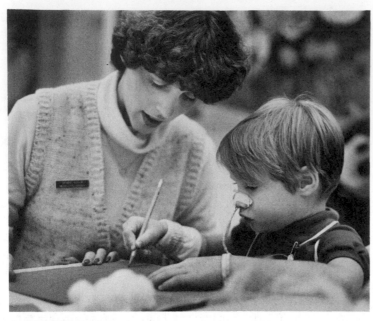

▲ FIGURE 10–9

Planned quiet activities aid the hospitalized child in gaining mastery and control following invasive procedures. (Courtesy of Blank Memorial Hospital for Children, Des Moines, Iowa.)

therapist may provide chest clapping and postural drainage exercise.

The nurse observes the patient for unfavorable symptoms such as a weak, rapid pulse; cyanosis; abdominal distention; constipation; and change in level of consciousness. Although recovery from uncomplicated pneumonia is dramatic today, recuperation takes time. Upon their child's discharge from the hospital, parents should receive written instructions concerning diet, activity, medication, return appointments, and so on. It is helpful if the parents repeat these instructions to the nurse to determine whether they have interpreted them correctly.

Urinary System

NEPHROTIC SYNDROME (NEPHROSIS)

Description. *Nephrotic syndrome* refers to a number of different types of kidney conditions that are distinguished by the presence of marked amounts of protein in the urine. *Nephrosis*, a minimal lesion form, is discussed here.

Nephrosis is more common in boys than in girls and is seen most often in children between 2 and 7 years of age. The cause is not known. The prognosis of children with nephrosis is usually very positive. The large majority of children will have repeated relapses until the disease resolves itself. Children with types other than minimal change nephrotic syndrome do not have as good a prognosis. They may develop renal failure and require dialysis or transplantation.

Symptoms. The characteristic symptom of nephrosis is *edema*. This occurs slowly; the child does not appear to be sick. It is noticed at first about the eyes and ankles, but later becomes generalized. The edema shifts with the position of the child during sleep. The patient gains weight because of the accumulation of this fluid. The abdomen may become so distended that *striae*, or stretch marks similar to those that appear on the skin of a pregnant woman, may occur. The child is pale, irritable and listless and has a poor appetite. Urine examination reveals albumin. The *glo-*

meruli, the working units of the kidneys that filter the blood, become damaged and allow albumin and blood cells to enter the urine. There is a fall in the level of protein in the blood, termed *hypoalbuminemia*, and a rise in cholesterol content, termed *hyperlipidemia* (*hyper*, above + *lipos*, fat + *emia*, blood). Vomiting and diarrhea may also be present. Renal biopsy and the examination of the tissue under the light and electron microscopes provide valuable information.

Treatment

Control of Edema. Steroid therapy is initiated to induce diuresis. Prednisone is safest, cheapest, and the drug of choice. When the urine is free of protein for more than 5 days, the child is put on an every-other-day dose of prednisone for approximately 3 to 6 months (Behrman and Vaughan, 1987). Since hormones mask the signs of infection, the patient must be watched closely for more subtle symptoms of illness. Study blood reports carefully. Children are prone to infection when absolute granulocyte counts fall below 1000 cells per cu mm. This is called *neutropenia*. Examine the child's skin at sites of punctures, wounds, pierced ears, catheters, and so on. Watch for temperature variations and changes in behavior. Report suspicions promptly, as septicemia is life-threatening. Prompt antibacterial therapy is begun when an acute infection is recognized. Diuretics have not generally been effective in reducing nephrotic edema. Immunosuppressive therapy (i.e., Cytoxan, chlorambucil) has shown promise for some steroid-resistant children.

Diet. A well-balanced diet high in protein is desirable because protein is constantly being lost in the urine. The carbohydrate and fat content of the diet should be high enough to prevent protein from being used for energy. If either dietary protein or body protein is used for energy, the waste product urea is excreted through the kidneys, which increases their workload. Low sodium diets may be ordered for short periods during the course of the disease, but they are generally not appealing to the child. Normal amounts of water are given unless otherwise ordered.

Ascites. *Ascites*, an abnormal collection of fluid in the peritoneal cavity, is seen in advanced cases of nephrosis. This fluid causes pressure on the heart and the organs of respiration. The doctor removes some of this fluid by a procedure known as an *abdominal paracentesis* (*para*, beside + *kentésis*, puncture). Fluid may also accumulate in the chest. This is termed hydrothorax (*hydro*, water + *thorax*, chest). The procedure used to remove fluid from the chest is called *thoracentesis* (*thorax*, chest + *kentésis*). The advent of corticosteroid diuresis has greatly reduced the need for these procedures.

Mental Hygiene. The doctor gives supportive care to the parents and child through the long course of this disease. Whenever possible the child is treated at home and brought to the hospital for special therapy only. Parents are instructed to keep a daily record of the child's weight, urinary proteins, and medications. Signs of infection, such as abnormal weight gain, and increased protein in the urine must be reported promptly. The child is allowed to be up and about after the acute stage of the illness subsides to participate in normal childhood activities.

Nursing Care

The nursing care of the patient with nephrosis is of the greatest significance because this disease is one that requires long-term therapy. The patient is hospitalized periodically and becomes a familiar personality to hospital personnel. The following factors are important in determining nursing care plans for the individual child.

Care of the Skin. Good skin care is especially important during periods of marked edema. The skin is bathed daily and whenever necessary. Special attention is given to the neck, underarms, groin, and other moist areas of the body. The patient is handled gently to prevent the skin from being injured. The male genitals may become edematous; they are bathed, and an antiseptic powder is applied. When necessary, the scrotum is supported with a soft pad held in place by a T binder. Cotton is used to separate the skin surfaces to prevent a rash from forming. Children who are not potty trained require meticulous care of the diaper area because urine acidity predisposes to breakdown of the skin.

Position. The patient is repositioned frequently to prevent respiratory infection. A pillow placed between the knees when the patient is lying on the side prevents pressure on edematous organs. The child's head is elevated from time to time during the day to reduce edema of the eyelids and to make the patient more comfortable. Swelling impairs the circulation of the lacrimal secretions. It may therefore be necessary to bathe the eyes to prevent the accumulation of exudate.

Diet. The appetite of the patient is poor. Serve small quantities of food, attractively arranged on brightly colored dishes. Colored straws may also be used. Serve favorite foods if they are nutritious. Sit by the patient during the feeding. Relax and allow plenty of time. If the child is able to feed the self, encourage this. Whenever possible, remain with the patient during meals, for it is more enjoyable for the patient, particularly if in a private room. If the parents are available, the child can enjoy their company during meals.

The child will be on strict intake and output charting. All intake and output must be recorded. The nurse should remember that the parents may be doing much of the feeding and caring for the child, and important information about intake and output will be lost if the parents are not informed. The importance of keeping *proper fluid balance sheets* (i.e., *intake and output records*) for patients with diseases of the kidneys cannot be overemphasized.

Urine. As stated previously, the patient's urine must be carefully measured. This is difficult with the toddler who is not toilet trained or who has had a regression in urinary habits. Diapers may be weighed on a gram scale before applying and after removal (1 g = 1 ml). Mark the weights on the diaper. A careful check of the number of voidings is of particular value. The character, odor, and color of the urine are also important.

Specific gravity of the urine is measured, and the urine is also examined for albumin—that is, protein. Normally little or no albumin is found in the urine of a healthy child. Reagent strips especially intended for this purpose are available. The nurse dips the end of the strip into urine and compares it with a special color chart. Specific instructions accompany test materials.

Additional Nursing Care. The patient is weighed daily to determine changes in the degree of edema. The child is weighed on the same scale each time and at about the same time of day.

Abdominal girth (circumference) should also be measured every day.

Nurses make every effort to protect the patients from exposure to upper respiratory tract infections. They wash hands carefully before caring for them. Children who are up and about must not be allowed to wander into areas where they would be in danger of contracting an infection. *No vaccinations or immunizations should be administered while the disease is active and during immunosuppressive therapy.*

The vital signs of a patient with nephrosis are taken regularly. Ordinarily, there is no elevation of temperature unless an infection is present. Blood pressure remains normal. An increase in blood pressure must be reported. A reading that remains high over a period of time is a grave sign.

Parental guidance and support should be given by all members of the nursing team. Family education about weighing, measuring abdominal girth, and determining urinary specific gravity and urinary albumin is necessary. Rooming-in is encouraged when possible. The parents should be allowed to visit the patient as often as they can. The child with nephrosis is kept under close medical supervision over an extended period. Prognosis is considered favorable but is dependent on the patient's response to drug therapy.

WILMS TUMOR

Description. Wilms tumor, or nephroblastoma (*nephro*, kidney + *blasto*, bud + *oma*, tumor), is one of the most common malignancies of early life. It is an embryonal adenosarcoma (*adeno*, glandular + *sarcoma*, cancer of connective tissue) that is now known to be associated with certain congenital anomalies, particularly of the genitourinary tract. During the early stages of growth, as with some other malignancies, there are few or no symptoms. About two thirds of these growths occur before the child is 3 years old. A mass in the abdomen is discovered generally by the mother or by the physician during a routine checkup. X-ray films of the kidneys (most importantly intravenous pyelograms) indicate a growth and verify the fact that the remaining kidney is normal. Chest radiograph, ultrasonography, bone surveys, liver scan, and computed tomography also may be indicated. Wilms tumor seldom affects both kidneys.

Treatment and Nursing Care

The treatment consists of a combination of surgery, radiation therapy, and chemotherapy. The kidney and tumor are removed as soon as possible after the diagnosis has been confirmed. It is important to prepare the parents and the child for the extent of the incision, which is considerable. The National Wilms' Tumor Study lists several categories of effective treatment. Five states of tumor activity are cited, and appropriate refinements in radiation therapy and chemotherapy are suggested. Children with localized tumors (stage I and stage II) stand a 90 per cent chance of cure. Prognosis also depends on the histological character of the tumor and evidence of recurrence. Patients younger than 2 years of age have a higher response to therapy.

General nursing measures for the comfort of the patient are accomplished. When the diagnosis of Wilms tumor has been made or is suspected, the abdomen should not be palpated. This is explained to the parents, and a sign is placed on the crib or child—"Do not palpate abdomen." The nurse must consider this extremely important. Drugs and irradiation may cause toxic reactions such as nausea, vomiting, anorexia, and general malaise. Ulceration of the mouth, hair loss, and peeling of the skin may also be seen. The student should anticipate such problems and should immediately report their appearance to the team leader or the nurse in charge of the unit.

The lungs are the most common site of metastasis for this disease. Observations of bloody urine, elevated blood pressure, and symptoms of infection, especially during chemotherapy, should be reported immediately. Helping the family and patient face the possibility of a fatal illness is discussed on page 70.

The Ear

DEAFNESS

Description. Deaf children present special challenges to the nursing team. They may be hospitalized for direct evaluation and treatment of hearing loss, or they may have other medical or surgical problems that are or are not related to the deafness. The student should have a basic knowledge of the problems that confront deaf children in order to give them comprehensive nursing care.

The inner ear is fully formed during the first months of prenatal life. If an expectant mother contracts German measles or another virus infection during this period, the child may be born with a hearing loss, which is termed *congenital deafness*. Deafness can also be *acquired*. Infectious diseases such as measles, mumps, chickenpox, or meningitis can result in various degrees of hearing loss. The common cold, some medications, certain allergies, and ear infections may also be responsible. Deafness also can be temporary owing to wax accumulation.

The old adage "An ounce of prevention is worth a pound of cure" is particularly applicable to the invisible handicap, deafness. Excessive cleansing of the ear can be damaging, especially if one probes into the canal with objects such as a hairpin. If a foreign object is trapped in the ear, consult a doctor. Trying to remove it yourself may cause further damage.

The nurse must stress the importance of proper immunization during childhood to prevent many of the communicable diseases. Vaccines against measles (rubeola), mumps, and German measles (rubella) are now available. The child should be taken to the doctor for periodic health examinations. Early diagnosis and treatment of the deaf child are important to prevent adverse physical and mental complications from developing. Members of the health team concerned with the child who is hard of hearing include the physician, otologist, audiologist, speech therapist, specially trained teacher, social worker, psychologist, nurse, and the child's family.

The various degrees of deafness range from complete bilateral hearing loss to a loss so mild that the problem is never discovered. *Bilateral* deafness affects both ears. If this is complete, the child misses all the pleasures that sound brings to life and has difficulty in communication, since children learn to talk through imitating what they hear. Behavior problems arise because the children do not understand directions. They may become aggressive with other children in their attempts to communicate with them. If they are ridiculed by playmates, their personality development will be affected. Unless helped, they will become socially isolated and unable to attend school.

Partial bilateral deafness may be responsible for behavior problems and poor progress in school. This may be caused by chronic infections such as otitis media or by blockage of the eustachian tube. It may be a warning signal of more serious defects in later life. Children who are deaf in one ear are less handicapped if the hearing in the other ear is normal.

Treatment and Nursing Care

Early diagnosis and prompt treatment are primary requisites, regardless of the patient's age. The use of *evoked response audiometry* permits testing of neonates and other children who cannot be tested otherwise. Complete bilateral deafness is usually discovered during infancy. Partial deafness may be unrecognized until the child begins school. Many hearing problems are detected then by the use of standard hearing tests. A machine called an *audiometer* is used. The child puts on an earphone that is connected to the audiometer. When the audiometer is turned on, it makes various noises and pitches of sound. The child raises the hand upon hearing the tones. The results of these tests are interpreted by specialists in this field. Children who are found to have a hearing loss are referred to an otologist (ear specialist). A child should be screened two times before a referral is made to avoid unnecessary referrals.

Children who suffer a severe loss of hearing need more extensive help from personnel at special hearing and speech centers. Whether the child should be placed in special classes in a regular school or attend a school for the deaf is decided on an individual basis. Some children who spend a few years in a school for the deaf can be advanced to a regular school. These children need to begin their education early, to aid them in catching up on what they have missed since infancy.

Various methods are used to bring the child into the world of sound. Lip reading, sign language, writing, visual aids, music, and amplified sound are but a few examples. Today, the deaf child is taught to speak so that others in the environment can comprehend. This is not accomplished over-

night. If a hearing aid is indicated, the child is equipped with one and taught how to use it. Regular checkups assure that the aid is working properly. A malfunctioning hearing aid may cause a child to lose interest in its use. The parents are instructed in means of communication that will coincide with those used by the teachers. New surgical procedures with implants are also being utilized successfully.

Role of the Nurse. The nurse must be aware of the symptoms of deafness in the child. Neonates are observed for their response to auditory stimuli. The Brazelton Neonatal Behavioral Assessment Scale evaluates the infant's orientation response to the sound of a voice. Persistence of the Moro reflex beyond 4 months may also be an indication of deafness. The infant who makes no verbal attempts by the 18th month of life should undergo a complete physical examination. Indifference to sound, behavior problems and, later, poor school performance may also be signs of deafness.

Since the prevention of this disorder is so important, the nurse should take advantage of opportunities to demonstrate and teach proper hygiene of the ears to the child and family. Stress the importance of infant immunization to parents with newborn babies. Proper safety measures must be taken to prevent injury to the ears from trauma to the head, especially during the toddler period. Mothers are instructed to avoid *ototoxic* drugs during pregnancy. Nurses should maintain a high index of suspicion in chronically ill children who may be on medications such as streptomycin, kanamycin, neomycin, and others. Sensorineural hearing loss also can be caused by noise pollution such as loud rock music or target shooting. Symptoms include buzzing of the ears and muffled dull sounds immediately following exposure.

The deaf child in the hospital needs the same opportunities to develop a healthy personality as does the child who does not have this handicap. When nurses approach a deaf child, they should smile. Their manner relates many things to this patient, especially if there is a severe communication problem. Face the child when you speak, and position yourself so that you are at eye level. Use short sentences rather than separate words. Speak clearly in a natural tone. It is not necessary to exaggerate speech. The nurse who is relaxed in manner with the patient will create an atmosphere that others will follow.

The older child who is able to write can use this as a means of communication. Have the patient read aloud what has been written. In this way you will become better accustomed to the child's speech. Regression in speech patterns may occur during hospitalization. Do not assume that because a child is not talking a great deal he or she does not understand what is being said. Repeat or reword certain statements as you would with any child.

Determine whether or not deaf patients fully understand what you ask of them. Deaf people tend to answer "yes" or "no" before they have caught the complete meaning of a question. When you have finished explaining a procedure to patients, question them to be sure that they understand what is expected of them. This is a good point to bear in mind in relation to all small children who are in the hospital. Children respond to nurses who are interested and patient enough to listen to what they say.

The nurse is often called upon to assist the physician in an ear examination. Hold a toddler in your lap with the head pressed against your chest. Place one hand on the child's forehead and the other securely around the body. The head is held still so that the delicate ear canal will not be injured by the *otoscope*. The doctor may need cotton swabs to remove excess secretions from the external ear. The ear *speculum* (a funnel-shaped device that comes in direct contact with the ear) must be washed and disinfected following each use.

A hearing aid is expensive and invaluable to the patient. See that it is put in a safe place when it is not in use. When the patient goes to surgery it should be placed in the hospital safe. Check the pockets of hospital gowns before putting them in the laundry chute. Sometimes a patient puts a hearing aid there for convenience. The nurse can gain valuable information concerning the use of the particular hearing aid from the parents of the child.

Poisoning

Specific poisons of pediatric concern are listed in Table 10–8.

Prevention. Nurses play a major role in the prevention of poisoning in children. As nurses use their knowledge of growth and development in teaching anticipatory guidance, they must focus the attention of the parent on the dangers of each age. Children are naturally curious, and as they become mobile they can climb and reach any hiding place and open almost any bottle. Parents are encouraged to have the poison control center telephone number posted in a prominent place. The use of safety caps has been effective in reducing the number of ingestions. Detailed coverage of prevention in poisoning is found in the individual chapters on growth and development.

Emergency Care (see Table 10–9). Most poisonings can be managed in the home. Certain steps should be taken when a poisoning victim has been identified. The nurse initially assesses the child for any signs of either impending or current respiratory or cardiac distress. Cardiorespiratory support is initiated if needed. The poison must be removed through the use of syrup of ipecac, gastric lavage, activated charcoal, or all three. Induction of vomiting is contraindicated when corrosives or hydrocarbons have been ingested or if the child is comatose. Specific antidotes may be used in some poisonings (such as acetaminophen).

The Family. The nurse should give special attention to the family. The parents may feel guilty and blame themselves for the child's condition. The nurse must not reinforce this belief through either verbal or nonverbal communication. The parents should be kept informed about their child's condition, allowed to be with the child if at all possible, and given a chance to vent their feelings. The nurse should listen and support them through this difficult period. Preventive teaching should not be done until the acute stage has passed.

ACETAMINOPHEN POISONING

Description. Acetaminophen (Tylenol) has become the most common drug poisoning in children. As aspirin is used less frequently, mainly because of the link with Reye syndrome, acetaminophen has replaced it in the home medicine cabinet. Consequently children are ingesting this medication. Acetaminophen poisoning occurs from acute ingestion, not long-term overdose as may be seen in aspirin toxicity. Acetaminophen is metabolized in the liver. Therefore, hepatic dam-

Table 10–8. SUMMARY OF SPECIFIC POISONS OF CONCERN IN PEDIATRICS

ACIDS
Toilet bowl cleaners
Swimming pool pH adjustment solutions
Concentrated acids in hardware and paint stores

ALKALIES
Clinitest tablets
Drain cleaning crystals
Dishwasher soaps
Industrial cleaners (brought home in unlabeled
   containers)

MEDICATIONS
Diet pills
Sleeping pills
Sedatives
Cold remedies
Birth control pills
Vitamin supplements, iron
Diarrhea remedies (Lomotil)
Menstrual pain relievers
Antipyretics (aspirin, acetaminophen)
Oil of wintergreen
Camphorated oil

CYANIDE
Pesticides
Metal polishers
Photographic solutions
Fumigating products

ETHANOL
Alcoholic beverages
Cold remedies
Perfumes
Mouth wash
Aftershave lotions

PETROLEUM DISTILLATES
Heavy greases, oils,
Turpentine
Furniture polishes
Gasoline, kerosene
Lighter fluid

INSECTICIDES
Home gardening products
Recently sprayed lawns

CARBON MONOXIDE
Accidental
Suicidal

LEAD
Paint
Air
Food
Ant poison
Unglazed pottery
Colored news print
Curtain weights
Fishing sinkers
Lead water pipes
Acid juices in leaded pottery

ARTHROPODS, INSECT STINGS
Spiders (brown recluse, black
   widow)
Certain scorpions
Insects (bees, wasps, hornets)

SNAKES
Rattlesnakes
Moccasins
Copperheads
Others

POISONOUS PLANTS
Boston ivy
Split leaf philodendron
Umbrella plant
Azalea
Daffodil
Foxglove
Mistletoe
Tulip
Others

Data from Gellis, S., and Kagan, B. (1990). *Current Pediatric Therapy.* Philadelphia, W. B. Saunders Company, and other sources.

Table 10–9. ACUTE POISONING—NURSING ALERT

Anticipate. Removal of poison (lavage, ipecac, activated charcoal)
CNS: restlessness, agitation, seizures, coma
Respiratory: airway obstruction, hypoventilation, hypoxia, oxygen therapy, respiratory arrest, CPR (keep artificial airway handy), chemical pneumonitis
Cardiovascular: difficulties with electrolytes, BUN, creatinine, glucose; need for ECG monitor
Gastrointestinal: difficulty swallowing, abdominal pain, possible gastrostomy
Kidneys: urine specific gravity, intake and output, IVs
Methods to increase elimination: cathartic, forced diuresis, dialysis, hemoperfusion
Hypo- or hyperthermia: sponge baths, cooling blanket
Child: physical and psychological crises
Parents: guilt, anger, family dysfunction

age is the major concern. Children under 6 years of age are much less likely to develop significant toxicity than are older children and adults (Behrman and Vaughan, 1987).

Signs and Symptoms. Four stages occur in the clinical course of acetaminophen poisoning (Table 10–10). Signs and symptoms may be vague and diagnosis may be delayed. Most children will recover if treated promptly and correctly. Death may result if treatment is delayed in severe overdosage.

Treatment and Nursing Care

The stomach is emptied by lavage or induced emesis from syrup of ipecac. N-acetylcysteine (Mu-comyst) is the antidote and is given depending upon the serum acetaminophen level. Active charcoal absorbs acetaminophen but should not be given if Mucomyst is used because it will bind the Mucomyst and make the antidote ineffective.

If the antidote is given, the nurse assists and supports the child in taking the offensive smelling Mucomyst (it smells like rotten eggs). It may be given by nasogastric tube or mixed with a carbonated drink. Vital signs are monitored, intake and output are observed and recorded, and laboratory work is monitored and reported if abnormal.

SALICYLATE POISONING

Description. Although the incidence of aspirin ingestion has decreased as the use of acetamino-

Table 10–10. STAGES IN THE CLINICAL COURSE OF ACETAMINOPHEN TOXICITY

STAGE	TIME FOLLOWING INGESTION	CHARACTERISTICS
I	0.5–24 hr	Anorexia, nausea, vomiting, malaise, pallor, diaphoresis
II	24–48 hr	Resolution of above; upper quadrant abdominal pain and tenderness; elevated bilirubin, prothrombin time, hepatic enzymes; oliguria
III	72–96 hr	Peak liver function abnormalities; anorexia, nausea, vomiting, malaise may reappear
IV	4 days–2 wk	Resolution of hepatic dysfunction

From Behrman, R., and Victor, V. (1987). *Nelson Textbook of Pediatrics*, 13th ed. Philadelphia, W. B. Saunders Company, p. 1497.

phen has increased, it is still a problem. Aspirin is used in most homes and often is stored carelessly on bedside stands or in mother's purse. This drug acts rapidly but is excreted slowly. Ingestion of 50 mg/kg will cause symptoms. Although aspirin overdoses are usually acute, they can also occur because of repeated small therapeutic doses. Salicylates are also an ingredient in some over-the-counter antihistamines and decongestants. Parents should be taught to read the labels and to use caution when giving these drugs in combination with aspirin.

Oil of wintergreen (methyl salicylate) is also extremely hazardous when mistakenly administered as cough medicine or swallowed by the curious child. It is sometimes used as a home remedy for arthritic pains. Even a dose as small as 1 teaspoon can cause the death of a child.

Symptoms. The symptoms of salicylate poisoning are varied. The peak action occurs about 2 hours after a single toxic dose. *In general, the younger the child, the more serious the overdose.* Mild poisoning may consist of ringing in the ears, dizziness, anorexia, sweating, nausea, vomiting, and diarrhea. *Hyperpnea* (*hyper*, above + *pnea*, breathing) is an early symptom of more serious trouble. The patient's respirations are faster and deeper than usual, much like the breathing evidenced after one exercises. This is because the respiratory center is stimulated by the drug. When carbon dioxide is eliminated, respiratory alkalosis quickly follows. Dehydration, metabolic acidosis, high fever, convulsions, and coma may follow. Bleeding is sometimes seen, since excessive levels of aspirin inhibit the formation of prothrombin, which is necessary for normal blood clotting. Hypokalemia often accompanies this condition because salicylates directly affect the renal tubular mechanism.

Treatment and Nursing Care

There is no specific antidote for salicylate poisoning; therefore, treatment is aimed at relieving the patient's symptoms. In mild cases of poisoning, the drug is discontinued and fluids are forced. When a child has swallowed an unspecified amount, gastric lavage is performed. A blood sample is taken to detect the level of salicylate poisoning. A positive ferric chloride urine test result is also highly indicative of poisoning. The doctor may request that the child be admitted to the hospital for observation. A sponge bath may be given to reduce fever. The patient's vital signs are closely observed and recorded. The nurse also determines the pH of the urine. When intravenous fluids are necessary to correct electrolyte imbalance and rid the body of toxins, the child's intake and output of fluid are charted hourly.

Vitamin K may be administered to correct bleeding tendencies. Sodium bicarbonate may be infused to promote excretion of salicylate through the urine. In severe cases, when the child does not respond to more conventional treatment, peritoneal dialysis, exchange transfusion, or hemodialysis may be used.

The nurse assists in monitoring the condition of the patient. Vital signs, intake and output, and the intravenous infusion are monitored closely. Sponging or cooling blankets may be used for the child with an uncontrolled fever. Seizure precautions are implemented. As with acetaminophen poisoning, the psychological needs of the family are a top priority.

LEAD POISONING (PLUMBISM)

Description. Lead poisoning results when a child repeatedly ingests or absorbs substances containing lead. The Agency for Toxic Substances and Disease Registry (ATSDR) (1990) reported that the major environmental sources of lead poisoning are paint, auto exhaust, food, and water. This includes ingestion of chips from lead-painted surfaces, inhalation of lead from automobile emissions, food from lead-soldered cans, drinking from lead-soldered plumbing, and medications in the form of folk remedies. The ATSDR (1990) noted that no economic or racial subgroup of children is free from the risk of having blood levels high enough to cause adverse health effects. However, the highest prevalence is among inner city, underprivileged children who live in deteriorating pre-1970s housing containing lead-paint surfaces.

Lead poisoning is more common in the summer months. The children chew on window sills and stair rails. They ingest flakes of paint, putty, or crumbled plaster. Food, particularly fruit juices

Table 10–11. CONTINUUM OF SIGNS AND SYMPTOMS ASSOCIATED WITH LEAD TOXICITY

MILD TOXICITY	MODERATE TOXICITY	SEVERE TOXICITY
Myalgia or paresthesia	Arthralgia	Paresis or paralysis
Mild fatigue	General fatigue	Encephalopathy—may abruptly lead to seizures, changes in consciousness, coma, and death
Irritability	Difficulty concentrating	Lead line (blue-black) on gingival tissue
Lethargy	Muscular exhaustibility	Colic (intermittent, severe abdominal cramps)
Occasional abdominal discomfort	Tremor	
	Headache	
	Diffuse abdominal pain	
	Vomiting	
	Weight loss	
	Constipation	

From Agency for Toxic Substances and Disease Registry (1990). *Case Studies in Environmental Medicine: Lead Toxicity.* Atlanta, U.S. Department of Health and Human Services.

consumed from improperly glazed earthenware, is another source. Lead poisoning among Mexican-Americans may be due to azarcon, a bright orange powder containing approximately 93.5 per cent lead.

Signs and Symptoms. Signs and symptoms occur gradually and vary among children. As exposure increases, the child's blood and urine can be expected to increase in toxicity. Table 10–11 shows the signs and symptoms associated with the degrees of lead toxicity.

Treatment, Nursing Care, and Education of Parents

Blood and urine tests are performed to determine the amount of lead in the system. Lead is especially toxic to the synthesis of *heme* in the blood, which is necessary for hemoglobin formation, and to the functioning of renal tubules. The free erythrocyte protoporphyrin (FEP) and blood lead concentration tests are definitive. X-ray studies of the long bones show further deposits of lead. The history of the patient may reveal *pica.* This is a condition in which a child has a perverted appetite, eating a variety of things that most persons consider unpalatable, e.g., sand, grass, wool, glass, plaster, coal, animal droppings, and paint

from furniture. This tendency is sometimes seen in neurotic children and is common in the mentally retarded. An underlying nutritional disturbance and family dysfunction may also account for it.

Treatment is aimed at reducing the concentration of lead in the tissues and blood. First, the child is removed from the source of lead and is closely supervised. Family members should also be tested. In asymptomatic children with low toxicity levels, removal from the source may be the only treatment needed. Chelating agents which render the lead nontoxic and excrete it in the urine are given. All chelating agents can have potentially serious side effects. Calcium disodium edetate (CaEDTA) and British anti-lewisite (BAL) are the two most commonly used drugs. CaEDTA may be given either by deep intramuscular injection or by intravenous drip. BAL is given by deep intramuscular injection. D-Penicillamine is the only oral chelating agent, but it is still considered experimental for use in lead poisoning (ATSDR, 1990). The child may need repeated courses of chelating therapy before normal iron levels return.

The prognosis depends upon the degree and duration of the lead ingestion. Some children will not have any residual effects, and others may have severe encephalopathy. Fifty or more per cent of the survivors of encephalopathy treated *after* the onset of symptoms have severe, permanent brain damage (Behrman and Vaughan, 1987).

The nurse stresses the importance of continued treatment to prevent recurrence of lead poisoning symptoms. Infectious disease in these youngsters must be treated promptly to avoid reactivation of the process. Parents are taught to be suspicious of changes in the disposition of their child. Siblings and playmates should also be screened. All residents should be removed from homes being de-leaded to avoid exposure. Parents living in apartments owned by uncooperative landlords may need assistance in relating to the Housing Authority. Appropriate literature and explanations are provided at the "therapeutic moment" and thereafter.

Prevention of this condition is foremost. Lead paint should not be used on children's toys or furniture. Instead, use paint that is marked for indoor use. Close observation of children in this age group also acts as a deterrent. The nurse and the parents should provide opportunities for the toddler to suck and chew on safe objects such as a teething ring or wash cloth during the oral stage of development: this will meet the normal sucking and chewing needs.

Nursing care is symptomatic. Unnecessary handling of the patient is avoided to prevent stimulating the central nervous system. Injection sites are rotated and the skin is evaluated for thickness or fibrous lumps. Therapeutic syringe play is advised. Observation and charting of convulsions are discussed on page 145. Indications of respiratory distress are reported immediately. The services of the public health nurse are valuable in investigating the physical and emotional environment of the child and in continuing the education of the parents.

CORROSIVE STRICTURES

Description. Children who have ingested toxic substances such as lye, bleach, ammonia, and drain cleaners are frequently seen in hospital emergency rooms. The destruction varies from slight pharyngitis and esophagitis to death.

Symptoms. The first mouthful that is swallowed is painful and acts as a deterrent to some children; however, the damage is done. Swelling of the lips, chin, tongue, throat, and esophagus occurs. Ulcerations appear on the mucous membranes. The patient is unable to swallow. Edema may interfere with breathing; in this case a tracheotomy is necessary. If the patient survives, an esophageal stricture generally develops within a short time. This is evidenced by anorexia and difficulty in swallowing.

Treatment

The corrosive agent is usually diluted with water. Vomiting is contraindicated because of the danger of further damage being done to the mucosa. In severe damage the child is given nothing by mouth (NPO), and an intravenous infusion is started. Analgesics are given intravenously if they cannot be given by mouth. The child may eventually need surgery to correct an esophageal stricture.

Nursing Care

The nursing considerations, again, stress the importance of prevention through education of the public. Toxic substances should never be placed in food containers such as soda pop bottles or water glasses. Children should not be allowed to play in the family garage unless it has been made "child proof" or an adult is closely supervising the activity. The nurse should also stress the potential dangers of furniture polish, kerosene, ant traps, insecticides, and toilet bowl cleaners.

A gastrostomy is made for the purpose of introducing food directly into the stomach through the abdominal wall. This is done by means of a surgically placed tube. It is used in patients who cannot have food by mouth because of anomalies or corrosive strictures of the esophagus or who are severely debilitated or in coma. The nurse may be asked to administer such feedings. This procedure is presented on page 56.

Good oral hygiene is essential. It is administered gently to prevent injury to damaged tissues. The skin around the gastrostomy tube must be kept clean and dry to prevent excoriations. The psychological needs of the children are important, since they are not receiving satisfaction and contentment from ingestion of foods. A pacifier will provide sucking during tube feedings for infants. They should be given additional attention and love by cuddling and other forms of contact whenever feasible.

References

Agency for Toxic Substances and Disease Registry (1990). *Case Studies in Environmental Medicine: Lead Toxicity*. Atlanta, Division of Health Education.

Behrman, R., and Vaughan, V. (1987). *Nelson Textbook of Pediatrics*, 13th ed. Philadelphia, W. B. Saunders Company.

Mauro, R., and Poole, S. (1988). Is it croup? A guide to diagnosis and treatment. *Contemp. Pediatr.* 5:51–70.

Wisoff, J., and Epstein, F. (1985). Management of pediatric head trauma. *In* Zimmerman, S., and Gildea, J. (eds). *Critical Care Pediatrics*. Philadelphia, W. B. Saunders Company.

Zimmerman, S., and Gildea, J. (1985). *Critical Care Pediatrics*. Philadelphia, W. B. Saunders Company.

Bibliography

Foster, R., Hunsberger, M., and Anderson, J. (1989). *Family-Centered Nursing Care of Children*. Philadelphia, W. B. Saunders Company.

Gahart, B. (1991). *Intravenous Medications*. St. Louis, C. V. Mosby.

Gellis, S., and Kagan, B. (1990). *Current Pediatric Therapy*. Philadelphia, W. B. Saunders Company.

Hockenberry, M., and Coody, D. (1986). *Pediatric Oncology and Hematology*. St. Louis, C. V. Mosby.

Hockenberry, M., Coody, D., and Bennett, B. (1990). Childhood cancers: Incidence, etiology, diagnosis, and treatment. *Pediatr. Nurs.* 16:239–245.

Marlow, D., and Redding, B. (1988). *Pediatric Nursing*. 6th ed. Philadelphia, W. B. Saunders Company.

Needleman, H. (1988). Why we should worry about lead poisoning. *Contemp. Pediatr.* 5:34–56.

Rocky Mountain Poison Control Center (1985). *Overview Lead*. Denver.

Stretton, M., and Newth, C. (1990). Croup and epiglottitis: The critical early diagnosis. *J. Respir. Dis.* 11:1087–1097.

STUDY QUESTIONS

1. List and describe the three stages of separation anxiety.
2. What measures can the nurse take to prevent contractures from developing in the bedridden patient?
3. Define the following: Bradford frame; Croupette; brace; hyperkinetic.
4. What facilities are available in your community for the following handicaps: cerebral palsy, deafness, blindness, and mental retardation?
5. Johnny, age 2 years, fell from your front steps and struck his head on the pavement. He is crying loudly but you cannot see any visible cuts. What would you do immediately in this situation? Later on?
6. Ann, age 2 years, suffered a fractured femur in a fall from a tree. She has been hospitalized for 3 weeks in Bryant traction. What factors would you consider in planning her daily care?
7. Frank, age 2½ years, was hospitalized with a diagnosis of nephrosis. He has little interest in food. Discuss measures that would be effective in encouraging him to eat.
8. List the symptoms of croup. What is the purpose of the Croupette?
9. Define primary and secondary pneumonia. Discuss the nursing care of patients with pneumonia.
10. Anthony, age 7 years, is admitted for an appendectomy. You notice he is wearing a hearing aid. What additional information should you obtain from his parents to make his adjustment to the hospital a satisfactory one?
11. What measures can be taken to reduce acetaminophen poisoning in the home?
12. Define the following terms: gastrostomy; pica; plumbism.

C H A P T E R 1 1 _____

Chapter Outline

GENERAL CHARACTERISTICS
PHYSICAL, PSYCHOSOCIAL, AND COGNITIVE
   DEVELOPMENT
      The 3 Year Old Child
      The 4 Year Old Child
      The 5 Year Old Child
GUIDING THE PRESCHOOL CHILD
      Discipline, Setting Limits
      Bad Language
      Jealousy
      Thumb Sucking
      Masturbation
      Enuresis
NURSERY SCHOOL
      Evaluating the Preschool Child
DAILY CARE
PLAY IN HEALTH AND ILLNESS
      Value of Play
      The Nurse's Role
      Storing Toys
      Playmates
      Other Aspects of Play

Objectives

Upon completion and mastery of Chapter 11, the
student will be able to
- Define the vocabulary terms listed.
- Identify the developmental characteristics that
  predispose the preschool child to certain
  accidents and suggest methods of prevention for
  each type of accident.
- Describe the characteristics of a good nursery
  school.
- Discuss the value of play in the life of a child.
- Designate two toys suitable for the preschool
  child and provide the rationale for each choice.
- Describe the physical and psychosocial
  development of children from 3 to 6 years of
  age, listing age-specific events and guidance
  when appropriate.

THE PRESCHOOL CHILD

Terms

General Characteristics

The child from ages 3 to 6 years is often referred to as the *preschool child* (Fig. 11–1). This period is marked by a slowing down of the growth process. The infant who tripled birth weight at 1 year has only doubled the 1-year weight by the age of 6 years. For instance, the boy who weighs 20 pounds on his first birthday will probably weigh about 40 pounds by his sixth. The child between 3 and 6 years of age grows taller and loses the chubbiness seen during the toddler period. Appetite fluctuates widely. The normal pulse rate is 90 to 110. The rate of respirations during relaxation is about 20 per minute. The systolic blood pressure is about 85 to 90 mm Hg; the diastolic is about 60 mm Hg.

Preschool children have good control of their muscles and participate in vigorous play activities. They become more adept at using old skills as each year passes. They can swing and jump higher. Their gait resembles that of an adult. They are quicker and have more confidence in themselves than they did as toddlers. While the preschool age may seem more or less quiet and steady with respect to physical development, certain difficulties stem from increased independence, life in a social world, and an increase in cognitive ability.

The thinking of the preschool child is unique. Piaget calls this period the *preoperational phase*. It comprises the ages of 2 to 7 years and is divided into two stages, the *preconceptual* stage from 2 to 4 years and the *intuitive* thought stage from 4 to 7 years. Of importance in the preconceptual stage is the increasing development of language and symbolic functioning. Symbolic functioning is seen in the play of children who pretend that an empty box is a fort; they create a mental image to stand for something that is not there. Another characteristic of this period is *egocentrism*, a type of thinking in which children have difficulty seeing any point of view other than their own. Since children's knowledge and understanding are restricted to their own limited experiences, misconceptions arise. One of these misconceptions is *animism*. This is a tendency to attribute life to inanimate objects. Another is *artificialism*, the idea that the world and everything in it are created by human beings. Table 11–1 lists examples of all three characteristics of thought at this age.

A distinctive characteristic of intuitive thinking is *centering*, the tendency to concentrate on a single outstanding characteristic of an object while excluding its other features. With time and experience, more mature conceptual awareness is established. The process is highly complex, and the implications for practical application are numer-

SIGMUND FREUD emphasizes the notion that early childhood is critical in the socialization of the individual. In his view of the psychosexual stages of development, during early childhood the child's sensual pleasure is focused on the genitals, and the child's fantasies about gratifying these desires results in sexual conflict with the parent of the opposite sex. According to Freud, the conflict is resolved when the child comes to identify with the parent of the same sex, and this identification forms the basis for appropriate sex-role development. Whether the opposite-sexed parent responds with warmth and affection to the child, thereby indirectly satisfying the child's desires, affects his personality development. The same-sexed parent, with whom the child learns to identify, becomes the model for the values that will be part of the child's adult personality.

ERIK ERIKSON concurs with the view that peer and parental responses are important factors in socialization during early childhood. Appropriate sex-role behavior develops when a child identifies with his same-sexed parent and assimilates his parent's behavior into his own personal identity. In Erikson's theory, peer-group and parental support and encouragement when the child first attempts to acquire appropriate sex-role behavior can help the child achieve a positive self-image and a strong personal identity.

LAWRENCE KOHLBERG emphasizes cognitive development as the most important factor in socialization. He takes the position that identification with the same-sexed parent develops once a child understands sex roles rather than the other way around. Thus, once girls or boys begin to think of themselves as girls or boys, they want to talk, think, and act as others of their sex do; in the process, they come to identify with them. In this view, although parents and others are important in socialization because they provide models and approval, children socialize themselves as they discover how to behave in competent and prescribed ways.

▲ **FIGURE 11–1**

Summary descriptions of some major theoretical viewpoints on personality development during early childhood. (Modified from Schell, R., and Hall, E. [1979]. *Developmental Psychology Today*, 3rd ed. New York, CRM/Random House.)

Table 11–1. THE NATURE OF EARLY CHILDHOOD THOUGHT

Sample Questions	Typical Answers
EGOCENTRISM	
Why does the sun shine?	To keep me warm.
Why is there snow?	For me to play in.
Why is grass green?	Because that's my favorite color.
What are TV sets for?	To watch my favorite shows and cartoons.
ANIMISM	
Why do trees have leaves?	To keep them warm.
Why do stars twinkle?	Because they're happy and cheerful.
Why does the sun move in the sky?	To follow children and hear what they say.
Where do boats go at night?	They sleep like we do.
ARTIFICIALISM	
What causes rain?	Someone emptying a watering can.
Why is the sky blue?	It has been painted.
What is the wind?	A man blowing.
What causes thunder?	A man grumbling.

(From Helms, D., and Turner, J. [1978]. *Exploring Child Behavior: Basic Principles.* Philadelphia, W. B. Saunders Company, p. 447.)

ous. Interested students are encouraged to explore these concepts through further study.

COMMUNICATION ALERT ▶ ▶ ▶ ▶ ▶
Preschool children sometimes believe that they are being punished for something they thought or did. When a painful procedure is performed on the child, the nurse might say, "I am sorry that it hurt when I put the needle in your arm. I did that so we can give you medicine to make you feel better, not to hurt or punish you."

Physical, Psychosocial, and Cognitive Development

THE 3 YEAR OLD CHILD

Three year olds are a delight to their parents. They are helpful and can participate in simple household chores. They obtain articles upon request and return them to the proper place. Three year olds come very close to the ideal picture that parents have in mind of their child. They are living proof that their parents' guidance during the "terrible twos" has been rewarded. Temper tantrums are less frequent, and in general the 3 year old is a pretty good youngster. Of course, they are still their individual selves but they seem to be able to direct their primitive instincts better than previously. They can help dress and undress themselves, use the toilet, and wash their hands. They eat independently, and their table manners have improved.

The 3 year old talks in longer sentences and can express thoughts: "What are you doing?" "Where is Daddy?" They are more company to their parents because they can verbally share experiences with them. They are imaginative, talk to their toys, and imitate what they see about them. Soon they begin to make friends outside the immediate family. Since they can now converse with playmates, they find satisfaction in joining their activities. Three year olds do not play cooperatively for long periods of time, but at least it's a start. Much of their play still consists of watching others, but now they can offer verbal advice, should they feel the need. They can ask others to "come out and play." If 3 year olds are placed in a strange situation with children they do not know, they commonly revert to "parallel play" because it is more comfortable.

At this time, there is a change in the relationship of the child and the family. They begin to find enjoyment away from Mom and Dad (Fig. 11–2), although they want them to be right there when needed. They begin to lose some of their interest in Mother, who up to this time has been more or less their total world. Father's prestige begins to increase. Romantic attachment to the parent of the opposite sex is seen during this period. Johnny wants to "marry Mommy" when he grows up. They also begin to identify themselves with the parent of the same sex.

Preschool children have more fears than the infant or the older child. Some of the many causes of this are increased intelligence, which enables them to recognize potential dangers; the development of memory; and graded independence, which brings them into contact with many new situations. Toddlers are not afraid of walking in the street because they do not know any better. Preschool children realize that trucks can injure them, and therefore they worry about crossing the street. This type of fear is well founded, but many others are not. The fear of bodily harm is particularly peculiar to this stage. The little boy who discovers that baby sister is made differently worries that perhaps she has been injured. He wonders if this will happen to him. Masturbation is

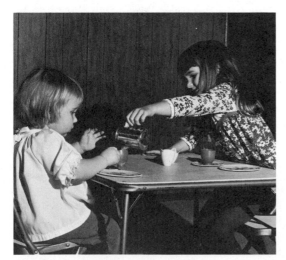

▲ **FIGURE 11–2**

Playmates promote social development.

common during this stage as children attempt to reassure themselves that they are all right. Other common fears include fear of animals, fear of the dark, and fear of strangers. A little night wandering is typical of this age group.

Preschool children become angry when others attempt to take their possessions. They grab, slap, and hang on to them for dear life. They become very distraught if toys do not work the way they should. Being disturbed from play is resented. They are sensitive, and their feelings are easily hurt. It is well to bear in mind that much of the disturbing social behavior seen during this time is normal and necessary to the children's total pattern of development.

THE 4 YEAR OLD CHILD

Four is a stormy age. Children are not as eager and willing as they were at 3 years, are more aggressive, and like to show off. They are eager to let others know they are superior and are prone to pick on their playmates, often taking sides and making life difficult for the child who does not measure up to their standards. Four year olds are boisterous, tattle on others, and may begin to swear if they are around children or adults who use profanity. Personal family activities are repeated with an amazing sense of recall, but where their bicycle has been left is forgotten. At this age, children become very interested in how old they are and want to know the exact age of each playmate. It bolsters their ego to know that they are older than someone else in the group. They also become interested in the relationship of one person to another. Timmy is a brother, but also Daddy's son, and so forth (Fig. 11–3).

Four year olds can use scissors with success. They can lace their shoes. Vocabulary has increased to about 1500 words. They run simple errands and can play with others for longer periods of time. Many feats are done for a purpose. For instance, they no longer run just for the sake of running. Instead, they run to get some place or see something. They are imaginative and like to pretend they are fire fighters or cowboys. They are beginning to enjoy playing with friends of the same sex better than those of the opposite sex.

The preschool child enjoys simple toys. Raw

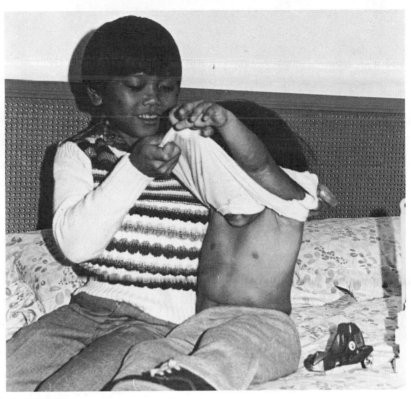

▲ **FIGURE 11–3**

The preschooler gets an assist from his older brother. (From Tackett, J., and Hunsberger, M. [1981]. *Family-Centered Care of Children and Adolescents.* Philadelphia, W. B. Saunders.)

materials are more appealing than toys that are ready made and complete in themselves. An old cardboard box that can be moved about and climbed into is more fun than a doll house with tiny furniture. A box of sand or colored pebbles can be made into roads and mountains. A small mirror becomes a lake. Parents should avoid showering their children with ready-made toys. Instead, they can select materials that are absorbing and stimulate the imagination of the child.

Stories that interest young children depict their daily experiences (Fig. 11–4). If the story has a simple plot, it must be related to what they understand to hold their interest. They also enjoy music; they like records they can march around to and simple instruments they can shake or bang. Make up a song about their daily life and watch their reaction.

Children's curiosity concerning sex continues to heighten. If the parents have answered questions simply, they should not be alarmed to find their children checking up on them. It is common for children of this age to take down their pants in front of friends of the opposite sex. They discuss their differences with their friends. Older children who are more sensitive about their bodies should be told that this is a natural curiosity seen in small children. This may rid them of guilt feelings that they might harbor, particularly if they participated in similar activities during the preschool period. Children are as matter-of-fact about these investigations as they would be about any other learning experience and are easily distracted to more socially acceptable forms of behavior.

Between ages 3 and 4 years, children begin to wonder about death and dying. They may be the hero who shoots the intruder dead, or they may witness a situation in which an animal is killed.

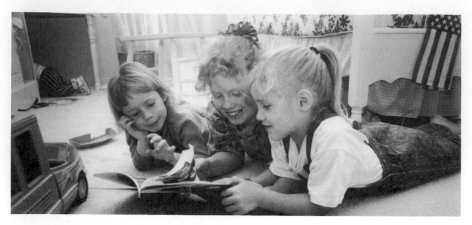

▲ FIGURE 11–4

The preschool child enjoys stories that depict daily experiences. (Photo by Vickie Ashwill.)

Their questions are very direct. "What is dead? Will I die?" There are no set answers to these inquiries. The religion of the family plays an important role regarding the interpretations of this complex phenomenon.

Perhaps children can become acquainted with death through objects that are not of particular significance to them. For instance, the flower dies at the end of the summer. It doesn't bloom any more. It no longer needs sunshine or water, for it is not alive. Usually young children realize that others die but do not relate this to themselves. If they continue to pursue the question of whether or not they will die, parents should be casual and reassure them that people do not generally die until they have lived a long and happy life. Of course, as they grow older they will discover that sometimes children do die. The underlying idea, nevertheless, is to encourage questions as they appear and gradually help them accept the truth without undue fear. Reality is often unpleasant, but children should be prepared to accept it.

THE 5 YEAR OLD CHILD

Five is a comfortable age. Children are more responsible, enjoy doing what is expected of them, have more patience, and like to finish what they start. Five year olds are serious about what they can and cannot do. They talk constantly and are inquisitive about the environment. They want to do things right and seek answers to their questions from those who they consider "know" the answers. Five year olds can play games governed by rules. They are less fearful because they feel their environment is controlled by authorities. The worries they do have are not as profound as they were at an earlier age.

The physical growth of 5 year olds is not particularly outstanding. Their height may increase 2 to 3 inches, and they may gain 3 to 6 pounds. The variations in height and weight of a group of 5 year olds are remarkable. They may begin to lose their deciduous teeth at this time. They can run and play games simultaneously, jump three or four steps at once, and tell a penny from a nickel or a dime. They can name the days of the week and understand what a week-long vacation is. They usually can print their first name.

Five year olds can ride a tricycle around the playground with speed and dexterity. They can use a hammer to pound nails. Adults should encourage them to develop motor skills and not be continually reminding them to "be careful." The practice children get will enable them to compete with others during the school age period and will increase confidence in their own abilities. As at any age level, children should not be scorned for failure to measure up to adult standards. Overdirection by solicitous adults is damaging. Children must learn to do tasks themselves in order for the experience to be satisfying.

The amount and type of television programs that parents allow preschool children to watch is a topic of current discussion. Although the children enjoyed television at 3 or 4 years of age, it was usually for short periods of time. They could not understand much of what was going on. Five year olds have better comprehension and may spend a great deal of time watching television. The plan of management differs with each family. Whatever is decided needs to be discussed with the children. Television should not be allowed to interfere with good health habits, e.g., sleep, meals, and physical activity. Most parents find that children do not insist on watching television if there is something better to do (see page 354).

Guiding the Preschool Child

DISCIPLINE, SETTING LIMITS

Much has been written on the subject of discipline, which has changed considerably with the passing of time. Today, authorities place a great deal of importance on the development of a continuous, warm relationship between the child and the parents. This, they feel, helps prevent many problems. The following is a brief discussion that may be helpful to the nurse in guiding parents.

Children need to have limits set to their behavior. Setting limits makes them feel secure, protects them from danger, and relieves them from making decisions that they may be too young to formulate. Children who are taught acceptable behavior have more friends and feel better about themselves. They live more enjoyably within the neighborhood and society. The manner in which discipline or limit setting is carried out varies from culture to culture. It also varies among different socioeconomic groups. Individual differences occur among families and between parents and according to the characteristics of each child. The purpose of discipline is to teach and to gradually shift control from parents to the child, i.e., self-discipline. Positive reinforcement for appropriate behavior rather than punishment for poor behavior has been cited as more effective in this regard (Levine et al., 1983). Expectations must be appropriate to the age and understanding of the child. The nurse en-

courages parents to try to be consistent, as mixed messages are confusing for the learner. "The facilitating family is one that loves and nurtures the child, encourages and admonishes appropriately, and provides a model of mutual caring and restrained behavior" (Offord and Waters, 1983).

Timing, Time Out. Most researchers agree that to be effective, discipline must be given at the time the incident occurs. It should also be adapted to the seriousness of the infraction. The child's self-worth must always be considered. Warning the preschool child who appears to be getting into trouble may be helpful. Too many warnings without follow-up, however, lead to ineffectiveness. Spankings, for the most part, are not productive. The child associates the fury of the parents with the pain rather than the wrong deed, because anger is the predominant factor in the situation. Thus, the real value of the spanking is lost. Beatings administered by a parent as a release for his or her own pent-up emotions are totally inappropriate and can lead to child abuse charges. In addition, the parent serves as a role model of aggression. Whether a parent is affectionate, warm, or cold (uncaring) also plays a role in the effectiveness of child rearing. Cold mothers who spanked their children found it less effective than warm mothers who also spanked. Time-out periods, such as sitting for 5 minutes in a chair or corner, are one alternative to inappropriate punishment. Parents need to be taught to resist the use of power and authority for its own sake. As the child understands more, privileges can be withheld. The reasons for such actions are carefully explained.

Reward. Rewarding the child for good behavior is a positive and effective method of discipline. This can be done by the use of hugs, smiles, tone of voice, and praise. Praise can always be tied with the act: "Thank you, Suzy, for picking up your toys." The encouragement of positive behavior eliminates many of the undesirable effects of punishment.

Consistency and Modeling. Being consistent is difficult for parents. It is realistically something to be strived for, as no parent is consistent all the time. Consistency must exist *between* parents as well as within each parent. It is suggested that parents establish a general style in terms of what, when, how, and to what degree punishment is appropriate to misconduct. Parents who are lax or erratic in their discipline and who alternate such procedures with punishment have children who experience increased behavioral difficulties.

The influence of modeling or good example has been widely explored. Such studies show that adult models significantly influence the education of children. Children identify and imitate adult behavior, both verbal and nonverbal. Parents who are aggressive and repeatedly lose control demonstrate the power of action over words. Those who communicate, show respect and encouragement, and use appropriate limit setting serve as more positive role models. Finally, parents need assistance in reviewing their own childhood in regard to parental discipline in order to recognize destructive patterns that may be carried into adulthood.

BAD LANGUAGE

Parents express astonishment at the words that flow from the mouths of their sweet little children during the preschool period. Bad language is inevitable. Caretakers should suppress their desire to emphatically shout their disapproval. The small child delights in attention, and it does not matter, unfortunately, whether this attention is good or bad. Swearing at this age is not particularly meaningful, since children are merely imitating what they hear, and it does not have any real significance to them. They use swearing as a way of identifying themselves with the older children in the neighborhood and to shock adults. One mother dealt with this problem by saying, "Johnny, Mommy doesn't mind if you hear or know what that word means, but we don't use it in our home any more than you would think of going outdoors without your clothes on." Johnny felt free to discuss what he heard with his mother, and shortly thereafter his interest was taken up by other subjects.

JEALOUSY

Jealousy is a normal response to actual, supposed, or threatened loss of affection. Children or adults may feel insecure in their relationship with the person they love. The closer children are to their mothers, the greater their fear of losing mother. Only children envy a new baby. They love the sibling, but at the same time resent its presence. They cannot understand the turmoil that is taking place within themselves (Fig. 11–5). Jealousy of a new baby is strongest in children under 5 years of age and is shown in various ways. Children may be aggressive and may bite or pinch, or they may be rather discreet and hug and kiss the baby with a determined look on their faces. Another common situation occurs when children attempt to identify with the baby. They revert to wetting the bed or want to be powdered after they urinate. Some 4 year olds even try the bottle, but it is usually a big disappointment to them.

Preschool children may be jealous of the attention that mother gives father. They may also envy the children they play with if they have bigger and better toys than they do. School age children more often are jealous of those who are more athletic or popular. There is less jealousy in only children since they are the center of attention and have only a minimum of rivals. Children of varied

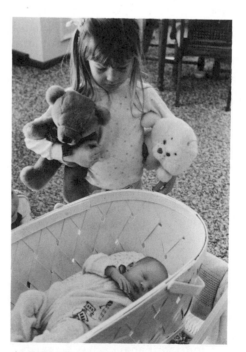

▲ **FIGURE 11–5**

An additional family member creates a lot of new feelings for the preschool child.

ages in one family are apt to feel that the younger ones are "pets" or that the older ones have more special privileges.

Parents can help reduce jealousy by the early management of individual occurrences. Preparing young children for the arrival of the new baby will lessen the blow. They should not be made to think that they are being crowded. If the new baby is going to occupy their crib, it is best to get older children happily settled in a large bed before the baby is born. Children should feel that they are helping with the care of the infant. Parents can inflate their ego from time to time by reminding them of the many activities they can do that the new baby cannot. If it is convenient, the new baby is given a bath or feeding while the older child is asleep. In this way the older sibling will avoid one of the occasions in which the mother shows the newborn infant affection for a relatively long period of time. Some persons feel that giving the child a pet to care for at this time helps. Many hospitals offer sibling courses that assist the parents in helping the child to overcome jealousy.

If the child intends to hit the baby or another child, both children must be separated, but the one who has caused or is about to cause the injury needs as much attention as the victim, if not more. Aggressiveness similar to this is seen when the child is made to share toys. It is even more difficult to learn to share the mother, so the child must be given time to adjust to new situations. Children should be assured that they are loved but also should be told that they cannot injure others.

THUMB SUCKING

From 1914 to 1921, the U.S. Children's Bureau pamphlet entitled *Infant Care* cautioned mothers that thumb sucking would deform the mouth and cause drooling. It also suggested that the thumb or fingers be consistently removed from the mouth while diverting the baby's attention (Levine et al., 1983). Today we recognize that thumb sucking is an instinctual behavioral pattern that is considered normal. Finger sucking or thumb sucking will not have a detrimental effect on the teeth as long as the habit is discontinued before the second teeth have erupted. Most children give up the habit by the time they reach school age, although they may regress during periods of stress or fatigue. Man-

agement includes education and support of the parents to relieve their anxiety and prevent secondary emotional problems in their children. The child who is trying to stop thumb-sucking is given praise and encouragement.

Treatment is not recommended in the child over the age of 4 years unless physical or emotional problems are evident or the child requests help in quitting (Friman and Schmitt, 1989).

MASTURBATION

Masturbation is common in both sexes during the preschool years. The child experiences pleasurable sensations, which lead to repetition of the behavior. It is beneficial to rule out other causes of this activity, such as rashes or penile or vaginal irritation. Masturbation is also exhibited in the child who feels emotionally isolated or anxious. A variety of interpretations of masturbation have been postulated; however, it appears that there are still many questions left unanswered in regard to the significance of this behavior for the child. Masturbation at this age is considered harmless if the child is outgoing, sociable, and not preoccupied with the activity. One common anxiety in boys that should be explored is fear of castration.

Education of the parents consists of assuring them that this behavior is normal and not harmful to the child, who is merely curious about sexuality. The cultural and moral background of the family must be considered when assessing the degree of discomfort in relation to this experience. A history of the time and place of masturbation and the parental response is helpful. Punitive reactions are discouraged, as these can be potentially harmful to the child. Parents are advised to try to ignore the behavior and to distract the child with some other activity. The child needs to know that masturbation is not acceptable in public; however, this must be accomplished in a nonthreatening manner. Children who masturbate excessively and who have experienced a great deal of disruption in their lives will benefit from ongoing counseling.

ENURESIS

Description. The term *enuresis* is derived from the Greek word *enourein*, to void urine. Bedwetting is an occurrence that has been around for generations and affects many cultures. There are two types—primary and secondary. Primary enuresis refers to bedwetting in the child who has never been dry. Secondary enuresis refers to a recurrence in a child who has been dry for a period of 1 year or more. *Diurnal,* or daytime, wetting is less common than nocturnal episodes. It is more common in boys than in girls; there is a higher incidence among the poor; and there appears to be a genetic influence. In many children a specific cause is never determined. The age when most children learn not to urinate in their sleep varies from 3 to 6 years for 90 per cent of children (Schmitt, 1990). Some organic causes of nocturnal enuresis are urinary tract infections, diabetes mellitus, diabetes insipidus, seizure disorders, obstructive uropathy, abnormalities of the urinary tract, and sleep disorders. Sudden onset may be due to psychological stress, such as a death in the family or divorce. Giggling may also precipitate wetting. Maturational delay of the nervous system has also been suggested as a cause. Other causes include small bladder, inability to delay voiding, and not awakening to the sensation of a full bladder (Table 11–2).

Treatment and Nursing Care

A detailed history is obtained. Such factors as the pattern of wetting, number of times per night or week, number of daytime voidings, type of stream, dysuria, amount of fluid taken between dinner and bedtime, family history, stress, and the reactions of the parents and child are documented. It is also important to determine any medications that the child may be taking and the extent to which social life is inhibited by the problem, e.g., inability to spend the night away from home. Developmental landmarks, including toilet training, are reviewed. If there appears to be an organic cause, appropriate blood and urine studies are undertaken. In most cases physical findings are negative.

Education of the family is extremely crucial to prevent secondary emotional problems. It is important to reassure parents that many children experience enuresis and that it is self-limited in nature. Power struggles, shame and guilt are fruit-

Table 11–2. WHAT CAUSES ENURESIS?
NONPATHOLOGIC CAUSES (97%)
Small functional bladder capacity
Inability to delay micturition urge
Nighttime polyuyria because ADH levels fail to rise at night
Nighttime polyuria because child drinks too much in the evening
Child doesn't wake up when bladder feels full
DISEASE STATES (3%)
Medically Treatable
Urinary tract infection
Diabetes insipidus
Diabetes mellitus
Fecal impaction or constipation
Surgically Treatable
Ectopic ureter
Lower urinary tract obstruction
Neurogenic bladder
Bladder calculus or foreign body
Sleep apnea secondary to large adenoids

From Schmitt, B. (1990). Nocturnal enuresis: Finding the treatment that fits the child. *Contemp. Pediatr. 7*:72.

less and destructive. Reassurance and support by the nurse are of great help.

Therapies for bedwetting are subject to controversy. Some modalities include counseling, hypnosis, behavior modification, and pharmacotherapy. Moisture-activated conditioning devices are also available commercially (an alarm rings when the child wets). These have had limited success. Bladder training exercises, in which the child is asked to withhold the urine for as long as possible, may serve to stretch the bladder and increase its size. The child's bedroom should be as close to the bathroom as possible and a night light employed. Limiting fluids at bedtime and awakening the child during the night have not been highly successful. A spontaneous cure may occur with little or no intervention or after other types of treatment have failed. The nurse prepares the parents for relapses, which are common.

The response to various therapies is highly individual. Overzealous treatment is to be avoided. A nonpunitive, matter-of-fact attitude appears prudent. It is necessary to involve children in any routine that is instigated and to allow them the responsibility of caring for themselves as much as possible.

Imipramine (Tofranil) has been found to decrease enuresis in controlled studies. It is administered before bedtime and is used only on a short-term basis. Imipramine has a variety of side effects, including mood and sleep disturbances and gastrointestinal upsets. It can be toxic and potentially lethal in low doses. Overdose can lead to cardiac arrhythmias, which may be life-threatening. Therefore, dosage and administration should be closely supervised. Imipramine should not be given to children under 6 years of age. Desmopressin (DDAVP) also has been used with some success. It is an antidiuretic hormone that inhibits urine production.

Nursery School

The change from home to nursery school is a big step toward independence. At this age the child is adjusting to the outside world as well as to the family group. Some children have the complicating factor of a new baby in the house. The child also finds at this time that parents are beginning to expect more in regard to neatness and cooperative play with others. This transition period is troublesome.

A good nursery school provides the child with opportunities to get rid of some pent-up emotions. There is plenty of room to run and shout. The toys are sturdy, and children can manipulate them because they are their own size. Since they are not their own, they find them easier to share. Children are not as emotionally involved with the teacher as they are with the parents. They feel more able to express their negative and positive feelings, and the teacher is able to be more objective about them. The teacher expects the child to decide what materials to play with and with whom to play (Fig. 11–6). Children take responsibility for their own belongings.

Children are accepted into nursery schools between the ages of 2 and 5 years. Most sessions last about 3 hours. This may be a child's first exposure to different cultures. A good nursery school should challenge the child's imagination and creativity. It is also an attempt to acquaint children with this social world in such a way that

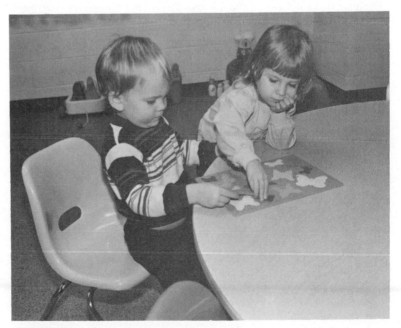

▲ FIGURE 11–6

Although home is cozier, children soon discover that nursery school is fun.

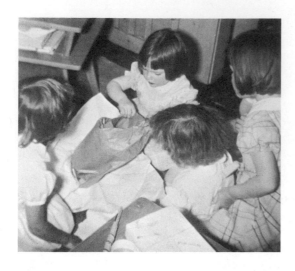

▲ FIGURE 11–7

Socialization is an important phase of the preschool period. Children begin to understand the meaning of friendship.

Table 11–3. OBSERVING THE NURSERY SCHOOL CHILD

Objective: To observe the behavioral characteristics of the preschool child

Watch for and evaluate the following in terms of a child's security and independence:

Physical Development
Ability to walk, run, jump, use play equipment
General health: easily fatigued, etc.

Emotional Development
Easily excited
Whines, cries frequently
Evidence of temper tantrums
Persistence in a task
Aggressive
Shy
Reaction to failure

Social Development
Talkative
Quiet
Plays with others
Plays near others
Special friends
Tends to lead
Tends to follow
Friendly toward other children and adults
Ability to share
Ability to take turns
Behavior when an object or attention of the teacher is desired

Degree of Independence
Removing coat, hat, boots; putting them away
Attending to toilet needs
Getting a drink
Amount of time going from one activity to another
Dependence on adult suggestions and help

Relaxation
Relaxes during rest periods
Sits and listens to stories
Is restless, in constant motion

Specific Routines
Music period: sings, plays games
Snacks: Eats lunch, takes other children's food, wanders about, disturbs others, plays with food
Free play period: toys preferred, amount of skill using hands, span of interest, evidence of destructive play, plays with others or alone, has imaginary friend

it will add to their security and increase independence (Fig. 11–7).

Parents who are considering nursery school for their child should evaluate the following factors: How many teachers are there? What is their educational background? Are the physical facilities adequate? How many children are there per teacher? What is the cost? Is the child ready for nursery school? Parents will also want to visit the school and talk with the person in charge. They may also wish to talk with parents whose children are attending the program.

The student nurse may have the opportunity to visit a nursery school during studies of the well child. This can be a rewarding experience if nurses use their powers of observation. When observing an individual child, they should compare him or her with others in the age group and not merely with one other child. The types of behavior to be observed are outlined in Table 11–3.

EVALUATING THE PRESCHOOL CHILD

The Preschool Readiness Experimental Screening Scale (PRESS) is intended to measure a child's general readiness to perform the usual tasks necessary in the school setting. It is easily administered by the physician or pediatric nurse practitioner during the physical examination. Figure 11–8 shows the general outline and record form used for the PRESS. A description of the administration and scoring of the PRESS follows (from Rogers and Rogers, 1972, 1975).

Administration and Scoring of the Preschool Readiness Experimental Screening Scale (PRESS)

ADMINISTERING THE ASSESSMENT

As the child is placed on the examining table and the records and equipment are organized, the following is said (the test questions are in italic type):

1. "Mrs. Smith, as I examine Johnny I will be asking him a few questions, so please don't talk to him for a few minutes. O.K.? [with a smile]."

2. "Johnny, I hear you're going to start kindergarten soon. Do you think you'll like that?"

Knowledge of Colors. These questions are asked during the EENT examination.

1. "I hear your teacher will want you to know colors. Do you know any colors yet?"
2. "If she asks you to color a house, what color should you make the grass?"
3. *"And what color should you make the sky if there are no clouds?"*

Knowledge of Numbers. Asked during the heart and lung examination.

1. "If the teacher tells you some numbers, could you remember them and repeat them back to her?"
2. *"I'm going to tell you some numbers. Now you remember them and say the same numbers right back to me."* (4-1-7-3) and (3-8-6-4)
3. "If the teacher asks you to count, could you count?"
4. *"Tell me, how many tongue blades are there?"* At this point place four tongue blades on the table beside the patient.

General Knowledge. As the abdomen, genitalia, and extremities are examined.

1. "I'm going to examine your tummy. You know where your tummy is, don't you?" or "Do you have a tickly tummy?"
2. *"Tell me, does Christmas come in the winter or in the summer?"*
3. *"Can you show me where your heel is?"*

Drawing Coordination. This is usually done at the end of the examination.

1. "If the teacher asked you to draw a square like this one [indicate the sample square], *let's see you draw one just like it right beside mine. Take your time and make a good one."*

General Assessment: Performance and Maturity. These are best evaluated following the hearing and visual acuity tests when everything else is finished.

SCORING

Colors. 1 point for knowing grass is green, 1 point for knowing the sky is blue. Any other answer, such as white, blue and white, black, gets no point.

Numbers. 1 point for repeating the four numbers in the same sequence. If the child misses the

NAME _____   BIRTHDATE _____

SCHOOL _____   DATE _____

1. a. What color is grass?   _____
    b. What color is the sky if there are no clouds?   _____

2. a. Repeat four numbers (one success in two tries): 4-1-7-3 or 3-8-6-4.   _____
    b. Recognize four tongue blades.   _____

3. a. Does Christmas come in the winter or the summer?   _____
    b. Where is your heel?   _____

4. Draw a square (best success in two tries).   _____

5. a. Comprehension and performance.   _____
    b. Personal-social maturity.
                                                              TOTAL   _____

Comments

▲ **FIGURE 11–8**

PRESS General Outline and Record Form. The children are asked to reproduce a standard 1-inch square. (From Rogers, W. B. Jr., and Rogers, R. A. [1972]. A new simplified preschool readiness experimental screening scale [the PRESS]. A preliminary report. *Clin. Pediatr.* 11:558.)

first set of numbers, try the second set. Score 1 point for *either* set of numbers repeated back correctly. 1 point for answering the correct number of tongue blades as four. If the child only counts "one, two, three, four," this is not given a point. You may then ask the child *one time only,* "Yes, but how many are there all together?" If the child does not answer four at this time, score 0.

General Knowledge. 1 point for answering winter. It is important to suggest winter first. Most children will give the second of two choices if they do not know the correct answer. 1 point for knowing the heel. The child must point to the heel or the Achilles tendon, not to the malleolus.

Drawing Coordination. Allow the child to draw a second square if the first one is poorly done. Encourage him to make the second more like the sample. Choosing the best square, score in the following manner:

2 points for drawing a good, readily recognizable square.

1 point for drawing a fairly recognizable square. 0 points for drawing a poor, unrecognizable square.

Comprehension and Performance. 1 point for those who reply promptly and follow instructions well (e.g., during the hearing and visual acuity tests). 0 points for those who have to be coaxed, need frequent repetition of instructions, or need repeated clarification of what you ask.

Personal-Social Maturity. 1 point if the child seems reasonably mature and self-confident. 0 points for:

Excessive silliness or playing around.
Overtalkative or hyperactive.
Uncooperative, evasive, no interest.
Unduly attached to mother.
Generally immature compared with most 5 year olds you see.

It should be evident that the PRESS is not so much a standardized test with strict rules of administration as it is a set of standardized questions that can be blended into a physical examination. One should note that it includes a few questions that are asked but not scored. These questions establish rapport and put the child at ease. They also serve as a lead-in to the test questions and serve indirectly in assessing the child's general maturity. The physician (or nurse) may intersperse or substitute other lead-in questions if it is felt they would better express a personal method of dealing with children. It is important to ask the parent not to speak, else an oversolicitous mother may interfere by offering help and encouragement.

RATING SYSTEM

1. *A score of 9 or 10 indicates high-average to above-average school readiness.* A child in this score range should have no difficulty doing average or above-average school work.

2. *A score of 7 or 8 indicates average school readiness.* A child in this score range should have little difficulty doing average school work.

3. *A score of 6 indicates borderline school readiness.* About half the boys and about a fourth of the girls with this score may have difficulty in school. It is recommended that close liaison be maintained with the teacher. If at any time the child is not functioning at class level, further study should be made at once.

4. *A score of 5 or less indicates insufficient school readiness.* Such children should be referred to a school psychologist or diagnostic center for further psychologic evaluation.

Draw-A-Person Test (D-A-P)

Another test that is frequently used to evaluate cognitive function in children is the *Goodenough Draw-A-Person Test.* The child is given pencil and paper and requested to "draw a picture of a person." When this is completed, the child is often requested to draw a person of the opposite sex from that in the picture. Clinicians can gain additional knowledge of the child by requesting information about the figures, such as what the person is feeling, thinking, or doing. The test is specifically scored by each item included in the drawing.

Daily Care

The child between 3 and 6 years of age does not require the extensive physical care given to a baby, but still needs a bath each day (more than ever) and a shampoo at least once a week. It is best to keep hair styles simple. A little girl fares the worst in this area, particularly if her mother expects her to sit still for an elaborate coiffure.

The child needs to visit a dentist regularly, at least every 6 months. The deciduous teeth are important for the proper formation of the permanent teeth and should not be neglected. The first visit may be merely for an examination. In this way the child becomes acquainted with the dentist and the appearance of the office. When calling for the appointment, the mother should tell the receptionist that this is Susie's first visit. It will also help to tell Susie a little in advance that she is going and that the dentist will look into her mouth. Too much detail may frighten the imaginative preschool child. The child's diet should continue to emphasize milk, vegetables, and fruits. Excess sweets, which contribute to dental decay, are restricted. Children must be reminded to brush their teeth regularly.

Preschool children like to do things for themselves. Simple clothes make it easy for them to dress. A hook nailed on the door within reach is helpful. They should dress and undress themselves as much as they can. Mother or father can assist but should not take over. They must be reminded to use the toilet from time to time. Some 3 year olds may still need assistance to get up onto the seat. There are occasional spills that embarrass preschool children. A stool kept next to the bathroom sink enables them to wash their hands.

The children need simple, nourishing meals. Their appetites fluctuate and they should not be bribed, scolded, or coaxed. Mealtimes should be happy. Parents who use good table manners set an example. The milk glass must be unbreakable and not filled completely. A waterproof tablecloth is useful. Children are included in the conversations but not allowed to take over. A nourishing dessert such as a custard pudding eases the apprehension about what has been left on the child's plate.

Preschool children need periods of active play both in and out of doors. Their clothes should be loose enough to prevent restriction of movement. Parents who see that their children are having a particularly good time should ask themselves whether it is necessary to interrupt them right at that moment. When children have verbal arguments, parents should avoid rushing in to defend their child. Growth can be painful, but children need to do it at their own rate.

Sleep habits at this time vary. Toward the end of this stage, children may balk at taking a nap. Instead of insisting that they sleep, parents should see that they engage in something interesting, but restful, such as reading a story together or playing with a simple puzzle. They need an opportunity to relax. Bedtime rituals are still important, and children may use these to put off going to bed. Also, preschool children may awaken frightened during the night. Parents should attend to their needs and reassure them that they are safe and that they are close by. A night light may be helpful. If they persist in awakening and are usually frightened, this is discussed with the doctor during one of the checkups. Children of this age should have a complete physical examination each year. Booster injections of the various immunizations are given when required.

Accidents are still a major threat during the years from 3 to 5. At this age children may suffer injuries from a bad fall. Preschool children hurtle up and down stairs. They climb trees and stand up on swings. They play hard with their toys, particularly those that they can mount. Stairways must be kept free from clutter. Shoes should have rubber soles, and new ones are bought when the thread becomes smooth. When buying toys, parents must be sure they are sturdy and can take a beating. Preschool children are not usually asked to do anything that is potentially dangerous, such as to carry a glass container or sharp knife to the kitchen sink.

Automobiles continue to be a threat. Children should be taught where they can safely ride their tricycles and where they can play ball, and they should not be allowed to use a sled on streets that are not blocked off for this purpose. They must not play in or around the car. Children this age must never be left alone in the car, either asleep or awake. In an attempt to "drive like Mommy," they can quickly set a car into motion. Accidents also have been caused by children left in cars who find matches or play with the cigarette lighter.

Burns that occur at this age frequently are due to children's experimentation with matches. Children are also intrigued by fancy cigarette lighters and coffee pots. These items are common hazards for this age group; they should be kept well out of reach, and their dangers should be explained.

Poisoning is still a danger. Children try to imitate adults and are apt to sample pills, especially if they smell good. Their increased freedom brings them into contact with many interesting containers in the garage or basement.

Preschool children are also taught the dangers of talking to or accepting rides from strangers. If they are stopped by a driver, they should run to a house where they know the people. Parents should make it clear to children in nursery school that they will never send a stranger to call for them. Children must know the dangers of playing in lonely places and of accepting gifts from strangers. Children should always know where to go if mother or father cannot be found.

Preschool children still require a good deal of unnoticed supervision to protect them from dangers that arise from their immature judgment or social environment.

Play in Health and Illness

VALUE OF PLAY

It has often been said that play is the business of children. Investigations stress the importance of play to both the well and the sick child's physical, mental, emotional, and social development. Children climbing on a jungle gym develop coordination of muscles and exercises all parts of the body. They use up energy and develop feelings of self-confidence. Their imaginations may take them to the jungle where they are swinging from limb to limb. They mentally face fears and solve problems that would be much more trying, if not impossible, in reality. They communicate with the other children and take a further step in the development of moral values, i.e., taking one's turn and consideration of others. Other types of play help them learn colors, shapes, sizes, and textures and teach them to be creative. This natural and readily available outlet must be tapped by institutional personnel. Preschool children may be unfamiliar with every facet of the hospital, but they know how to play, and playing is a good way for the nurse to establish rapport with them (Fig. 11–9).

THE NURSE'S ROLE

Some hospitals have well-established Child Life programs supervised by play therapists. Play ex-

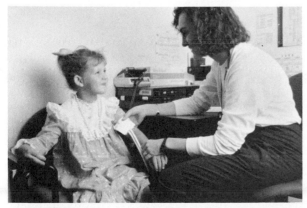

▲ **FIGURE 11–9**

The preschool child likes to please and is usually cooperative when noninvasive procedures are performed. (Courtesy of Cook–Fort Worth Children's Medical Center, Fort Worth, Texas.)

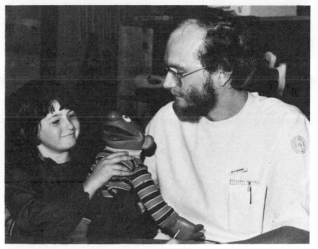

▲ **FIGURE 11–10**

Puppets are a universal means of communicating with children. (Courtesy of New Hampshire Vocational-Technical College, Claremont, New Hampshire.)

perience may be included during the nurse's education. It is not necessary to be an expert in manual dexterity, art, or music. To be of assistance one must be able to understand the needs of the child. Play is not just the responsibility of those who are assigned to it nor is it confined to certain times or shifts.

Many factors are involved in providing suitable play for children of various ages in the hospital (Fig. 11–10). The patient's state of health has to be considered. This will determine the amount of activity in which one can participate. The nurse can provide many activities that will relieve stress and provide enjoyment for the patient on bed rest. Overstimulation, nevertheless, would be hazardous for the severely ill child, e.g., the child with a heart disorder, who needs to conserve strength. Nurses should always be on guard for signs of fatigue in a patient and should use their judgment accordingly.

Basically, toys should be safe, durable, and suited to the child's developmental level (Table 11–4). Toys should not be sharp or have parts that are easily removed and swallowed. Too many toys at one time are confusing to the child. Complicated toys are frustrating and disappointing. Well-selected toys, such as balls, blocks, and dolls, are useful throughout the years. Each child needs sufficient time to complete the activity. In general,

Table 11–4. CHOOSING TOYS

AGE	TOYS	GENERAL CONSIDERATIONS
Infant	Soft stuffed animals and dolls Cradle gym Soft balls Bath toys Rattles Pots and pans	Baby likes to pat and hug. Toys should be brightly colored, of different textures, washable. Large enough so that they can't be aspirated. Smooth edges. Attention span is short. The infant looks at, reaches, grabs, chews
Toddler	Nest of blocks Push-pull toys Dolls Toy telephone Rocking horse or chair Wooden pegs and hammer Cloth books Pots and pans Ball	May have favorite toy. Enjoys exploring drawers and closets. Likes to place things in containers and dump them out. Parallel play. May injure others
Preschool	Crayons Simple puzzles Paints with large brushes Finger paints Dolls Dishes, housekeeping equipment Sand box, playground equipment Floating boats for water play Trucks Horns, drums, simple musical instruments Books about familiar circumstances Records	Shifts from solitary to parallel to beginning cooperative play. Exchanges ideas with others. Active play—climbs, runs, and hammers. Imitative play—firefighter, teacher. Imaginative play—let's pretend. Creative and dramatic play. Toys that do not require fine hand coordination. Games that teach safety in everyday life

quiet play should precede meals and bedtime for both the well and the sick child. Investigations have shown that the toys that are enjoyed by both boys and girls are more similar than dissimilar.

The nurse can entertain the child during routine procedures by nursery rhymes, stories, nonsense games, songs or finger play (Fig. 11–11). Often the other children on the unit can be included for "I'm thinking of something blue, red, and green," and so forth. Simple crafts are fun. The nurse may find various instructions from children's magazines or the local public library. Scrapbooks are entertaining. The child may even want to make a storybook about the hospital experience. The nurse who is involved in enrichment programs for children can make a definite contribution. A younger student may have helped out at a summer camp, babysat, or assisted at Sunday school. Surprise boxes in which a gift is opened every day provide anticipation for the patient. Collections of scrap material containing bright ribbons, bits of string, old popsicle sticks, pipe cleaners, paper bags, newspapers, or bits of cotton can be started in the classroom. Since the turnover of patients is fairly rapid, many projects can simply be repeated with different children.

Music is provided by the radio, record player, and piano. Sending messages to friends via a tape deck is enjoyed by older children. Special children's recordings are available. Drawing materials, finger paints, and modeling clay foster expression and creativity. They require merely a flat surface, such as the overbed table, and the particular medium. The bedridden child can participate in

Table 11–4. CHOOSING TOYS *Continued*

AGE	TOYS	GENERAL CONSIDERATIONS
School	Dolls and doll house Toy housewares Handicrafts Jump rope Skates Construction sets Trains Dress-up materials Table games Books for self-reading Bicycles Puppets Music	Attention span increases. Play is more organized, more competitive. Interested in hobbies or collections of things
The convalescent child	Ball on string that can be dropped from bed and returned Telephone Easy puzzles Large beads to string Record player close to bed Goldfish bowl Miniature autos, trains, dolls, farm animals Stick'ems, paper dolls Hand puppets Lap blackboard Alphabet boards Cutouts (Many toys previously listed are also applicable)	Play should not require a great expenditure of energy. Offer a wide variety because the child's interest span is decreased. Consider bed limitation. Toys should not require long continuous focusing of eyes. Consider toys that will be a little easier than those liked when well. Pay attention to special interests of individual child.

messy projects, too. The bed linens are protected by newspapers or plastic. Children in cribs need adequate back support for such projects. This is done by elevating the mattress or using pillows.

STORING TOYS

The hospital playroom may house many of the toys. Toys should be available for all shifts and should not be locked up at the end of the day. Children may have a durable washable bag tied to the bed for their own possessions. Closets, open shelves, toy chests, cupboards, and bins on rollers may be utilized in the hospital or home. Pegboards for hanging items frequently used are effective. Sturdy boxes, plastic ice cream contain-

ers, and laundry baskets are other suggestions for housing articles of various sizes and shapes. Children need to be taught how to care for toys following play. If children open and close drawers, they should use the handles so that their fingers will not get pinched.

PLAYMATES

Children need playmates to promote social development. The 1 year old plays near other children. The 2 year old grabs, pushes, and cannot share but in an individual way acknowledges other children. The older preschool child shows a beginning readiness for cooperative play. The ability to play with others increases during the school years,

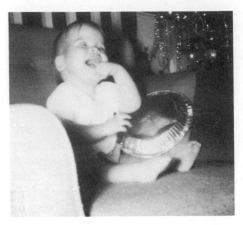

▲ FIGURE 11–11

Improvised games and songs amuse Kelly.

and in late elementary years girls prefer to play with girls and boys prefer to play with boys. This preference changes during adolescence. Playmates can be provided in the hospital playroom or on the unit. Children who are ambulatory can visit and play table games with bedridden patients. Of course the type of illness that each child has must be considered for everyone's protection. If there is a question as to the advisability of a particular type of play, ask your head nurse to obtain permission from the physician.

Factors that would be applicable to the healthy child at home should also be considered during hospitalization. Occasional play with younger children offers relief from competition with peers. However, continuous association with younger children tends to make a child immature in interests and behavior. Eventually this child could fall behind peers in physical skills and language. On the other hand, the child who is in the constant company of older children might feel inferior. This sets the pattern of submission to others. Older children tend to dominate and interfere with the friendships of younger children, which leads to bickering and disruption of play. When this is pronounced, younger children lose their friends and are unable to develop effective relationships with their peers.

Also, potential dangers are created by adults through domination, indifference, and overconcern. The nurse or parent who directs all the child's activities, chooses the friends, and plans and thinks for the child is doing a grave injustice. If one is indifferent to the social needs of preschool children, they will be lonely in the hospital, avoid their peers, and remain friendless. Overly concerned adults cannot bear to have children mistreated in any way during the normal give-and-take of childhood play. They scold the supposed offender and separate the children. This eventually isolates children, making it impossible for them to make the necessary social relationships needed for a healthy personality.

OTHER ASPECTS OF PLAY

Therapeutic Play. Play and toys can be of therapeutic value in the retraining of muscles, in the improvement of eye-hand coordination, and in helping children crawl and walk (push-pull toys). A musical instrument such as the clarinet promotes flexion and extension of the fingers. Blowing is an excellent prerequisite for speech therapy. Therapists supervise such activities. They leave specific instructions if they wish their work reinforced on the unit.

Play Therapy. The nurse may also hear the term *play therapy* used. This technique is used for the child under stress (Fig. 11–12). A well-equipped playroom is provided. The child is free to play with whatever articles she or he chooses. A counselor may be in the room observing and talking with the child, or the child may be observed through a one-way glass window. By using these as well as other methods the therapist obtains a better understanding of the patient's struggles,

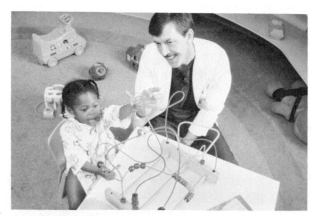

▲ FIGURE 11–12

The playroom should provide the child with opportunities to express feelings through play. (Courtesy of Cook–Fort Worth Children's Hospital, Fort Worth, Texas.)

fears, resentments, and feelings toward self and others. When the child acts out feelings through "dramatic play," they are externalized and provide a relief from tension. The interpretation of child behavior is complex and requires a great deal of time, study, and sensitivity before it can be fully understood.

Art Therapy. Art has been defined by Elinor Ulman as "the meeting ground of the world inside and the world outside." Art therapy is a process that is useful in communicating with children and adults. It is becoming more widely utilized. The art therapist is especially trained to assist children to express their feelings through drawings, clay, and other media. Some hospitals with inpatient mental health units have art therapy departments. An example of art work created by a sexually abused child is depicted on page 217.

Role of the Nurse. The nurse who is with children daily can describe their behavior. It is important to describe good as well as poor behavior, conversations that you may feel are pertinent, and the relationships with other children in the hospital. What is the approach to play? Do they join in freely or linger outside the group? Do they prefer active or quiet activities? Do they seem to be able to tolerate frustrations? Can they talk with their playmates and get their ideas across? What kind of attention span do they have? This type of charting is meaningful and should be used to describe the activities of pediatric patients so that they may be better understood.

References

Friman, P., and Schmitt, B. (1989). Thumb sucking: Pediatricians' guidelines. *Clin. Pediatr.* 28:438–440.

Levine, M., Carey, W., Crocker, A., and Gross, R. (1983). *Developmental-Behavioral Pediatrics.* Philadelphia, W. B. Saunders Company.

Offord, D., and Waters, B. (1983). Socialization and its failure. *In* Levine, M., et al. (eds.): *Developmental Behavioral Pediatrics.* Philadelphia, W. B. Saunders Company.

Rogers, W. B. Jr., and Rogers, R. A. (1972). A new simplified preschool readiness experimental screening scale (the PRESS): A preliminary report. *Clin. Pediatr.* 11:558.

Schmitt, B. (1990). Nocturnal enuresis: Finding the treatment that fits the child. *Contemp. Pediatr.* 7:70–97.

Bibliography

Foster, R., Hunsberger, M., and Anderson, J. (1989). *Family-Centered Nursing Care of Children.* Philadelphia, W. B. Saunders Company.

Herman-Giddens, M., Jellinek, M., Jonides, L., et al. (1989). *The Age of Mastery: A Multi-Disciplinary Roundtable Discussion on Toilet Training and Enuresis.* Educational grant from Kimberly-Clark Corp. New York.

Howard, B. (1990). Growing together: Learning independence in the preschool years. *Contemp. Pediatr.* 7:11–26.

Levine, M., Carey, W., Crocker, A., and Gross, R. (1983). *Developmental Behavioral Pediatrics.* Philadelphia, W. B. Saunders Company.

Lewis, M. (1989). Emotional development in the preschool child. *Pediatr. Ann.* 18:316–327.

Marlow, D., and Redding, B. (1988). *Textbook of Pediatric Nursing,* 6th ed. Philadelphia, W. B. Saunders Company.

Vaughan, V., and Litt, I. (1990). *Child and Adolescent Development.* Philadelphia, W. B. Saunders Company.

STUDY QUESTIONS

1. In what ways do the needs of the preschool child differ from those of the infant? The toddler?
2. Debbie, age 3, has a new baby brother. Discuss how you would prepare her for this situation.
3. What is meant by the term *discipline*? How do you feel about bodily punishment? Be prepared to discuss your answer in class.
4. Mrs. Welsh is wondering what to do with 4 year old Freddie. She states, "Lately he just never bothers to come into the house to urinate." What do you think would be the most effective way to handle this situation?
5. How do you feel the preschool child would react to hospitalization? Give reasons for your answer.
6. Henry is 5 years old. His father died unexpectedly. What special problems would this present to the preschool child?
7. What are the characteristics of a good nursery school?
8. You have been observing nursery school children during the past week. How will this experience help you during your assignment to the pediatric ward?
9. Sandy, age 3, and Joan, age 2, are playing in the living room. There is a squabble, and when you appear Sandy is snatching a book from Joan. Joan starts to cry. What would you do?
10. Of what value is play to the child? Why is play so important to the hospitalized child?
11. What accidents in particular are common with the preschool child?
12. Discuss the fears of a child of 3, 4, and 5 years. What measures can adults take to prevent them?
13. Define the following: *play therapy, art therapy, chronological age, PRESS.*

CHAPTER 12 _____

Chapter Outline

Objectives

Upon completion and mastery of Chapter 12, the student will be able to

- Define the vocabulary terms listed.
- Describe two milestones in the psychosocial development of the preschool child that contribute either positively or negatively to the adjustment during hospitalization.
- List and define the more common disorders of the preschool years.
- Identify the pathological changes that cause the following manifestations in a preschool child with leukemia: anemia, bone pain, proliferation of immature (blast) white cells, petechiae.
- Summarize the preoperative and postoperative nursing care for a preschool child scheduled for surgical removal of the tonsils and adenoids.
- Differentiate among the following types of seizures: tonic-clonic, absence, akinetic.
- List the nursing measures required for a patient during and following a tonic-clonic seizure.
- Describe the symptoms and nursing considerations in two communicable diseases seen in childhood.

Disorders of the Preschool Child

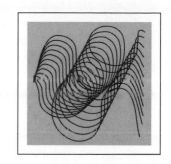

Terms

alopecia (309)
cytochemistry (305)
epicanthal fold (334)
hyperkalemia (322)
idiopathic (326)
myelosuppression (307)
prodromal (346)
thrombocytopenia (308)

Hospitalization is not as threatening to the preschool child as it is to the toddler, and it is easier for patients who have had more outside contact such as nursery school and kindergarten than for those who have never been separated from their parents. Since children of this age understand more, they can be better prepared for what will occur. They should be made to realize that hospitalization is not a punishment for something they have done wrong. They may feel guilty, particularly if an accident happens because of some mischief on their part, as in the case of burns or falls.

Although preschoolers tend to have less separation anxiety than do younger children, as their stress increases their tolerance for separation decreases.

The child may continually ask about the parents, refuse to eat, have difficulty sleeping, or withdraw. Nurses should use their communication skills to assist the child in dealing with feelings. The nurse might say, "Sometimes when I am in a strange place I feel afraid." This assists the child in expressing fears. The nurse and the parents must not tell a child that they will return unless they intend to do so.

> **COMMUNICATION ALERT ▶ ▶ ▶ ▶ ▶**
> Preschool children do not have a concept of time as it relates to the clock. If the child asks a question regarding time, the nurse might reply, "We will do that after cartoons," or "Mommy will come back after you eat your lunch."

Rivalry within a unit or in the playroom is common because the ages of the children are so varied. Younger children may wish to have the games or privileges that are allotted to the older children. They should be made to understand that certain rights come with age. The nurse deals with each child according to needs. Some require more emotional support than others.

At this age, the child is afraid of bodily harm, particularly invasive procedures. The surgical patient needs to be shown the part of the body that requires surgery. The nurse can sketch a body outline and draw a circle around the operative site, giving simple information about the system that will be affected, and stressing that this is the only area of the body that will be involved. Preschool boys also have a fear of castration. The nurse must be mindful of this if any procedure involves the genital area. When possible, the child should be allowed to look at his penis after the

303

procedure to reassure himself that the penis has been fixed and not cut off.

Patients also worry about other children on the unit who have physical deformities and wonder if this will happen to them. Questions concerning other children should not be ignored. Compliment those who shows inquisitiveness; listen to them and correct any misinterpretations that they may have. Help patients increase their self-esteem through praise. The child relieves tension through role playing. Tongue depressors, Band-Aids, and other materials related to everyday hospital life are relished by the sick child.

Children this age are pre-logical in their thinking and have difficulty distinguishing between fantasy and reality. They may believe that their illness was caused by something they did or thought. The nurse should tell preschoolers that their illness or the treatment is not a punishment. Also, words such as "dye," "cut off," "take out," or "draw" may be taken literally and may confuse the child (Whaley and Wong, 1987) (Fig. 12–1).

The nurse must be aware of nonverbal cues from children this age. The child may withdraw or act in an aggressive manner. Parents may tell their children to "be brave" or to "act like a man." This may stop the child from verbalizing fears and discomfort. A knowledge of growth and development guides the nurse in the assessment of the child.

The family is also affected by the child's hospitalization. If the caregiver stays with the child in the hospital, then normal duties at home are neglected. The parent may be concerned with small children who are being kept by relatives or friends. If the parents are unable to stay at the hospital, they may feel guilty about leaving the child and may attempt to rearrange their schedules to spend as much time as possible with the hospitalized child. Whatever the situation, the parents' needs should be identified by the nurse and attempts made to decrease the anxiety the parent is experiencing.

Preschool children may regress in their behavior when they are ill. They may also be irritable and demanding when they are discharged. The parent should be assured that these behavior changes are temporary and they will soon return to their "old self."

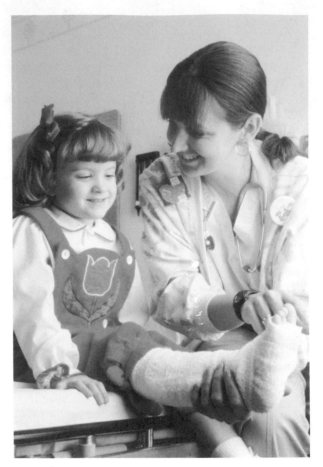

▲ **FIGURE 12–1**

Explanation of procedures can lessen a preschooler's anxiety. (Courtesy of Cook–Fort Worth Children's Medical Center, Fort Worth, Texas.)

The Blood

LEUKEMIA

Description. Leukemia (*leuko*, white + *emia*, blood) is a malignant disease of the blood-forming organs of the body that results in an uncontrolled growth of immature white blood cells. It is the most common type of cancer in children. There are several types of white blood cells. Some are produced in the red marrow of the bone; others are produced in the spleen and lymph nodes. The immature cells are called *blasts*, or stem cells (the suffix "blast" comes from the Greek *blastos*, meaning germ or formative cell). The white blood cell count may range from 5000 to as high as 100,000 cells per cu mm. In some cases the overall white blood cell count is normal, but the differential count may show a predominance of blast cells. The pathology of the disease lies in its ability to infiltrate and compete for metabolic elements. The reticuloendothelial system (liver, spleen, lymph glands) is most severely affected.

The classification of childhood leukemia has aided in the identification of prognostic factors and methods of treatment (Table 12–1). Various subtypes are now recognized on the basis of cell membrane markers and the reaction of the body cells to different chemical agents. This science is termed *cytochemistry*. About 75 per cent of childhood cases are *acute lymphocytic leukemia* (ALL); 15 to 20 per cent, *acute myelogenous leukemia* (AML); and the remainder, other forms of *acute nonlymphocytic leukemia* (ANLL).

The incidence of leukemia is highest in children between 3 and 4 years of age, and it occurs more commonly in boys than in girls. The cause of the disease is unknown. Current research on the relationship of viruses to leukemia is well under way. There also seems to be a genetic correlation,

as the incidence of leukemia is higher in children who suffer from Down syndrome and in twins. Investigators have associated leukemia with disorders of the immune mechanisms of the body. All tissues of the body are affected, either by direct infiltration of cancer cells or by the change in the blood that is carried to them. There is a reduction in the number of red blood cells, which produces anemia. The platelet count is also reduced, and since platelets are essential for the clotting of blood, hemorrhage occurs. Intracranial bleeding, if it occurs, can cause immediate death. Hemorrhage from other vital organs may occur. As cancer cells invade the bone marrow, bone and joint pain is experienced. Physiological fractures may occur. Leukemia that occurs outside the bone marrow is referred to as *extramedullary* (*extra*, outside + *medulla*, marrow). The most common sites for this are the central nervous system and the testicles. Increased evidence of extramedullary leukemia is being seen because children with this disorder are surviving longer.

Symptoms. The most common symptoms during the initial phase of the illness are low-grade fever, pallor, tendency to bruise, leg and joint pain, listlessness, and enlargement of lymph nodes. Abdominal pain, often attributed to other

Table 12–1. SOME PROGNOSTIC FEATURES OF ACUTE LYMPHOCYTIC LEUKEMIA IN CHILDREN

FACTOR	FAVORABLE	LESS FAVORABLE
Age	3–7 years	< 2 years and > 10 years
Race	White	Black
Sex	Female	Male
Initial white blood cell count	< 20,000/cm mm	> 50,000/cu mm
Mediastinal mass	No	Yes
T-cell markers on lymphocytes	No	Yes
Morphology—lymphocyte type	L1	L2, L3
Central nervous system involvement (at diagnosis)	No	Yes
Massive adenopathy	No	Yes
Massive enlargement of liver and spleen	No	Yes
Early diagnosis	Yes	No
Length of first remission	Long	Short

illnesses or even constipation, is a common symptom of leukemia. These symptoms may develop gradually or may be sudden in onset. As the disease progresses, the liver and spleen become enlarged. *Petechiae*—pinpoint hemorrhagic spots beneath the skin—and *purpura*—hemorrhage into the skin—may be early objective symptoms. Anorexia, vomiting, weight loss, and dyspnea are also common. The kidneys and testicles may become enlarged, and the patient may develop hematuria.

Because the white blood cells are not functioning normally, bacteria easily invade the body. Ulcerations develop about the mucous membranes of the mouth and anal region and have a tendency to bleed. Anemia becomes severe despite transfusions. The child may die as a direct result of the disease or from secondary infection. The symptoms are the same regardless of the type of white blood cell affected, and they vary widely with each patient, depending on the parts of the body involved.

Diagnosis. The diagnosis of leukemia is based on the history and symptoms of the patient and the results of extensive blood tests that demonstrate the presence of leukemic blast cells in the blood, bone marrow, and/or other tissues. Because the bone marrow is where many white and red blood cells are formed, a bone marrow aspiration is performed. Bone marrow is removed from the sternum or iliac crest by the use of a special needle and is studied in the laboratory. X-ray films of the long bones show changes in the bones. After the diagnosis has been confirmed, a spinal tap will determine any central nervous system involvement. Kidney and liver function studies are also performed, because normal function of these organs is absolutely necessary for the chemotherapy to be used in treating the disease.

NURSING BRIEF ▷ ▷ ▷ ▷ ▷ ▷ ▷ ▷
Repeated blood tests, especially in anemic infants and small children, can deplete blood volume, which could lead to hypoxia and shock unless the withdrawn blood is replaced.

Treatment

The development of specific chemotherapeutic agents for acute leukemia has changed the survival time significantly. In most cases of acute lymphoblastic leukemia, it is now possible to induce remissions that may be maintained for prolonged periods (more than 3 years). There is mounting optimism that some of these patients may never relapse and that the chemotherapy may thus represent a complete cure. Other acute varieties show a less predictable response to therapy. Untreated leukemia results in death from infection or hemorrhage in about 6 months. Components of therapy include (1) an induction period, (2) central nervous system prophylaxis, (3) maintenance, (4) reinduction therapy (if relapse occurs), and (5) extramedullary disease therapy.

The list of medications useful in the treatment of this disease is growing. A combination of drugs that is used to induce remissions includes prednisone, vincristine, and daunorubicin or L-asparaginase. They work within 4 to 6 weeks in about 95 per cent of children with ALL. The therapeutic effects of these drugs are of short duration, however, so that it is necessary to use additional drugs that help maintain the remissions. The steroid prednisone has the side effects of masking the symptoms of infection, increasing fluid retention, inducing personality changes, and causing the child's face to appear moon-shaped. Methotrexate and 6-mercaptopurine are useful in maintaining remissions, since they act against chemicals vital to the life of the white blood cell. These powerful medications produce side effects of varying degrees, such as nausea, diarrhea, rash, hair loss (alopecia), fever, anuria, anemia, and bone marrow depression. Peripheral neuropathy may be signaled by severe constipation due to decreased nerve supply to the bowel. Footdrop and difficulty with coordination may be seen. These complications are reversed once the offending drug is discontinued. The nurse should consult a pharmacology text for information concerning the particular drugs used for the patient in order to anticipate potential problems.

Intrathecal chemotherapy is given for central nervous system prophylaxis. Cranial radiation is no longer given unless the child has central nervous system relapse.

The various drugs used in treating leukemia may be given in cycles. Antibiotics are administered to prevent or control infection, and transfusions of whole blood or packed cells are given to correct anemia. Sedatives necessary for the patient's comfort are also administered. A pain reliever such as Percodan, codeine, Demerol, acetaminophen, or morphine may be ordered if the disease worsens; a Brompton cocktail is also useful. Medications should be administered before pain is too severe.

Bone Marrow Transplants and Immunotherapy. Bone marrow transplant is not recommended for children with ALL during the first remission because of their excellent prognosis with the use of chemotherapy. However, it is a consideration for children with ANLL during their first remission and children with ALL who have relapsed and are in their second remission (Trigg, 1988). Improvements in transplantation and supportive care, which involve specialized nursing care, have increased the number of long-term survivors of this procedure.

Immunotherapy, although still in the research stages, is another area of therapeutics. Immunotherapy may be passive or active, specific or nonspecific. The main objective of treatment is to strengthen the immune response of the patient to cancer cells and, it is hoped, prevent cancer by use of immunization.

Nursing Care

The child suffering from acute leukemia has many needs, both physical and psychological. These will vary in intensity according to exacerbations and progression of the disease. The diagnosis has such an impact on the patient's family that they are unable to focus on anything other than the child and the illness. Suppression of their own needs mounts if the disease is prolonged and can lead to illness and broken marital ties. Support groups such as those provided in Ronald McDonald Houses and various hospice programs aid parents in expressing and examining their concerns and give both the child and the family freedom to hurt but still remain whole.

Children's anxieties often center on their symptoms. They fear that the treatments necessary to correct their problems may be painful, as indeed some of them are—for example, venipunctures, bone marrow aspirations, and blood transfusions. Their trust in others is in a precarious balance. It is very important that nurses inform preschoolers of what they are about to do and why it is necessary. Their explanations should be made in terms the children will understand (Fig. 12–2).

It may be the nurse of whom the child asks the inevitable question, "Am I going to die?" One suggestion is to reply with a question such as "Why do you ask that? Do you feel sick today?" This may encourage the child to verbalize feelings. The pediatric nurse who gives a patient permission to discuss these concerns will find opportunities to clear up misconceptions and decrease the child's feelings of isolation. The element of hope is conveyed because it is indispensable to continued functioning, although the nature of hope may change from that of being cured to that of additional time to live. Further information on the holistic care of the dying child is presented on page 70. The following discussion focuses on the intense physical care necessary for the child with leukemia.

Remission Induction Period. Upon establishment of diagnosis, induction therapy is begun. The goal is to reduce the number of and preferably to eradicate leukemic cells. Careful explanations should be given to the child and family before any procedure is instigated. The disease and many of the necessary medications cause myelosuppression (*myelo*, marrow + suppression), which de-

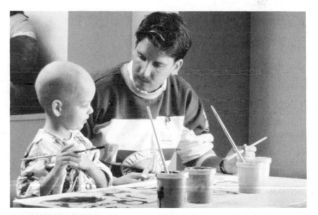

▲ **FIGURE 12–2**

The child life specialist plays an important role in helping meet the psychological needs of the child with cancer. (Courtesy of Cook–Fort Worth Children's Medical Center, Fort Worth, Texas.)

presses the normal function of the bone marrow as well as destroys cancer cells. The patient becomes anemic, may hemorrhage, and is highly susceptible to infection (even from harmless environmental flora).

Preventing Infection. Some of the organisms that may be hazardous to the child with leukemia are listed in Table 12–2. The choice of medication used to combat these infections varies according to the physician's protocol and the causative organism. When fever occurs, broad-spectrum antibiotics are begun until the offending agent is identified. Septra or Bactrim is administered to prevent the development of *Pneumocystis carinii* pneumonia, which is life-threatening. White blood cell transfusions may also be used. Laminar flow patient isolation (LFPI) rooms are available in some centers. These provide a protective environment for the highly susceptible patient.

In most hospitals patients are placed in a private room for their own protection. The nurse limits visitors and any auxiliary or medical personnel who appear unhealthy. All persons must meticulously adhere to handwashing techniques. Teaching parents concurrently will help prepare them for home care, i.e., protecting the patient from children with communicable diseases, handwashing, and so on. The nurse explains to the child the purpose for the various procedures utilized.

Observe the patient frequently for signs of infection. Particular attention is paid to potential infected sites such as the patient's mucous membranes and puncture breaks in the skin from laboratory or therapeutic procedures. Observe pierced ears for inflammation. Vital signs are observed for subtle variances, as steroid therapy may mask these indicators. Turn the patient often and observe for skin breakdown, particularly in the perianal area. Offer nutritious meals and supplemental feedings high in protein and calories. Teach parents and the child what to look for and to report. Chickenpox and other communicable diseases are a particular hazard to the child approaching school age. *Varicella-zoster immune globulin* (VZIG) may lessen the severity of the disease upon exposure. Open communication among the school nurse, family, clinic nurse, and physician is paramount.

Hemorrhage. Thrombocytopenic bleeding is a frequent complication of leukemia. The nurse observes the patient's skin for petechiae and ecchymosis. Nosebleeds are common and are treated by application of cold and pressure.

The mouth is inspected daily for ulcerations and hemorrhage from the gums. It may be rinsed with a prescribed solution of one part hydrogen peroxide to four parts saline solution. Commercial mouthwashes are used with caution, as they may alter normal flora and may cause fungal overgrowth. A Water-Pik is helpful in massaging and toughening the gums. A soft sponge toothbrush is helpful. The nurse may also clean food particles from the patient's teeth with a piece of gauze wrapped around the finger. Apply petroleum jelly to dry, cracked lips.

Hemorrhagic cystitis is not uncommon, as some drugs irritate the mucosa of the bladder. The nurse is alert to complaints of burning on urination or

Table 12–2. SOME INFECTIOUS AGENTS HAZARDOUS TO THE CHILD WITH LEUKEMIA

TYPE	ORGANISM
Bacterial	*Pseudomonas, Escherichia coli, Staphylococcus aureus, Klebsiella, Proteus*
Viral	Cytomegalovirus, varicella-zoster (chickenpox)
Protozoan	*Pneumocystis carinii* (prophylactic drugs—Septra, Bactrim)
Fungal	*Candida albicans, Histoplasma*

Note: Overwhelming infection can lead to death in children with leukemia. The possibility of infection is high during induction therapy, immediately following radiation therapy, and during maintenance.

feelings of pressure, which may indicate infection. Attention is given to providing plenty of fluids and encouraging frequent voidings. The physician is notified of complications immediately so that proper adjustment in medications can be made.

The nurse observes the patient for gastrointestinal bleeding. This is evidenced by *hematemesis* (*hema*, blood + *emesis*, vomiting) and bloody or tarry stools. Hemarthrosis (*hema*, blood + *arthron*, joint + *osis*, condition of), or effusion of blood into a joint cavity, may develop. This makes moving about painful; therefore, nursing intervention is necessary for the comfort of the patient when in or out of bed. The nurse manipulates catheters and suction drainage gently to avoid irritation of the sensitive mucosa. Scanning the patient's unit for environmental hazards is also of importance. Emergency procedures for control of bleeding are reviewed.

NURSING BRIEF ▷ ▷ ▷ ▷ ▷ ▷ ▷ ▷
Bleeding from the nose or mouth may be evidenced by a soiled pillowcase or sheet.

Transfusions. Platelet and packed red blood cells may be given to patients with anemia and thrombocytopenia (decrease in platelets in blood). If student nurses are asked to assume responsibility for the leukemic child receiving a *blood transfusion*, they request explicit directions from the team leader or charge nurse. Hemolytic reactions caused by mismatched blood are rare. Nevertheless, the registered nurse should positively identify donor and recipient blood types and groups on labels and the patient's chart with another professional. Blood is administered *slowly*. The patient is observed for *signs of transfusion reaction*, which include chills, itching, rash, fever, headache, and pain in the back or elsewhere. If such reactions occur, the student nurse clamps off the tubing immediately and reports to the nurse in charge. *Do not* remove the needle unless specifically instructed to do so. Save subsequent voiding of urine for hemoglobin determination.

Transfusions with piggyback setups are preferred. Blood and normal saline or other suitable intravenous solutions are connected by a stopcock. When blood must be stopped, tube patency can be maintained by opening the saline line. Neces-

sary emergency medications can thus be administered, and the vein is preserved for future infusions. Some facilities use an autosyringe to deliver small amounts of a blood product. When this is used, the line is flushed with normal saline before and after the infusion.

Circulatory overload is always a danger with children. The use of an infusion pump to regulate flow is routine. Dyspnea, precordial pain, rales, cyanosis, dry cough, and distended neck veins are indicative of this complication. Apprehension can also be a warning signal of air emboli or electrolyte disturbance. The nurse must maintain a high level of alertness for such signs, particularly in children whose conditions warrant repeated transfusions. If a reaction occurs, save the blood bag and tubing and return them to the blood bank. Most transfusion reactions occur within the first 10 minutes of administration; nevertheless, the patient is carefully monitored throughout this treatment.

Establish baseline data (temperature, pulse, respiration, and blood pressure) before transfusion and monitor for changes. It is helpful if the parents can remain with the child during this time. Suitable diversions will minimize boredom.

Elimination. Constipation is a common side effect of vincristine. Special care to promote normal bowel patterns is essential during the period children receive drug.

Skin and Hair Care. The skin is bathed daily and whenever necessary. Observe thoroughly for petechiae and bruising. Careful attention is given to the rectal mucosa, which is observed for fissures and ulcerations. Cleanse well after each bowel movement. Avoid using a rectal thermometer. Stool softeners may be necessary for relief of constipation, which frequently accompanies chemotherapy. Sitz baths promote relaxation and may lessen discomfort. The use of dry heat will promote healing.

The child's hair is combed daily and whenever necessary. Hair loss (*alopecia*) because of drug therapy is not unusual. Psychological preparation of the child and family will lessen its impact. Hair will return in a period of time, and meanwhile a wig suitable to the child's preference and age may be worn. If this is not acceptable, a cap is necessary during cold weather. Cleansing of the scalp will prevent cradle cap from forming.

Positioning the Patient. Repositioning of the patient is necessary to promote circulation and avoid pressure sores. Bone pain can be acute, and whenever possible coordinating administration of pain relievers with posture change is helpful. The patient is handled gently. A bean bag chair, a water bed, or a flotation mattress may be employed for comfort. Use a footboard to prevent footdrop due to peripheral neuropathy.

Nutrition. The patient is served well-balanced meals consisting of preferred foods. Since food may not be appealing to children with leukemia, nurses must use their ingenuity to interest them. Mealtimes are kept pleasant. The companionship of a nurse or attendant is preferable. The nurse should note individual preferences and report them to the dietitian. Food from home may be relished. When the child is too tired or irritable to eat, between-meal feedings are given. When parents understand this, they will be less anxious about what the child consumes at a particular meal. Steroid therapy often increases appetite, which is heartening but temporary. High-calorie commercial foods are tasty and can be used as an adjunct. A low-salt diet may be ordered during chemotherapy cycles containing prednisone to reduce the side effects of the steroid.

Small amounts of fluid are offered frequently. If the nurse places the fingers over the end of a drinking tube after it is in a glass of water, a suction can be created that will hold the water in the tube until it is placed in the child's mouth. Removing the finger allows the water to flow out of the tube. In this way the listless child can be given fluids. The child who is listless may receive a combination of oral and intravenous fluids. These children can be expected to have Hickman lines or Mediports for easy access. When parenteral fluids are given, they must be carefully observed (see page 54). A record is kept of all fluid intake and output.

Care of the child with leukemia is described in Nursing Care Plan 12–1.

HEMOPHILIA

Description. Hemophilia is one of the oldest hereditary diseases known. It has been called "the disease of kings" because it has occurred in children of several royal families in Russia and Europe. It is a sex-linked congenital disorder that primarily affects males. The male inherits the bleeding disorder from the mother who is the carrier. In hemophilia, the blood does not clot normally, and even the slightest injury can cause severe bleeding.

There are two types of hemophilia: hemophilia A and hemophilia B. Hemophilia A is five times more common than hemophilia B. For our purposes this discussion will be limited to classic hemophilia, or hemophilia A, which accounts for about 84 per cent of cases. The incidence of hemophilia A is about one in every 10,000 persons. The mechanism of blood formation is very complex. Defects in the synthesis of protein may lead to deficiencies in any of the factors in blood plasma needed for clotting to occur. The treatment of each type consists of replacing the deficient factor as it is isolated. The nursing care for all types is similar.

Hemophilia is due to a deficiency of coagulation factor VIII, or antihemophilic globulin (AHG). The severity of the disease depends on the level of factor VIII in the plasma of the patient's blood. Hemophilia is classified as severe, moderate, and mild. In mild hemophilia, bleeding is usually only a problem after surgery or major trauma. The child with moderate hemophilia can expect bleeding episodes after trauma. Children with severe hemophilia may bleed without apparent cause. The degree of severity tends to remain constant within a given family. The aim of therapy is to increase the level of factor VIII to assure clotting. It is possible to determine the level of factor VIII in the blood by means of a test called the *partial thromboplastin time* (PTT). This aids in the diagnosis and assessment of the child's condition. In some cases women who are carriers also can be identified.

Signs and Symptoms. Hemophilia is usually not apparent in the newborn infant unless abnormal bleeding occurs at the umbilical cord or following circumcision. As the child grows older and becomes more subject to injury, it is found that the slightest bruise or cut can induce extensive bleeding. Normal blood clots in about 3 to 6 minutes. In a patient with severe hemophilia, the time required for clotting may extend for an hour or more. Anemia, leukocytosis, and a moderate increase in platelets may be seen in the hemorrhaging child, who may show signs of shock. Hema-

Text continued on page 315

CARE PLAN 12–1

THE CHILD WITH LEUKEMIA

Nursing Diagnosis	Goals/Outcome Criteria	Nursing Interventions
Potential for infection, related to immunosuppression	Child will remain free of infection, as evidenced by normal vital signs, absence of respiratory changes, and normal laboratory values (blood, urine, wound cultures)	Good handwashing
		Prevent exposure to others who are ill
		Place child in private room or with child who is noninfectious
		Use scrupulous aseptic technique with all procedures
		Monitor vital signs for signs of infection
		Auscultate breath sounds for any abnormal signs
		Assess for any ulcerations of mucosa (mouth and anus)
		Assess for any breaks in skin integrity
		Axillary temperatures to prevent injury to rectal mucosa
		Observe IV site for signs of infection
		Report cloudy or foul-smelling urine
		Educate parents that they must notify the physician if the child develops a fever
		Communicate with school nurse, teacher, and family the importance of child not being exposed to communicable diseases (varicella) and the need to contact the physician immediately if exposure takes place

Care Plan continued on following page

CARE PLAN 12–1 *Continued*

THE CHILD WITH LEUKEMIA

Nursing Diagnosis	Goals/Outcome Criteria	Nursing Interventions
Injury, potential for bleeding, related to decreased platelets and breaks in skin	Child will show no signs of bleeding, as evidenced by lack of bruising, stable vital signs, and negative testing for blood in urine	Axillary temperatures to prevent injury to rectal mucosa Limit activity level when platelet count drops Monitor vital signs for signs of blood loss (tachycardia, hypotension) Monitor laboratory results (platelet count) Observe for hematuria (burning and pain on urination) Force fluids and encourage frequent voiding, including during the night Hematest emesis, urine, and stools Assess for petechiae and bruising Handle child gently Use toothettes to clean mouth and teeth
Knowledge deficit, related to disease process and treatment of disease	Family members demonstrate understanding of treatment and care of child.	Evaluate level of understanding Document teaching Provide written materials about disease and treatment Prepare child and family for procedures and treatments Plan and teach family regarding medications, laboratory results, procedures, side effects of treatments, and expected hospital admissions Encourage all to ask questions Involve child and family whenever possible in care of child

THE CHILD WITH LEUKEMIA

Nursing Diagnosis	Goals/Outcome Criteria	Nursing Interventions
Altered nutrition: less than body requirements, related to anorexia and nausea and vomiting	Child will consume adequate amounts of solids and liquids to maintain growth (based on child's needs)	Allow any food child will eat Assess for food preferences Obtain dietary consultation Small, frequent meals Make food appealing (small portions, attractively placed) Add food supplements to milkshakes (caution should be used if these distort the taste of a food the child is taking) Encourage parents to bring foods from home Intake and output recording Daily weights Administer antiemetics as ordered
Potential for impaired skin integrity, related to immobility and effects of treatment	Child's skin will remain intact	Provide meticulous skin care (especially mouth and perianal regions) Change position frequently Supply good nutrition Eggcrate or flotation mattresses
Anxiety, related to hospitalization, disease process, and treatment	Family and child will express feelings concerning illness	Encourage verbalization of fears and feelings Provide for a consistent nurse to care for child Keep parents and child informed of care Orient to hospital and the care child will receive Allow time for parents to ask questions Involve parents and child, if appropriate, in care Refer to social services Refer to support group
Pain, related to disease process and treatment of disease	Child will verbalize comfort, rest quietly, show no signs of distress (grimacing, crying, restlessness)	Assess for pain (nonverbal cues) Use distraction Provide for a quiet room and comfortable temperature Administer pain medication as ordered Document response to pain medication Avoid pressure on painful areas or bony prominences Sit with child, hold child

Care Plan continued on following page

Nursing Diagnosis	Goals/Outcome Criteria	Nursing Interventions
Body image disturbance, related to side effects of treatment and disease process (loss of hair, moon face, weight changes)	Child will discuss body changes and participate in activities with friends	Encourage older children to try different things to cover their head (wigs, hats, scarfs, turbans)
		Suggest short hair to make styling easier
		Integrate child with peers as soon as possible to avoid marked changes in appearance
		Provide opportunities for child to discuss changes taking place with body
		Introduce to other children with cancer
		Utilize child therapist to assist child in working through feelings about changes in body appearance (play therapy, art, role playing)
		Reassure that changes are temporary
		Reassure hair will regrow in 3 to 6 months and may be slightly different in color and texture (alopecia during a second treatment is usually less)
Altered family process, related to child with life-threatening disease	Family will discuss feelings and participate in care of child	Encourage the family to discuss feelings concerning disease and treatment
		Explain hospital routine, expected treatment, and procedures
		Provide for a consistent nurse to care for child
		Prepare family for expected physical and psychological changes from the disease and treatment
		Involve parents in care when possible
		Encourage family to allow the child to lead as normal a life as possible (school, peers, discipline)
		Discuss needs of siblings and their involvement with the ill child
		Refer to support groups and social services

turia is occasionally seen. Death can result from excessive bleeding anywhere in the body, but particularly when hemorrhage occurs into the brain or neck.

The circumstances leading to diagnosis may be the inability of a parent to stop a child's bleeding from a cut about the mouth or gums. A tooth extraction may precipitate problems in an unknown bleeder. An injured knee, elbow, or ankle presents particular problems for this patient. Hemorrhage into the joint cavity, or hemarthrosis, is considered a classic symptom of hemophilia. The *effusion* (*ex*, out + *fundere*, to pour) into the joint is very painful because of the lack of space. Repeated hemorrhages may cause permanent deformities that could cripple the child. The nurse may hear this deformity referred to as an *ankylosis* (*ankyle*, stiff joint + *osis*, condition of).

Treatment

The patient's family history is of particular importance in the diagnosis of hemophilia. When hemophilia is present and the patient has had periods of abnormal bleeding from early childhood, the determination is relatively easy. However, in many cases the family history may be vague or unobtainable. In some instances, even careful scrutiny produces no evidence of the disease in the family. Researchers believe that such cases result from new gene *mutations*. The cause of the mutations is not known, although exposure to excess radiation may be one possibility. Prenatal diagnosis can be made by fetoscope.

> **COMMUNICATION ALERT ▶ ▶ ▶ ▶ ▶**
> The preschool child can be included in the admission interview by saying, "Jimmy, tell what happened when you fell off the swing." After the child recounts the incident, the nurse can direct the interview by asking specific questions if the child has not already answered them.

Current treatment of hemophilia is the administration of concentrated preparations of factor VIII

(Pierce and colleagues, 1989). These are currently manufactured from fresh frozen plasma and cryoprecipitate, which are from single blood donors and require special freezing, and "freeze-dried" factor VIII and factor IX concentrates. They may be kept at room temperature or in the refrigerator. In the past, the risk of hepatitis and AIDS has been high in this population because there can be as many as 20,000 donors in one lot of factor VII concentrate. Currently all blood donors are tested for blood-borne viruses, and all blood products are tested for hepatitis and the virus that causes AIDS. All concentrates are also specially treated and purified to reduce the risks of these diseases. Recombinant factor VIII is a new product, not derived from human blood, that should be available in the near future (Eckert, 1990). Only then will the risk of hepatitis and AIDS to this population be totally eliminated.

The concept of comprehensive care for hemophilia was introduced in the mid-1970s. This is advantageous because the patient sees professionals who are experienced in seeing many patients with the same illness (Hockenberry and Coody, 1986). Patients or their parents are taught how to administer the prescribed concentrate so that treatment can be done at home. The nurse assists the patient and family in learning about and understanding the disease. The goal is for the patient to become independent and for the health care center to be available as a backup when a need arises.

Nursing Care

An open wound is treated immediately by the use of cold and pressure. When possible, elevate the bleeding area above heart level to decrease blood flow. The child or parents can sometimes sense when a bleed is occurring. Parents should have ice packs available at all times. Nosebleeds can be controlled by tilting the head forward and applying firm pressure to the nose for 15 to 30 minutes. Mouth bleeding is usually minor, but if it cannot be controlled, Amicar, an antifibrinolytic agent, may be used to promote clot formation. *Hemarthrosis* (bleeding into a joint) is the most common type of hemorrhage and the most debilitating associated with hemophilia. It occurs most frequently in the knees, elbows, and ankles. The deficient factor should be given and the joint immobilized. Cold packs should be applied to decrease the pain, and analgesics such as acetaminophen can be given as ordered. Aspirin should be avoided as it has a depressive effect on platelet function. The joint may be placed in a splint. When the bleeding has ceased, passive exercises are performed by the physical therapist.

When the patient with hemophilia is an infant, the crib sides require padding and all toys must be checked for sharp edges. The nurse carefully observes the skin at bath time for bruises or hematomas. The patient's nails are kept short. Good oral hygiene is essential. Select a toothbrush with soft bristles. The dentist needs to be consulted early in the preschool years to establish a program of preventive therapy. The patient requires well-balanced meals. Excessive weight gain is to be avoided, as it places additional strain on the joints. If the child is receiving medication by injection or if blood work has been ordered, pressure is applied to the site. The site is carefully observed by the patient's nurse to ensure that all is well. The patient's stools and urine are observed for blood. The vital signs are taken routinely to detect concealed bleeding. Patients are instructed to wear a Medic-Alert bracelet.

Home care programs are the treatment of choice. This greatly reduces the cost of treatment and decreases the risk of psychological trauma. Teaching is done by the physician and nurse in the specialty clinic. Instruction includes an exact explanation of the illness, with emphasis on the signs and treatment of hemorrhage. Specific procedures include the storage and preparation of replacement factors, venipuncture, transfusion management and transfusion reactions, and record keeping. Signs of complications are reviewed and emergency numbers and other protocols are spelled out.

Having a child with hemophilia provides a challenge to the family. The family needs to create a positive environment that allows the child to be independent. It is natural for parents to be overprotective. Parents need to understand that they can create a "safe environment" while still allowing the child to develop to full capabilities. The National Hemophilia Foundation is a resource for financial, psychological, and medical support for the family.

NURSING BRIEF ▷ ▷ ▷ ▷ ▷ ▷ ▷ ▷
Instruct parents of the hemophiliac child to avoid administration of medications that inhibit platelet function, e.g., aspirin. Explain the importance of contacting their physician or pharmacist before giving any over-the-counter drugs to the child.

The Respiratory System

TONSILLITIS AND ADENOIDITIS

Description. The tonsils and adenoids, located in the pharynx, or throat, are made of lymph tissue and act as part of the body's defense mechanism against infection. The tonsils and adenoids formerly have been blamed for causing many assorted illnesses, and for a time it was thought that having them removed was part of growing up. Today, doctors stress that not *all* children need to have them removed. A careful physical examination and an evaluation of the patient's history are done to rule out other diseases. The fact that tonsils are enlarged is not sufficient evidence for removal. These structures are normally larger in early childhood than in later years. The current trend is to treat the conditions as separate problems, according to individual criteria.

Treatment

The removal of the tonsils and adenoids, referred to as a *T and A,* is not usually recommended for the child three or four years of age or younger. It is felt that if surgery is postponed until later, the condition may correct itself, since the tissues become smaller as the child grows. It is also easier for the child to cope with hospitalization when older. Fears are not as intense, especially those of abandonment.

The decision as to whether or not surgery is required is perhaps the most important single factor from a medical standpoint. Same-day surgery is becoming common. The use of antibiotics during acute infections has reduced the need for surgery. The patient should be free of symptoms for 2 to 3 weeks before an operation is attempted.

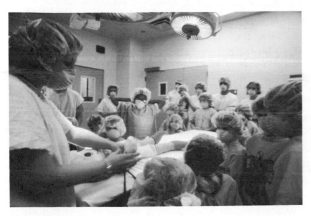

▲ FIGURE 12–3

Children visit an operating room prior to surgery. Familiarization with equipment and the setting reduces fear. (Courtesy of Cook–Fort Worth Children's Medical Center, Fort Worth, Texas.)

Nursing Care

Preoperative Care. Many T and As are done in the day surgery, and the child is sent home the night of surgery. The child is prepared in advance for hospitalization. Children need to know that the tonsils are two small lumps located in the back of the mouth. Since they are causing the throat to be sore (or whatever symptoms the children are experiencing), they need to be fixed. The doctor will do this by taking them out. The doctor will not operate on any other part of the body. Children are also informed that they will receive a special medicine that will make them go to sleep and will keep them asleep until the operation is over. Then *they will wake up.* Medical personnel and parents must be alert to the young child's fantasies and anxieties and answer questions honestly and at a level suitable to the age of the child.

One concern uncovered by television personality Mister Rogers is that many young children fear that an operation will change them into a completely different person (Rogers and Head, 1983). Children need to know that medical personnel understand their feelings. It is also important that someone they know and trust is close by. Include the child's parents in discussions and encourage them to stay with the child. Many hospitals have special programs to prepare children for surgery. These include videotapes, prehospital tours, and opportunities to handle supplies (Fig. 12–3).

A complete physical examination and urinalysis are performed before surgery. Blood work includes hemoglobin, hematocrit, prothrombin time (PT), and partial thromboplastin time (PTT). The latter tests are done because bleeding is anticipated. These procedures are usually performed prior to admission (Fig. 12–4). The child is inspected for loose teeth and signs of upper respi-

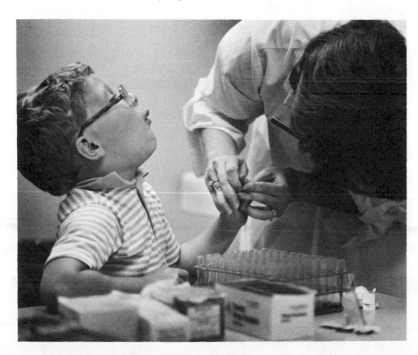

▲ FIGURE 12–4

Laboratory work for same-day surgery is performed on an outpatient basis. (Courtesy of Raymond Blank Memorial Hospital for Children, Des Moines, Iowa.)

ratory tract infection. It is also important to determine any family bleeding tendencies, any history of chronic illness (such as rheumatic fever), elevations in temperature, and recent exposure to communicable diseases. The child is encouraged to drink fluids the evening before surgery to maintain hydration; however, food and fluids are withheld for several hours prior to surgery to prevent aspiration from vomitus. If the child is hospitalized, the child's bed is tagged with an NPO sign. In some hospitals, a sign is attached directly to the child's clothing. The nurse should check the patient's bedside stand for candy or gum and remove them. The nurse checks to see that the child's identification band is securely attached to the wrist. The patient should void before leaving the unit. The child may or may not receive a preoperative injection. Some facilities use rectal induction, which allows the child to go to sleep in the parent's arms. Many hospitals like to have parents in the recovery room to decrease children's anxiety by providing a familiar face and arms to welcome them when they awaken. Review postoperative procedures with the parents, including what to expect when the child returns to the room (e.g., color, bleeding, possible use of an IV, vomiting, irritability).

NURSING BRIEF ▷ ▷ ▷ ▷ ▷ ▷ ▷ ▷

In differentiating sleep from death to a young child, one points out that in sleep the insides of the body slow down, whereas in death they stop completely.

Postoperative Care. Immediately following surgery, to facilitate drainage, the child is placed partly on the side and partly on the abdomen, with the knee of the uppermost leg flexed to hold the position. The child is watched carefully for evidence of bleeding, i.e., an increase in pulse and respirations, restlessness, frequent swallowing, and vomiting of bright red blood. An ice collar may be applied for comfort. Some children prefer not to have an ice collar. If wearing the collar causes the child to be upset, it should be discarded. More damage could be done by a crying child than the good done by an ice collar. An emesis basin and tissues are provided. The child's face and hands are wiped with a warm face cloth, and the hospital gown and linen are changed whenever necessary. Small amounts of clear liq-

uids are given when the vomiting has ceased. Synthetic fruit juices are used because they are not as irritating as natural juices. A popsicle may appeal to the child. If these are tolerated well, progression to a soft diet is begun. The child is kept quiet for the remainder of the day. A small child may nestle on a parent's lap.

Hemorrhage is the most common postoperative complication. The nurse should not assume that because surgery is minor it does not involve certain risks. Because bleeding after this type of surgery is concealed, the nurse must watch carefully for evidence of hemorrhage. When bleeding is suspected, packing and sometimes ligation are indicated. Lung abscesses and pneumonia are infrequent complications.

Hospital Discharge. Written instructions are given to the parents when the child is discharged. The child should be kept quiet for a few days and should receive nourishing fluids and soft foods. After this, children may continue to take a nap or have a rest period so that they have a sufficient convalescent time. Acetaminophen (Tylenol) may be given to reduce discomfort in the throat. The child needs to be protected from exposure to infections. Fresh bleeding, chest pain, or persistent cough should be reported to the physician. Earache may follow a T and A, and slight fever (37.2 to 37.8° C, or 99 to 100° F) may occur for one or two days. A follow-up appointment is made, since the surgeon will wish to check the operative site after it has healed.

ASTHMA

Description. Asthma is the most common chronic illness in childhood. It is also the leading cause of emergency room visits, hospital admissions, and school absenteeism. Eighty per cent of cases of asthma occurs before the age of 5 years. Prior to puberty it is more common in boys; after puberty the sex incidence is equal.

Asthma is a reversible obstruction of the large and small airways, caused by mucosal edema, smooth muscle constriction, and thick, tenacious mucus. The onset of asthma may be precipitated by allergens such as pollens, foods, dust mites, and animal dander. Asthma also may be triggered by temperature changes, cold air, viral infections,

Table 12–3. ADRENERGIC BRONCHODILATORS

Name	Trade Name	Dose Form	Duration
Albuterol	Proventil Ventolin	MDI/solution Syrup/powder	4–6 hours
Isoetharine	Bronkosol Bronkometer	MDI/solution	3 hours
Metaproterenol	Alupent Metaprel	MDI/solution Syrup	4 hours
Terbutaline	Brethine Brethaire Bricanyl	MDI Solution (injection)	4–6 hours
Pirbuterol	Maxair	MDI	4–6 hours

MDI, metered-dose inhaler.
From Green, N., and Haggerty, R. (1990). *Ambulatory Pediatrics.* Philadelphia, W. B. Saunders Company.

and exercise. Although emotional stress may aggravate asthma, it is probably more likely that asthma may precipitate stress (Goldenhersh and Rachelefsky, 1989).

A family history of allergies is often seen, although the patient may have different manifestations. Although asthma can be fatal, most children with onset before the age of 5 years will go into remission when they are in their teens. Children with severe chronic asthma and those with onset in adolescence often continue to have recurrent asthma in adulthood (Behrman and Kliegman, 1990). In *status asthmaticus,* an episode of asthma does not respond to ordinary therapeutic measures. Hospitalization is required, and the child may be in the intensive care unit.

Treatment

The goals of treatment are to minimize symptoms, prevent acute exacerbations, maintain optimal function, avoid side effects of therapy, and help the child maintain a normal lifestyle (Traver and Martinez, 1988). Treatment has four foci: (1) control of allergens, (2) immunotherapy, (3) drug therapy, and (4) self-management.

The physician obtains the child's history in detail. Skin tests may be administered to determine whether allergy is a cause. It is then necessary to eliminate the offender, whether it is an environmental agent or a food. Special measures may be

taken to reduce dust, humidity, and tobacco smoke in the home.

Table 12–3 lists the common bronchodilators used in the management of asthma. The preferred route of administration of these medications is by aerosol inhalation. This provides delivery directly to airway receptors and allows a lower dosage, a more rapid onset, a longer duration of effects, and fewer side effects (Green and Haggerty, 1990). These drugs may also be given by metered-dose inhaler (Table 12–4). Cromolyn sodium is administered in the inhaled form and can be given alone or in conjunction with the aforementioned drugs.

Whereas albuterol blocks early response to antigen inhalation, cromolyn blocks late asthmatic response. Theophylline is still a safe and effective choice for children who need daily instead of as-

Table 12–4. METERED-DOSE INHALER: OPEN-MOUTH TECHNIQUE

1. Open mouth with tongue forward.
2. Hold MDI 2 inches from mouth.
3. Begin slow inspiration.
4. Activate MDI as inspiration begins.
5. Hold breath for 10 seconds.
6. Wait 2 to 5 minutes between inhalations.

From Green, N., and Haggerty, R. (1990). *Ambulatory Pediatrics.* Philadelphia, W. B. Saunders Company.

needed treatment. Theophylline can cause nausea, vomiting, abdominal discomfort, headache, nervousness, and behavioral changes such as attention deficit. Obviously, these can cause problems with compliance. Serum levels are monitored to insure a therapeutic dose. Finally, steroids may be used in the oral or inhaled form. For long-term treatment they should be used by the inhaled route because they produce fewer side effects.

The patient and parent are taught home management. Educational materials and instruction about the disease are given. The child is encouraged to have a planned exercise program. Instruction is also given in taking the medication, methods of administration, and possible side effects. Finally, the child and the family should be aware of early signs of an asthma attack and the methods of limiting such an attack.

A child is hospitalized with asthma when there is significant airway obstruction and inadequate response to initial treatment. The treatment of the hospitalized child is different from the maintenance management. Nebulized albuterol may be given while breath sounds and the heart rate are monitored. An intravenous solution is started, and oxygen is given by nasal prongs, hood, or mask. Aminophylline is given in a loading dose, followed by a continuous infusion of the medication. Dosage is adjusted by assessing the response of the patient and monitoring the serum theophylline levels. Intravenous steroids are administered to control the inflammatory response. Before discharge the child is changed to oral medication.

Nursing Care

The child who is hospitalized with asthma will have an intravenous infusion started. If the child is not in acute respiratory distress, oral fluids also should be offered. The child has increased needs for fluids because of loss through dyspnea and diaphoresis. Fluids also aid in liquefying secretions. Fluids offered should not be cold, for these may cause bronchospasm. The child is placed on intake and output measurement. If aminophylline is given, vital signs are monitored closely. Check with your institution how often this is done, for the time varies from setting to setting. Vital signs, breath sounds, and a respiratory assessment are done at least every 4 hours. Children in acute distress are assessed more frequently.

Place the child in high-Fowler position. Some children may prefer to have a pillow placed on the over-bed table and to extend their arms over it. This allows maximal utilization of the accessory muscles of breathing. The child may be placed in a mist tent or may receive oxygen by mask or cannula. An oxygen mask is not used if it causes the child anxiety. The nurse should organize care to provide for periods of uninterrupted rest. The child may be apprehensive due to the respiratory distress. The nurse should display a calm manner and remain with the child during periods of distress.

Prior to discharge, the older child and parent are taught self-care. The patient is taught to recognize early signs of difficulties and "personal triggers" that can serve as forewarnings of an attack. The importance of following directions in the administration of medications is stressed, as is being aware of side effects. The use of nebulizers or aerosol devices is also taught. Specific information about how often and when to use a particular inhaler is also emphasized. Exercise is stressed. Swimming is an excellent sport for asthmatics. The child needs to be seen regularly by the physician to evaluate progress and adjust medications as needed. Review signs of respiratory infection and where, when, and whom to call for help. Listen to and provide support for the patient, parents, and siblings. Refer the family to social services for additional support and to the Asthma and Allergy Foundation of America or the American Lung Association.

The Muscular System

DUCHENNE MUSCULAR DYSTROPHY (PSEUDOHYPERTROPHIC)

Description. The muscular dystrophies are a group of disorders in which progressive muscle degeneration occurs. The childhood form (Duchenne muscular dystrophy) is the most common type, with an incidence of about 0.14 per 1,000 children. It is a sex-linked inherited disorder occurring only in boys. Mothers are likely carriers for the disease; however, spontaneous mutations also occur. Individuals at risk in the female bloodline may choose to be evaluated and counseled about the carrier state.

Symptoms. The onset is generally between 2 and 6 years of age; however, a history of delayed motor development during infancy may be evidenced. A waddling gait, slowness in running or climbing, and enlarged, rubbery muscles are indicative of this disorder. The calf muscles in particular become hypertrophied. Other signs include frequent falling, clumsiness, contractures of the ankles and hips, and Gower maneuver (a characteristic way of rising from the floor) (Fig. 12–5). Laboratory findings show marked increases in blood creatine phosphokinase (CPK). Muscle biopsy reveals degeneration of muscle fibers and replacement of these fibers by fat and connective tissue. An *electromyogram* (a graphic record of muscle contraction as a result of electrical stimulation) shows decreases in amplitude and duration of motor unit potentials. Electrocardiographic abnormalities are also common. The disease becomes progressively worse, and wheelchair confinement occurs when the child is about 12 years old. Seventy-five per cent of these patients die before 20 years of age (Behrman and Vaughan, 1987). Death is usually due to cardiac failure or respiratory infection. Mental retardation may occur.

Treatment and Nursing Care

Treatment at this time is mainly supportive. This consists of passive exercises to prevent joint contractures, bracing, weight control, surgery for joint contractures, and referrals to appropriate social agencies. Psychological considerations revolve about the chronic and progressive nature of the disease and its fatal outcome. Family denial of the diagnosis is common early in the disease, when symptoms are fairly benign. If the patient

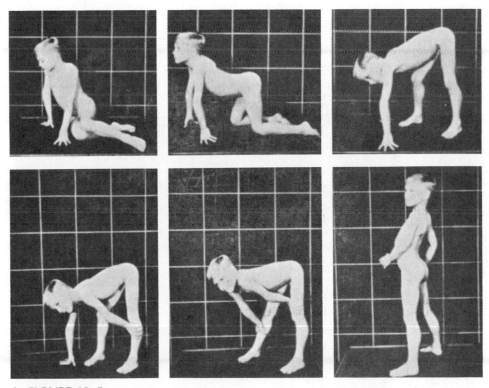

▲ **FIGURE 12–5**

A child 7 years of age with pseudohypertrophic muscular dystrophy, showing the characteristic manner of rising from the floor (Gowers sign). The last picture shows the standing position with the severe lordosis. (From Behrman, R., and Vaughan, V. (1987). *Nelson Textbook of Pediatrics*, 13th ed. Philadelphia, W. B. Saunders.)

is hospitalized for diagnosis, parents and child are prepared for muscle biopsy and electromyography. During the biopsy a small piece of muscle is removed for examination. Vital signs and drainage from the incision are monitored following the procedure. During electromyography small needles are placed in the muscles to record contractions. Muscles examined may ache slightly following the test, but this is temporary. There is no special preparation preceding electromyography. Whenever possible, the nurse should plan to remain with the child during the test.

Compared with other children with disabilities, the child with muscular dystrophy may appear passive and withdrawn. Early on, he may become very depressed, as he is unable to compete with his peers. Social and emotional pressures on the child and his family are great. Financial pressures become magnified as medical and surgical costs escalate. In addition, expensive alterations to the family, home, and vehicles are sometimes necessary.

Nurses function as team members along with personnel from many other disciplines in the care of the child with muscular dystrophy. They encourage the child to be as active as possible in order to delay muscle atrophy. They provide support for the many daily issues that occur by placing parents in touch with other parents, camp programs, respite care, the Muscular Dystrophy Association, public health nurses, home health agencies, family therapists, and eventually hospice care.

The Urinary System

ACUTE GLOMERULONEPHRITIS

Description. Acute glomerulonephritis seems to be an allergic reaction (antigen-antibody) to an infection in the body. The infection is generally caused by a nephritogenic strain of group A beta-hemolytic streptococci infecting the throat. It may appear after the patient has had scarlet fever or skin infections. The body's immune mechanisms appear to be important in its development. Antibodies produced to fight the invading organisms also react against the glomerular tissue. Glomerulonephritis is the most common form of nephritis

in children and occurs most frequently in boys between 3 and 7 years of age. It has a seasonal incidence with peaks in winter and spring. Both kidneys are affected.

From a study of the urinary system one may recall that the nephron is the working unit of the kidneys. Nephrons number in the millions. Within the bulb of each nephron lies a cluster of capillaries called the glomerulus. It is these structures that are affected, as the name implies. They become inflamed and sometimes blocked, permitting red blood cells and protein, which are normally retained, to enter the urine. The kidneys become pale and slightly enlarged.

The prognosis is excellent. Patients with mild cases of the disease may recover within 10 to 14 days. Patients with protracted cases may show urinary changes for as long as a year but have complete recovery. Chronic nephritis is seen in a small number of children, death generally being the result of renal failure or heart failure. These severe complications, plus hypertensive changes in the blood supply of the brain, necessitate careful observation and care of each patient.

Symptoms. Symptoms range from mild to severe. From 1 to 3 weeks after a streptococcal infection has occurred in the child, the mother may notice that the urine is smoky brown in color or bloody. This is frightening to the mother and child; medical advice is immediately sought by most parents. *Periorbital edema* (mild swelling about the eyes) may also be present, with fever (high at first but gradually leveling off to about 37.8° C, or 100° F), headache, diarrhea, and vomiting. Urinary output is decreased. The urine specific gravity is high, and albumin, red and white blood cells, and casts may be found upon examination. The blood urea nitrogen (BUN) level is elevated, as are the serum creatinine and sedimentation rates. The serum complement level is usually reduced. *Hyperkalemia* (excess potassium in the blood) may produce cardiac toxicity. Hypertension may occur. Complications such as heart failure and encephalopathy may occur.

Treatment

Although the child may feel well, he is confined to bed until gross hematuria subsides. The urine is examined regularly. Every effort is made to prevent the child from becoming overtired, chilled, or exposed to infection. As renal function is impaired, there is a danger of accumulation of nitrogenous wastes and sodium in the body. Sodium is restricted until symptoms disappear; then the patient is returned to a regular diet. Protein restriction is not usually required. Fluid restriction may be necessary for some patients. A liquid diet is instituted and is followed by a soft to full diet as tolerated. Penicillin is given during the acute phase and may be continued orally for a period of time to prevent renewed activity before healing is complete. Second attacks of glomerulonephritis are rare.

Nursing Care

The nurse should try to make the period of bed rest as pleasant as possible for the patient by providing quiet diversions. She should protect the child from being chilled during the bed bath and trips to various departments. Sufficient blankets are provided at night. When the child is allowed up, the nurse observes him frequently for signs of fatigue. He should be protected from contact with persons with infections.

The patient's vital signs are taken regularly, preferably with the same apparatus. A rise in blood pressure is reported immediately. Between readings the nurse should be alert for symptoms such as headache, drowsiness, vomiting, and blurring of vision. If any of these are noticed, the child is returned to bed and the cribsides or rails are raised. Since convulsions can occur, someone should remain with the child until medication is given. Hypotensive drugs may be ordered by the physician. These reduce the blood pressure rapidly, and the cerebral symptoms subside. If cardiac failure is evidenced by an electrocardiogram or chest radiograph, sedation, oxygen, and digitalis may be required.

An *accurate* record is kept of the patient's fluid intake and urine output. Fluids may be restricted, especially if the urinary output is scant. The physician will order the oral intake allowed, for example, 650 ml daily. This must be distributed throughout the 24-hour period. Each shift should know the specific amount of fluids the patient is to receive so that an excess amount is not given. The greater amounts of fluid are allotted to the

day and evening shifts when thirst is more pronounced. The individual needs of the child should be observed and incorporated into the day's events. Daily weighing of the patient will also help to determine progress. Persistent anuria may require dialysis by the artificial kidney.

Although glomerulonephritis is generally benign, it can be a source of anguish for parents and child. If the patient is treated at home, the parents must plan activities to keep the child occupied while confined to bed. They must understand the importance of continued medical supervision, as follow-up urine and blood tests are necessary to ensure that the disease has been eradicated.

The Nervous System

MENTAL RETARDATION

Description. The national organization for professionals and paraprofessionals working with the retarded, the American Association on Mental Deficiency (AAMD), defines mental retardation as "significantly sub-average general intellectual functioning existing concurrently with deficits in adaptive behavior and manifested during the developmental period" (Grossman, 1983). The AAMD emphasizes both intelligence and behavior as criteria. Tests to measure intelligence are numerous. One test that is frequently given to children and adolescents is the Stanford-Binet Intelligence Scale. These tests differ somewhat depending on the age of the subject. Intelligence testing of children is difficult to evaluate and is best done on an individual basis. Personality tests such as picture story tests, inkblot tests, drawing tests, and sentence completion tests may also be administered. All such tests have their limitations and, of course, are subject to the abilities of the person interpreting them. The tests, nonetheless, are of value when used in conjunction with a thorough study of the child's physical, mental, emotional, and social development.

There are many causes of mental retardation. Some conditions that can develop during the prenatal period are phenylketonuria, Down syndrome, fetal alcohol syndrome, malformations of the brain (such as microcephaly, hydrocephalus, craniostenosis), maternal infections, and anoxia.

Birth injuries or anoxia during or shortly after delivery may also cause retardation. Diseases such as meningitis, lead poisoning, neoplasms, and encephalitis can cause mental retardation in a child or adult at any age. Heredity is a factor in mental retardation. It is also possible for children to live in such a physically and emotionally deprived environment that they become mentally retarded.

The diagnosis is determined after a thorough study is made by a team of experts, including a pediatrician, psychologist, psychiatrist, nurse, and social worker. Conditions such as epilepsy, cerebral palsy, severe malnutrition, emotional disturbances, blindness, deafness, and speech disorders must be ruled out. Severe mental retardation may be noticeable at birth (Table 12–5). *The nursery nurse must be alert for the following symptoms:* failure to suck, feeding difficulties, spasticity, listlessness, twitching or convulsions, vomiting, jaundice, unusual-looking stools, unusual odor of urine, enlarged tongue, oriental appearance to Caucasians. Early recognition in certain cases can lessen or prevent brain damage. Other symptoms are associated with landmarks of the growth process. A child who does not smile, sit, climb stairs, stand, or walk within the usual age limits may be retarded. A child may also be slow in speech, in learning to help himself or herself, in toilet training. Unusual clumsiness and failure to respond to stimuli are early indications. Sometimes this handicap is not discovered until the child enters school.

For purposes of clarification, mental retardation is classified in groups. Each case must be frequently re-evaluated according to the child's individual progress. No patients should be kept stagnant merely because they happen to fall within a certain category.

Management and Nursing Goals

For nurses to be of substantial help to the retarded child and the family, they must face their own feelings and develop a positive attitude toward the problem. It is helpful for students to discuss their personal views in a group where ideas and feelings can be exchanged. They should realize that the experienced personnel who work with these patients see them entirely differently from the casual observer.

The parents of a retarded child need support, compassion and understanding, not pity. It should be clear to them that the nurse does not regard the child's condition as a disgrace. Usually the problems confronting the parents become greater as the child develops physically and chronologically but still requires constant supervision. The decision to institutionalize the patient is a difficult one. Many things must be taken into consideration, such as the health of the parents, the effect on other children in the family, the community services available, and the financial status of the family. Even when the decision is made, there are long waiting lists in many places. Facilities are overcrowded, and the tendency is to take the most severely retarded first.

The current trend in dealing with retarded people is toward deinstitutionalization and admittance

---

Table 12–5. SUMMARY OF SYMPTOMS THAT MAY SUGGEST COGNITIVE HANDICAP IN NEWBORN PERIOD AND EARLY INFANCY

Failure to suck	Jaundice
Feeding difficulties	Unusual-looking stools
Spasticity	Unusual odor of urine
Convulsions	Enlarged tongue
Listlessness, irritability	Oriental appearance in Caucasians
Floppy, hypotonic muscles	Stubby fingers or toes
Decreased alertness	Failure to master milestones of development
Unresponsive to eye contact	(smile, roll over, sit, etc.)
Unusual clumsiness	

to the mainstream of society. In 1975, the United States Congress passed the Education for All Handicapped Children Act X (PL 94-142), which assures that the retarded, as well as other handicapped persons, have the right to receive education at public expense. Currently these children are in programs in their local public schools. Many communities also have "sheltered workshops" in which retarded adults can work. These centers provide an opportunity for individuals to be more independent and increase their self-esteem.

It is important that nurses be familiar with the resources of their communities so they can direct the family to them. The local chapter of the National Association for Retarded Citizens (NARC) may provide information and support. The child guidance clinic or the psychological services of a nearby college or hospital may be tapped. The visits of the public health nurse are invaluable in many cases. Patients also may be eligible to obtain help from their local vocational and rehabilitation agency. Respite care workers afford needed rest and increased mobility for parents. In some communities parent groups meet to discuss mutual problems. Arrangements for proper dental health must be made, as in some cases dental care must be given under anesthesia.

Retarded infants should be started in infant stimulation programs as soon as possible. The training of retarded children is similar to that of the child with normal intelligence, only slower. They do, however, lack the ability to think abstractly, so they cannot transfer learning from one situation to another. They must learn by habit formation, which involves routine, repetition, and relaxation. The nurse working with these patients must have a good understanding of the growth and developmental process. It is important that the child show a *readiness* for the task, whether it is toilet training, feeding self, or dressing. The atmosphere should be one of friendliness, and directions should be kept simple. (Like other children, the retarded child must have limits set on behavior.) The adult must be firm and consistent. Correction must directly follow the offense. Love, liberal praise, respect, and infinite patience are essential in helping this child to develop to fullest capacity (Fig. 12–6).

The nurse caring for retarded children in the hospital needs to know their stage of maturation and abilities. A detailed history, including a habit

and care sheet, is completed. Self-help activities are documented. Communicating with the patient may be difficult. It is important to follow home routines as closely as possible. The progress the child has made should not be allowed to slip during hospitalization. Good communications between parents and nurse will help to make the transition from home to hospital as smooth as possible for the child. In obtaining information about the child from the parents, a positive approach is recommended. A request such as "Tell me about Tom's eating habits" is preferable to "Does Tom feed himself?" and is likely to yield more helpful information.

NURSING BRIEF ▶ ▶ ▶ ▶ ▶ ▶ ▶ ▶
A list of words, sounds, and gestures and their meanings posted on the retarded child's bed will aid personnel in communicating with the patient.

ENCEPHALITIS

Description. Encephalitis (*encephalo*, brain + *itis*, inflammation) is an inflammation of the brain. When the spinal cord is also infected, the condition is known as *encephalomyelitis* (*myelo*, spinal cord). This disorder can be caused by arboviruses (RNA viruses) and herpesvirus types 1 and 2; it can be the aftermath of disorders such as upper respiratory tract infections, German measles, or measles, or, rarely, an untoward reaction to vaccinations such as DPT (diphtheria, pertussis, tetanus); or it may result from lead poisoning. Other less common etiological agents are bacteria, spirochetes, and fungi. More than half the cases of encephalitis in the United States are caused by unknown complexes.

This disease also affects horses, and during epidemics, newspapers specify equine variety if this is the case. If the specific virus is determined, it is given the name of the geographic location in which it is found, e.g., eastern (U.S.), western (U.S.), St. Louis, and California. The infection is transmitted to horses and humans by mosquitoes and ticks.

Symptoms. The symptoms of encephalitis result from the central nervous system's response to irritation. In general, the viruses invade the lymphatic system and multiply. The blood stream becomes affected, and consequently various organs are also involved. Characteristically, the history is that of a headache followed by drowsiness, which may proceed to coma. Because coma is sometimes prolonged, encephalitis is sometimes referred to as "sleeping sickness." Convulsions are seen, particularly in infants. Fever, cramps, abdominal pain, vomiting, stiff neck, delirium, muscle twitching, and abnormal eye movements are other manifestations of the disease. The patient's history is of particular significance. Recent illness, injections, travel, and geographical location are recorded.

Treatment and Nursing Care

At this time no specific medication is known, with the exception of the use of adenine arabinoside or acyclovir for herpesvirus encephalitis. Mosquitoes and ticks should be destroyed in known infested areas where encephalitis is prevalent. A brain scan, electroencephalogram (EEG), and computed tomography (CT) may be useful in determining the diagnosis. Intracranial monitoring may also be employed. The treatment is supportive and is aimed at providing relief from specific symptoms. Sedatives also may be prescribed. Adequate nutrition and hydration via gavage or IV, control of convulsions, and catheterization for urinary retention may be required. Antipyretics are given as ordered, and seizure precautions are instituted. An oral airway may be kept at the bedside. The nurse provides a quiet environment, good oral hygiene, skin care, and frequent change of position. Oxygen is given as needed, and the mouth and nose are kept free of mucus by suctioning. Bowel movements are recorded daily, as the patient may be constipated from lack of activity. Preventing this and other secondary effects of immobility is paramount. Physical therapy may also be indicated. The nurse closely observes the patient for neurological changes.

Fatality rates and residual effects are higher among infants than older children. Speech, mental processes, and motor abilities may be slowed, and permanent brain damage and mental retardation can result. Parents are encouraged to help with the care of the child as soon as the condition is stable. They are instructed in the nursing procedures required for home care. In long-term cases,

the services of the home health care nurse and related agencies are invaluable.

RECURRENT SEIZURE DISORDERS (EPILEPSY)

Description. The term *epilepsy* (chronic recurrent convulsions) comes from the Greek *epilepsia,* which means seizure. It is the name of a very old and misunderstood disease. Between 3 and 5 per cent of children will have at least one seizure. Most of these seizures are associated with a fever, but 0.5 per cent of children will have epilepsy (Green and Haggerty, 1990). Depending upon the type of epilepsy, a child may require treatment for only a period of time. Others will require lifetime treatment.

Three of four new cases begin in childhood. Education of the patient and family is a prime consideration in developing nursing care plans. In the past, words such as "fit," "spell," and "blackout" were used to describe this entity. These are nonspecific and create confusion. Children who state that they are subject to seizures indicate that they are aware of their condition, and this encourages others to relate to them in a mature way.

Epilepsy is characterized by recurrent paroxysmal attacks of unconsciousness or impaired consciousness that may be followed by alternate contraction and relaxation of the muscles or by disturbed feelings or behavior. It is a disorder of the central nervous system in which the neurons or nerve cells discharge in an abnormal way. These discharges may be focal or diffuse. The site of general discharge can sometimes be ascertained by observing the patient's symptoms during the attack. The international classification of epileptic seizures is condensed in Table 12–6. It provides a framework upon which medical therapy may be instigated. When the cause is unknown, the term *idiopathic* (spontaneous) or *cryptogenic* (hidden) is used. If a cerebral abnormality is found, the patient may be said to have *organic* or *symptomatic* epilepsy.

Idiopathic epilepsy is the most common cause of recurrent convulsions in children more than 3 years of age. It is possible that some specific genetic defect in cerebral metabolism is responsible in many children. It has been pointed out that electroencephalographic abnormalities (cerebral

Table 12–6. EPILEPSY: RECOGNITION AND FIRST AID

SEIZURE TYPE	WHAT IT LOOKS LIKE	WHAT IT IS NOT	WHAT TO DO	WHAT NOT TO DO
Generalized tonic-clonic (also called grand mal)	Sudden cry, fall, rigidity, followed by muscle jerks, shallow breathing or temporarily suspended breathing, bluish skin, possible loss of bladder or bowel control, usually lasts a couple of minutes. Normal breathing then starts again. There may be some confusion and/or fatigue, followed by return to full consciousness.	Heart attack. Stroke.	Look for medical identification. Protect from nearby hazards. Loosen ties or shirt collars. Protect head from injury Turn on side to keep airway clear. Reassure when consciousness returns. If single seizure lasted less than 5 minutes, ask if hospital evaluation wanted. If multiple seizures, or if one seizure lasts longer than 5 minutes, call an ambulance. If person is pregnant, injured, or diabetic, call for aid at once.	Don't put any hard implement in the mouth. Don't try to hold tongue. It can't be swallowed. Don't try to give liquids during or just after seizure. Don't use artificial respiration unless breathing is absent after muscle jerks subside or unless water has been inhaled. Don't restrain.
Absence (also called petit mal)	A blank stare, beginning and ending abruptly, lasting only a few seconds, most common in children. May be accompanied by rapid blinking, some chewing movements of the mouth. Child is unaware of what's going on during the seizure, but quickly returns to full awareness once it has stopped. May result in learning difficulties if not recognized and treated.	Daydreaming. Lack of attention. Deliberate ignoring of adult instructions.	No first aid necessary, but if this is the first observation of the seizure, medical evaluation should be recommended.	

Table continued on following page

Table 12–6. EPILEPSY: RECOGNITION AND FIRST AID *Continued*

SEIZURE TYPE	WHAT IT LOOKS LIKE	WHAT IT IS NOT	WHAT TO DO	WHAT NOT TO DO
Simple partial	Jerking may begin in one area of body, arm, leg, or face. Can't be stopped, but patient stays awake and aware. Jerking may proceed from one area of the body to another, and sometimes spreads to become a convulsive seizure.	Acting out, bizarre behavior.	No first aid necessary unless seizure becomes convulsive, then first aid as above.	
	Partial sensory seizures, may not be obvious to an onlooker. Patient experiences a distorted environment. May see or hear things that aren't there, may feel unexplained fear, sadness, anger, or joy. May have nausea, experience odd smells, and have a generally "funny" feeling in the stomach.	Hysteria. Mental illness. Psychosomatic illness. Parapsychological or mystical experience.	No action needed other than reassurance and emotional support. Medical evaluation should be recommended.	
Complex partial (also called psychomotor or temporal lobe)	Usually starts with blank stare, followed by chewing, followed by random activity. Person appears unaware of surroundings, may seem dazed and mumble. Unresponsive. Actions clumsy, not directed. May pick at clothing, pick up objects, try to take clothes off. May run, appear afraid. May struggle or flail at restraint. Once pattern established, same set of actions usually occurs with each seizure. Lasts a few minutes, but post-seizure confusion can last substantially longer. No memory of what happened during seizure period.	Drunkenness. Intoxication on drugs. Mental illness. Disorderly conduct.	Speak calmly and reassuringly to patient and others. Guide gently away from obvious hazards. Stay with person until completely aware of environment. Offer to help getting home.	Don't grab hold unless sudden danger (such as a cliff edge or an approaching car) threatens. Don't try to restrain. Don't shout. Don't expect verbal instructions to be obeyed.

Table 12–6. EPILEPSY: RECOGNITION AND FIRST AID *Continued*

SEIZURE TYPE	WHAT IT LOOKS LIKE	WHAT IT IS NOT	WHAT TO DO	WHAT NOT TO DO
Atonic seizures (also called drop attacks)	A child or adult suddenly collapses. After 10 seconds to a minute he recovers, regains consciousness, and can stand and walk again.	Clumsiness. Normal childhood "stage." In a child, lack of good walking skills. In an adult, drunkenness, acute illness.	No first aid needed (unless he hurt himself as he fell), but the child should be given a thorough medical evaluation.	
Mycoclonic seizures	Sudden brief, massive muscle jerks that may involve the whole body or parts of the body. May cause persons to spill what they were holding or fall off a chair.	Clumsiness. Poor coordination.	No first aid needed, but should be given a thorough medical evaluation.	
Infantile spasms	These are clusters of quick, sudden movements that start between 3 months and 2 years. If a child is sitting up, the head will fall forward, and the arms will flex forward. If lying down, the knees will be drawn up, with arms and head flexed forward as if the baby is reaching for support.	Normal movements of the baby. Colic.	No first aid, but doctor should be consulted.	

From Epilepsy Foundation of America (1989). *Seizure Recognition and First Aid.* Landover, Maryland.

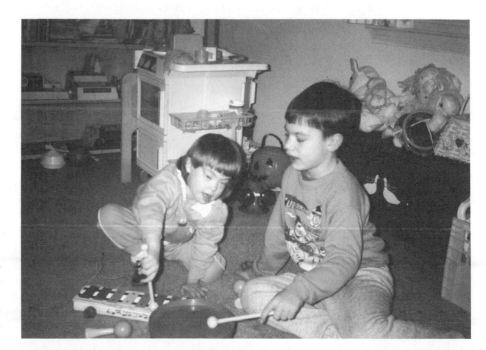

▲ FIGURE 12–6

The child who is retarded is stimulated through play with an older sibling. This environment increases the child's abilities.

dysrhythmias) are more likely to be found in parents and siblings of affected children than in the population at large.

Organic epilepsy may be caused by a number of conditions or injuries that have impaired the brain. Many genetically determined conditions, such as phenylketonuria (PKU), hydrocephalus, and tuberous sclerosis, are associated with seizures. Convulsions may also occur as a result of brain injury during prenatal, perinatal, or postnatal periods. Acute infections may be responsible for epilepsy in infants and toddlers. There are also contributing conditions that can alter the convulsive threshold. If the patient becomes overtired or overexcited or if faced with a stressful situation, a seizure may be experienced. Alteration in serum and brain concentrations of sodium, potassium, and water due to fluid retention can be a precipitating factor. Hormonal changes during puberty, excess fluid intake, and photogenic stimulation have also been suggested as causes.

Prevention of organic epilepsy is fostered by nurses who promote good prenatal and postnatal care and healthful living for children. Parents need to be educated about the importance of providing a safe environment and supervision for small children. Play areas need to be properly supervised, poisonous substances must be stored away from little hands, and proper seat belts should be utilized in automobiles to prevent head injury. Early diagnosis and treatment for such conditions as PKU, meningitis, Reye syndrome, and encephalitis are also crucial in minimizing irreversible brain damage. Children must be immunized against childhood diseases that could foster epilepsy. The abuse of drugs, including alcohol, and drug combinations, by teenagers can result in cerebral anoxia and convulsions, and this danger should be stressed in comprehensive health teaching for this age group. It is not possible or desirable to shield children from every stressful situation, but adults can assist growing children by helping them make wise decisions at their level of competency and by being supportive. The response of parents and nurses in stressful situations is also of importance in role modeling.

Types and Symptoms. Symptoms vary according to the type of seizure. Mixed seizures may also occur in epileptics. Seizures may be convulsive or nonconvulsive.

Tonic-Clonic (Grand Mal) Seizures. This is the most common type of seizure and probably the most dramatic. It is a generalized convulsion, usually with *tonic* and *clonic* phases. Onset is abrupt. During the *tonic* phase the body stiffens; patients may lose consciousness simultaneously and may drop to the floor if they have been sitting or standing. This may be preceded by an *aura*, which is a particular sensation such as dizziness, visual images, nausea, headache, or an ascending feeling of abdominal discomfort. This phenomenon is not as well established in children, who may be unable to describe it. The face becomes pale at first and then cyanotic owing to arrest of respiratory movements. The eyes roll upward or to one side. The child may utter a brief cry as air is forced out of the lungs across tightly closed vocal cords. The head, back, and legs stiffen. This phase lasts about 20 to 40 seconds and is followed by the *clonic* phase, which lasts for variable periods. Jerking movements of the trunk and extremities begin. Frothing at the mouth, biting of the tongue, and urinary or fecal incontinence may occur. Muscle contraction and relaxation gradually subside, and the child enters the *postictal* (*post*, after + *ictus*, a sudden stroke) state. The patient appears dazed and confused and generally sleeps for a while. Upon awakening patients may complain of a headache and may perform more or less automatic acts. This is believed to be due to malfunctioning of the neurons, which may not be fully recovered. The patient has no recollection of the seizure. *Status epilepticus* is a series of convulsions rapidly following one another. The most common cause is abrupt withdrawal of anticonvulsant medication. It is an emergency situation because death can result from respiratory failure and exhaustion.

Table 12–6 describes the first aid treatment for various types of seizures. The nurse observes and records the following: the child's activity immediately before the seizure; body movements; changes in color, respiration, or muscle tone; incontinence; and the parts of the body involved. When possible, the seizure is timed. The child's appearance, behavior, and level of consciousness following the seizure are also documented.

Absence (Petit Mal) Seizures. These seizures are characterized by transient loss of consciousness. They originate from the central portion of the brain and cortex and last less than 30 seconds. There may be associated upward rolling of the eyes, rhythmic nodding of the head, or slight quivering of the limbs. This condition is rarely seen in children less than 3 years old and often disappears by puberty. The patient seldom falls but may drop articles being held. These episodes are often referred to by parents as "lapses," "absences," or "dizzy spells." This condition is more common in females. Attacks vary in frequency. Following the attack the child is alert and appears normal, as if nothing had happened.

Atonic (Akinetic) Seizures. Also called "drop seizures," akinetic seizures are characterized by a sudden loss of postural muscle tone. The patient loses consciousness momentarily and if standing may fall to the ground. Some patients experience only a dropping forward of the head and neck. The episodes may occur frequently during the day.

Myoclonic Seizures. These are brief, shocklike contractions that may involve the entire body or be confined to the face, trunk, or extremities.

Infantile Spasms. Infantile spasms usually have their onset within the first 6 to 8 months of life (Hrachovy and Frost, 1989). There may be a sudden dropping of the head and flexion of the arms. Clonic movements of the extremities may also be seen. The episodes last only a few seconds and vary in frequency. They are the most common type of seizure seen in infancy, with the exception of febrile convulsions. When spasms occur before 4 months of age, a congenital cerebral defect is most likely. There may be significant developmental retardation. Infantile spasms disappear at about 4 years of age but are often replaced by major motor seizures.

Simple Partial Seizures. Focal or partial cortical seizures may arise from any area of the cerebral cortex but usually affect the frontal, temporal, or parietal lobe. They may be either motor or sensory in nature. Focal seizures may sometimes become generalized. Minor one-sided tonic or clonic seizures are more common in children than are true *jacksonian* seizures, which begin in one muscle group and proceed to other groups in a fixed manner. This pattern or "jacksonian march" proceeds from thumb to fingers, to wrist, to arm, to face, and then to the leg of the same side. They are typically clonic in nature.

Complex Partial (Psychomotor) Seizures. This type of seizure is more common in adults but is also seen in children over 3 years of age. It is localized to the temporal lobe of the cerebrum and is characterized by an altered state of consciousness. The patient appears to be in a dreamlike state. The child may perform *automatisms,* such as lip smacking, grimacing, or repetition of words. The young child may cry out and run to an adult. There are generally no clonic or tonic movements, although the patient may gently collapse to the floor. A brief period of unconsciousness may follow. Upon awakening, the patient resumes normal activities. Some patients sleep for a period of time. These seizures are very difficult to recognize and control. Electroencephalographic patterns remain normal except when the EEG is taken during an attack.

Treatment and Nursing Care

Initially, treatment is aimed at determining the type, site, and/or cause of the disorder. Diagnostic measures include a complete history and physical and neurological examinations. Skull radiography and CT are employed to establish the presence or absence of tumors, skull abnormalities, hematomas, and intracranial calcifications. Magnetic resonance imaging (MRI) is also used in some areas as it is technically superior to the CT scan. The EEG is also a valuable tool in evaluating seizures. It is especially helpful in differentiating between an absence seizure and a complex partial seizure. Video EEG recordings can detect more subtle manifestations and provide a permanent record for playback. Prolonged ambulatory EEG monitoring (24 hours) is another advanced technique. Laboratory studies such as complete blood count (CBC) and determinations of serum calcium and blood urea nitrogen (BUN) may detect acute infections, lead poisoning, or other metabolic disorders. A spinal tap may be ordered when encephalitis or meningitis is suspected. If the seizure is related to any such underlying cause, appropriate therapy is begun. Anticonvulsive drug therapy is begun only after all such causes have been excluded.

Some common anticonvulsants and their side effects are listed in Table 12–7. The duration of therapy is individual. Initially the doctor pre-

Table 12–7. SOME COMMONLY USED ANTICONVULSANT DRUGS

DRUG	SIDE EFFECTS	COMMENTS
Luminal (phenobarbital)	Drowsiness, irritability, hyperactivity	Safest overall medication; bitter, often combined with other drugs
Dilantin (phenytoin)	Ataxia, insomnia, motor twitching, gum overgrowth, hirsutism (hairiness), rash, nausea, vitamin D and folic acid deficiencies	Generally effective and safe; regular massaging of gums decreases hyperplasia; is used in combination with phenobarbital or primidone
Depakene (valproic acid)	Gastrointestinal disturbance, altered bleeding time, liver toxicity	Monitor blood counts; take with food or use enteric-coated preparations; potentiates action of phenobarbital and other drugs
Mysoline (primidone)	Ataxia, vertigo, anorexia, fatigue, hyperirritability, dermatitis	May be used alone or in combination; side effects minimized by starting with small amounts
Valium (diazepam)	Headache, tremor, fatigue, depression	Used in combination or alone
Clonopin (clonazepam)	Behavior changes, ataxia, anorexia, nystagmus	Effective for most minor motor seizures
Tegretol (carbamazepine)	Blurred vision, diplopia, drowsiness, vertigo	Few side effects; fewer sedative properties

The physician determines the child's medication by the type of seizure and other factors. The goal is to achieve the best control with the minimum dosage and the least number of side effects. An important aspect of nursing intervention includes reinforcing the need for drug supervision and compliance.

scribes the lowest dose likely to control the seizures. He or she may have to experiment with a combination of drugs. Drowsiness, a common side effect of many anticonvulsants, can interfere with the child's activities and requires regulation. Careful recording of seizure activity and adherence to the drug regimen are of particular importance in determining a suitable program. The medication is not addictive when used as prescribed. Tablet form is preferable to suspensions, which are more expensive and tend to separate if not shaken well. Most small children can ingest the tablet when it is administered in a teaspoon with a small amount of applesauce. Medication is given at the same time each day, generally with meals or at bedtime. Parents need to work with the physician to find the medication that works best with their child. Noncompliance can be a problem because of the side effects (hyperactivity, drowsiness). Parents

should be told that children often will reach a level where they adjust to the medication and side effects may not be as severe.

If it is necessary for the child to take medication during school hours, the parents sign a consent form so that the school nurse may monitor administration. This provides the child and the nurse opportunities to get acquainted and share their knowledge of the disease. Nurse and teacher response, particularly during and after a seizure, will have a significant effect on the attitude of classmates toward the disease.

It is important that medication be reduced gradually under a physician's supervision, because abrupt withdrawal of medications is the most common cause of status epilepticus. In the hospital, the nurse consults the physician as to whether anticonvulsants are to be withheld if the patient is to consume nothing by mouth (NPO). As in any long-term drug therapy, periodic blood and urine tests should be performed to detect subtle side effects. When children are old enough, they can assume responsibility for their own medications. They should wear a Medic-Alert bracelet. During puberty and adolescence, dosages may have to be adjusted to meet growth needs. Premenstrual fluid retention in girls can sometimes trigger seizures.

The *ketogenic diet* is sometimes prescribed for children who do not respond well to anticonvulsant therapy. It is high in fats and low in carbohydrates and produces ketoacidosis in the body, which appears to have a calming effect. The use of medium-chain triglycerides (MCT) is more flexible and palatable. It simulates fasting, which has been used for years to control grand mal seizures. Reduction of fluid intake tends to increase its ketogenic effect. The diet has an extraordinary effect, but it is unpalatable, expensive, and is so strict it causes social isolation (Lockman, 1989).

Seizure precautions include padding siderails and having oropharyngeal suction, oxygen, and an oral airway at the bedside. The child's bed should be kept at the lowest position with the rails up at all times. During a seizure, the nurse protects the child from injury, maintains an airway, observes the seizure activity, and records the data observed. Any tight clothing is loosened, and the child's head is turned to the side with the neck extended to maintain the airway and aid in drainage from the mouth. Attempts to insert objects into the mouth after a seizure begins are contraindicated. Severe damage can be done to the mouth and teeth. The nurse's goal is to protect from injury, not restrain. Remain with the child after the seizure and provide a quiet environment for rest.

Rebellion against medical routine is not uncommon during adolescence. Some states do not allow controlled epileptics to obtain a driver's license, which is disheartening to the patient. Other states have stipulations about the amount of seizure-free time required before licensure. Excess intake of fluids, particularly alcoholic beverages, can be a source of contention. Parents can obtain valuable information and support from the Epilepsy Foundation of America.

The well-controlled patient can lead a normal life with a few safety restrictions. Too much atten-tion to seizures by well-meaning adults can make control difficult. The child will also learn to use the threat of a seizure to manipulate those caring for her or him. Patients can participate in selected athletic and recreational activities. Death or serious injury rarely occurs from a seizure, and it does not cause mental deterioration. Careful evaluation and placement of the child with a learning disorder are essential. Patients under proper treatment can lead full and productive lives. A family assessment is helpful in establishing rapport and setting realistic short-term and long-term goals.

The Eyes

AMBLYOPIA

Description. Amblyopia ("lazy eye") is a decrease in or loss of vision in an eye that is otherwise normal. If both retinas do not receive a clearly defined image, bilateral amblyopia may result. However, it is more common for one eye to be affected. Prognosis depends on how long the eye has been affected and the age of the child when treatment is instigated. The earlier the treatment, the better the results. There are various types of amblyopia. Strabismus is the most common; however, dissimilar refractory errors can also result in this condition.

Treatment and Nursing Care

The goal of treatment is to obtain normal and equal vision in each eye. Treatment consists of glasses for significant refractive errors (hyperopia, myopia) and patching (occlusion) of the good eye. In an infant, amblyopia often can be corrected in days or weeks. With an older child, the treatment may take months or years. In most cases the patch covers the eye throughout the waking hours, although partial occlusion is used in maintenance therapy and with low-grade amblyopia (Friendly, 1987). Occlusion therapy is often difficult to maintain. The nurse can be of help by explaining the importance of the procedure and by offering support. The child may be subject to ridicule by peers. Providing a safe place for children to express their feelings about this is important in promoting a healthy self-image.

Strabismus

Description. Strabismus (cross-eye), also known as *squint*, is a condition in which the child is not able to direct both eyes toward the same object. There is a lack of coordination between the eye muscles that direct movement of the eye.

There are several kinds of strabismus. In *monocular* squint (*mono*, one + *oculus*, eye), one eye is used continuously for vision and the other is turned inward or outward. In *alternating* squint, either eye may be used singly for vision, with the other eye crossed. Strabismus may be present at birth or may be acquired after a disease.

Two simple tests can be done to detect strabismus. They are the corneal light reflex test and the cover, uncover, and cross-cover tests. In the corneal light reflex test, the examiner shines a penlight into the patient's eyes from a distance of about 18 inches. If the child is looking directly at the light, the reflection should be at the same point in each pupil. In the cover test, the eyes are observed for compensatory or adjustment movements. When quickly uncovered, the eye should not move; if it has to shift to focus on the light, malalignment is present. *Epicanthal folds*, the vertical folds of skin on either side of the nose that are frequently seen in children of Asian descent, can give a false impression of strabismus.

Treatment. When strabismus is seen during early infancy, the doctor may recommend that the unaffected eye be covered by a patch until the baby is old enough to wear glasses. The affected eye may improve through use and often becomes normal. Eye exercises and glasses are effective ways of treating the condition medically. If this does not help, surgery should be considered. It is generally performed when the child is 3 or 4 years old; the condition should be corrected before children start school to prevent them from becoming the subject of ridicule. Early correction is necessary to prevent amblyopia (see preceding discussion). If strabismus is left untreated, blindness may result, since the brain tends to obliterate the confusing double image.

NURSING CARE

The child undergoing surgery for strabismus is hospitalized for only a brief period. Some doctors prefer not to have the child restrained following surgery, since it is frightening and the child's struggles may increase. The surgery involves structures outside the eyeball; therefore, the child is allowed to be up and about postoperatively. Eye dressings are kept at a minimum, and elbow restraints may be all that is needed to keep the child from touching the dressings.

If the doctor feels that it is necessary to cover the eyes and restrain the patient's movements following surgery, the patient is told this before surgery and is assured that the bandages and restraints will be removed as soon as possible. Since this is frightening for children, it is best that the parents remain with them. Since they cannot move or see, diversions such as stories and records are necessary. When nausea has ceased, the child is put on a regular diet. Tell the patients what they are about to eat when you are feeding them. Speak to the children before you touch them so that they will not be startled.

Care of the Eyes

Children should have a thorough ophthalmic examination by the age of 3 to 4 years. These are crucial years for detecting and treating amblyopia, strabismus, high refractive errors, and certain tumors in childhood (Behrman and Vaughan, 1987).

The nurse may be asked to perform various eye screening procedures. The Denver Eye Screening Test (DEST) is useful in detecting appropriate visual development in children 2.5 years or older. The Snellen alphabet chart and the Snellen E version, for preschoolers who have not learned the alphabet, are important tools for detecting *visual acuity*, or the ability to see near and far objects. Picture cards are also useful for children who do not know letters. The Titmus machine is frequently used for school children and adolescents. Directions for testing are standardized and must be carefully adhered to for proper results.

Prevention of Eyestrain. The nurse should stress the importance of proper care of the eyes in work and daily life. Little children who are beginning to read need books with large type in which the letters are spaced far apart. The lighting provided must be adequate and without glare. Chairs and desks must be of proper height.

Symptoms that may indicate eyestrain include inflammation, aching or smarting of the eyes, squinting, a short attention span, frequent headaches, difficulties with school work, or inability to see the blackboard. They may occur suddenly. The child between 6 and 10 years of age often becomes nearsighted and has to hold books very close to the eyes to read. An eye examination and in some cases a complete physical examination are indicated.

The Integumentary System

BURNS

Description. Burns are a leading cause of accidental death in children. Most burns are minor and can be treated on an outpatient basis. However, some burns are quite severe and require hospitalization. Toddlers may pull hot liquids upon themselves. Older children sometimes misuse matches and flammable materials. One common, preventable burn, is caused by the child being burned by a curling iron. Burns are categorized as thermal, radiation, electrical, or chemical.

The burn wound is usually classified according to depth, per cent of body surface involved, location of the injury, and association with other injuries. The age of the child and the presence of respiratory involvement are also important factors.

First degree burns (superficial burns) involve the epidermis and are red, dry, and painful (sunburn). *Second degree burns* are partial thickness burns involving the epidermis and the outermost portion of the dermis. This burn forms blisters, is painful, and, depending upon the severity, may need grafting. A full thickness burn, *third degree*, involves total destruction of the epidermis and dermis and may also involve underlying tissues. The wound is leathery, tan, dark red or brown, and not as painful as the partial thickness burn. It should be noted that although the patient may not experience pain at the actual wound site, there is pain along the edges of the wound where nerve endings are intact.

A method for determining the percentage of skin surface area in children at various ages is presented in Figure 12–7. The "rule of nines" which is used with the older adolescent and the adult is not applicable in the infant and small child because of the difference in body proportions (Fig. 12–8).

Partial thickness burns of the face, hands, feet, or perineum are considered to be *severe*. Burns in children under the age of 2 years and those having respiratory complications also come under this category.

Treatment. *Minor burns* usually do not require hospitalization. The wound can be cleaned with a mild soap and cool water and then rinsed with sterile normal saline. A dry dressing or fine-mesh gauze lightly lubricated with water-soluble antiseptic or antimicrobial cream is placed over the area, and it is then wrapped with a bulky gauze dressing. Parents are taught to change the dressing twice daily and to force fluids. Blisters are left intact and allowed to break under the dressing. The goal of care is to prevent infection in the wound. Tetanus antitoxin should be given if the child is not current in this immunization. Acetaminophen (Tylenol) should be sufficient to relieve pain.

The primary goal in the treatment of *major burns* is the maintenance of an airway and the prevention of shock. Airway obstruction should be suspected if the child has inhaled smoke or the burn involves the face. The child may be placed in a Croupette or under an oxygen hood. An endotracheal tube is inserted if the child is in respiratory distress. An intravenous infusion is started and a Foley catheter is inserted. The type of fluids used is controversial and depends on the philosophy of the institution. The child may be NPO for the first 24 to 48 hours if the burn is severe and bowel sounds are absent. A nasogastric tube may be inserted.

Metabolism increases and there is severe protein and fat wasting in response to severe burns. The child requires a high-protein, high-caloric diet. Oral feedings are preferred, although it may be necessary to supplement with nasogastric feedings. Many of these children have poor appetites and intake is a challenge.

Morphine sulfate is the drug of choice for severely burned patients. It should be given intravenously. Intramuscular or subcutaneous drugs should be avoided for the first 72 hours. Poor tissue perfusion and the danger of pooling of the drugs could later cause an overload when circu-

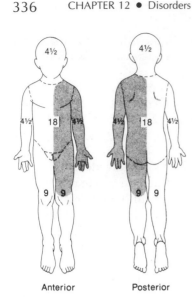

Calculation of Extent of Burn			
Body Part	Ant.	Post.	Total
Head	4½	4½	9
Rt. Upper Extremity	4½	4½	9
Lt. Upper Extremity	4½	4½	9
Trunk	18	18	36
Perineum	1		1
Rt. Lower Extremity	9	9	18
Lt. Lower Extremity	9	9	18
			Total 100%

Anterior   Posterior

▲ FIGURE 12–7

Estimation of the size of a burn by rule of nines. The head and each entire upper extremity (shoulder to fingertips [glove fashion]) are given the value of 9 per cent of the body surface. The anterior trunk and posterior trunk are each valued at 18 per cent, as is each leg. The sum of these parts is 99 per cent and the perineum is 1 per cent, totaling 100 per cent. This method may be used visually at the accident scene or in the emergency room to estimate the size of a burn quickly; however, it does not allow for the difference in proportion of head and lower extremities of the various ages. (From Foster, R., Hunsberger, M., and Anderson, J. (1989). *Family-Centered Nursing Care of Children*. Philadelphia, W. B. Saunders.)

lation and absorption return to normal. Special attention should be given to respiratory rates when morphine is given. Acetaminophen with codeine may be given for less severe pain.

Wound Care

Goals of wound care include

1. Prevention of infection
2. Development of granulation tissue
3. Promotion of re-epithelialization
4. Preparation for grafting
5. Reduction of scarring and contractures (Bayley, 1990)

The wound can be cleansed several ways. At the bedside, sterile water or saline can be used with a mild antibacterial cleansing agent (Betadine). Cleansing can also take place in a hydrotherapy tank or on a spray table where water is sprayed over the wounds. Wounds are usually cleansed at least once daily. All traces of topical agents should be gently removed from the wound.

Burn wounds must be debrided in order to remove tissue contaminated by bacteria and to remove dead tissue. There are three means of debridement: surgical, commercial topical enzymes, and mechanical (Gordon, 1990). Mechanical debridement includes the use of scissors and forceps and is usually done during the daily dressing change and cleansing procedure. Soaking in the hydrotherapy tank aids in the loosening of tissue, eschar exudate, and topical medication. The old dressing can be removed while in the tank. Debridement is painful and should be preceded by the administration of analgesics.

Burn wound sepsis is best controlled by the application of antibacterial agents to the burn wound. The most common topical agent used is silver sulfadiazine (Silvadene). Other agents used include Sulfamylon, Betadine, and silver nitrate. These creams can be applied with a sterile gloved hand and dressed with a sterile dressing. It is important to remove all residue from previous applications and any exudate before applying a new layer of topical agent (Bayley, 1990).

The wound may be left open after the applica-

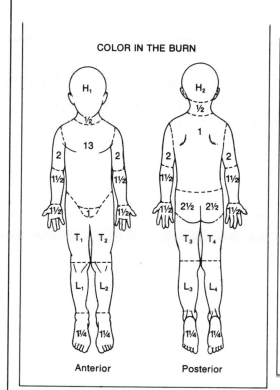

COLOR IN THE BURN

Anterior

Posterior

CALCULATE EXTENT OF BURN

	Anterior	Posterior
	H₁	H₁
Head	H_1	H_1
Neck		
Rt. Arm		
Rt. Forearm		
Rt. Hand		
Lt. Arm		
Lt. Forearm		
Lt. Hand		
Trunk		
Buttock	(R)	(L)
Perineum		
Rt. Thigh	T_1	T_4
Rt. Leg.	L_1	L_4
Rt. Foot		
Lt. Thigh	T_2	T_3
Lt. Leg.	L_2	L_3
Lt. Foot		
Subtotal		
% Total Area Burned		%

CIRCLE AGE FACTOR	Percentage of Areas Affected by Growth					
	Age					
	0	1	5	10	15	Adult
H(1 or 2) = ½ of the Head	9½	8½	6½	5½	4½	3½
T(1,2,3, or 4) = ½ of a Thigh	2¾	3¼	4	4¼	4½	4¾
L(1,2,3, or 4) − ½ of a Leg	2½	2½	2¾	3	3¼	3½

▲ FIGURE 12–8

Estimation of the size of a burn by per cent. 1. Shade in the diagram to represent the extent of burn, as viewed anteriorly and posteriorly. 2. Circle the age closest to that of the patient and use those percentages for the head, thigh, and leg to calculate the extent of the burn. 3. The percentage of total body surface is printed on the diagram for those areas that do not vary with age. The areas that do vary with age are marked with H (head), T (thigh), and L (leg). The extent of the burn is calculated by adding the percentages of each affected area. If a portion of a body part is burned, an approximate fraction of the percentage should be used. (Redrawn from Feller, I., and Jones, C.A.: *Emergency Care of the Burn Victim*. National Institute for Burn Medicine, Ann Arbor, Michigan, 1977.)

tion of topical ointments. This can cause increased hypothermia but has the advantage of easy visualization of the wound and simplicity of wound care. Various types of dressings may be used, from net coverings to multiple layers of gauze. When dressing the wound, no two burn surfaces should touch, fingers and toes should be wrapped separately, and burned ears should not touch the back of the head. This prevents webbing of these areas. Dressings are usually changed twice daily. As mentioned, these changes may take place in the hydrotherapy tank.

In full thickness burns where re-epithelialization does not take place, grafting (skin transplant) is required. Temporary grafts may be needed until permanent grafting can take place. Permanent grafts are obtained from an undamaged area of the patient's body (autografts).

Nursing Care

NURSING DIAGNOSES

1. Potential for infection, related to destruction of skin
2. Impaired skin integrity, related to thermal injury
3. Pain, related to dressing changes, debridement, wound
4. Altered nutrition: less than body requirements, related to anorexia
5. Fluid volume deficit, related to loss through body surface
6. Potential ineffective airway clearance, related to edema
7. Body image disturbance, related to disfigurement secondary to burn
8. Altered process, related to child with severe burn

The care of a child with a severe burn requires a team approach. In the acute phase of care, the nurse monitors vital signs, urinary output, respiratory status, and the general condition of the patient. Fluid management is crucial during this period, and nurses must be vigilant in monitoring the intravenous infusion. They must be aware of the psychological needs of the family and the child at this time. Families may be dealing with guilt, anger, grief, denial, and fear.

The nurse is usually responsible for the daily care of the wound. Dressing changes are almost always painful, and the child should receive pain medication prior to the procedure. The nurse maintains strict aseptic technique during this procedure. Outer dressings are removed before the child is placed in the tub, but adherent dressings are more easily removed after soaking in water. Loose tissue, exudate, and remaining topical medication are removed. The child is encouraged to move about and exercise movable parts of the body while in the tub. Topical creams can be applied with a sterile gloved hand or sterile tongue blade. They can be applied directly to the wound or they can be impregnated into fine-mesh gauze. Burn wounds to which topical creams have been applied may be treated open or they may be covered with various types of gauze dressings (Bayley, 1990).

Because of the increased nutritional needs of such patients and their accompanying anorexia, the nurse must be creative. Procedures should be planned away from meals. Small, frequent feedings of favorite foods should be provided. Supplements may be added to foods to meet the high protein and calorie needs. Parents may be able to bring favorite foods from home. Daily weights and intake and output are recorded.

Sterile gloves, mask, and gown are worn when handling the wound. The environment is kept clean, and good handwashing is imperative. Exposure to infectious persons is avoided. The wound is assessed for any signs of infection (purulent drainage, odor, redness). Any other areas of potential infection are also observed closely (IV site, Foley catheter, tracheostomy).

The child should be encouraged to be as independent as possible. Range of motion exercises are implemented, and the child is allowed to walk, condition permitting. In bed, the child should be positioned in extension to prevent flexion contractures. Splints may be applied to maintain position.

Psychological care of the child and family is a priority goal. Encourage parents to spend as much time as possible with the child. Since this may be a long-term admission, they may not be able to be with the child at all times. Activities appropriate for the child's age and condition should be provided. Schooling needs should be met when the child is of school age. Encourage the child to help with bath, dressing change, feeding, and other self-care activities. Provide opportunities for fam-

Text continued on page 346

Table 12–8. COMMUNICABLE DISEASES

DISEASE	COMMUNICABILITY PERIOD AND ROUTE	CLINICAL MANIFESTATIONS	TREATMENT AND NURSING CARE	COMPLICATIONS
CHICKENPOX (vari-cella) *Incubation Period:* 10–21 days	1 day before onset to 6 days after first vesicles appear *Route:* 1. Air-borne: droplet infection 2. Direct or indirect contact 3. Dry scabs are not infectious	General malaise, slight fever, an-orexia, headache. Successive crops of macules, papules, vesicles, crusts. These may all be present at the same time. Itching of the skin. Generalized lymphadenopathy	Symptomatic. Prevent child from scratching. Keep fingernails short and clean. Sedation may be necessary. Use soothing lotions to al-lay itching. If second-ary infections occur, antibiotics or chemo-therapy may be given. *Do not give aspirin* due to high risk of Reye syndrome	Bacterial superinfec-tion; thrombocyto-penia, arthritis, en-cephalitis, nephritis, Reye syndrome (with aspirin use)
DIPHTHERIA *Incubation Period:* 2–6 days or longer	Several hours before onset of disease un-til organisms disap-pear from respira-tory tract *Route:* Droplets from respira-tory tract of infected person or carrier	Local and systemic manifestations. Membrane over tis-sue in nose or throat at site of bac-terial invasion. Hoarse, brassy cough with stridor. Toxin from organ-isms produces mal-aise and fever. Toxin has affinity for renal, nervous, and cardiac tissue	Aims of treatment are to inactivate toxins, kill the organism, and pre-vent respiratory ob-struction. Antitoxin is given against toxin, IV administration pre-ferred. Antimicrobial therapy with erythro-mycin or procaine pen-icillin is given for 14 days in addition to an-titoxin. Toxoid is given to asymptomatic im-munized contacts who have not had a booster dose in 5 years. Speci-mens from all close contacts taken. Strict bedrest. Prevent exer-tion. Cleansing throat gargles may be or-dered. Liquid or soft diet. Gavage or paren-teral administration of fluids may become necessary. Observe for respiratory obstruction. Equipment for suction-ing should be avail-able. Oxygen and emergency tracheos-tomy may be necessary	Vary with severity of disease: broncho-pneumonia, circula-tory or cardiac fail-ure. Degenerative changes may occur in kidneys

Table continued on following page

Table 12–8. COMMUNICABLE DISEASES Continued

DISEASE	COMMUNICABILITY PERIOD AND ROUTE	CLINICAL MANIFESTATIONS	TREATMENT AND NURSING CARE	COMPLICATIONS
EPIDEMIC INFLUENZA *Incubation Period:* 1–3 days	Not known, possibly during febrile stages *Route:* Air-borne droplet infection, direct contact	Manifestations in respiratory tract. Sudden onset with chills, fever, muscle pains, cough. If infection is severe and spreads to lower respiratory tract, air hunger may develop	Symptomatic. Provide bedrest and increased fluid intake. Antibiotics and sulfonamides may prevent secondary infection. Acetaminophen (antipyretic), drugs to control cough, and analgesics for pain may be given. *Do not give aspirin* because of high risk of Reye syndrome	In severe cases, pulmonary edema and cardiac failure. Secondary invaders may produce bacterial infections of respiratory tract
ERYTHEMA INFECTIOSUM (fifth disease) *Incubation Period:* 4–14 days	Uncertain *Route:* Infected persons	Three-stage rash: 1. Erythema on face, mostly on cheeks (disappears in 1–4 days) 2. 1 day after face rash, maculopapular red spots appear on upper and lower extremities, progressing proximal to distal 3. Rash subsides but reappears if skin is irritated (sun, heat, cold); may last 1–3 weeks	Reinforce benign nature of the condition to parents. No treatment indicated	Arthritis, pneumonitis, encephalopathy seen rarely
EXANTHEMA SUBITUM (roseola) *Incubation Period:* 5–15 days *Causative Agent:* Probably virus	Unknown *Route:* Unknown	Persistent high fever for 3–4 days in child who appears well. Precipitous drop in fever to normal with appearance of rash. Rash: discrete rose-pink macules appearing first on trunk, then spreading to neck, face, and extremities. Nonpruritic, fades on pressure, lasts 1–2 days.	Antipyretics to control fever. Anticonvulsants to child having history of febrile seizures Teach parents measures for combating high temperature. Reinforce benign nature of illness	Febrile seizures

Table 12–8. COMMUNICABLE DISEASES *Continued*

DISEASE	COMMUNICABILITY PERIOD AND ROUTE	CLINICAL MANIFESTATIONS	TREATMENT AND NURSING CARE	COMPLICATIONS
HEPATITIS TYPE A *Incubation Period:* 15–50 days *Causative Agent:* Hepatitis A virus (HAV)	Few days before to 1 month or more after onset *Route:* 1. Oral contamination by intestinal excretions 2. Contaminated food, milk, or water 3. Hepatitis A is a major potential health problem in day care centers	Manifestations occur rapidly and vary from mild to severe, from mild fever, anorexia, generalized malaise, nausea, vomiting, unpleasant taste in mouth, abdominal discomfort, and nonexistent or mild jaundice to severe jaundice, coma, and death. Early leukopenia is seen. Bile may be detected in urine; bowel movements are clay colored. Liver function tests are useful for diagnosis	Symptomatic. No specific therapy for uncomplicated HAV infection. Enteric precautions are necessary for 1 week after onset of jaundice. Persons caring for those who are not toilet trained, have diarrhea, or are incontinent should use disposable gloves when carrying fecal waste Prevention: in day care centers, thorough washing of hands after changing diapers and before preparing and serving food. Because HAV may survive on objects in the environment for weeks, adequate environmental hygiene is essential; e.g., infant changing tables	Liver damage, recurrence of symptoms Maybe a source of chromosomal damage
HEPATITIS TYPE B *Incubation Period:* 50–180 days *Causative Agent:* Hepatitis B virus (HBV)	Few days before to 1 month or more after onset *Route:* Person-to-person by percutaneous introduction of blood, direct contact with secretions or blood contaminated with HBV. May be spread by contaminated blood products. In the pediatric population, more common in children on hemodialysis, children receiving blood or blood products including those with hemophilia, and intravenous drug users	Manifestations occur slowly. See Hepatitis A for clinical manifestations	Symptomatic. The child should be allowed to regulate own activity. Diet should be high protein, high caloric, high carbohydrate, and low fat. Food should be served in small, attractive, frequent feedings. Chief reasons for hospitalization are persistent vomiting and toxicity. Fluids may be given parenterally. Enteric precautions are necessary. Prevention: Thorough washing of hands after changing diapers or bowel movements, adequate cleansing of toilets, decontamination of food and water before use	Acute fulminating hepatitis characterized by rapidly rising bilirubin, encephalpathy, edema, ascites, and hepatic coma Chronic active hepatitis with hepatic dysfunction and cirrhosis of liver

Table continued on following page

Table 12–8. COMMUNICABLE DISEASES Continued

DISEASE	COMMUNICABILITY PERIOD AND ROUTE	CLINICAL MANIFESTATIONS	TREATMENT AND NURSING CARE	COMPLICATIONS
MEASLES (rubeola) *Incubation Period:* 8–12 days *Causative Agent:* Virus	From 4 days before to 5 days after rash appears *Route:* 1. Direct contact 2. Air-borne by droplets and contaminated dust	Coryza, conjunctivitis, and photophobia are present before rash. Koplik spots in mouth, hacking cough, high fever, rash, and enlarged lymph nodes. Rash consists of small reddish-brown or pink macules changing to papules; fades on pressure. Rash begins behind ears, on forehead or cheeks, progresses to extremities, and lasts about 5 days	Symptomatic. Keep child in bed until fever and cough subside. Light in room should be dimmed. Keep hands from eyes. Irrigate eyes with physiologic saline solution to relieve itching. Tepid baths and soothing lotion relieve itching of skin. Encourage fluids during fever. Immune serum globulin maybe given to modify illness and reduce complications within 6 days of exposure. Antibacterial therapy given for complications	Vary with severity of disease: otitis media, pneumonia, tracheobronchitis, nephritis. Encephalitis may occur Subacute sclerosing panencephalitis (SSPE), a rare degenerative central nervous system disease, may occur. The mean incubation period is 7 years following measles illness
MEASLES, GERMAN (rubella) *Incubation Period:* 14–21 days *Causative Agent:* Virus	During prodromal period and for 5 days after appearance of rash *Route:* 1. Direct contact with secretions of nose and throat of infected persons 2. Air-borne by contaminated dust particles	Fetus may contract measles in utero if mother has the disease Slight fever, mild coryza. Rash consists of small pink or pale red macules closely grouped to appear as scarlet blush that fades on pressure. Rash fades in 3 days. Swelling of posterior cervical and occipital lymph nodes. No Koplik spots or photophobia as in measles	Symptomatic. Bedrest until fever subsides. Children should be excluded from school or day care for 7 days after onset of rash Infants with congenital rubella should be considered contagious until 1 year old	Chief danger of disease is damage to fetus if mother contracts infection during first trimester of pregnancy. Neonate may have *congenital rubella syndrome* with permanent defects (cataracts, cardiovascular anomalies, deafness, microcephaly, mental retardation, etc.). Virus can be isolated from blood, urine, throat, cerebrospinal fluid, lens, and other involved organs Infants may shed virus for 12 to 18 months Severe complications rare. Encephalitis may occur

Table 12–8. COMMUNICABLE DISEASES Continued

DISEASE	COMMUNICABILITY PERIOD AND ROUTE	CLINICAL MANIFESTATIONS	TREATMENT AND NURSING CARE	COMPLICATIONS
MUMPS (infectious parotitis) Incubation Period: 16–18 days Causative Agent: Virus	1–6 days before symptoms appear until swelling disappears Route: Direct or indirect contact with salivary secretions of infected person	Salivary glands are chiefly affected. Parotid, sublingual, and submaxillary glands may be involved. Swelling and pain occur in these glands either unilaterally or bilaterally. Child may have difficulty in swallowing, headache, fever, and malaise	Local application of heat or cold to salivary glands to reduce discomfort. Liquids or soft foods are given. Foods containing acid may increase pain. Bedrest until swelling subsides	Complications are less frequent in children than in adults Meningoencephalitis, inflammation of ovaries or testes, or deafness may occur
PERTUSSIS (whooping cough) Incubation Period: 7–10 days Causative Agent: Bordetella pertussis	4–6 weeks from onset Route: 1. Direct contact 2. Air-borne by droplet spread from infected person	Coryza, dry cough which is worse at night. Cough occurs in paroxysms of several sharp coughs in one expiration, then a rapid deep inspiration followed by a whoop. Dyspnea and fever may be present. Vomiting may occur after coughing. Lymphocytosis occurs	Symptomatic. Erythromycin may limit communicability. Protect child from secondary infection. Sulfonamides and antibiotics may be given to prevent secondary infections. Provide mental and physical rest to prevent paroxysms of coughing. Provide warm, humid air. Oxygen may be necessary. Avoid chilling. Offer small, frequent feedings to maintain nutritional status. Refeed if child vomits. Small amounts of sedatives may be given to quiet the child	Very serious disease during infancy because of complication of bronchopneumonia Otitis media, marasmus, bronchiectasis, and atelectasis may occur. Hemorrhage may occur during paroxysms of coughing. Encephalitis may occur

Table 12–8. COMMUNICABLE DISEASES *Continued*

DISEASE	COMMUNICABILITY PERIOD AND ROUTE	CLINICAL MANIFESTATIONS	TREATMENT AND NURSING CARE	COMPLICATIONS
POLIOVIRUS INFECTION (poliomyelitis) *Incubation Period:* 3–6 days *Causative Agent:* Virus types 1 (Brunhilde), 2 (Lansing), and 3 (Leon)	During period of infection, latter part of incubation period, and the first week of acute illness *Route:* Oral contamination by pharyngeal and intestinal excretions	Acute illness. Initial symptoms of upper respiratory tract infection, headache, fever, vomiting. Types of poliomyelitis include abortive, nonparalytic, spinal paralytic, and bulbar paralytic. Clinical manifestations may vary from mild to very severe after symptomless period following initial symptoms.	Both parents and child need support and reassurance, for they are fearful of the term *polio*. Treatment and nursing care are symptomatic. Avoid overfatigue. Place child on firm mattress with support for feet. Prevent pressure on the toes when child is on abdomen by pulling mattress away from foot of bed and letting feet protrude over the edge; when child is on back; use a foot board for support of the feet. Change position frequently. Maintain good body alignment. Encourage oral intake of food and fluids appropriate to degree of illness. Administer mild sedative to relieve anxiety and promote rest. Provide physiotherapy (applications of moist head to alleviate muscular pain). Catheterization of a distended bladder may be necessary. Since the stools contain the virus, they should be considered infectious. In bulbar poliomyelitis, therapy is directed toward suctioning of the pharynx and postural drainage to prevent aspiration of secretions, feeding by gavage, parenteral fluids, tracheostomy, use of respirator, oxygen, and prevention of intercurrent infection. Prolonged rehabilitation may be necessary, including braces, splints, or surgery	Emotional disturbances, gastric dilatation, melena, hypertension, or transitory paralysis of bladder may occur

Table 12–8. COMMUNICABLE DISEASES *Continued*

DISEASE	COMMUNICABILITY PERIOD AND ROUTE	CLINICAL MANIFESTATIONS	TREATMENT AND NURSING CARE	COMPLICATIONS
ROCKY MOUNTAIN SPOTTED FEVER *Incubation Period:* 3–12 days *Causative Agent:* *Rickettsia rickettsii*	Not communicable from person to person *Route:* Spreads by wood ticks or dog ticks from animals to humans. (If tick is found, it should be removed without crushing)	Sudden onset of non-specific symptoms: headache, fever, restlessness, anorexia. 1–5 days after onset, pale, discrete, rose-red macules or maculo-papules appear	Early diagnosis and prompt use of chloramphenicol or tetracyclines (tetracycline not given to child under 9 years of age). Corticosteroid therapy may be given. Supportive therapy, parenteral fluids, oxygen, and sedatives may be necessary for seriously ill children	Central nervous system symptoms, electrolyte disturbances, peripheral circulatory collapse, and pneumonia may occur
LYME DISEASE *Incubation Period:* 3–32 days *Causative Agent:* Borrelia burgdorferi	Not communicable from person to person; patients with active disease should not donate blood *Route:* Spread by ticks. Most common hosts are the white-tailed deer and white footed mice	Begins with a skin lesion at the site of a recent tick bite. The red macule expands to form a large papule with a raised border and a clear center. Systemic manifestations include malaise, lethargy, fever, headache, arthralgias, stiff neck, myalgias, and lymphadenopathy. Late manifestations involve the joints and the cardiac and neurological systems	Early treatment is tetracycline for children 9 years and older. Children under 9 years: penicillin V. Later-stage disease is treated with high-dose intravenous pencillin. Prevention by teaching parents to observe for signs of disease during tick season. Protective clothing should be worn in areas where tick exposure is likely. Ticks should be removed	Chronic arthritis may develop. Transplacental infection has resulted in fetal death, prematurity, and congenital anomalies

Table continued on following page

Table 12–8. COMMUNICABLE DISEASES *Continued*

DISEASE	COMMUNICABILITY PERIOD AND ROUTE	CLINICAL MANIFESTATIONS	TREATMENT AND NURSING CARE	COMPLICATIONS
STREPTOCOCCAL IN-FECTION, GROUP A HEMOLYTIC (streptococcal sore throat, scarlet fever, scarlatina) *Incubation Period:* 2–5 days *Causative Agent:* Beta-hemolytic strep-toccci, group A strains	Onset to recovery *Route:* 1. Droplet infection 2. Direct and indirect transmission may occur	Initial symptoms of streptococcal sore throat are seen in pharynx. The source of this organism may also be in a burn or wound. Toxin from site of infection is absorbed into blood-stream. The typical symptoms of scarlet fever are headache, fever, rapid pulse, rash, thrist, vomit-ing, lymphadenitis, and delirium. Throat is injected, and cel-lulitis of throat oc-curs. White tongue coating desqua-mates, and red-strawberry tongue results. Other mani-festations may in-clude otitis media, mastoiditis, and meningitis	Penicillin G is the drug of choice. Erythromycin is used for penicillin-sen-sitive individuals. Ade-quate fluid intake, bed-rest, pain-relieving drugs, and mouth care are important. Diet should be given as the child wishes: liquid, soft, or regular. Warm saline throat irrigations may be given to the older child. Increased humidity for severe in-fection of upper respi-ratory tract. Cold or hot applications to painful cervical lymph nodes	Complications are caused by toxins, the streptococci, or secondary infection. Complications of pneumonia, glomer-ulonephritis, or rheumatic fever may occur

Modified from Marlow, D., and Redding, B. (1988). *Textbook of Pediatric Nursing.* Philadelphia, W. B. Saunders Company.

ily and child to talk about feelings and changes in body appearance. Provide for visits by siblings and friends. Accept negative behaviors expressed by the child. Assist in ventilating these feelings through play therapy and the use of a play ther-apist, social worker, or psychologist.

Communicable Diseases

Prevention and control are key factors in com-municable disease. Prevention is obtained mainly through immunization. Control is through the early identification and isolation of cases.

When a communicable disease is suspected, a thorough history must be obtained. The nurse asks if the child has recently been exposed to a communicable disease, has been immunized, or has had the disease. The nurse may inquire whether the patient has experienced any of the *prodromal symptoms* (symptom indicating the onset of a disease).

Most communicable diseases can be treated at home unless the child is immune suppressed or complications occur. The child may be given tepid baths or have lotions (calamine) applied to relieve itching. Nails should be kept short and mittens may be worn by younger children who persist in scratching. Benadryl may be given if the child cannot be soothed. Acetaminophen is given for an elevated temperature. Aspirin should be avoided because of its connection with Reye syndrome. Older children may gargle with saline rinses, or use lozenges for sore throat relief. Anorexia is common, but children tend to increase their intake if they are limited to liquids and bland foods.

Quiet activities should be provided to allow for rest and provide diversion.

Table 12–8 summarizes nursing care of several often-seen communicable diseases.

References

Bayley, E. (1990). Wound healing in the patient with burns. *Nurs. Clin. North Am.* 25:205–222.

Behrman, R., and Vaughan, V. (1987). *Nelson Textbook of Pediatrics.* 13th ed. Philadelphia, W. B. Saunders Company.

Eckert, E. (1990). *Your Child and Hemophilia.* New York, The National Hemophilia Foundation.

Friendly, D. (1987). Amblyopia: Definition, classification, diagnosis, and management considerations for pediatricians, family physicians, and general practitioners. *Pediatr. Clin. North Am.* 34:1389–1413.

Goldenhersh, M., and Rachelefsky, G. (1989). Childhood asthma: Overview; Management. *Pediatr. Review* 10:227–234; 259–267.

Gordon, M. (1990). Mechanical debridement. *J. Burn Care Rehab.* 10:271–275.

Green, M., and Haggerty, R. (1990). *Ambulatory Pediatrics.* Philadelphia, W. B. Saunders Company.

Grossman, H. (1983). *Manual on Terminology and Classification in Mental Retardation.* Washington, D.C., American Association on Mental Deficiency.

Hockenberry, M., Coody, D., and Bennett, B. (1990). Childhood cancers: Incidence, etiology, diagnosis, and treatment. *Pediatr. Nurs.* 16:239–245.

Hrachovy, R., and Frost, J. (1989). Infantile spasms. *Pediatr. Clin. North Am.* 36:311–329.

Lockman, L. (1989). Absence, myoclonic, and atonic seizures. *Pediatr. Clin. North Am.* 35:331–341.

Pierce, G., Lusher, J., Brownstein, A., et al. (1989). The use of purified clotting factor concentrates in hemophilia. *J. Am. Med. Assoc.* 261:3434–3438.

Rogers, F., and Head, B. (1983). *Mister Rogers Talks with Parents.* New York, Berkeley Books.

Traver, G., and Martinez, M. (1988). Asthma update. *J. Pediatr. Health Care* 2:227–233.

Trigg, M. (1988). Bone Marrow transplantation for treatment of leukemia in children. *Pediatr. Clin. North Am.* 35:933–945.

Whaley, L., and Wong, D. (1987). *Nursing Care of Infants and Children.* St. Louis, C. V. Mosby.

Bibliography

Beard, S., Herndon, D., and Manu, D. (1989). Adaptation of self-image in burn-disfigured children. *J. Burn Care Rehab.* 10:550–554.

Behrman, R., and Kliegman, R. (1990). *Nelson Essentials of Pediatrics.* Philadelphia, W. B. Saunders Company.

Catalano, J. (1990). Strabismus. *Pediatr. Ann.* 19:289–297.

Foster, R., Hunsberger, M., and Anderson, J. (1989). *Family-Centered Nursing Care of Children.* Philadelphia, W. B. Saunders.

Hobdell, E. (1988). Infantile spasms. *Pediatr. Nurs.* 14:207–209.

Hockenberry, M., and Coody, D. (1986). *Pediatric Oncology and Hematology.* St. Louis, C. V. Mosby.

Mott, S., James, S., and Sperhac, A. (1990). *Nursing Care of Children and Families.* Redwood City, Cal., Addison-Wesley.

Shapiro, G. (1990). Let's help kids with asthma lead normal lives. *Contemp. Pediatr.* 7:105–123.

Stager, D., Birch, E., and Weakley, D. (1990). Amblyopia and the pediatrician. *Pediatr. Ann.* 19:301–315.

Vessey, J., Braithwaite, K., and Wiedmann, M. (1990). Teaching children about their internal bodies. *Pediatr. Nurs.* 16:29–33.

Wynn, S. (1989). Alternative approaches to asthma. *J. Pediatr.* 115:846–849.

Zahr, L., Connolly, M., and Page, D. (1989). Assessment and management of the child with asthma. *Pediatr. Nurs.* 15:109–114.

STUDY QUESTIONS

1. Review the composition of blood. What is the normal number of red blood cells? Of white blood cells? Of platelets? What are the functions of each of these components?
2. Gown technique is being utilized for 6 month old Tracy. Her sister Cassie, who is 4 years old and is visiting her, inquires. "Do you have ghosts in this hospital?" What fears predominate in the preschool years? How could the nurse assist Cassie to master her "ghostly" fear?
3. Define the following terms: communicable disease; immunity; serum; gamma globulin; incubation period; epidemic; virulence.
4. Discuss the postoperative care of a child who has had tonsils and adenoids removed.
5. Billy, 4 years of age, has alternating strabismus. What are the cause and treatment of this condition? List two methods of detection.
6. What is the cause of the bleeding from mucous membranes that is seen in leukemia? List two skin manifestations of bleeding.
7. Describe the nursing observations necessary for the child receiving a blood transfusion.
8. You are requested to give a talk on epilepsy to a group of school children aged 10 through 12. What facts about this disease would you emphasize? Why?
9. List the symptoms of the following diseases: mumps; chickenpox; measles; German measles; roseola.
10. Define acute glomerulonephritis. What nursing measures are specific to the condition?
11. What factors might conceivably precipitate an attack of asthma?

CHAPTER 13 _____

Chapter Outline

Objectives

Upon completion and mastery of Chapter 13, the student will be able to

- Define the vocabulary terms listed.
- Plan a diet that will provide adequate nutrition for the school age child.
- List two ways in which school life influences the growing child.
- Discuss how to assist parents in preparing a child for school entry.
- Describe the physical and psychosocial development of children from 6 to 12 years, listing age-specific events and type of guidance where appropriate.

THE SCHOOL AGE CHILD

Terms

ACT (354)
age of industry (349)
latchkey child (354)
latency (350)
self-image (350)
sibling rivalry (349)

General Characteristics

School age children, from ages 6 to 12 years, differ from preschool children in that they are more engrossed in fact than in fantasy. They have an ardent thirst for knowledge and accomplishment and admire their teachers and adult companions, whom they consider wise. They use the skill and knowledge they obtain to attempt to master the activities they enjoy—music, sports, art, and so on. Thus, the phase is referred to by Erikson as the "age of industry" (Fig. 13–1). Unsuccessful adaptations at this time can lead to a sense of inferiority. Children in school learn that they must cooperate with others. Participation in group activities heightens, and loosely knit gangs appear. Romantic love for the parent of the opposite sex diminishes, and children identify with the parent of the same sex. The type of acceptance they receive at home and at school will affect the attitudes they develop about themselves and their roles in life.

The child of this age is aware that parents are human and make mistakes. Conflicts may appear, particularly if what the child learns in school is different from what is practiced at home. Between ages 6 and 12 years, children prefer friends of their own sex and usually would rather be in the company of their friends than of their brothers and sisters. Outward displays of affection by adults are embarrassing to them. Sibling rivalry is common.

PHYSICAL GROWTH

Growth is slow until the spurt directly before puberty. Weight gains are more rapid than increases in height. The average gain in weight per year is about 7 pounds or 3 to 3.5 kg. The average increase in height is approximately 2.5 inches or 6 cm. Growth in head circumference is slower than before; between the ages of 5 and 12 years, the circumference increases from 20 to 21 inches. At the end of this time, the brain has reached approximately adult size (Behrman and Vaughan, 1987).

Muscular coordination is improved, and the lymphatic tissues become highly developed. The skeletal bones continue to ossify. The body is supple, and sometimes skeletal growth is more rapid than growth of muscles and ligaments. The child may appear gangling. There is a noticeable change in facial structures as the jaw lengthens. The sinuses are frequently sites for infection. The 6-year molars (the first permanent teeth) erupt. The gastrointestinal tract is more mature and the stomach is upset less often. The heart grows slowly and is now smaller in proportion to body size than at any other time of life.

349

SIGMUND FREUD considers later childhood to be a period of sexual latency in contrast to early childhood when, in his view, the child's sexual fantasies resulted in a conflict between him and his parents. During later childhood, the repression (or exclusion from conscious thought) of the child's sexuality permits him to form relationships with children of the same sex and allows him to assume the role of either leader or follower. According to Freud, both the child's peers and the authority figures in his world, such as his parents and teachers, have a continuing influence, especially in strengthening the child's self-image or in causing him further to repress his sexual urges.

ERIK ERIKSON places great emphasis on the influence of others in role development during later childhood. The child's learning takes place in the context of school and society, and Erikson suggests that popularity and the potential for leadership are a function of the child's relative success in learning to exert control over his environment. Successful control enables him to make positive contributions to those around him. The child acquires a positive self-concept from his ability to be productive, self-directing, and accepted.

▲ **FIGURE 13–1**

Some major theoretical viewpoints regarding personality development during later childhood. (From Schell, R., and Hall, E. [1979]. *Developmental Psychology Today*, 3rd ed. New York, CRM/Random House. Reproduced with permission of McGraw-Hill, Inc.)

The shape of the eye changes with growth. The exact age at which 20/20 vision occurs is subject to discussion. Prior to research done in the 1970s, it was generally thought that visual acuity did not reach an adult level until age 7 years or later. The best evidence currently available indicates that 20/20 or 20/30 vision is achieved by the age of about 3 years (Behrman and Vaughan, 1987). This rather drastic revision has come about as the result of new and improved techniques of measurement. The capabilities of the child's sense organs, including hearing, have an important bearing on learning abilities.

The vital signs of the child of school age are near those of the adult. Temperature is 37°C (98.6°F); pulse is 85 to 100 per minute; and respiration is 18 to 20 per minute. The systolic blood pressure ranges from 90 to 108 mm Hg and the diastolic from 60 to 68 mm Hg. Boys are slightly taller and somewhat heavier than girls until changes indicating puberty appear. The differences among children are greater at the end of middle childhood than at the beginning.

SEX EDUCATION

Sexuality refers to the physical, psychological, social, emotional, and spiritual makeup of an individual (Miller and Keane, 1987). Freud believed the school age period was a time of sexual latency, when the child's energy was directed toward cognitive and physical skills. This does not mean to imply that there is a complete lack of sexual activity at this age.

Young school age children continue to be curious about their bodies. This is sometimes evident in their play (doctor or nurse). As children grow and develop, so does their desire for knowledge about male and female roles. No longer can adults answer questions in three or four words.

Sex education is a lifelong process. Parents convey their attitudes and feelings about all aspects of life, including sexuality, to the growing child. Teaching is not so much a matter of talking or formal instruction as the whole climate of the home, particularly the respect shown to each family member. Sexuality is only one of the child's capacities and is not a fearful, isolated, episodic kind of experience.

Children's questions about sex should be answered simply and at their level of understanding. Correct names are used to describe the genitals. The hospitalized child who complains "My penis hurts" is understood by all. Private masturbation is normal and is practiced by both sexes at various times throughout their lives. It does not cause acne, blindness, insanity, or impotence. The young boy needs to be prepared for erections and nocturnal emissions (wet dreams), which are to be expected and are not necessarily due to masturbation. The young girl is prepared for menarche and is provided with the necessary articles in anticipation of this event. This is of particular importance to the early maturer, as an elementary school may not provide sanitary napkin machines in the restrooms. Both sexes are concerned during the school years with the disproportion of their bodies, and they may be self-conscious when undressing. They may compare themselves with their friends. They need reassurance about their feelings concerning awakening sexuality, which affects their thoughts and behavior.

Sex education programs in the schools are still subject to various group and community pressures. Most are fragmented and provide only basic anatomy and physiology with a general discussion of hygiene. When this is the case, and if school age children realize that their parents are uncomfortable with the subject, they turn to their peers, who often can supply only erroneous and distorted information. Some school programs emphasize that with each new freedom comes a responsibility. In addition, decision making skills are taught. Children are taught that when they do not make a decision, they have made a decision.

Regardless of their practice setting, nurses can aid in the sex education of parents and children through careful listening and anticipatory guidance. When it is appropriate, they review normal developmental behavior and explain age-specific information, e.g., sexual curiosity and masturbation. They provide families with useful written information that stresses sexuality as a healthful rather than an illness-related concept. Cultural differences should be taken into account when counseling. Teenagers frequently share their concerns, and the nurse must be prepared to assess their level of knowledge and assist in solving problems. An unexpected pregnancy in adolescence, although traumatic, can also serve as framework for continued sex education.

NURSING BRIEF ▷ ▷ ▷ ▷ ▷ ▷ ▷ ▷
When discussing sexuality with the school age child, it is necessary to identify slang or street terms. Most children hear the terms but may be confused about their meanings.

INFLUENCES FROM THE WIDER WORLD

School

Schools have a profound influence on the socialization of children. Children bring to school what they have learned and experienced in the home. Although some children come from healthy, intact families that are financially secure, many do not. Children themselves may be disabled, retarded, or abused or may suffer from a chronic illness. Parents may be abusers of alcohol or other drugs, may be unemployed, or may suffer from numerous other physical or stress-related conditions. These factors are important for nurses to remember, as they surface continually with this population. In addition, children may be unable to verbalize their needs; therefore, the caretakers must become particularly astute in their observations.

Children may look similar, but what each one will be able to absorb intellectually is directly related to their emotional health and, more often than not, to the emotional health of the family (Fig. 13–2). Schools reflect the social values and economic standing of the community that support them. If a community has various ethnic and

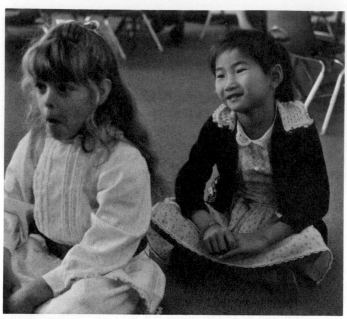

▲ **FIGURE 13–2**

The school age child is capable of logical reasoning, but it is limited to his or her own experience.

economic groups, conflicts may appear in the schools. School children are exposed to many new adults and peers whose values and expectations may be different from what they have experienced thus far.

Wright and Nader (1983) identified certain common stages or transitions in which predictable developmental crises may occur. These are school entry, the beginning of academic reading instruction, reading to learn at about third grade, start of middle school, and the period from junior to senior high school. In addition, the child can no longer be protected from prejudices because of beliefs, color, or ethnic background. The teacher becomes an important role model and influence, as do fellow students. The sensitive nurse can assist parents by affirming the individuality of children and by encouraging parents to share with children the pride they are experiencing as the children learn and progress through the elementary grades. Table 13–1 is a summary of parental guidance that the nurse may find useful in preparing children for the beginning of school.

By the time a child reaches middle school, anticipatory guidance should include dealing with peer abuse, organization of time, and the increased hazards of substance abuse. The nurse can assess patterns of communication between parents and child and assist with specific behavioral problems. Parents may have a problem in letting go. The nurse can be supportive of their endeavors in accordance with the child's maturity. The transition to junior high school generally means multiple classrooms, a series of teachers, and a change of buildings. The child is developing adult characteristics and has new feelings about the body and about parents, teachers, and peers. Anticipatory guidance includes a review of normal physiology and how it changes with puberty. Information concerning sexuality is reviewed, and the child is encouraged to ask questions at the time they arise. A warm, ongoing relationship between parents and child helps provide a safe atmosphere of caring. Adults should develop a heightened awareness for such things as school attendance problems, tardiness, and signs of loneliness or depression. They should continue to encourage children to discuss their school problems and worries. It is important that parents and children set realistic goals. A good question for

Table 13–1. SUMMARY OF PARENTAL GUIDANCE FOR THE CHILD STARTING SCHOOL

Encourage parents to
    Review normal growth and development of 5 to 6 year old children
    Anticipate regression such as thumb sucking, clinging behavior, occasional soiling
    Encourage children to express what they think school will be like
    Arrange for child to meet children who will be entering school at the same time
    Tour school with child
    Introduce child to school crossing-guard, bus driver
    Teach child the family name and telephone number
    Teach safety precautions about crossing street, strangers, "blue star" homes*
    Allow sufficient time in the morning to prepare for school
    Provide a cheerful send-off
    Instruct child about where to go in case of emergency at home, e.g., neighbor or relative
    Walk child to school until route is understood, or designate a bus stop
    Listen to child at end of day; become interested in school life
    Get to know the child's teacher, take an interest in the school
    Inform the teacher of sudden or unusual stresses in the child's life

*Community-established "safe homes" for children in an emergency. Such houses are designated by a blue star or other symbol.

(Data from Rogers, F., and Head, B. [1983]. *Mister Rogers Talks with Parents*. New York, Berkley Books, and other sources.)

Television

Television has a powerful influence on children. The amount of time children watch television has declined since 1980. However, this is misleading because it does not include the time children spend playing video games. Television has been called the "great babysitter" of our time. Some of the criticisms leveled at television viewing by children are (1) it does not challenge the imagination, (2) it interferes with solitude and play, and (3) it promotes materialism and passivity. People on television are frequently stereotyped. Schorr (1983) suggests that heavy television watching can have these effects:

1. Increased aggressive behavior and acceptance of violence.

2. Difficulty in distinguishing between reality and fantasy.

3. Trivialization of sex and sexuality.

4. Negative effects on cognitive learning.

5. Increased passivity.

Table 13–2 suggests ways in which the nurse can guide parents in regard to television viewing by children. Some programs are educational and sensitive to the needs of children. Fred Rogers suggests that children's fears can be diminished by watching and discussing television with them. He also suggests that we teach children to focus on "the helpers" of the story. Thus, they see volunteers and friends, which provides balance (Rogers and Head, 1983). The American Academy of Pediatrics recommends that parents limit their children's television viewing to 1 to 2 hours per day (American Academy of Pediatrics, 1990) (Fig. 13–3). Concerned parents and educators can obtain more information about how they can help to minimize television's harmful effects from such

adults to contemplate periodically is "When was the last time this child had a success?" Homework should be the child's responsibility, with a minimum of assistance from the parents.

Table 13–2. PARENTAL GUIDANCE FOR TELEVISION VIEWING BY CHILDREN

Encourage parents to
  Establish limits on viewing by day or week
  Establish limits on circumstances regarding viewing (no viewing during meals, no
    private sets in bedroom)
  Refrain from using television as reward or punishment
  Be good role models
  Supervise or consult with children concerning various programs available
  Spend time watching television with child, discuss feelings aroused
  Teach children to be critical of programs, help distinguish fact from fantasy
  Teach small children differences between program and commercials
  Encourage other activities such as imaginative play, reading, active games

organizations as Action for Children's Television (ACT), and the National Council for Children and Television. As video games become more and more important to children, questions will be raised about the influence of this medium.

Latchkey Children

A recent development of this generation is the large number of children who are left unsupervised after school closes. Many are asked to as-

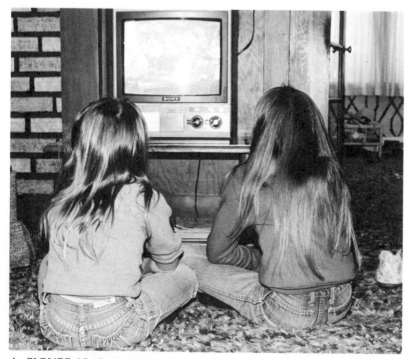

▲ FIGURE 13–3

Parents need to supervise the amount and type of television programs viewed by children.

sume responsibilities for which they are not ready. Several factors contribute to this trend, most of which revolve around the changing nature of the family. There has been an increase in single parent families headed predominantly by women whose income is at or near the poverty level. The high cost of living makes it necessary for both parents to work in order to make ends meet. In addition, the nuclear family is often separated geographically from the extended family; therefore, relatives are not available for child care. There is a lack of assistance for intact families who are poor (McClellan, 1984).

These children are at increased risk for accidents due to mischief or immature judgment. They also show heightened evidence of fear and loneliness. They have fewer opportunities to socialize with friends, as they may be instructed to remain alone in the house.

Box 13–1 shows parental and child guidance for latchkey children. Nurses should become aware of local resources such as "Prepared for Today," a program sponsored by the National Boy Scouts of America, and YMCA and YWCA after-school activities. They can also assist in developing innovative programs such as co-op babysitting, in which parents exchange child care services. It is also important for the nurse to spend time with parents, lend support, and help them explore their options.

Biological and Psychosocial Development

Table 13–3 describes the development of various competencies in the school age child.

SIX YEARS

Children of 6 years burst with energy and are on the go constantly. They soon become overtired, and it is necessary to set limits to their activities. They like to start tasks but do not always finish them, for their attention span is fairly brief. They tend to be bossy and sometimes rude, but they are very sensitive to criticism. Sex investigations begun in earlier years may persist. Their conscience is active, and they find it difficult to make decisions.

One of the most obvious physical changes at this age is the loss of the temporary teeth (Fig. 13–4). The important 6-year molars also erupt. The child can jump rope, throw and catch a ball, and tie shoe laces. They also perform numerous other feats that require muscle coordination. Their language differs from that of the preschool child. They use it for a purpose rather than for the pure joy of talking. Vocabulary consists of about 2500 words. They require 11 to 13 hours of sleep a night.

Boys and girls play together at this age, although there is the beginning preference to associate with children of the same sex. Certain activities, such as imaginative play, are common to both sexes (Fig. 13–5). Most children enjoy collecting objects that catch their fancy, such as leaves, stones, and shells. Play at this time usually reflects events that occur in the immediate environment.

Children of 6 years need time and support to help them adjust to school (see page 352). If they have nursery school or kindergarten experience, the transition may be more comfortable. Most children go to school expecting the same reception that they are accustomed to in the home. If parents are critical or overprotective, children will assume that the teacher will be too. When this differs markedly from their expectations, they begin to feel insecure and may even be hostile toward the teacher. Parents need to observe children for signs of fatigue and stress. Not all children are ready for school merely because they have reached the proper age. Even those who are need time and support from parents and teachers before they can settle down to the job at hand. Being in school exposes the child to infection more frequently than at home. Preschool immunizations and a physical examination are indicated.

SEVEN YEARS

Children at 7 years are generally less of a problem than they were at 6. It is a quieter age, and the child does not go looking for trouble. Some educators have noted that second graders are the easiest to teach. They set high standards for themselves and for their family, have a good sense of humor, tend to be somewhat of a tease (wiggle loose teeth to annoy adults), and are a little more modest than they were at an earlier age. They enjoy being active but can also appreciate periods Text continued on page 361

Table 13–3. COMPETENCY DEVELOPMENT OF THE

AGE (YEARS)	PHYSICAL COMPETENCY	INTELLECTUAL COMPETENCY	EMOTIONAL-SOCIAL COMPETENCY
General: 6–12	Gains an average of 2.5 to 3.2 kg/year (5.5 to 7 pounds/year). Overall height gains of 5.5 cm (2 inches) per year; growth occurs in spurts and is mainly in trunk and extremities. Loses deciduous teeth; most of permanent teeth erupt. Progressively more coordinated in both gross and fine motor skills. Caloric needs increase with growth spurts	Masters concrete operations. Moves from egocentrism; learns he or she is not always right. Learns grammar and expression of emotions and thoughts. Vocabulary increases to 3000 words or more; handles complex sentences	Central crisis; industry vs. inferiority; wants to do and make things. Progressive sex education needed. Wants to be like friends; competition important. Fears body mutilation, alterations in body image; earlier phobias may recur; nightmares; fears death. Nervous habits common
6–7	Gross motor skill exceeds fine motor coordination. Balance and rhythm are good—runs, skips, jumps, climbs, gallops. Throws and catches ball. Dresses self with little or no help	Vocabulary of 2500 words. Learning to read and print; beginning concrete concepts of numbers, general classification of items. Knows concepts of right and left; morning, afternoon, and evening; coinage. Intuitive thought process. Verbally aggressive, bossy, opinionated, argumentative. Likes simple games with basic rules	Boisterous, outgoing, and a know-it-all; whiny; parents should sidestep power struggles, offer choices. Becomes quiet and reflective during 7th year; very sensitive. Can use telephone. Likes to make things; starts many, finishes few. Give some responsibility for household duties
8–10	Myopia may appear. Secondary sex characteristics begin in girls. Hand-eye coordination and fine motor skills well established. Movements are graceful, coordinated. Cares for own physical needs completely. Constantly on move; plays and works hard; enforce balance in rest and activity	Learning correct grammar and to express feelings in words. Likes books he or she can read alone; will read funny papers, scan newspaper. Enjoys making detailed drawings. Mastering classification, seriation, spatial, temporal, and numerical concepts. Uses language as a tool; likes riddles, jokes, chants, word games. Rules guiding force in life now. Very interested in how things work, what and how weather, seasons, etc., are made	Strong preference for same-sex peers; antagonizes opposite-sex peers. Self-assured and pragmatic at home; questions parental values and ideas. Has a strong sense of humor. Enjoys clubs, group projects, outings, large groups, camp. Modesty about own body increases over time; sex-conscious. Works diligently to perfect skills she or he does best. Happy, cooperative, relaxed and casual in relationships. Increasingly courteous and well-mannered with adults. Gang stage at a peak; secret codes and rituals prevail. Responds better to suggestion than dictatorial approach
11–12	Vital signs approximate adult norms. Growth spurt for girls; inequalities between sexes are increasingly noticeable; boys greater physical strength. Eruption of permanent teeth complete except for third molars. Secondary sex characteristics begin in boys. Menstruation may begin	Able to think about social problems and prejudices; sees others' points of view. Enjoys reading mysteries, love stories. Begins playing with abstract ideas. Interested in whys of health measures and understands human reproduction. Very moralistic; religious commitment often made during this time	Intense team loyalty; boys begin teasing girls and girls flirt with boys for attention; best friend period. Wants unreasonable independence. Rebellious about routines; wide mood swings; needs some time daily for privacy. Very critical of own work. Hero worship prevails. "Facts of life" chats with friends prevail; masturbation increases. Appears under constant tension

Adapted from Foster, R., Hunsberger, M., and Anderson, J. (1989). *Family-Centered Nursing Care of Children.* Philadelphia, W. B. Saunders Company.

SCHOOL AGE CHILD

NUTRITION	PLAY	SAFETY	IMMUNIZATIONS
Fluctuations in appetite due to uneven growth pattern and tendency to get involved in activities. Tendency to neglect breakfast in rush of getting to school. Though school lunch is provided in most schools, child does not always eat it	Plays in groups, mostly of same sex; "gang" activities predominate. Books for all ages. Bicycles a must. Sports equipment. Cards, board and table games. Most of play is active games requiring little or no equipment	Enforce continued use of safety belts during car travel. Bicycle safety must be taught and enforced. Teach safety related to hobbies, handicrafts, mechanical equipment	
Preschool food dislikes persist. Tendency for deficiencies in iron, vitamin A, and riboflavin. 100 ml/kg of water per day, 3 gm/kg protein daily.	Still enjoys dolls, cars, and trucks. Plays well alone but enjoys small groups of both sexes; begins to prefer same sex peer during 7th year. Ready to learn how to ride a bicycle. Prefers imaginary, dramatic play with real costumes. Begins collecting for quantity, not quality. Enjoys active games such as hide-and-seek, tag, jump rope, roller skating, kickball. Ready for lessons in dancing, gymnastics, music. Restrict TV time to 1–2 hours/day	Teach and reinforce traffic safety. Still needs adult supervision of play. Teach to avoid strangers, never take anything from strangers. Teach illness prevention and reinforce continued practice of other health habits. Restrict bicycle use to home ground; no traffic areas; teach bicycle safety. Teach and set examples re harmful use of drugs, alcohol, smoking	TOPV and DPT boosters if not received at age 5 years
Needs about 2100 calories/day; nutritious snacks. Tends to be too busy to bother to eat. Tendency for deficiencies in calcium, iron, and thiamine. Problem of obesity may begin now. Good table manners. Able to help with food preparation	Likes hiking, sports. Enjoys cooking, woodworking, crafts. Enjoys cards and table games. Likes radio and records. Begins qualitative collecting now. Continue restriction on TV time	Stress safety with firearms. Keep them out of reach and allow use only with adult supervision. Know who the child's friends are; parents should still have some control over friend selection. Teach water safety; swimming should be supervised by an adult	TD vaccine if series not previously received
Boy needs 2500 calories/day; girl needs 2250 (70 cal/kg/day). 75 ml/kg of water per day; 2 gm/kg protein daily)	Enjoys projects and working with hands. Likes to do errands and jobs to earn money. Very involved in sports, dancing, talking on phone. Enjoys all aspects of acting and drama	Continue monitoring friends. Stress bicycle safety on streets and in traffic	Measles, mumps, rubella, primarily to boost measles and mumps immunity

BOX 13–1. PROBLEMS AND NEEDS OF LATCHKEY CHILDREN

SAFETY

1. Teach children not to display keys and always to lock doors. Teach children what to do if a key is lost.

*2. Tell children not to go into the house after school if the door is ajar, a window is open, or if anything looks unusual. Teach child not to open the door to anyone unless the person has been approved by the parent.

*3. Walk through the after-school routine with the child. Some children have keys but cannot reach the locks. Teach child not to get in cars with strangers.

*4. Consult with fire and police officials about burglar-proofing and fire-proofing the home. Teach child what to do if a burglary attempt occurs.

5. Teach children what to do in case of accidents; how to call for help.

*6. Prepare a safety kit.

7. Teach safety rules to children who are expected to cook. Microwave ovens are the safest.

8. Emphasize such fire safety rules as:
   a. Leave the house and do not return to it if a fire starts.
   b. Practice fire drills and evacuation at home, including a safe place to meet outside the home.

9. Teach children about weather-related safety.

10. Prevent drowning. Children *should never swim without adult supervision.*

11. Use *locked* storage for firearms. Never store guns and ammunition together. Instruct children that firearms are to be handled by adults only.

TELEPHONE USE

1. Teach children to tell callers that their parents are "busy," rather than saying "They're not here."

*2. Keep police, fire department, and other important telephone numbers by the phone. Be sure child knows how to report emergencies.

3. Be sure children know their own telephone numbers, addresses, and parents' names.

AFTERSCHOOL ACTIVITIES

*1. Arrange for the child to spend some afternoons with friends.

*2. Provide structured activities, such as art projects.

*3. Have the child go to a public library—sponsored activity rather than watching television at home.

4. Establish clear rules with child as to what may/may not be done until parent gets home.

*5. Offer children a choice of activities.

6. Discuss with all children in a class what they do after school. Recommend specific activities other than television.

7. Teach children that independence and resourcefulness are virtues, but don't demand too much.

8. Help children feel successful in taking care of themselves.

*9. Counsel parents regarding the potential problems of having older children care for younger ones when not developmentally ready.

LONELINESS

1. Talk to children about their experiences of being alone after school.

*2. Be punctual. Children's anxiety escalates when parents don't return home as promised.

*3. Call the child when parents will be late.

*4. Leave a tape-recorded message for children to play when they arrive home.

*5. Form a group of parents with flex-time so that their children can be cared for by one of the group after school.

NETWORKING

*1. Parents, teachers, and nurses can help develop a supportive network of working parents.

2. Families may find church memberships helpful.

---

*Items specifically for parents.

(Adapted from Foster, R., Hunsberger, M., and Anderson, J. [1989]. *Family-Centered Nursing Care of Children.* Philadelphia, W. B. Saunders Company.)

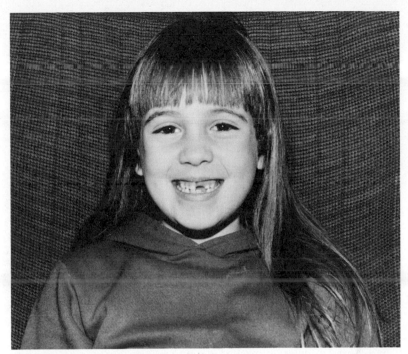

▲ **FIGURE 13–4**

Still smiling!

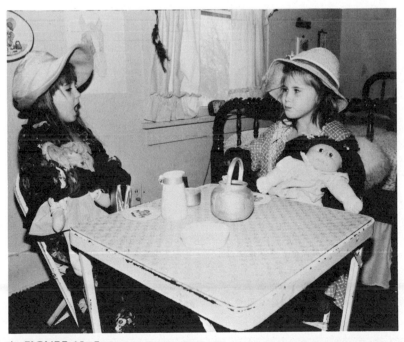

▲ **FIGURE 13–5**

Young children prepare for various roles through imaginative play.

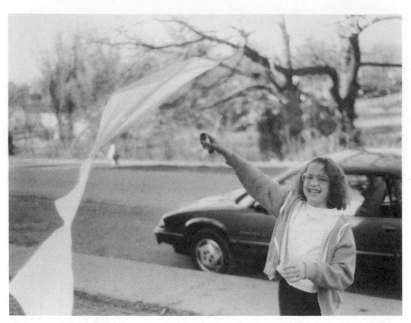

▲ **FIGURE 13–6**

The 8 year old child enjoys projects and active play.

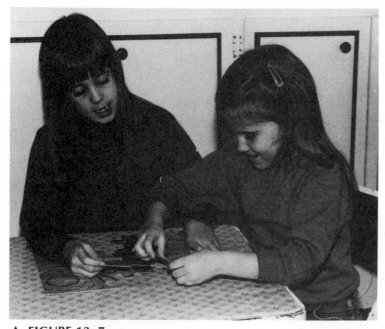

▲ **FIGURE 13–7**

Competition between siblings is common in the school years.

of rest. The second grader may acquire a "crush" on a friend of the opposite sex.

These children know the months and seasons of the year and begin to tell time. They have a beginning concept of arithmetic, can count by twos and fives, and know that money is valuable. Their hands are steadier. Interest in God and heaven is heightened.

Active play is still important to both sexes (Fig. 13–6). The boys are more apt to tease the girls rather than to participate in such games as jump rope or tag. Both sexes enjoy bike riding and table games. Realistic toys, such as dolls that can be bathed and fed and trains that back up and whistle, appeal to the 7 year old. Comic books are also popular. Becoming increasingly independent, the children imagine themselves accomplishing feats more adventuresome than those of their parents (Fig. 13–7). They cannot understand how Mom and Dad ever chose to lead such dull lives.

Stealing. One problem that may arise at about this age is stealing. This is generally a signal that some need of the child is not being met. It may be actual or perceived. In many cases the child steals only to distribute the loot to neighborhood friends. This may in actuality be an attempt to buy friendship. Children's independence has separated them to a degree from the parents; if they cannot establish good relationships with their friends, they may feel left out. When children steal something, parents should tell them that they are aware of the fact and should insist on some form of restitution. They should not humiliate the child, but they must make it clear that such actions cannot be permitted. As always, accept the child but not the deed, and then try to understand the circumstances that are causing such behavior.

NURSING BRIEF ▷ ▷ ▷ ▷ ▷ ▷ ▷ ▷ ▷
Before the age of 3 years, small children frequently take things that don't belong to them. This is not stealing, as the child does not know any better.

EIGHT YEARS

The eight year old wants to do everything and can play alone for longer periods than the child of 7 can. Work is usually creative. Group activities such as Brownies and Cub Scouts are enjoyed, and companions of the same sex are preferred. Group fads begin to be seen. Eight year olds like

to be considered important, particularly by adults. They may behave better for company than for the family. Hero worship is evident.

The arms and hands of the 8 year old seem to grow faster than the rest of the body. The large and small muscles are better developed, and movements are smoother and more graceful. The child can write rather than print and understands the number of days that must pass before special events such as Christmas, birthdays, and discharge from the hospital.

Competitive sports are enjoyed, but the child is generally a poor loser. Long, involved arguments occur over decisions made by referees. Wrestling is frequent, and dramatic play is popular. Most children like to be the hero or heroine of their favorite program. Neighborhood secret clubs are organized, and all members must pay strict attention to the rules.

NINE YEARS

The 9 year old is dependable and is not as restless as the child of 8 years. More interest is shown in family activities, more responsibility is assumed for personal belongings and for younger brothers and sisters, and tasks are more likely to be completed (Figs. 13–8 and 13–9). Children resist

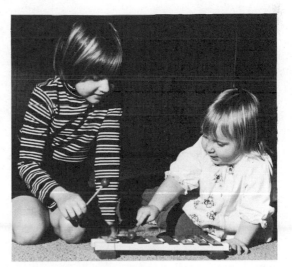

▲ FIGURE 13–8

The child of school age entertains younger members of the family.

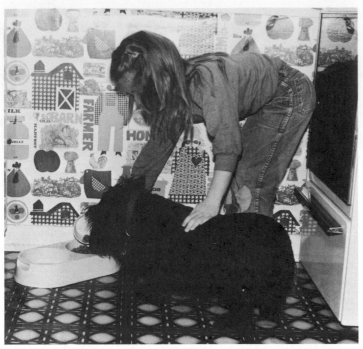

▲ **FIGURE 13–9**

The 9 year old is capable of caring for the family pet.

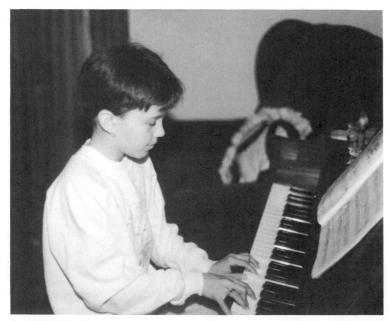

▲ **FIGURE 13–10**

Outlets such as music help the child express feelings in a positive way.

adult authority if it does not coincide with the opinions or ideals of the group. They are, however, more able to accept criticism for their actions. Individual differences are very pronounced.

Worries and mild compulsions are common. Children avoid cracks in the pavement: "Step on a crack, break your mother's back." They realize that these actions are senseless but still feel obliged to repeat them. Nervous habits, sometimes referred to as "tics," may also appear and may vary widely. Eye blinking, facial grimacing, and shoulder shrugging are but a few examples. The child cannot help such actions and should not be scolded for them because they are due mainly to tension; they usually disappear when home and social life become more relaxed.

Hand-and-eye coordination is well developed, and manual activities are managed with skill. The child works and plays hard and becomes overtired. About 10 hours of sleep a night are needed. The permanent teeth are still erupting.

Competitive sports are still popular, as are reading, listening to the radio, and watching television and movies. Contact sports should be limited to minimize permanent growth-related injuries. Girls play for long periods of time with dolls. An interest in music is shown, and the child may desire to take lessons (Fig. 13–10). The children know the date, can repeat months of the year in order, and can multiply and do simple division. They takes care of their bodily needs, and by now table manners are considerably improved.

PREADOLESCENCE

10 Years

This marks the beginning of the preadolescent years. Girls are more physically mature than boys. The child begins to show self-direction, is courteous to adults, and thinks quite clearly about social problems and prejudices. The 10 year old wants to be independent and resents being told what to do but is receptive to suggestion. The ideas of the group are more important than individual ideas. Interest in sex and sex investigations continues.

Girls in general are more poised than boys. Both sexes are fairly reliable about household duties (Fig. 13–11). Slang terms are used. The 10 year

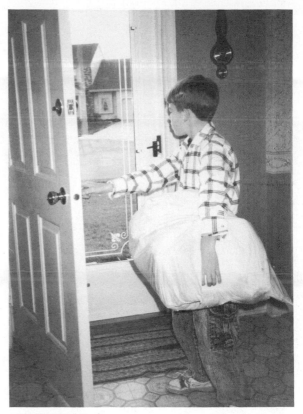

▲ FIGURE 13–11

The school age child helps with chores to earn an allowance.

old can write for a relatively long period of time and maintains good writing speed. The child uses fractions and knows numbers over 100. Boys and girls begin to identify themselves with skills that pertain to their particular sex role. There is an intolerance of the opposite sex. The play enjoyed by the 10 year old is similar to that enjoyed by the 9 year old. In addition, the child takes more interest in appearance.

11 to 12 Years

Adjectives that describe this age group include intense, observant, all-knowing, energetic, meddlesome, and argumentative. This period before the onset of puberty is one of complete disorganization. Its beginning comes earlier in some children; the onset and rate of physical maturity vary

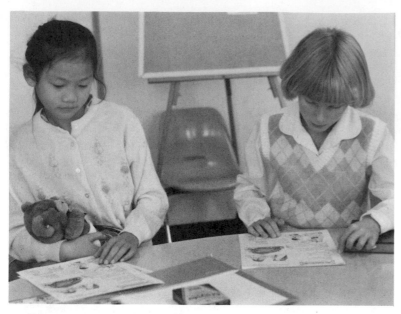

▲ **FIGURE 13–12**

Getting acquainted is scary and takes time.

greatly. Before the end of this period, the hormones of the body begin to influence physical growth. Posture is poor. There are 24 to 26 permanent teeth.

The child has an overabundance of energy and is on the go every minute. Girls become "tomboyish" in their actions. Table manners are a thing of the past, and the refrigerator is constantly emptied. Children this age are less concerned with appearance. They seem to be preoccupied a great deal of the time, and this, along with physical activities and numerous anxieties, accounts for some of the decline seen in school grades. Ability to concentrate decreases, and parents complain that the children "never hear anything." When asked to do a new task, they moan and groan.

Gangs are still important. They are not ready to stand alone, but they cannot bear the thought of depending on parents. They must overcome the problems that confront them without parental help (Fig. 13–12). Their attitude implies, "Can't you see that I'm not a child anymore?"

During prepuberty, they are very much interested in the body and watch for signs of growing up. Girls look forward to menstruation and wearing their first bra. Boys and girls tend to ignore the opposite sex, but in reality they are much aware of them. There is a tendency to tease one another. Their descriptions of each other are far

from complimentary—"stupid, crazy, nerd." Both sexes enjoy earning money by obtaining odd jobs. Preadolescents often seek an adult friend of the same sex to idolize.

Guiding preadolescents is not easy. They need freedom within limits and recognition that they

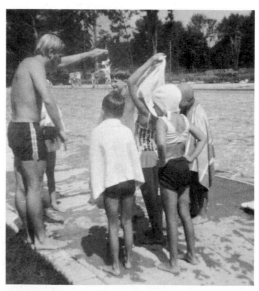

▲ **FIGURE 13–13**

Children should be taught how to swim and should learn the rules of water safety.

are no longer a baby (Fig. 13–13). They should know why parents make a decision. They should not be expected to follow household rules blindly. Their conscience enables them to understand and accept reasonable discipline. Constant verbal nagging is ignored. They should be provided with constructive opportunities to aid in getting rid of pent-up emotions and energies. Their irritating behavior is more easily accepted when one realizes that much of it is indeed "just a phase."

Physical Care

HYGIENE

Children of school age are gradually able to accept more responsibility for personal hygiene. They need reminders and, in some instances, demonstrations of how to do a task correctly. They are able to dress, brush the teeth, comb the hair, and wash face and hands. (Most children of this age tend to forget that they have ears and a neck.) They must be taught how to care for fingernails and toenails.

CLOTHING

Clothing need not be expensive but it should be simple in design and durable. Children must be taught the proper way to care for their clothes, but parents should anticipate temporary regressions in this area. Shoes must be sturdy and of the proper size. Boots and raincoats are necessary to protect the child from inclement weather. Stockings should fit properly to prevent irritation of the feet. All coats, sweaters, hats, boots, and gloves worn to school should be labeled.

SLEEP

Children of this age are so active during the day, both physically and mentally, that they soon become exhausted. Children from 6 to 8 years average approximately 11 to 13 hours of sleep a night. As they grow older, a little less is required. The 9 to 12 year old averages about 10 hours per night. Parents can judge the amount of sleep a child needs by the behavior. If a child is eating and playing well and keeping up with schoolwork, chances are that sleep is sufficient.

HEALTH EXAMINATIONS

The yearly preschool physical examination is given in the spring preceding admission. This allows time for correction of any problems that are found. Booster immunizations are given as needed (see Table 13–4); the child's teeth are examined and dental work completed.

School health programs aimed at maintaining and promoting health are provided in most school systems. The nurses and other professional persons who take part in such programs can play an important role in counseling parents. They also help in meeting the needs of handicapped children enrolled in their schools. A carefully taken health history provides the nurse with much-needed information (Fig. 13–14).

The eating habits of a child of this age should be basically good, as long as a variety of nutritious foods are offered. See Table 13–4 for the recommended food intake for school age children. A good breakfast is important. The chief breakfast foods necessary are fruit, cereal, and milk. Eggs add variety. Menus centered on these foods are more substantial than those consisting of doughnuts or sweet rolls and coffee.

The federal government has established the school breakfast program in many areas. The National School Lunch Program has been ongoing. Summer lunch programs are also available in some communities. These lunches must provide certain nutritional standards (the goal is to provide one third of the recommended daily allowance of foods).

Guidance

Children in school are continuously in need of understanding from persons concerned with their care. The types of relationships they have had previously are reflected in their behavior. They must know that they are wanted and loved and that their parents are proud of them and of their accomplishments, both in and out of school. They need approval for tasks well done and a minimum of criticism. They need assistance in recognizing

Table 13–4. RECOMMENDED FOOD INTAKE FOR GOOD NUTRITION ACCORDING TO FOOD GROUPS AND THE AVERAGE SIZE OF SERVINGS AT DIFFERENT AGE LEVELS

FOOD GROUP	SERVINGS PER DAY	AVERAGE SIZE OF SERVINGS					
		1 year	2–3 years	4–5 years	6–9 years	10–12 years	13–15 years
Milk and cheese (1.5 oz cheese = 1 C milk) (C = 1 cup = 8 oz or 240 gm)	4	½ C	½–¾ C	¾ C	¾–1 C	1 C	1 C
Meat group (protein foods)	3 or more						
Egg		1	1	1	1	1	1 or more
Lean meat, fish, poultry (liver once a week)		2 Tbsp	2 Tbsp	4 Tbsp	2–3 oz (4–6 Tbsp)	3–4 oz	4 oz or more
Peanut butter			1 Tbsp	2 Tbsp	2–3 Tbsp	3 Tbsp	3 Tbsp
Fruits and vegetables Vitamin C source (citrus fruits, berries, tomato, cabbage, cantaloupe)	At least 4, including: 1 or more (twice as much tomato as citrus)	⅓ C citrus	½ C	½ C	1 medium orange	1 medium orange	1 medium orange
Vitamin A source (green or yellow fruits and vegetables)	1 or more	2 Tbsp	3 Tbsp	4 Tbsp (¼ C)	¼ C	⅓ C	½ C
Other vegetables (potato and legumes, etc.) *or*	2	2 Tbsp	3 Tbsp	4 Tbsp (¼ C)	¼ C	½ C	¾ C
Other fruits (apple, banana, etc.)		¼ C	⅓ C	½ C	1 medium	1 medium	1 medium

Table 13–4. RECOMMENDED FOOD INTAKE FOR GOOD NUTRITION ACCORDING TO FOOD GROUPS AND THE AVERAGE SIZE OF SERVINGS AT DIFFERENT AGE LEVELS *Continued*

FOOD GROUP	SERVINGS PER DAY	AVERAGE SIZE OF SERVINGS					
		1 year	2–3 years	4–5 years	6–9 years	10–12 years	13–15 years
Cereals (whole-grain or enriched)	At least 4						
Bread		½ slice	1 slice	1½ slices	1–2 slices	2 slices	2 slices
Ready-to-eat cereals		½ oz	¾ oz	1 oz	1 oz	1 oz	1 oz
Cooked cereal (including macaroni, spaghetti, rice, etc.)		¼ C	⅓ C	½ C	½ C	¾ C	1 C or more
Fats and carbohydrates	To meet caloric needs						
Butter, margarine, mayonnaise, oils: 1 Tbsp = 100 calories (kcal)		1 Tbsp	1 Tbsp	1 Tbsp	2 Tbsp	2 Tbsp	2–4 Tbsp
Desserts and sweets: 100-calorie portions as follows: ⅓ C pudding or ice cream 2–3" cookies, 1 oz cake, 1⅓ oz pie, 2 Tbsp jelly, jam, honey, sugar		1 portion	1½ portions	1½ portions	3 portions	3 portions	3–6 portions

(From Behrman, R., and Vaughan, V. [1987]. *Nelson Textbook of Pediatrics*, 13th ed. Philadelphia, W. B. Saunders Company. Prepared in collaboration with Mildred J. Bennett, Ph.D., From "Four Food Groups of the Daily Food Guide," Institute of Home Economics, U.S.D.A., and Publication #30, Children's Bureau of the United States Department of Health, Education, and Welfare.)

and keeping in touch with their feelings. At this age, they are quite critical of themselves. They need help in self-acceptance. Their judgment improves with age. Their decision-making capabilities need encouragement, e.g., "I feel you can make that decision yourself." Some of their decisions will reflect their immaturity, and it may be necessary for parents to intervene if these are life-threatening or may cause injury. However, they will learn from making minor mistakes. Parents and nurses who have empathy with school children can better understand their views.

Preadolescents want to be accepted by their group; they imitate their speech, manner of dress, and actions. Interest in organizations is at its peak. Children enjoy scouting programs and young people's groups affiliated with their church. Parents

should encourage such group activities because they are both physically and morally strengthening.

These children need time and a place to study. They should have a desk of their own or at least a private area of the house where they are able to concentrate. Furniture should be of the proper size; lighting should be adequate. They must learn to take responsibility for their assignments and school supplies and to keep their room orderly. Parents can encourage them by showing interest in what they are learning, by joining parent-teacher organizations, and by visiting the teacher periodically. They must also vote on civic matters that will benefit the school system in their community.

At this age, an allowance or at least a means of

I. GENERAL INFORMATION

Name_____ Date_____
Age and birth date _____ Language _____
Grade _____ Informant _____
Sex _____ Parents' home and business
Religion _____   phones _____

II. FAMILY PROFILE (health history of family members)

Mother _____
Father _____
Siblings _____
Paternal grandparents _____
Maternal grandparents _____
Life change events: death, divorce, new baby, moves of family, illness, separation, etc.
_____
_____

III. CHILD PROFILE

Newborn status: Did baby leave hospital with you? _____
Birth defects _____
Developmental history: Age for crawling_____sitting_____
   walking _____speech _____toilet training _____
Immunizations _____
Habits, general behavior in school _____ Home _____
Sleeping patterns _____ Fears _____
Exercise _____ Friends _____
Interests _____ Special skills _____
_____
Previous illness or accidents _____
Is child taking any medications? _____
Hearing aid _____ Glasses _____
Dental care _____ Allergies _____
Typical foods consumed:
   breakfast _____
   lunch _____
   supper _____
   snacks _____
Eating problems _____ Elimination _____
Menses _____ Sexual maturation _____
Sex education _____ Personal hygiene _____
Review of systems _____
_____

IV. NURSE'S OBSERVATIONS AND COMMENTS

General physical description _____
_____
Results of screening procedures: vision _____ audiometer _____
Scoliosis _____ Other _____
Individual health education and guidance _____
_____
Problem-solving plan _____
_____

                              Interviewer _____

▲ FIGURE 13–14

Health assessment summary of the school age child.

earning money provides them with opportunities to learn its value. It will take time and encouragement for them to learn to spend money wisely. Such experiences aid in making the school child a more responsible person.

Girls and boys need information and reassurance in advance about the changes that will take place in their bodies at puberty. This information is discussed in Chapter 15.

Safety. Table 13–5 presents a guide for parents

Text continued on page 375

Table 13–5. AGE-APPROPRIATE ADVICE FOR INJURY PREVENTION

The following guide is designed to help you tailor anticipatory guidance about injury prevention to the age of each patient. The left-hand column lists prevention strategies for various injuries. Some are aimed at the parent, some at the child. Appropriate ages at which to discuss each strategy are indicated by Xs in the "Child's Age at Visit" columns, which are based on the standard schedule of well-child visits. As you will see, many of the strategies are appropriate at all ages throughout the "middle years." (X) indicates that the individual child's maturity, experience, exposures, and locale as well as past counseling should be taken into account.

	Child's Age at Visit			
Prevention Strategies	**6 Y**	**8 Y**	**10 Y**	**12 Y**
MOTOR VEHICLE OCCUPANT INJURIES				
Parent				
Do not drink or take drugs and drive	X	X	X	X
Set a good example; wear your own seat belt	X	X	X	X
Check to see that your child's seat belt is buckled before you start the car	X	X	X	X
If the seat belt is unfastened, stop the car	X	X	X	X
Transport your child in the safest seating position possible (lap and shoulder belt is better than lap alone; rear seat is better than front)	X	X	X	X
Insist that your child wear a seat belt no matter whose car he or she is riding in	X	X	X	X
Never transport a child in the cargo area of a vehicle (back of station wagon, van, or truck)	X	X	X	X
Do not allow your child to operate a motor vehicle; this includes motorcycles, motorbikes, trail bikes, and other off-road vehicles, including farm vehicles	X	X	X	X
Be *very* cautious about allowing your child to ride as a *passenger* on a motorcycle, motor vehicle, or off-road vehicle (insist on helmet, slow speed, and a mature, sober driver)	(X)	(X)	X	X
Child				
Always wear a seat belt, no matter whom you ride with	X	X	X	X
Do not ride in the back of a station wagon, van, or truck	X	X	X	X
Do not drive *any* motor vehicle yourself	X	X	X	X

Table continued on following page

Table 13–5. AGE-APPROPRIATE ADVICE FOR INJURY PREVENTION *Continued*

	Child's Age at Visit			
Prevention Strategies	**6 Y**	**8 Y**	**10 Y**	**12 Y**
PEDESTRIAN INJURIES				
Parent				
When crossing the street, teach and model: Stop at the curb. Look (L,R,L) before entering the street	X	X		
Your child is too young to cross the street without supervision	X	(X)	(X)	
Plan walking routes that minimize crossings with heavy traffic			X	X
Child				
Never cross the street without a grown-up	X	(X)		
Don't play near or in the street	X	X	X	X
Always stop and look (L,R,L) before entering the street	X	X	X	X
DROWNING				
Parent				
Your child requires continuous adult supervision in, on, and around water	X	X	X	X
Prohibit swimming in fast-moving water (rivers, canals)	X	X	X	X
Permit diving only after training and only from an official board; hands, not head, should break water	(X)	X	X	X
All persons in a boat should wear a personal flotation device (PFD)	X	X	X	X
Your pool should have a tall, hard-to-climb fence around all four sides and be kept locked when not supervised	(X)	(X)	(X)	(X)
Keep rescue equipment at waterside	X	X	X	X
Child				
Don't swim or enter water without your parent's permission and an adult watching	X	X	X	X
Don't swim where water moves fast (rivers, canals)	X	X	X	X
Don't dive except from an official board; elsewhere enter water feet first	X	X	X	X
Wear a PFD when in a boat	X	X	X	X

Table 13–5. AGE-APPROPRIATE ADVICE FOR INJURY PREVENTION Continued

	Child's Age at Visit			
Prevention Strategies	6 Y	8 Y	10 Y	12 Y
FIRES AND BURNS				
Parent				
Install and maintain smoke detector near your child's room and in other appropriate locations in the house (check batteries monthly, replace batteries annually)	X	X	X	X
Teach your child what to do if the smoke alarm sounds	X	(X)	(X)	(X)
Make an escape plan in case of fire and practice it	X	X	X	X
Have heating system checked annually	X	X	X	X
No one in household should smoke in bed	(X)	(X)	(X)	(X)
Place matches and lighters off limits	X	X	X	X
Have a working fire extinguisher near the kitchen, but instruct your child not to use it; tell her or him to leave the house in case of fire	X	X	X	X
Do not permit your child to have or handle fireworks	X	X	X	X
Child				
If smoke alarm sounds or fire is obvious, leave the house, call fire department from a neighbor's house, meet your family at agreed upon spot	X	X	X	X
Don't play with matches or lighters	X	X	X	X
Firecrackers and fireworks cause many serious burns; do not handle or use them or watch as others do except at an official show	X	X	X	X

Table continued on following page

Table 13–5. AGE-APPROPRIATE ADVICE FOR INJURY PREVENTION *Continued*

	Child's Age at Visit			
Prevention Strategies	**6 Y**	**8 Y**	**10 Y**	**12 Y**
BICYCLE INJURIES				
Parent				
Buy a helmet that meets ANSI or Snell standards when you buy the first bike; update both helmet and bike as child grows	X	X	X	X
Your child is too young to ride in the street safely	X	(X)	(X)	
Make sure the bike is the right size (take the child along when you buy it)	X	X	X	X
When sitting on seat with hands on handlebars, the child should be able to reach ground with the balls of the feet When straddling center bar, both feet flat on ground, there should be at least 1-in clearance from bar to crotch				
Do not buy a bike with hand brakes until the child is able to grasp with sufficient pressure to stop the bike		X		
Teach and enforce the "rules of the road"		X	X	X
Do not allow night riding	X	X	X	X
Keep bike in good repair	X	X		
Teach child to maintain bike			X	X
Child				
Always wear a helmet when riding a bike	X	X	X	X
Two people don't belong on one bike	X	X	X	X
Ride off-road only	X	(X)	(X)	
Obey the "rules of the road"		(X)	(X)	X
Keep bike in good repair			X	X

Table 13–5. AGE-APPROPRIATE ADVICE FOR INJURY PREVENTION *Continued*

Prevention Strategies	Child's Age at Visit			
	6 Y	8 Y	10 Y	12 Y
INJURIES FROM FIREARMS				
Parent				
Pediatricians do not recommend nonpowder firearms (BB gun, pellet gun); they are too dangerous	X	X	X	X
Any guns kept in the home should be unloaded and locked up; ammunition should be locked in a separate location	X	X	X	X
Keeping a handgun for "protection" is dangerous to your family	X	X	X	X
Child				
Do not touch any gun; it might be real, and it might be loaded	X	X	X	X
Never play with a gun	X	X	X	X
If you see or hear about a gun at school, tell your teacher immediately	(X)	(X)	X	X
SUICIDE				
Parent				
If your child threatens to harm himself or herself, take it seriously; call pediatrician urgently			X	X
If your child's personality changes (seems depressed and withdrawn, school performance drops, etc.) get help			X	X
Prevent access to firearms, medications			X	X
Child				
Ask question: Do you ever feel like life is not worth living? Pursue affirmative answers			X	X

Table continued on following page

Table 13–5. AGE-APPROPRIATE ADVICE FOR INJURY PREVENTION *Continued*

Prevention Strategies	Child's Age at Visit			
	6 Y	8 Y	10 Y	12 Y
SPORTS INJURIES				
Parent				
Provide the protective equipment appropriate for any sport your child plays	(X)	X	X	X
Praise your child for progress and emphasize enjoyment, not winning	(X)	X	X	X
Child				
Wear the protective equipment your coach and your parents suggest—in practice as well as in competition	(X)	X	X	X
Wear a helmet for bicycling, skateboarding, batting, horseback riding, ice hockey	X	X	X	X
SUPERVISION				
Parent				
Make arrangements for mature supervision of your child when you are not present, including after school	X	X	X	X
EMERGENCY PROCEDURES				
Parent				
Learn Heimlich maneuver	X	(X)	(X)	(X)
Take a CPR course	X	(X)	(X)	(X)
Have ready access to a phone	X	X	X	X
Know emergency numbers (fire, police, ambulance, poison control); post near phone; teach them to your child	X	(X)	(X)	(X)
Child				
Memorize emergency phone numbers	X	(X)	(X)	(X)
Learn Heimlich maneuver			(X)	X

Strategies include, but are not limited to, those recommended in The Injury Prevention Program safety sheets and *Guidelines for Health Supervision II* of the American Academy of Pediatrics.

(From Wilson, M. [1989]. Preventing injury in the "middle years." *Contemp. Pediatr.* 6:48–51.)

and children to review for prevention of injuries and accidents in school age children.

Injury rates in school age boys are higher than those in girls of the same age. As the child becomes more mobile, the scope of possibilities of injuries increases. This age group tends to have a high incidence of cuts, abrasions, fractures, strains, and sprains.

References

American Academy of Pediatrics (1990). Children, adolescents, and television. *Pediatrics* 85:1119.

Behrman, R., and Vaughan, V. (1987). *Nelson Textbook of Pediatrics*. Philadelphia, W. B. Saunders Company.

McClellan, M. (1984). On their own: Latchkey children. *Pediatr. Nurs.* May–June, p. 198.

Miller, B., and Keane, C. (1987). *Encyclopedia and Dictionary of Medicine, Nursing, and Allied Health*. Philadelphia, W. B. Saunders Company.

Rogers, F., and Head, B. (1983). *Mister Rogers Talks with Parents*. New York, Berkley Books.

Schorr, L. (1983). Environmental deterrents: Poverty, affluence, violence and television. *In* Levine, M., Carey, W., Crocker, A., and Gross, R. (eds.). *Developmental-Behavioral Pediatrics*. Philadelphia, W. B. Saunders Company, pp. 293–311.

Wright, G., and Nader, R. (1983). Schools as milieux. *In* Levine, M., Carey, W., Crocker, A., and Gross, R. (eds.). *Developmental-Behavioral Pediatrics*. Philadelphia, W. B. Saunders Company, pp. 276–283.

Bibliography

Balk, S., and Christoffel, K. (1988). Advising the working mother. *Contemp. Pediatr.* 5:56–85.

Dworkin, P. (1989). Behavior during middle childhood: Developmental themes and clinical issues. *Pediatr. Ann.* 18:347–355.

Foster, R., Hunsberger, M., and Anderson, J. (1989). *Family-Centered Nursing Care of Children*, Philadelphia, W. B. Saunders Company.

Gil, D. (1979). *Child Abuse and Violence*. New York, AMS Press Inc.

Howard, B. (1990). Growing together: Making the grade from 6 to 12. *Contemp. Pediatr.* 7:13–37.

Mott, S., James, S., and Sperhac, A. (1990). *Nursing Care of Children and Families*. Redwood City, Cal, Addison-Wesley.

Rosenberg, L. (1990). Is video game violence harmful to children's health? *Contemp. Pediatr.* 7:80–98.

Sieving, R., and Zirbel-Donisch, S. (1990). Development and enhancement of self-esteem in children. *J. Pediatr. Health Care* 4:290–296.

STUDY QUESTIONS

1. Identify the average range of vital signs for the school age child.
2. Mrs. Thule has two children. Chris, age 6, is a girl and Brandon, age 9, is a boy. Select two games that might be enjoyed by both children and contrast their ability to use these games.
3. Melody, age 6, will be separated from her family for an overnight visit with friends. Suggest two ways in which her family might manage this experience so that it will be less threatening to her.
4. Leroy, age 11, is criticized by his siblings for cheating in a game. How would you advise parents to handle this situation?
5. Spencer, age 10, lied to his parents in regards to his whereabouts after school. Discuss how you would advise his parents to handle this situation.
6. You are working the evening shift and visiting hours are over. When you enter the boys' unit, you find Freddie, age 10, and Don, age 12, engaged in a pillow fight. From your knowledge of this age group, would you consider this unreasonable behavior? How would you deal with this situation?
7. Discuss activities enjoyed by the child of 8. What diversions would you suggest for the long-term patient of this age?
8. Plan a day's menu for the school age child. What foods should be included?
9. Nicole, age 7, is caught stealing change from her mother's purse. Discuss how you would advise parents to handle this situation.
10. Plan an interview with a teacher in an elementary school. Determine what health needs he or she feels are being met and what areas could use improvement. Determine what resources are available in providing age-related health guidance.

CHAPTER 14 _____

Objectives

Upon completion and mastery of Chapter 14, the student will be able to

- Define the vocabulary terms listed.
- List three major and two minor manifestations of rheumatic fever as determined by the modified Jones criteria.
- List the symptoms of appendicitis and discuss what modifications in treatment and postoperative nursing care are necessary if a 9 year old girl suffers a ruptured appendix.
- Devise a nursing care plan for a 12 year old boy with juvenile rheumatoid arthritis, including discharge plans and home teaching.
- Discuss two ways in which the nurse can help an 8 year old girl with a brain tumor adjust to her return to the community.
- Differentiate between Type I and Type II diabetes.
- Outline the educational needs of the diabetic child and the parents in the following areas: nutrition and meal planning, exercise, urine tests, administration of insulin, and skin care.
- Identify the structures involved in Legg-Calvé-Perthes disease.

DISORDERS OF THE SCHOOL AGE CHILD

Terms

Aschoff bodies (380)
DSM-III (412)
fecalith (383)
hirsutism (381)
iridocyclitis (406)
nystagmus (410)
papilledema (410)
Russell traction (402)
Somogyi phenomenon (397)

Children of school age are able to accept hospitalization more readily than the preschool child. They can endure separation from parents if it is not prolonged. Children who have been cherished from birth can tolerate brief interruptions in their lives more easily than those who come from dysfunctional homes. If nurses are to help, they should find out as much about the child as possible. This enables the nurse to individualize the care of the child.

One of the fears these children may have is that their peers will "forget" them while they are away from school. Teachers should be notified if a child will be out of school for any length of time, and classmates are encouraged to send cards, draw pictures, and call and visit if appropriate. The nurse should assist the child in displaying the cards and pictures. Care should be planned around the visit of a friend (Fig. 14–1).

A child this age may also fear bodily harm and loss of control. The child should be prepared for all procedures and allowed to participate in care.

Privacy should be provided. Care should be taken either to include the child in conversations or, if inappropriate, to talk with parents away from the child. The older school age child also may fear death. Opportunities should be provided for verbalization of fears and the acting out through role playing, drawing, dolls, and so on. The child life therapist is consulted when available.

The nurse will come in contact with many school age children who are handicapped and are long-term patients. Unfortunately, some of them come from an unstable home environment, or because of their illness or poor family relationships have been unable to proceed along the lines of healthy emotional development. They need your help. Anyone can care for the cute, cooperative, well-adjusted patient. It takes an *exceptional* nurse to establish good rapport with a sulky, unruly, unhappy child.

> **COMMUNICATION ALERT** ▶ ▶ ▶ ▶ ▶
> Playing a board game with a school age child often facilitates communication with a child who may be uncomfortable talking with an adult. As the two participants become involved in the game, therapeutic conversation can be directed and begin to flow.

At this age, children are trying to establish their own identity. They like to talk with adults and to feel that their opinions are respected and that they are important. Children seldom respond to direct questions from strangers. The new nurse might

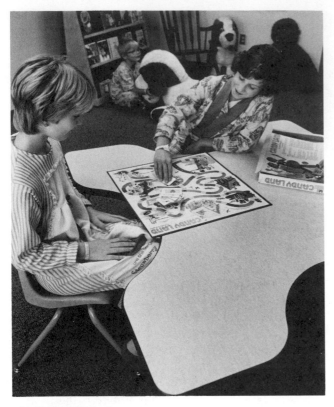

▲ **FIGURE 14–1**

Socializing with peers is an important aspect of hospitalization for the school age child. Furniture, games, and toys need to be appropriate for the child's age. (Courtesy of Raymond Blank Memorial Hospital for Children, Des Moines, Iowa.)

consists of subjective and objective data, problem definition, assessment plan, suggested intervention, and evaluation. Common behavioral problems are addressed by many disciplines in a wide variety of ways. Nurses who work with children should keep abreast of current trends that identify various approaches to discipline. Positive direction and consistency are tools of particular importance in the pediatric nurse.

The education of the school age child must continue throughout any illness. This gives the child a sense of continuity with the outside world, provides periods of socialization, and may reinforce weak academic areas. It involves the parents, who may act as liaisons between school and hospital. The teacher needs to be informed of the child's physical and emotional health in order to deal effectively with the patient. The nurse provides the children with opportunities to study undisturbed so that they will be prepared for their classes. Diagnostic tests and treatments should be scheduled around established school routines whenever possible.

It is common for a school age child to be "brave," showing little, if any, fear in situations that actually may be quite upsetting. Observation of body language may provide some clues to a child's emotional state. The nurse's presence during unfamiliar procedures is comforting. Following the event, encourage the child to draw and to talk

try to establish contact by engaging the patient in a competitive table game (Fig. 14–2).

When student nurses first enter a noisy unit and see school age children bursting with pent-up energies, they may be at a complete loss as to how to proceed in establishing some kind of order. They should reject their first impulses to utilize negative discipline. Instead, they should attempt to foster harmony through mutual cooperation. Knowledge of the processes of growth and development in the school age child will assist in anticipatory guidance. They can also enlist the assistance of parents to determine what, if any, successful approaches they use in guiding the child. For specific patients whose behavior is unacceptable, it would be beneficial to utilize the nursing process to establish a plan of care. This

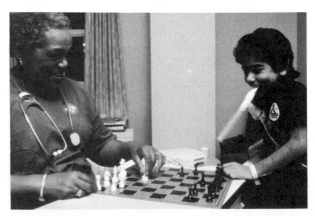

▲ **FIGURE 14–2**

Discussing feelings about having a chronic disease can be difficult for a child. Therapeutic communication often takes place over a board game. (Courtesy of Cook–Fort Worth Children's Medical Center, Fort Worth, Texas.)

about the drawing or to get in touch with feelings through puppet play. The child is given permission to cry and is told when the procedure is going to be uncomfortable. Trust can be built only if the nurse is truthful. The nurse may offer a hand to squeeze, tell a story, count, or use other methods of diversion. The child is praised for cooperative behavior.

NURSING BRIEF ▷ ▷ ▷ ▷ ▷ ▷ ▷ ▷ ▷
Observation of nonverbal cues, such as facial grimaces, squirming about, finger tapping, and so on, is important in determining support for the child.

Circulatory System

RHEUMATIC FEVER

Description. Rheumatic fever is a systemic disease involving the joints, heart, central nervous system, skin, and subcutaneous tissues (Fig. 14–3). It is rare in the first 3 years of life but reaches its peak incidence between the ages of 5 and 15. The first attacks occur most often between 6 and 8 years of age. Rheumatic fever has a high family incidence and is more common worldwide in lower income groups and where overcrowded conditions exist. It is more prevalent in late winter and spring, and carrier rates among school children are believed to be increased during these seasons. Genetic factors also have been implicated.

Rheumatic fever typically follows an upper respiratory infection (tonsillitis, pharyngitis). Throat cultures done at the time of diagnosis of rheumatic fever are not always positive for streptococci. This is because there is a *latent* period of 2 to 5 weeks between the respiratory infection and the onset of rheumatic fever. The body becomes sensitized to the organism after repeated attacks and develops an allergic or autoimmune response to it. Although there has been a decline in the incidence and severity of this disease in recent years, rheumatic fever remains important because it can lead to serious heart damage.

Symptoms. Symptoms range from mild to severe and may not occur for several weeks after a streptococcal infection. The classic symptoms are *polyarthritis* (wandering joint pains), *erythema marginatum*, *Sydenham chorea* (a nervous disorder), and

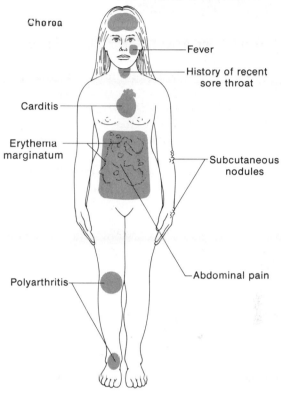

MAJOR MANIFESTATIONS MINOR MANIFESTATIONS AND LATER FINDINGS

Chorea
Fever
History of recent sore throat
Carditis
Erythema marginatum
Subcutaneous nodules
Polyarthritis
Abdominal pain

▲ **FIGURE 14–3**

Manifestations of rheumatic fever. (From Foster, R., Hunsberger, M., and Anderson, J. J. [1989]. *Family-Centered Nursing Care of Children*. Philadelphia, W. B. Saunders Company.)

rheumatic carditis. Subcutaneous nodules appear in a small percentage of patients. They are hard, painless swellings and occur most frequently over bony prominences (scalp, spine, joints). Abdominal pain, often mistaken for appendicitis, sometimes occurs. Fever varies from slight to very high. Pallor, fatigue, anorexia, and unexplained nose bleeds may be seen. Rheumatic fever has a tendency to *recur*, and each attack carries the threat of further damage to the heart. The recurrences are most frequent during the first 5 years following the initial attack and decline rapidly thereafter.

Polyarthritis. The polyarthritis (*poly*, many + *arthr*, joint + *itis*, inflammation of) seen in rheumatic fever is distinctive in that it does not result in permanent deformity to the joint. It involves mainly the larger joints: the knees, elbows, ankles, wrists, and shoulders. The joints become painful, tender, warm, red, and swollen. The symptoms last for a few days, disappear without treatment, and frequently return in another joint. This pattern may continue for a few weeks. The symptoms tend to be more severe in older children. The joint may be visibly swollen and inflamed. Relief is obtained by the administration of salicylates after the diagnosis is confirmed.

Erythema Marginatum. This consists of small red circles and wavy lines on the trunk and extremities that appear and disappear rapidly. The rash may come and go for several months.

Sydenham Chorea (St. Vitus Dance). This is a disorder of the central nervous system characterized by involuntary, purposeless movements of the muscles. It may occur as an acute rheumatic involvement of the brain. Sydenham chorea is seen primarily in prepubertal girls.

Attacks of chorea, which begin slowly, may be preceded by increased tension and behavioral problems. The child may stumble and spill things, and may have difficulty buttoning clothes and writing. When the facial muscles are involved, grimaces occur. The child may laugh and cry inappropriately. In severe cases, the patient may become completely incapacitated, and deterioration in speech may be noticeable. Treatment of Sydenham chorea is directed toward the relief of symptoms by physical and mental rest.

Chorea is self-limited and a full recovery is expected. It can last as little as 2 weeks or more than a year.

Rheumatic Carditis. Inflammation of the heart, a manifestation of rheumatic fever, can be fatal. It occurs more often in the young child. The tissues that cover the heart and the heart valves are affected. The heart muscle—the myocardium—may be involved, as well as the pericardium and endocardium. The *mitral valve*, located between the left atrium and left ventricle, is frequently involved. Vegetations form that interfere with the proper closing of the valve and disturb its normal function. When this valve becomes narrowed, the condition is called *mitral stenosis.* Myocardial lesions called *Aschoff bodies* are also characteristic of the disease. The burden on the heart is great because it has to pump harder to circulate the blood. As a result, it may become enlarged. Symptoms of poor circulation and heart failure may occur.

The patient has an irregular low-grade fever, is pale and listless, and has a poor appetite. Moderate anemia and weight loss are apparent. The child may experience dyspnea upon exertion. The most common heart murmur heard is an apical systolic murmur.

Diagnosis. The diagnosis of rheumatic fever is difficult to make, and for this reason the *Jones criteria* have been developed and modified over the years (Table 14–1). The presence of two major manifestations or of one major and two minor manifestations listed in the criteria, supported by evidence of recent streptococcal infection, indicates a high probability of rheumatic fever. A careful physical examination is done and a complete history of the patient is taken. Certain blood tests are helpful. The erythrocyte sedimentation rate (ESR) is elevated. Abnormal proteins, such as C-reactive protein (CRP) may also be evident in the serum. Leukocytosis may occur but is not regularly present. Antibodies against the streptococci (measured by antistreptolysin-O titer) may also be detected. Additional studies may include chest radiograph, throat culture, and lung tests. The electrocardiogram, a graphic record of the electrical changes caused by the beating of the heart, is very useful. Changes in conductivity, particularly a prolonged P-R interval (first-degree heart block), may indicate carditis. These tests are repeated throughout the course of the disease so that the doctor may determine when the active stage has subsided.

Treatment and Nursing Care

Treatment is aimed at preventing permanent damage to the heart. This is accomplished by antibacterial therapy, physical and mental rest, relief of pain and fever, and management of cardiac failure should it occur. Initial antibacterial therapy is directed toward elimination of the streptococcal infection. Penicillin is the drug of choice unless the patient is sensitive to it; if so, erythromycin is substituted.

Elimination of infection by antibacterial therapy is followed by long-term *chemoprophylaxis* (prevention of disease by drugs). Intramuscular benzathine penicillin G is given monthly to patients with a history of rheumatic fever or evidence of rheumatic heart disease to prevent recurrence.

Table 14–1. CLINICAL AND LABORATORY MANIFESTATIONS OF ACUTE RHEUMATIC FEVER (MODIFIED JONES CRITERIA)

MAJOR MANIFESTATIONS	MINOR MANIFESTATIONS	SUPPORTING EVIDENCE OF STREPTOCOCCAL INFECTION
Carditis	Fever	Recent scarlet fever
Polyarthritis	Arthralgia*	Throat culture positive or group A
Chorea	Previous rheumatic fever or rheumatic	streptococci
Erythema marginatum	heart disease	Increased ASO or other streptococcal
Subcutaneous nodules	Positive acute phase reactants:	antibodies
	Increased erythrocyte sedimentation rate	
	C-reactive protein	
	Leukocytosis	
	Prolonged P-R interval†	

*Should not be counted as a minor manifestation in patients in whom polyarthritis is counted as a major manifestation.
†Should not be counted as a minor manifestation in patients in whom carditis is counted as a major manifestation.
(From Behrman, R., and Vaughan, V. [1987]. *Nelson Texbook of Pediatrics*, 13th ed. Philadelphia, W. B. Saunders Company. Adapted from the recommendations of the Committee of the American Heart Association [*Circulation* 32:664, 1965]. By permission.)

Oral administration is considered for patients with minimal involvement whose reliability about medications can be ascertained. The duration of therapy is from 5 years to the lifetime of the patient. Preparation of the child and family for such long-term compliance is extremely important. Sulfadiazine is recommended for long-term therapy for patients who cannot tolerate penicillin. Financial assistance is available to patients on long-term chemotherapy. Local heart associations and crippled children's services, as well as state and municipal health departments, are among sources of such aid.

Anti-inflammatory drugs are used to decrease fever and pain. Aspirin is the drug of choice for joint disease. The use of steroids is controversial and is reserved for patients with severe carditis and congestive heart failure (CHF). Important concerns during therapy include aspirin toxicity and the effect of aspirin therapy on clotting time. Mild signs of Cushing disease, such as moonface, acne, and hirsutism (increased hairiness), should be anticipated with the use of steroids. More severe reactions such as gastric ulcer, hypertension, overwhelming infection, and psychic disturbances should be guarded against.

Bed Rest. Bed rest during the initial attack is recommended, especially if carditis is present. The amount of work the heart has to do must be limited by resting the entire body. In this way the circulation through the heart is slower and the heart does not have to work as fast or as hard as it does when a patient is active. The nurse must make sure that the physician's orders specifically state any limitations on activity. This issue has added importance now that more patients with rheumatic fever are being treated at home.

A schedule of daily events is reviewed with the child and parents, and the importance of bed rest is discussed frankly. To minimize boredom, parents and siblings might set aside a special time daily to spend with the patient. They should be prepared for periods of withdrawal or rebellion, which is common to all children whose activities are curtailed. In the hospital, the patient may benefit from having a roommate who is similarly confined. Upon recovery, no restrictions on physical activity are usually required except in cases of cardiac enlargement.

Nursing procedures are carried out quickly and skillfully to minimize discomfort. They should be organized to assure as few interruptions as possible to prevent tiring the patient. A bed cradle is used to prevent pressure on painful extremities. The nurse supports the joints with the hands when moving the patient. Care includes special attention to the skin, especially over bony prominences, back care, good oral hygiene, and small, frequent feedings of nourishing foods. Maintenance of healthy teeth and prevention of cavities are of special importance. The patient with rheumatic fever is particularly susceptible to *subacute bacterial endocarditis,* which can occur as a complication of dental or other invasive procedures likely to cause bleeding or infection.

NURSING BRIEF ▷ ▷ ▷ ▷ ▷ ▷ ▷ ▷
Nurses need to become skilled at providing quiet activities for the child who is ill.

Nutrition. During the initial stage of the disease, the child may experience anorexia. Caution parents not to pressure the patient at this time, as it may lead to feeding problems during recovery. Offer small amounts of foods frequently. As the child's appetite improves, encourage nutritive essentials with occasional "special treats." Consider ethnic food preferences. Refrain from overfeeding, which could lead to obesity in patients whose activities are restricted.

Fluid Intake. Keep a record of fluid intake and output. Although dehydration is to be avoided, excessive fluids will tax a congestive heart and lead to fluid retention. Overhydration is termed *hypervolemia* (*hyper,* excessive + *volumen,* volume + *emia,* blood). Monitoring fluids, observing skin turgor, and moisture of mucous membranes will prevent this complication. Assist the child in establishing regular bowel habits to guard against constipation. Vital signs are taken at regular intervals. An apical pulse should always be taken with special regard to any abnormalities, including pulse deficit, along with documentation of the type of activity the child was engaged in at the time the abnormality was observed.

Safety Measures. Special nursing considerations are necessary for the patient suffering from Sydenham chorea. The patient must be protected against injury from spasms and convulsions. Siderails are padded, and mittens and head protection are improvised as needed. A chair restraint may be required. The environment should be free of bright lights and excessive noise. The patient may have to be fed or plastic utensils used. Permitting children to select the menu and the order in which they eat will allow them some feeling of competence at a time when they are otherwise dependent on others. Fingernails are trimmed for protection,

and body temperature is measured rectally. The nurse observes and records any increase or decrease in choreic movements. Sedatives may be required, although in some cases they tend to increase agitation. Children with this condition tend to be moody and require much patience from their caretakers. Choreic movements are aggravated by anxiety; therefore, the nurse should suggest activities that do not require fine motor coordination of the hands, which may cause frustration.

Prevention. The nurse may be involved in the prevention of rheumatic fever through recognition of signs and symptoms of strep infections, screening, and referral for treatment. Any child with symptoms who has been exposed to scarlet fever or another person with a streptococcal infection requires investigation. Examination of family contacts is also important. Once a diagnosis is established, the nurse stresses the importance of completing antibiotic therapy; parents sometimes neglect this once the child's symptoms disappear. Parents should be made to realize that their child may have a relapse if the medication is not given for the full course of treatment. The absence of acute signs and symptoms may inaccurately be associated with the eradication of the organism.

School Work. Provisions must be made for the child to carry out school work as the condition permits. It is the nurse's responsibility to prepare the child for sessions with the teacher. If the patient does not feel well that day, the nurse notifies the team leader. The room is adequately ventilated and lighted. The patient rests for at least a half hour before instruction begins. The bedpan and nourishment are offered. The back rest is elevated, and the over-bed table is cleared and placed at a convenient level. A chair is provided for the teacher. The nurse should place a sign on the door so that no one will interrupt. Since a period of convalescence is needed upon discharge, a tutor will be required unless closed-circuit television or a school-to-home telephone is available.

Emotional Support. All efforts are made to provide emotional support for the child and family. When persons are ill, they tend to intensify the feelings of failure everyone experiences from time to time. They may brood and become obstinate. The child is prohibited from participating in many of the natural activities of childhood; therefore, return to the community may find the patient poorly coordinated and self-conscious. To prevent serious problems from arising, children need to be kept occupied within their capacity. They also need the companionship of friends via mail, telephone, and, when possible, visits. This and a close relationship with the rest of the family will keep the child from feeling left out. The spiritual needs of the patient should not be neglected.

Suggested passive diversions include an aquarium, a mirror hung so that the patient may see the activities in the corridor, plants of various types, stories, and quiet music. As the condition improves, part of the time may be taken up by doing simple self-care tasks. Hobbies such as needlework or stamp collecting are interesting and fun to start. Boys and girls can be encouraged to follow sports or popular series on television; this will help them keep up with peer interests.

Close medical supervision and follow-up care are essential. Persons caring for the long-term patient must try to instill positive attitudes toward overcoming the limitations of the disease and help the patient build feelings of self-confidence rather than dependence. The incidence of this disease appears to be rapidly declining; nevertheless, valvular heart disease is still prevalent in adults. When the disease is diagnosed, it is generally observed in children of the poor.

The prognosis in rheumatic fever is favorable. The immediate outlook is good for recovery without residual heart damage during the acute stage. Death from uncomplicated rheumatic fever is rare. Recurrent infections may cause further damage to the heart, however, and result in chronic disabilities. Recurrences happen frequently in children with rheumatic fever who are not protected by antistreptococcal prophylaxis.

Digestive System

APPENDICITIS

Description. Appendicitis occurs when the opening of the appendix into the cecum becomes obstructed. This may be due to a number of reasons: fecaliths (blockage by fecal matter), infection, or allergy. Diet has also been implicated.

Appendicitis is rare under the age of 2 years, but it is the most common cause of abdominal surgery during childhood. The incidence is higher in boys.

Symptoms. The symptoms in older children are similar to those in adults and include nausea, vomiting, abdominal tenderness, fever, constipation and/or diarrhea, and an elevated blood count. Pain, which is initially about the umbilicus, localizes in the right lower quadrant midway between the umbilicus and the iliac crest (McBurney point). The pain in younger children may not localize. Absent or diminished bowel sounds, rigid abdomen, and rebound tenderness are also indicative of appendicitis. Rebound tenderness in the right lower quadrant (RLQ), while classic for appendicitis, is not reliable in children. Since it can be falsely negative or positive, eliciting it in the child can cause needless pain. Rectal examination will elicit tenderness. Diarrhea may be present in retrocecal appendicitis. A chest film may be ordered to rule out lower lobe pneumonia, which sometimes mimics appendicitis. A careful history and physical examination are paramount. The presence of vomiting and the degree of change in the child's behavior are considered particularly significant. Children will almost always refuse solids and liquids. The child may "guard" the abdomen or voluntarily lie down. One position frequently seen in the child with pain of appendicitis is lying on the side with the knees flexed toward the abdomen.

The symptoms of appendicitis in the *young child* are more obscure. The patient has to be observed carefully over a period of time to determine the diagnosis. The child cries and is restless and runs a low-grade fever. Pain is more generalized and harder to pinpoint, and nausea and vomiting may occur. Since these symptoms are indicative of many childhood upsets, the diagnosis is more difficult to establish than in adolescents or adults.

Treatment

Appendicitis is treated by a surgical operation called an *appendectomy*. Surgery is performed immediately upon diagnosis unless the patient is dehydrated and needs rehydration. Antibiotic therapy is instituted prior to surgery in the patient with a perforated appendix. *Heat is never applied, as it might cause a rupture, leading to the possibility of peritonitis.*

Oral fluids and feedings are withheld pending surgery. As in other emergency situations, emotional support is given by the nurse and the patient's family. Cathartics are withheld when a patient has abdominal pain to prevent rupture of the appendix. The prognosis of uncomplicated appendicitis is good.

Nursing Care

A recovery bed is prepared to receive the child upon return to the unit. The furniture is arranged so that the stretcher can be wheeled easily to the bedside. The bed should be equipped with siderails. An emesis basin and tissues are placed on the bedside table, and an intravenous pole is brought into the room. The patient is transferred gently from the stretcher to the bed. Temperature, pulse, respirations, and blood pressure are taken upon arrival, and the dressing is observed for drainage. If an intravenous line is running, the type, amount, and rate are observed. The nurse records his or her observations, including the time the patient arrived on the unit, the state of consciousness (e.g., alert, groggy), the presence of nausea or vomiting, and the appearance of any drainage. The student nurse reports to the team leader or head nurse to review the postoperative orders left by the physician.

During the course of the day, the following nursing measures are carried out: The patient's position is changed frequently. Teach the patient to take deep breaths and to cough. Wash the patient's hands and face and help with putting on a clean hospital gown. An accurate record of intake and output is kept. The nurse reports the first voiding to the head nurse. If the child has not voided during the shift, the nurse should report this also. The physician's orders will indicate whether or not the child with nausea can have sips of water or ice chips.

As soon as the child is able to take and retain water and other fluids by mouth, intravenous feedings are discontinued. Vital signs and bowel sounds are monitored as ordered or according to institution policies. The patient is encouraged to move about in bed; reluctance to move and an-

orexia may be early signs of complications. Evidence of pain is reported and analgesics are administered as ordered.

Pediatric patients recuperate quickly from uncomplicated surgery. Ambulation is generally not a problem. Children usually can return to school in 1 or 2 weeks, but specific instructions concerning restriction of activity should be reviewed before hospital discharge.

COMMUNICATION ALERT ▶ ▶ ▶ ▶ ▶
The nurse can communicate to the school age child the need to hold still during a procedure by saying, "You can help by holding your arm still. I will help you by putting my hand on your arm." After the procedure the child should be praised for cooperation, "You were great. We could not have started that IV without your help."

Ruptured Appendix. Early recognition of appendicitis decreases the danger of perforation. Because diagnosis is difficult in children, the nurse may come in contact with more patients with a ruptured appendix on the pediatric unit than on adult divisions. In addition, the body systems of a child are less mature; thus, the progression of the condition is rapid. Parents may also be confused by the symptoms and hesitate to obtain medical attention. If the appendix ruptures, the infected contents spill into the abdominal cavity and a generalized infection called *peritonitis* results. This is often seen in younger children. Progression is rapid because the child's omentum is smaller and less effective in localizing the infection. In the older child a walled-off abscess may occur. Accessory organs of the digestive tract and the reproductive organs may also become infected. The child is acutely ill and the recovery period prolonged. After the appendix ruptures, the abdomen rapidly becomes rigid.

Preoperative Care. Medical management to prevent shock, dehydration, and infection is instigated. This usually includes intravenous administration of fluids and electrolytes, systemic antibiotics, nasogastric suctioning, and positioning in low Fowler position or the right side to facilitate drainage into the pelvic area. The patient is given nothing by mouth. Intermittent suction is maintained at appropriate negative pressure, and irrigations are carried out as ordered to ensure patency of the nasogastric tube. When a perforated appendix is suspected, triple antibiotic therapy of gentamicin, ampicillin, and clindamycin or cefoxitin may be ordered (Behrman and Vaughan, 1987).

Postoperative Care. Penrose drains are placed in the incision to drain exudate or abscess. Some surgeons prefer to leave the incision open and packed with Betadine or saline gauze. The nurse may do a wet-to-dry dressing change several times a day in which she removes the contaminated dressing and repacks the wound. Wound precautions are instigated according to hospital procedure. The area is kept clean and dry, and medication is applied if ordered. Administer analgesics for pain relief. Monitor intake, output, and bowel sounds. Supply nutritious foods as the diet is increased. Administer nursing care as described for the child with simple appendicitis, including appropriate modifications and interventions in nursing care plans. The child should be placed in semi-Fowler position to prevent spread of the infection. The child's hospital stay is increased, and intravenous antibiotic therapy is given.

The Skin

PEDICULOSIS

The infestation of humans by lice is termed pediculosis. There are three types: pediculosis capitis—head lice; pediculosis corporis—body lice; and pediculosis pubis—crab or pubic lice. The various types usually remain in the part of the body designated by their name. They are transmitted from person to person or from contaminated articles. Their survival is dependent on the blood they extract from the infected person. Severe itching in the affected area is the main symptom. Treatment in all cases is aimed at ridding the patient of the parasite, treating the excoriated skin, and preventing the infestation of others. The most common form seen in children is head lice. The child or parents may be embarrassed by the presence of lice, but infestations spread quickly in schools and do not reflect on hygiene of the families.

PEDICULOSIS CAPITIS

Description. *Head lice* affect the scalp and hair. The eggs, called nits, attach to the hair, become numerous, and hatch within 3 or 4 days. Head lice are more common in girls than in boys because of hair length. The parasite may be acquired from hats, combs, or hairbrushes. It is easily transferred from one child to another and is seen most frequently in the school age child and in preschool children who attend day care centers.

Symptoms. The child suffers from severe itching of the scalp. Scratching of the head can cause further irritation. The hair may become matted. Occasionally pustules and excoriations are seen about the face. Nurses admitting patients to pediatric units should be on the alert for head lice. In particular, inspect the hairline at the back of the neck and about the ears. Crusts, pediculi, nits, and dirt may cause matting of the hair and a foul odor.

Treatment and Nursing Care

Management is directed toward killing the lice, getting rid of the nits, and treating any infections of the face and scalp. Family members and playmates of the child should be examined and treated as necessary. Prescription shampoos such as pyrethrin are commonly used. Kwell has also been used; however, it has more reported side effects (consult circular). Nonprescription remedies (RID, NIX) are also available. Follow the manufacturer's directions carefully. Watch for an allergic response, particularly in children with a history of skin problems. If the eyebrows and eyelashes are involved, a thick coating of petrolatum (Vaseline) is applied, followed by removal of remaining nits. Nits on the head are removed by combing the hair with a fine-tooth comb dipped in hot vinegar. Be careful not to burn the child. The hair is then washed.

Charting includes date, time, condition of scalp and hair prior to treatment, odor (if noticeable), type of shampoo used, how the patient tolerated the procedure, and the amount of relief obtained. Any signs of systemic infection are also documented.

Clothing or bedding is laundered in hot water and dried for 20 minutes or aired in sunlight. Mattresses may be sprayed with a disinfectant. Wool clothing requires dry cleaning. Children should be cautioned against swapping caps, headscarfs, and combs. Parents are instructed to inspect the child's head regularly. Encourage parents to report infestations to the school nurse, as widespread outbreaks are encountered periodically.

The cutting of the child's hair is discouraged because it can be a source of stress to the child who is already being singled out as "the child with lice." Oral Benadryl may be given for the pruritus. Parents should be cautioned to watch for symptoms of secondary infection caused by breaks in the skin from scratching.

Endocrine System

DIABETES MELLITUS (TYPE I)

Description. Diabetes is a chronic metabolic condition in which the body is unable to utilize carbohydrates properly owing to a deficiency of insulin, an internal secretion of the pancreas. Insulin deficiency leads to impairment of glucose transport (sugar cannot pass into the cells) (Fig. 14–4). The body is also unable to store and utilize fats properly. There is a decrease in protein synthesis. When the blood glucose level becomes dangerously high, glucose spills into the urine and diuresis occurs. Incomplete fat metabolism produces ketone bodies that accumulate in the blood. Untreated diabetes can lead to coma and death.

Type I diabetes is the most common endocrine/metabolic disorder of childhood. It is found worldwide, affects every organ of the body, and is unique in that it requires a great deal of self-management by the person affected (Fig. 14–5). Patient education and compliance are extremely important. Morbidity and mortality are associated with chronic complications that affect small and large blood vessels, resulting in retinopathy, nephropathy, neuropathy, ischemic heart disease, and obstruction of large vessels.

Classification. It is now clear that diabetes is not a single entity but rather a syndrome. To help eliminate confusion in terminology, the National Institutes of Health appointed an international committee, the National Diabetes Data Group, to classify the carbohydrate intolerance syndromes (Table 14–2). As more is learned, no doubt further refinements will be necessary. Three of the categories pertinent to this discussion of pediatric diabetes are:

Type I, Insulin-Dependent Diabetes Mellitus (IDDM). This was formerly termed juvenile-onset

Table 14–2. CLINICAL FEATURES OF DIABETES

FEATURES	TYPE I (IDDM)	TYPE II (NIDDM)
Onset	Abrupt, frequently can date week of onset	Insidious, often found by screening tests
Body size	Normal or thin	Frequently obese
Blood sugar	Fluctuates widely with exercise and infection	Fluctuations are less marked
Ketoacidosis	Common	Infrequent
Sulfonylurea-responsive	Rare, except in "honeymoon" phase	Greater than 50%
Insulin required	Almost all	Less than 25%
Insulin dosage	Increases until total diabetes	May remain stable

(Adapted from Smith, D., and Marshall R. [1972]. *Introduction to Clinical Pediatrics.* Philadelphia, W. B. Saunders Company.)

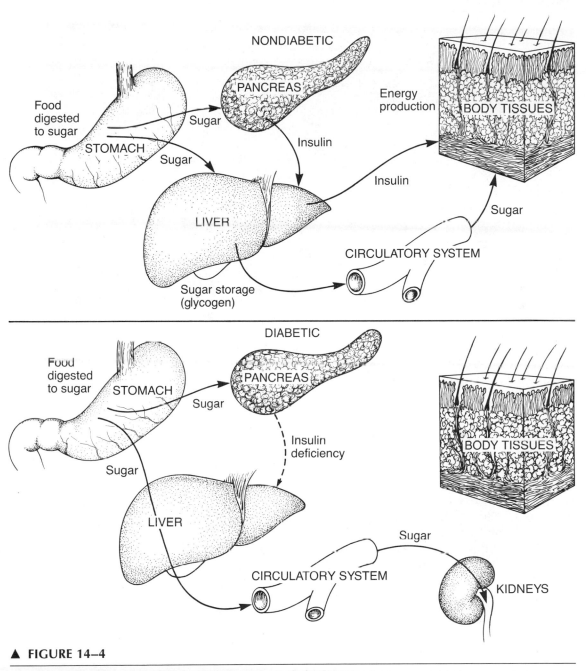

▲ **FIGURE 14–4**

Physiology of sugar utilization in diabetic and nondiabetic persons.

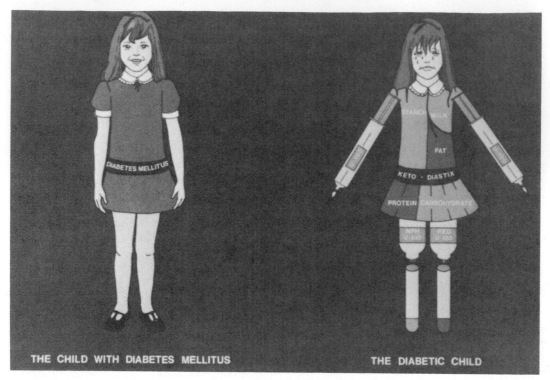

THE CHILD WITH DIABETES MELLITUS

THE DIABETIC CHILD

▲ FIGURE 14–5

This illustration, which Dr. L. B. Travis originally designed in 1968, is relevant today. The child with diabetes *(left)* represents how we wish such persons to be and to view themselves. But when professionals use the adjective "diabetic" to describe such persons, there is small wonder that many children see themselves as a composite of what they feel is the disease itself. (From Travis, L. B., Brouhard, B., and Schreiner, B. [1987]. *Diabetes in Children and Adolescents.* Philadelphia, W. B. Saunders Company.)

diabetes or brittle diabetes. It is characterized by partial or complete insulin deficiency. Childhood diabetes is usually of this type. Although there may be some insulin production during certain phases of the disease, patients eventually become insulin-deficient. They are prone to ketosis. Environmental as well as genetic factors are strongly implicated. Apparently, IDDM is sometimes set off by seemingly harmless viruses believed to provoke the immune system into mistakenly destroying its own islets. The presence of islet cell antibodies and reports associating IDDM with juvenile rheumatoid arthritis appear to support an autoimmune etiology. Mumps, congenital rubella, and Coxsackie B4 virus have also been implicated.

Type II, Non-Insulin–Dependent Diabetes Mellitus (NIDDM). This was formerly called adult-onset diabetes and is rare in the pediatric popu-

lation. These persons are not usually dependent on insulin and rarely develop ketosis. Although NIDDM may occur at any age, it generally develops after the age of 40 years.

Incidence. The exact incidence of Type I diabetes is unknown. In the United States, surveys indicate the prevalence to be about 1.9 per 1000 in school age children. The frequency increases with age. One of four families has a history of diabetes. Symptoms of IDDM may occur at any time in childhood, but the rate of occurrence of new cases is highest among 5 to 7 year old children and pubescents from 11 to 13 years of age. In the former, the stress of school and the increased exposure to infectious diseases may be responsible. The incidence increases following the viral illness seasons. During puberty, increased growth, increased emotional stress, and the insulin antagonism of sex hormones may be implicated. The sexual incidence of diabetes is equal. Socioeconomic correlations have not been seen. The disease is more severe in childhood because the patients are growing, they expend a great deal of energy, their nutritional needs vary, and they have to face a lifetime of diabetic management. Children with IDDM often do not present the typical textbook picture of the disorder; therefore, the nurse must be particularly astute in subjective and objective observations.

Symptoms. Children with diabetes present a classic triad of symptoms: polyuria, polydipsia, and polyphagia. The symptoms appear more rapidly in children. The patient complains of excessive thirst (polydipsia), excretes frequent large amounts of urine (polyuria), and is constantly hungry (polyphagia). An insidious onset with fatigue, nausea, lethargy, weakness, and weight loss is also quite common. Anorexia may be seen. The child who is toilet trained may begin wetting the bed or have frequent "accidents" during play periods, may lose weight, and is irritable. The skin becomes dry. Vaginal yeast infections may be seen in the adolescent girl. Abdominal cramps are common. There may be a history of recurrent infections. The symptoms may go unrecognized until an infection becomes apparent or coma results.

Laboratory findings indicate glucose in the urine (glycosuria or glucosuria). Hyperglycemia (*hyper*, above + *gly*, sugar + *emia*, blood) is also apparent.

Diagnosis. Diagnosis of diabetes mellitus should be considered in children who have a history suggestive of the disease (polyuria, polydipsia, polyphagia, weight loss), a transient or persistent glycosuria, or clinical manifestations of metabolic acidosis with or without stupor or coma (Behrman and Vaughan, 1987).

In addition to the history, several diagnostic blood tests may be ordered. A fasting blood glucose level greater than 140 mg/dl on at least two occasions and a blood glucose concentration greater than 200 mg/dl are positive signs. In most cases the diagnosis is not difficult.

> **COMMUNICATION ALERT ► ► ► ► ►**
> When parents dominate a conversation and the child is not given an opportunity to answer a question, the nurse directs the conversation to the child. For example, during an admission interview of a child admitted for diabetic ketoacidosis, the nurse says "Vin, can you tell me what happened yesterday before your mother found you in your bedroom?"

Diabetic Ketoacidosis (DKA). Diabetic ketoacidosis is also referred to as *diabetic coma*, although a person may have diabetic ketoacidosis with or without being in a coma. It may result if a diabetic patient contracts a secondary infection and does not take care of the self, or, as occurs fairly often in diabetic children, the disease proceeds unrecognized until coma occurs (Fig. 14–6). Even minor infections such as a cold increase the severity of diabetes. This occurs because infections may increase the metabolic rate, thus changing insulin demands. DKA may also occur in the child who has omitted the insulin dose, sometimes deliberately, or is under emotional stress. The symptoms range from mild to severe, and occur in hours to days. The skin is dry and the face flushed. Patients appear dehydrated. They are thirsty but may vomit if fluids are offered. They perspire and are restless. There may be generalized pain in the abdomen and throughout the body. A character-

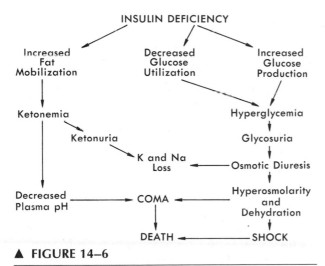

▲ **FIGURE 14–6**

The pathogenesis of diabetic ketoacidosis. (From Sodeman, W., and Sodeman, T. [1979]. *Sodeman's Pathologic Physiology: Mechanisms of Disease*, 6th ed. Philadelphia, W. B. Saunders Company.)

istic *fruity odor* of the breath is apparent because the patient expels acetone from the respiratory tree, and the lips are cherry-red. As the condition becomes worse, the patient becomes weak and drowsy. Breathing patterns are peculiar in that there is no normal period of rest between inspiration and expiration; this is termed *Kussmaul* breathing. The patient becomes unconscious. Death will result unless insulin, fluids, and electrolytes are administered.

The correction of depleted fluids, frequent checking of vital signs, hourly urine tests, blood chemistry measurements, and close observation of consciousness are necessary. Baseline studies include venous blood glucose, serum acetone, pH, total carbon dioxide (TCO_2), blood urea nitrogen (BUN), electrolytes, calcium, phosphate, white blood cell count (WBC), urinalysis, and appropriate cultures. Glucose levels in the blood and urine, electrolytes, and any other abnormal laboratory values are continuously monitored until the child stabilizes. Low doses of regular insulin, IV, SC, or IM, are administered, and the patient is observed. A cardiac monitor is helpful in determining changes in potassium levels. If the patient has an infection, this is treated. Cerebral edema, although rare, can be life-threatening. A diabetic flow chart at the bedside registers all pertinent information. Response to treatment is gradual, occurring over a period of hours.

Treatment and Nursing Care

The aims of treatment in juvenile diabetes are (1) to assure normal growth and development, through metabolic control, (2) to enable the child to have a happy and active childhood, and (3) to prevent complications (Table 14–3). Teaching ideally begins when the diagnosis has been confirmed. A planned educational program is necessary to provide a consistent body of information, which can then be individualized. The patient's age and financial, educational, cultural, and religious background must be considered. Many hospitals hold group clinics for diabetic patients and their relatives. These sessions are conducted by various professionals such as the physician, dietitian, and nurse. Patients who are living with the disease provide encouragement and help by shar-

Table 14–3. OVERALL GOALS OF MANAGEMENT

I. "Control" of Carbohydrate Metabolism, to Maximum Degree Possible
  A. Good health
     Freedom from most symptoms
     Feels and looks as good as most nondiabetic peers
  B. Normal functional capacity
     Able to compete on functional level with peers
     Normal school or work attendance
  C. Regulation of biochemical markers
     Blood (or urine) sugars as near nondiabetic as possible
     Blood glucose values 80 to 150 on >75% of checks
     Glycosylated hemoglobins as near nondiabetic as possible
     Lipid profile normal
  D. Adaptive coping pattern that is successful

II. Normal Growth, Development, Maturation
  A. Optimum statural growth
     Normal linear growth
     Normal height/weight ratio
     Normal physical potential
  B. Optimum psychosocial development
     Achieve intellectual and behavioral potential
     Attain maturity of mind and thought
     Preparation for "leaving home"

III. Prevention of Significant Acute Complications

IV. Delay or Prevention of Chronic Complications
  A. Microvascular disease
  B. Neuropathy
  C. Hyperlipidemia
  D. Macrovascular disease

(From Travis, L., Brouhard, B., and Schreiner, B. [1987]. *Diabetes in Children and Adolescents.* Philadelphia, W. B. Saunders Company.)

ing concerns. Health professionals become directly involved with the patient's progress and can offer necessary feedback and support. Continuous follow-up is extremely important.

Because diabetic children are growing, additional dimensions of the disorder and its treatment become evident. Growth is not steady but occurs in spurts and plateaus that have a bearing on treatment. Infants and toddlers may have hydration problems, especially during illness. Preschool children have irregular activity and eating patterns. School age children may grieve over the diagnosis and question "Why me?" They may use the illness to gain attention or to avoid responsibilities. The onset of puberty may require adjustments in insulin as a result of growth and the antagonistic effect of the sex hormones on insulin. Adolescents often resent this condition, which deviates from their conception of the "body ideal." They have more difficulty in resolving the conflict between dependence and independence. This may lead to rebellion against the parents and also the treatment regimen.

The impact of the disease on the rest of the family must also be considered. One mother commented, "I was so scared. I felt very strongly that whether my child lived or died depended on me. It was overwhelming. I couldn't allow myself mistakes. This was reinforced by all the do's and dont's of the instructions." Parents may also feel guilty for having passed on the disease. Siblings may feel jealous of the patient. The sharing of responsibility by parents is ideal but is not necessarily a reality. Everyone may have difficulty accepting the diagnosis and the more regimented lifestyle it imposes. Each family member must cope with a personal reaction to the stress of the illness.

It is important that the child assume responsibility for her or his care gradually and with a minimum of pressure. Overprotection can be as detrimental as neglect. Parents who have received satisfaction from their child's dependence on them may need help "letting go." Diabetic camp experience is helpful in this respect.

The nursing management of juvenile diabetes requires knowledge of pathophysiology, blood glucose self-monitoring, nutritional management, insulin management, insulin shock, exercise, skin and foot care, infections, effects of emotional upsets, and long-term care.

Pathophysiology of Juvenile Diabetes. The patient and the family are instructed about the location of the pancreas and its normal function. The nurse explains the relationship of insulin to the pancreas, differentiating between Type I and Type II diabetes. All information is given gradually and at the level of understanding of the child and the family. Audiovisual aids and pamphlets are incorporated into the session. Most newly diagnosed diabetic patients are hospitalized for varying periods of time for intense instruction.

Blood Glucose Self-Monitoring. Blood glucose self-monitoring has dramatically changed the approach to diabetes. Previously, blood tests for glucose could only be carried out in a doctor's office or laboratory. The patient had to rely on urine tests, which often presented a confusing picture, particularly when the urine had been in the bladder for several hours (glucose might turn up in the urine when the diabetic's blood sugar level was actually low). Only a blood check can show the actual amount of sugar in the blood at the time of the test. Technology has made it possible for patients to test their own blood sugar in the home. While still under the supervision and consultation of the physician, the patient can nonetheless make rational changes in insulin dosage, nutritional requirements, and daily exercise. This is of great psychological value to the child, teenager, and/or parents, as it reduces feelings of helplessness and complete dependence on medical personnel. Home glucose monitoring should be taught to all young patients and/or their caretakers (Fig. 14–7). It is important that the patient not only be skilled in the techniques but understand the results and how to incorporate them into the

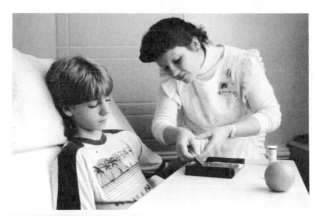

▲ **FIGURE 14–7**

The school age child can be taught home glucose monitoring, and also the meaning of the results and how it affects care. (Courtesy of Cook–Fort Worth Children's Medical Center, Fort Worth, Texas.)

daily regimen. This means involvement of the entire health-care team in ongoing supervision, demonstrations, and support. Although instructions come with the various products, it is highly recommended that patients receive individual training.

Obtaining blood specimens has been simplified by the use of capillary blood-letting devices such as the Autolet. This device automatically controls the depth of penetration of the lancet into the skin. Other brands include the Hamalet, Autoclix, and Monojector. The sides of the fingertips are recommended, as there are fewer nerve endings and more capillary beds in these areas. The best fingers to use are the middle, ring, or little finger on either hand. If the child washes hands in warm water for about 30 seconds, the finger will bleed easier. To perform the test a drop of blood is put on a chemically treated reagent strip (Chemstrip bG or Dextrostix). Meters are available for reading blood sugar determinations. The test strip with a drop of blood is inserted and the reading appears.

Cost, convenience, and lability of the disease are factors to consider when selecting devices. Most products can be obtained at the local pharmacy. Newer and more precise instruments are being developed constantly. Frequency of use is determined by the physician.

Nutritional Management. The triad of management of Type I diabetes includes a well-balanced diet, insulin, and regular exercise. The importance of glycemic control (tight blood sugars) in decreasing the incidence of symptoms and complications of the disease has been established. The advent of blood glucose self-monitoring is affecting food intake, in that diets can be fine tuned and more flexible, and yet the cornerstone of *consistency* (amount of food and time of feeding) remains. Contrary to popular belief, there is no scientific evidence that persons with diabetes require special foods. In fact, if it is good for the diabetic, it is good for the entire family. The nutrient needs of diabetic children are essentially no different from those of nondiabetic children with the exception of elimination of concentrated carbohydrates (simple sugars). These cause a marked increase in blood sugar and generally should be avoided.

The goals of nutritional management in children are to ensure normal growth and development, to distribute food intake so that it aids metabolic control, and to individualize the diet in accordance with the child's ethnic background, age, sex, weight, activity, family economics, and food preferences. Once a diet order is received from the physician, the dietitian calculates the distribution of carbohydrates, protein, and fat. Portion size is demonstrated by the use of food models and measuring cups and spoons. Regularly spaced meals and snacks are emphasized, and the family is taught how to read labels and the differences between carbohydrates, protein, and fat. The dietitian also explains the use of exchange lists.

Education of the patient is an ongoing process. Too much information given at one time may appear overwhelming to parents and discouraging to the child. Well-informed nurses can do much in the way of reinforcement and support. They can clarify such terms as dietetic, sugar-free, juice-packed, water-packed, unsweetened. Meal trays in the hospital provide an excellent opportunity for teaching. Children should bring their lunch to school. Teenagers need to be advised that alcohol will lower the blood sugar. It suppresses gluconeogenesis and is high in calories. Most cocktail mixes contain sugar; however, water, sugar-free pop, club soda, and tomato juice do not. Although the consumption of alcohol is to be discouraged, if the young person wishes to drink it is wise to drink after dinner or to consume the beverage with some type of food.

The Constant Carbohydrate Diet (CCHO Diet). The constant carbohydrate diet is a fairly new approach to meal planning. The goal is to maintain a consistent amount of carbohydrate at each meal and snack. Regularity of meals is stressed. The amount of carbohydrate may, and usually does, vary between meals. The initial carbohydrate pattern is determined by the individual's current food intake. To calculate the number of grams of carbohydrate in food, exchange lists that divide foods into six categories are used. This food plan appeals to young diabetics because of its ease in use and flexibility.

Fiber. The importance of fiber in diets is well documented. In the diabetic patient, fiber has been shown to reduce blood sugar levels, lower serum cholesterol values, and sometimes reduce insulin requirements (Cleland, 1983). Fiber appears to slow the rate of absorption of sugar by the digestive tract. Raw fruits and vegetables and whole grain breads and cereals are good sources of fiber.

Cholesterol, Artificial Sweeteners. As persons

with diabetes have an increased risk for heart disease, the reduction of serum cholesterol is another concern. These persons (like most of the general public) need to reduce their intake of animal fats or substitute vegetable fat for animal fat. The use of polyunsaturated fats in cooking is advised. The form of the food is also important. An apple, apple juice, or applesauce may precipitate different blood sugar responses. Portions, the type of processing, cooking, and combinations of foods have also been shown to have a bearing on these responses.

Aspartame (Nutra-Sweet) was approved by the Food and Drug Administration (FDA) in 1981. It is used in items that do not require cooking. Aspartame is made of two amino acids. Both contain insignificant amounts of carbohydrate. One granulation form is called Equal. Sorbitol, mannitol, and xylitol are sugars commonly found in foods called "sugar-free." These substances are absorbed more slowly into the blood stream. They are carbohydrates and must be calculated in the food plan.

Role of the Nurse. The student nurse has a number of responsibilities as a member of the team concerned with the patient and food management. This begins by preparing the child for meals. Blood glucose is usually checked before meals and at bedtime when the child receives a snack. The child's face and hands are washed, and distracting toys are removed for the time being. The child is served the meal tray in the crib on a bedtable or at the regular table suited to size. Small children require bibs. The tray is served *on time*. Patients who receive regular insulin before meals may have an insulin reaction if food is not taken within 20 minutes. If nurses are scheduled for lunch when diet meals are served, they should notify the team leader and should not assume that others will feed the child. No foods or liquids, with the exception of water, are given between meals unless authorized by the physician or dietitian. Be sure that the tray is served to the *right patient*. A mistake can occur, particularly if several children are on special diets. This can happen more easily on the pediatric unit where patients roam about freely. Food should be cut into small pieces. Toast or muffins are buttered, and eggs are removed from their shells. A child who is able to eat alone is encouraged to do so. The nurse uses powers of observation to determine when

help is needed. Foods the child especially enjoys or dislikes are noted.

When the child has finished, the tray is removed. The nurse observes the types and amounts of foods that the patient refused, charts them in the nurses' notes, and also informs the nurse in charge. These are brought to the attention of the dietitian, who determines the number of calories that need to be made up and orders a between-meal snack such as orange juice to compensate. Anorexia or vomiting is reported promptly. After the meal, the nurse washes the child's hands and face, straightens the crib, and returns the toys.

Insulin Management. Insulin is used principally as a specific drug for the control of diabetes mellitus. It is a specially prepared extract obtained from the pancreas of cattle or pigs. When injected into the diabetic patient, it enables the body to burn and store sugar.

Current data emphasize the importance of blood sugar control in the prevention of microvascular disease. Insulin pumps are being used in carefully selected children. More highly purified insulins are being developed to reduce complications. *Human insulin*, produced biosynthetically in bacteria using recombinant DNA technology, is now available and widely used. One example is Humulin, manufactured by the Eli Lilly Company. Human insulin is used most frequently and is associated with a lesser incidence of allergies.

The dosage of insulin is measured in units, and special syringes are used in its administration. U-100 (100-unit) insulin is the standard form. Each marking on the 1-ml (100-unit) syringes represents *two* units of insulin. The 50-unit disposable syringe is intended for small doses. All vials of U-100 insulin have color-coded orange caps, and all labels bear black print on a white background. Bold letters indicate type: "R" for regular, "P" for PZI, "N" for NPH, "L" for lente, "U" for ultralente, and "S" for semilente. Table 14–4 presents the usual insulin programs.

Insulin is administered *subcutaneously*. Parents and children must be taught why it is necessary to take the hormone and how to administer it by injection. A child can generally be taught to give self-injections after the age of 7. The earlier this is learned, the better. Proper instruction of the patient is one of the most important aspects of the treatment of diabetes. The doctor prescribes the type and amount of insulin and specifies the time

Table 14–4. INSULIN PROGRAMS IN COMMON USE

I. One injection per day (usually in A.M. before breakfast)
  A. Intermediate-acting insulin *alone*
  B. Intermediate-acting and regular insulin *together*
  C. Long-acting, intermediate-acting, and regular insulin *together*
II. Two injections per day
  A. Intermediate-acting insulin before breakfast and supper
  B. Addition of regular insulin to one or both of IIA
  C. IC plus intermediate-acting insulin at bedtime
III. Three (or more) injections per day
  A. Long-acting insulin in A.M.; regular before meals
  B. Long-acting insulin before breakfast and supper; regular before meals
  C. Intermediate and regular insulin before breakfast; regular before supper; intermediate before bedtime
  D. Regular insulin before meals; intermediate-acting before bedtime
  E. Long-acting insulin at bedtime; regular before meals
IV. Continuous subcutaneous insulin infusion (CSII) Various methods

(From Travis, L., Brouhard, B., and Schreiner, B. [1987]. *Diabetes in Children and Adolescents.* Philadelphia, W. B. Saunders Company.)

of administration. The site of the injection is rotated to prevent poor absorption and injury to tissues (Fig. 14–8). Injection model forms made from construction paper and site rotation patterns are useful. One suggested site rotation is to use one area for a week. Move to a different site within that area for each injection. Each injection should be about 1 inch apart. The young child can use a doll for practice. Parents usually find the experience of injecting their own child difficult. One mother stated that for the first few months she gave the injection in the child's hips so that her daughter could not see the expression on her face.

Allergic responses to insulin can be divided into those that occur locally at the injection site, the rare systemic sensitivity (true insulin allergy), and immunological reactions. Lipoatrophy (*lipo*, fat + *atrophy*, loss of) and lipohypertrophy (*lipo*, fat + *hypertrophy*, increase of) refer to changes in the subcutaneous tissue at the injection site. Proper rotation of sites and the availability of the newer purified insulins have helped eliminate these conditions. The child is taught to "feel for lumps" every week and to avoid using any sites that are suspicious. The nurse should ascertain what brand of insulin the patient is using. In general, it is not wise to switch brands of insulin (e.g., Eli Lilly, Squibb), because they may be made slightly differently. Questions should be directed to the hospital pharmacist. It is no longer necessary to refrigerate insulin in order to prevent deterioration. Avoid extremes in temperature and check expiration dates.

The various types of insulin and their action are listed in Table 14–5. The main difference is in the amount of time required for effect and the length of protection given. One must bear in mind that the values listed in Table 14–5 serve only as guidelines and that the response of each diabetic to any given insulin dose is highly individual and depends on many factors, such as site of injection, local destruction of insulin by tissue enzymes, and insulin antibodies. Regular or crystalline insulin is a purified form of regular insulin and is less likely to cause allergic reactions. Both NPH, an intermediate type, and PZI, a long-lasting insulin, have had small amounts of chemicals added to prolong their action and to make them more stable. They offer protection over a period of hours, enabling the patient to do without repeated injections of unmodified insulin. They are cloudy and require mixing before being withdrawn from the vials (Fig. 14–9). This is done by rolling the bottle gently between the palms of the hands. Insulin is not used if it is discolored.

Frequently the doctor will order a combination of a short-acting insulin and an intermediate-acting one; e.g., "Give 10 units of NPH insulin and 5 units of regular insulin at 7:30 A.M." This offers the patient immediate and longer-lasting protection. A two-dose schedule has also been used with success (Fig. 14–10). NPH or lente insulin may be given in the same syringe as regular or crystalline insulin. Long-acting types of insulin are seldom

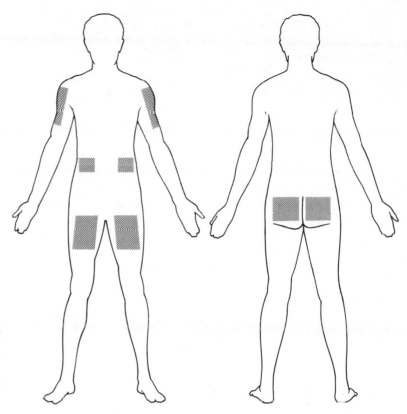

▲ FIGURE 14–8

Sites of injection of insulin. The site of injection should be changed daily to prevent poor absorption and injury to tissues. Rotation occurs both within and among body areas.

Table 14–5. CHARACTERISTICS OF UNITED STATES INSULIN PREPARATIONS

| CLASS/NAME | MANUFACTURER* | SPECIES† | APPROX. ACTION CURVES (hrs) | | |
			Onset	*Peak*	*Duration*
Rapid-acting					
Regular	L, S/N	B, P, B-P, H	0.5	2–4	4–6
Velosulin	Nd	P	0.5	1–3	4–8
Semilente	L, S/N	B, B-P	0.5–1.0	5–10	4–10
Biphasic					
Mixtard	Nd	P	0.5–1.0	3–4/4–8	16–24
Intermediate-acting					
NPH	L, S/N	B, P, B-P, H	1.5–2	6–12	16–24
Lente	L, S/N	B, P, B-P, H	1.5–2	6–12	16–24
Insulatard	Nd	P	1.5–2	4–12	16–24
Long-acting					
PZI	L	B, P, B-P	4–8	14–24	36+
Ultralente	L, S/N	B, B-P	4–8	18–24	36+

*L = Lilly Laboratories, S/N = Squibb-Novo, Nd = Nordisk-USA.
†B = beef, P = pork, B-P = beef-pork, H = human.
(From Travis, L., Brouhard, B., and Schreiner, B. [1987]. *Diabetes in Children and Adolescents.* Philadelphia, W. B. Saunders Company.)

1. Wash hands.
2. Gently rotate intermediate insulin bottle.
3. Wipe off tops of insulin vials with alcohol sponge.
4. Draw back amount of air into the syringe that equals total dose.

5. Inject air equal to NPH dose into NPH vial. Remove syringe from vial.

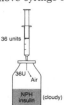

6. Inject air equal to regular dose into regular vial.

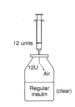

7. Invert regular insulin bottle and withdraw regular insulin dose.

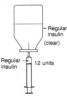

8. Without adding more air to NPH vial, carefully withdraw NPH dose.

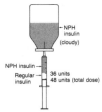

▲ FIGURE 14–9

Mixing insulin. This step-order process avoids the problem of contaminating the regular insulin with the intermediate insulin. If contamination of the regular insulin does occur, the rapid-acting effect of this drug would be dampened, and it would be unreliable as a quick-acting insulin in an acute situation such as diabetic ketoacidosis. (From Price, M. [1983]. *Nurs. Clin. North Am.,* Dec., 1983, p. 692.)

given to children because of the danger of hypoglycemia during sleep. Stable premixed insulins are now being introduced by some manufacturers.

Insulin Shock. Insulin shock, also known as *hypoglycemia* (*hypo*, below + *glyco*, sugar + *emia*, blood) occurs when the blood sugar level becomes abnormally low. This condition is caused by too much insulin. Factors that may account for this imbalance include poorly planned exercise, reduction of diet, improvement of the condition so that the patient requires less insulin, and errors made because of improper knowledge of insulin and the insulin syringe.

Children are *more prone* to insulin reactions than adults because (1) the condition itself is more unstable in young people, (2) they are growing, and (3) their activities are more irregular. *Poorly planned exercise* is frequently the cause of insulin shock during childhood. Hospitalized patients

who are being regulated must be observed frequently during naptime and at night. The nurse becomes suspicious of problems if unable to arouse the patient or if the child is perspiring a great deal.

The symptoms of an insulin reaction, which range from mild to severe, are generally noticed and treated in the early stages. They appear *suddenly* in the *otherwise well* person. Examination of the blood reveals a lowered blood sugar level. The child becomes irritable and may behave poorly, is pale, and may complain of feeling hungry and weak. Sweating occurs. Symptoms related to disorders of the nervous system arise, since glucose is vital to the proper functioning of nerves. The child may become mentally confused and giddy, complain of a headache, and the muscular coordination is affected. If insulin shock is left untreated, coma and convulsions can occur.

The immediate treatment consists of administering sugar in some form such as orange juice, cola beverages, ginger ale, hard candy, or a commercial product such as Glutose. The patient begins to feel better within a few minutes, at which time he or she may eat a small amount of protein or starch (sandwich, milk, cheese) to prevent another reaction. *Glucagon* is recommended for the treatment of severe hypoglycemia. It acts quickly to restore the child to consciousness in an emergency situation; the child is then able to consume some form of sugar. Glucagon is a hormone produced by the pancreatic islets that also produce insulin. Normally, a fall in blood sugar will make the body release this substance. It causes a rapid breakdown of glycogen to glucose in the liver. Glucagon is packaged commercially in individual dose units that are very stable in powdered form. When it is diluted, it can be given subcutaneously, intramuscularly, or intravenously. Families of patients on insulin can be instructed to administer it subcuta-

neously or intramuscularly. It acts quickly to restore the child to consciousness in an emergency situation. If the patient does not respond rapidly, contact the physician. When the patient is unconscious, keep the child warm by covering with a blanket. Do not give anything by mouth; get medical attention immediately.

The *Somogyi phenomenon* is described as a hyperglycemic surge that occurs in the early morning hours in response to nocturnal hypoglycemia that causes counterregulatory hormones to be released. Behrman and Vaughan (1987) describe this phenomenon as "hypoglycemia begetting hyperglycemia." The *dawn phenomenon* is early morning hyperglycemia in the absence of hypoglycemia preceding it. In order to adjust insulin, blood glucose must be monitored in the early morning hours. The evening intermediate-acting insulin dose is increased in the presence of the dawn phenomenon and decreased in the Somogyi phenomenon.

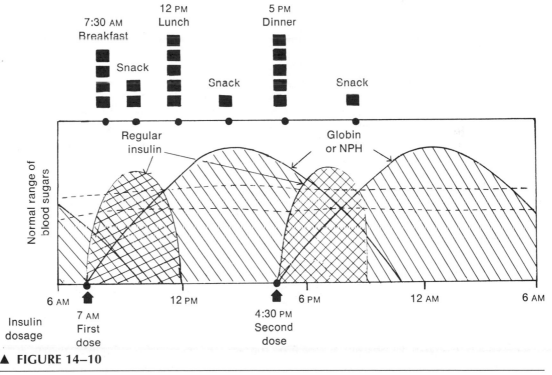

▲ FIGURE 14–10

The 24-hour insulin action on a two-dose schedule using regular and NPH insulin. (From Whaley, L., and Wong, D. [1979]. *Nursing Care of Infants and Children*. St. Louis, The C. V. Mosby Company.)

Exercise. Exercise is important for the patient with diabetes because it causes the body to use sugar and promotes good circulation. It lowers the blood sugar, and in this respect acts like more insulin. The diabetic patient who has planned vigorous exercise should carry extra sugar to avoid insulin reactions. The patient should also carry money for candy or a drink or to use a telephone. The blood sugar level is high directly after meals, so active sports can be participated in at such times. Less active games should be enjoyed directly before meals. The diabetic child is able to participate in almost all active sports. Poorly planned exercise, however, can lead to difficulties. The diabetic child should not be allowed to swim unsupervised.

Skin Care. The patient should be instructed to bathe daily and dry well. Cleansing of the inguinal area, axillae, perineum, and inframammary areas is especially important, as yeast and fungal infections tend to occur there. Inspect skin for cuts, rashes, abrasions, bruises, cysts, or boils. Treat promptly. If the skin is very dry, an oil such as Alpha-Keri may be used in the bath water. Adolescents are taught to use electric razors. Avoid exposing the skin to extremes in temperatures. Inspect injection sites for lumps.

Foot Care. Although circulatory problems of the feet are less common in children, proper habits of foot hygiene need to be established. Instruct the patient to wash and dry the feet well each day. Inspect for interdigital cracking and check the condition of the toenails. Trim nails straight across. Do not use corn remedies, iodine, or alcohol. Change socks daily; avoid tight socks or large ones that bunch up. Replace shoes often as the child grows. Wear boots only for short periods to minimize sweating. The patient should not go barefoot. If problems arise, consult a physician or podiatrist.

Infections. Obtain immunizations against communicable diseases. Cystitis, subcutaneous nodules, and monilial vulvitis occur with greater frequency in diabetic patients. During late adolescence females should see a gynecologist yearly.

Emotional Upsets. These can be as disturbing to the patient as an infection and may require food and/or insulin adjustments. Early detection of and intervention in deteriorating personal relationships and rebellion against diabetic management will decrease the severity of the effects on the diabetic. The nurse should be attuned to "little problems," which are frequently veiled requests for help. Family therapy and other forms of psychotherapeutic help may be required. Support by caretakers helps in prevention of difficulties. See Table 14–6 for stresses of the diabetic child and possible nursing interventions.

Urine Checks. Routine urine checks for sugar are being replaced by the more accurate glucose blood monitoring. However, this procedure does not test for acetone, which the patient may need to determine, particularly when the blood sugar level is high and during illness. Daily checks may also be advocated for some patients. The term "urine check" rather than "test" is less confusing to young children. During hospitalization, urine testing may be ordered. The two-drop method, using a second voided specimen, is frequently used. It is not always possible to obtain a second specimen from a child; therefore, it may be prudent to test the one you have. If this occurs, record as first or second voiding. The nurse reads the manufacturer's directions and reviews the directions with the child. Regardless of which method is used, *exact timing* is important. The dipstick method is used more frequently than tablets because it is convenient and simple. Clinitest tablets are poison and must be kept away from children and confused adults. Test results may be affected by large doses of aspirin, antibiotics, and other medications. Check expiration dates on the carton or bottle. Instruct the child to wash hands before and after the procedure. Record results. Quantitative urine collection is sometimes ordered. All voided specimens over a period of time are collected in a receptacle. The results show how many grams of glucose are eliminated during the time allocated (generally 24 hours).

Glucose-Insulin Imbalances. The patient is taught to recognize the signs of insulin shock and ketoacidosis. Early attention to change and daily record keeping are stressed. Many excellent teaching films and brochures are available. The child should wear an identification bracelet. Wallet cards are also available. Teachers, athletic coaches, and guidance officers should be informed about the disease and should have the phone numbers of the patient's parents and physician.

Travel. With planning, children can enjoy travel

Table 14–6. SUMMARY OF PREDICTABLE STRESS ON CHILD WITH TYPE I DIABETES AND HIS FAMILY

AGE	ISSUE	NURSING INTERVENTION
Infant	Trust vs. mistrust Onset and diagnosis particularly difficult during infancy; anxiety can be transmitted to baby	Stress consistency in need fulfillment Involve both parents in education Avoid information overload Instill hope and confidence Focus on child rather than disease Review normal growth and development of infancy Assist in problem solving (babysitters, difficulty in obtaining specimens, baby food exchange lists, etc.)
Toddler	Autonomy vs. shame and doubt Is this a temper tantrum or high or low blood sugar?	Prepare child for procedures and/or separations Encourage exploration of environment Stress limit setting as a form of love Admit it is difficult to distinguish temper tantrums from symptoms If worsens or is prolonged or physical symptoms appear, check blood sugar Provide 24-hour telephone number
Preschool child	Initiative vs. guilt May view injections as punishment May view denial of sweets as lack of love "Picky eater"	Foster sense of competence Educate parents to provide consistent warmth, reassurance, and love Discuss feelings about personal life and diabetes Avoid negative connotation by words, e.g., "bad blood test," "cheating" Help parents sort out child's fantasies Plan favorite party dishes on occasion Invite a playmate for lunch Suggest alternative nutritious snacks
Elementary school pupil	Industry vs. inferiority May feel hospitalization will be cure Grief over lack of cure Rebellion over treatment regimen Rebellion over food plan Anxiety about disclosure of condition to friends Embarrassed about reactions in school, missed days Unpredictable effects of exercise	Assist child in how to respond to teasing from peers ("Ick, needles!") Explain "honeymoon stage" of disease Accept child's disappointment Gradually assume self-management of insulin and specimen tests; this increases feelings of mastery and control Provide lists of fast-food exchanges Group-related education with diabetic peers Open dialogue between health personnel and teachers, school nurse, fellow students Continual reinforcement of treatment principles with specific regard to hypo- or hyperglycemia and emergencies

Table continued on following page

Table 14–6. SUMMARY OF PREDICTABLE STRESS ON CHILD WITH TYPE I DIABETES AND HIS FAMILY *Continued*

AGE	ISSUE	NURSING INTERVENTION
At puberty	Bouncing blood sugars may make child feel out of control	Explain that growth and sex hormones affect blood sugars Girls, in particular, experience difficulties about the time of menstruation Adjustments in insulin and food are common for most diabetics at this stage
	Anger at the disease, "Why must I be different?"	Assist patient in acceptable ways of expressing anger; discuss anger with parents, as they are often the target of it
	More frequent hospitalizations	Provide encouragement and support; be alert to marital stress and sibling deprivation
Teenager	Threatens sexual identity and body image	Encourage teenager to meet other adolescents with diabetes (camps, support groups, if not tried earlier); this helps decrease isolation
	Surge toward independence, risk taking or greater than usual need for security	Provide consistency with limit setting, avoid overcontrol—listen, listen, listen
	Worries about health, prospects for marriage and family	Adolescents need to have full instruction in regards to pregnancy risk and/or male potency; provide a safe environment for discussion, make appropriate referrals Encourage patient's interest in diabetic research
	Alcohol and drug abuse	Share concerns and dangers with teenager

with their families, and older adolescents can travel alone. Before leaving, the child should be seen by the physician for a check-up and prescriptions for supplies. A written statement and I.D. card identifying the child as a diabetic should be carried. Realize that time changes may affect meals. Keep additional supplies of insulin, sugar, and food with the child. Never check these with luggage, especially on an airplane. If foreign travel is planned, parents need to become familiar with the food in the area so that dietary requirements can be met. Local chapters of the American Diabetes Association or the Juvenile Diabetes Foundation can help vacationing families in an emergency.

Follow-up Care. The child needs to see the physician regularly and have a physical examination every 3 to 4 months. The patient also should be taught to visit the dentist regularly for cleaning of teeth and gums; schedule appointments for right after meals. Brushing and flossing daily are

important. Eyes should be examined regularly; blurry vision must not be disregarded. Magazines such as "Diabetes Forecast" and "Diabetes in the News" offer excellent suggestions and guidance.

Surgery. The diabetic person usually tolerates surgery well. Insulin may be given before or after operation. If the patient is restricted to NPO, calories may be supplied by intravenous glucose. Details vary according to the procedure and the patient's diabetes treatment. Careful review of the patient's history will help in formulating nursing care plans and provide a basis for teaching. The goal is to prevent hypoglycemia during the NPO period perioperatively as the body is stressed from the surgery.

The Future. Diabetic research is being conducted on many fronts. Geneticists are helping determine how diabetes is inherited so that one day they will be able to predict who will inherit the disease. If a virus is involved, a vaccine may help in its prevention. Pancreas transplantation has been performed and the success rate is improving. Beta cells have been transplanted in animals, with the result that the animals have been cured. Another possibility is that of an artificial pancreas. Its precursors might be the insulin pumps being refined today. The laser beam has aided in the treatment of complicated eye conditions. Such advances hold promise for the hope of resolving or eradicating the dilemma of diabetes.

Musculoskeletal System

LEGG-CALVÉ-PERTHES DISEASE (COXA PLANA)

Description. This disease is one of a group of disorders called the *osteochondroses* (*osteo*, bone + *chondros*, cartilage + *osis*, disease), in which the blood supply to the *epiphyses*, or end of the bone, is disrupted. The tissue death that results from the inadequate blood supply is termed *avascular necrosis*. Legg-Calvé-Perthes disease affects the development of the head of the femur. Its cause and incidence are unknown. The disease is age-related and is seen most commonly in boys between the ages of 5 and 9 years, although children between the ages of 3 and 11 may be affected. It is more common in whites than in blacks. This disease is unilateral in about 85 per cent of cases. Healing occurs spontaneously over a period of 2 to 3 years; however, marked distortion of the head of the femur may lead to an imperfect joint or degenerative arthritis of the hip in later life. Symptoms include limping, pain that may be referred to the knee, and limitation of motion. A number of cases are diagnosed in sports clinics. Legg-Calvé-Perthes disease may or may not be preceded by trauma or infection. X-ray films and isotopic bone scans confirm the diagnosis.

Treatment

In general, the earlier the age of onset the better the results of treatment. In recent years extensive confinement of the child and weight-relieving methods have been replaced by allowing weight bearing and by keeping the femoral head deep in the hip socket while it heals. This is accomplished through the use of ambulation-abduction casts or braces that prevent *subluxation* (*sub*, beneath + *luxatio*, dislocation) and enable the acetabulum to mold the healing head in such a way that it does not become deformed. This treatment may be preceded by bedrest and traction. Newer surgical reconstruction and containment methods show promise in shortening the length of treatment. The prognosis in Legg-Calvé-Perthes disease depends on age of onset, stage of the disease at diagnosis, and type of treatment instigated.

Nursing Care

Nursing considerations depend on the age of the patient and the type of treatment. When immobilization of the child is necessary, the general principles of traction, cast, and brace care are employed. Teaching and counseling are directed toward a holistic understanding of and interest in the individual child and the family. Total or partial mobility is particularly trying for children. Braces and casts hinder the patients' movement toward independence and deprive them of many natural outlets for relieving stress. The natural inclination to compete physically is thwarted. When the child is hospitalized, environmental stimuli and peer interaction are limited. The danger that the child might develop a sense of inferiority and inadequacy is heightened unless thoughtful nursing intervention is employed. The nurse should also provide support for the parents and should include their input when designing care plans. Inquiring about the welfare of siblings at home may aid parents in understanding the impact of one child's illness on the total family.

TRAUMATIC FRACTURES AND TRACTION

The active school child is often subject to traumatic injury to the extremities due to bicycle accidents, sports injuries, or falls on the playground. The various types of fractures, emergency care, and Bryant traction (Fig. 14–11) are discussed on page 257. *Traction* is used when the immobilization required is more than what could be obtained by casting. Skeletal muscles act as a splint for the

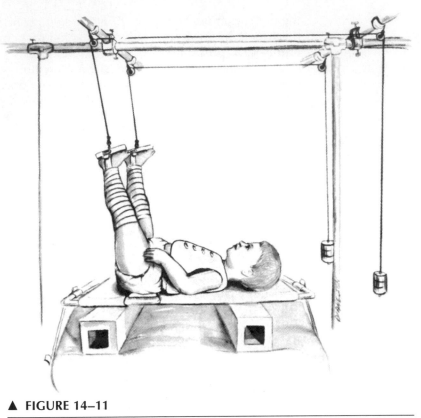

▲ **FIGURE 14–11**

Bryant direct overhead traction. (From Tachdjian, M. [1972]. *Pediatric Orthopedics*. Philadelphia, W. B. Saunders Company.)

fracture. Traction extends the injured extremity by the use of weights and countertraction. Immobilization is maintained until the bones fuse (Fig. 14–12).

Buck extension is a type of skin traction used in fractures of the femur and in hip and knee contractures. It pulls the hip and leg into extension. Countertraction is supplied by the child's body; therefore, it is essential that the patient not slip down in bed. Buck extension is sometimes used preoperatively either unilaterally or bilaterally to reduce pain and muscle spasm associated with a slipped capital femoral epiphysis. *Russell traction* is similar to Buck extension; however, in the former a sling is positioned under the knee, which suspends the distal thigh above the bed. Skin traction is applied to the lower extremity. Pull is in two directions—vertical from the knee sling and longitudinal from the footplate. This prevents posterior subluxation of the tibia on the femur, which

can occur in children in traction. *Split Russell traction* uses two sets of weights, one suspending the thigh and the other exerting a pull on the leg.

In *skeletal traction* a pin is inserted into the bone, and traction is applied to the pin. *Crutchfield or Cone-Barton tongs* may be used in the skull to provide cervical traction. With skeletal traction there is the added risk of infection from skin bacteria that may cause osteomyelitis. *Suspension therapy* elevates or suspends an extremity above the bed. It can be utilized by itself or with skin or skeletal traction. Suspension therapy reduces edema and increases the comfort of the patient. Balanced suspension employing the *Thomas splint and Pearson attachments* is used to treat diseases of the hip as well as fractures in older children and adolescents (Fig. 14–13). It may be used both before and after surgery.

Nursing Care Plan 14–1 describes care for the child in traction.

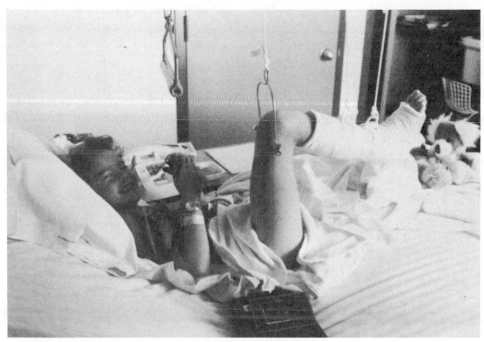

▲ **FIGURE 14–12**

A child with a fractured femur in skeletal 90-90 traction. (Photo by Stephanie Wright, *in* Foster, R., Hunsberger, M., and Anderson, J. J. [1989]. *Family-Centered Nursing Care of Children.* Philadelphia, W. B. Saunders Company.)

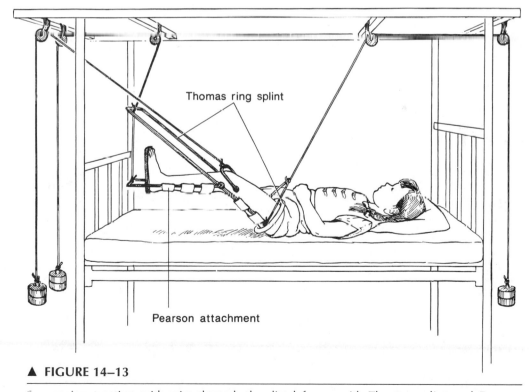

▲ **FIGURE 14–13**

Suspension traction with wire through the distal femur with Thomas splint and Pearson attachment. (Drawing modified from Tachdjian, M. [1972]. *Pediatric Orthopedics.* Philadelphia, W. B. Saunders Company.)

SELECTED NURSING DIAGNOSES FOR THE CHILD IN TRACTION

Nursing Diagnosis	Goals/Outcome Criteria	Intervention
Mobility, impaired physical activity, related to fixation devices	Child will remain free of complications of immobility Child will not develop complications of immobility, as evidenced by intact skin and absence of respiratory and urinary infections Child will have a bowel movement each day or according to previous routine	Draw picture of fracture for child, explain Explain fraction apparatus Designate call bell Change position as traction allows q 2 hr Encourage exercise through play (throwing foam balls, bean bags, pull-ups on trapeze) Instigate range of motion exercises to avoid muscle atrophy or contractures Encourage self-care Provide roughage foods to prevent constipation Provide adequate fluids; monitor intake and output Encourage blowing of harmonica, bubbles, as lung exercise Anticipate urinary tract infection
Comfort, alternations in pain, related to tissue trauma	Child will show no signs of pain Child will be comfortable, as evidenced by the absence of crying, restlessness, body posturing, and anorexia Older child will verbalize relief of pain	Administer pain medication before pain begins or escalates Allow child to choose method of pain relief, if possible Encourage child to hold favorite possession Provide pacifier for toddler Distract with music box, tapes, as age-appropriate Listen and communicate with child Use touch as a comfort measure Involve family in supporting child's ability to cope with pain Consider cultural background in relation to pain expression Determine vital signs; heart rate and respirations increase with pain, should improve after medication or comfort measure Evaluate pain management techniques daily Anticipate patient's pain as a stressor for family members

CARE PLAN 14–1 *Continued*

SELECTED NURSING DIAGNOSES FOR THE CHILD IN TRACTION

Nursing Diagnosis	Goals/Outcome Criteria	Intervention
Potential for skin irritation or breakdown, related to immobility, traction, poor circulation	Skin integrity will be maintained Circulation of affected extremity is adequate as evidenced by normal capillary refill, peripheral pulses equal and strong, and sensation and motion present in extremity	Inspect skin regularity Check capillary refill of nailbeds in affected extremity q 4 hr or as ordered Measure peripheral pulses when checking refill Have child wiggle toes or fingers of affected extremity to determine sensation and motion Utilize sheepskin, egg carton, underneath hips and back Assess restraining devices and elastic bandages for wrinkles or looseness Monitor traction and pulleys for intractness, rubbing on skin surfaces, patient comfort Maintain body alignment; massage skin to stimulate circulation Inspect pin sites for redness, bleeding, infection
Diversional activity deficit, related to boredom and restriction of activity by treatment apparatus	Child's developmental level will be maintained Child will participate in one enjoyable activity	Allow child to choose age-appropriate games, regulate the daily schedule Promote self-care activities as appropriate Encourage peer contact and interaction with new hospital friends Assist in decorating direct environment Involve child life specialist, play therapist, volunteers to visit and interact with child

JUVENILE RHEUMATOID ARTHRITIS

Description. Juvenile rheumatoid arthritis (JRA) is the most common arthritic condition of childhood. It is a systemic inflammatory disease that involves the joints, connective tissues, and viscera. JRA is not a rare disease, as there are an estimated quarter million children in the United States with this disorder (Behrman and Vaughan, 1987). The exact cause is unknown, but infections and an autoimmune response have been implicated.

Symptoms and Types (Table 14–7). This disease varies from one patient to the next and has three distinct methods of onset: systemic (or acute febrile), polyarticular, and pauciarticular. The *systemic* form is manifested by fever, rash, abdominal pain, pleuritis, pericarditis, and an enlarged liver and spleen. It occurs most frequently in children 1 to 3 and 8 to 10 years of age. Joint symptoms may be absent at onset but will develop in most patients. The *polyarticular* form can involve any of the joints, which become swollen, warm, and tender. This form occurs throughout childhood and adolescence and affects predominantly girls. Approximately 40 per cent of patients with JRA have the polyarticular type. The *pauciarticular* form is limited to four or fewer joints, generally the larger ones such as the hips, knees, ankles, and elbows. It occurs in children under age 3 years (mostly in girls) and in those aged 13 years (mostly in boys). Approximately 35 per cent of patients with JRA have the pauciarticular form.

Iridocyclitis. Children with pauciarticular disease are at risk for iridocyclitis (*irido*, iris + *cycl*, circle + *itis*, inflammation), an inflammation of the iris and ciliary body of the eye. Symptoms include redness, pain, photophobia, decreased visual acuity, and nonreactive pupils. This disease occurs most frequently in young girls. The course is unpredictable. All children with pauciarticular arthritis need slit-lamp eye examinations periodically. Distortion of the pupil and cataracts may occur. The long-term visual prognosis is uncertain.

Treatment

There are no specific tests or cures for JRA. The duration of the symptoms is important, particularly when they have lasted longer than 6 weeks. Diagnosis is determined by clinical manifestations, x-ray studies, laboratory results, and the exclusion of other disorders. Aspirated joint fluid is yellow to green and cloudy and has a low viscosity. The goals of therapy are to reduce pain and swelling, to promote mobility, to preserve joint function, to educate the patient and family, and to help the child and family adjust to living with a chronic disease.

Treatment is supportive. Drug therapy and exercise are the mainstays of therapy. The three principal medications used in this condition are aspirin, the corticosteroids, and nonsteroidal anti-inflammatory agents such as naproxen (Naprosyn). Gold compounds are used when other measures prove ineffective. Regular monitoring of all medications is imperative. Aspirin is given with meals to avoid gastric irritation. Parents are informed of the side effects of aspirin, which include tinnitus, lethargy, hyperventilation, dizziness, headaches, nausea, and vomiting. Aspirin is discontinued if the prothrombin time is prolonged excessively. The corticosteroids have to be closely screened. Opportunistic infections may occur, as advanced warning of serious infections may be masked by steroids. Gold compounds are given intramuscularly. The effect of these compounds occurs slowly. Liver function tests, blood urea nitrogen, creatinine, complete blood count, platelet count, and urinalysis are checked prior to initiation of gold compounds. The patient is warned about avoiding exposure to strong sunlight. The skin and mucous membranes are inspected before each injection for rash, stomatitis, or itching. The nurse reads the manufacturer's circular carefully, as test doses are required.

Nursing Care

The nurse functions as a member of a team that includes the pediatrician, rheumatologist, social worker, physical therapist, occupational therapist, psychologist, ophthalmologist, and school and community nurses. The child may be hospitalized during an acute episode or for an unrelated illness. Treatment consists of the administration of medications, warm tub baths, joint exercises, and rest. The physical therapist oversees the type and amount of exercise performed. Daily range of motion exercises and play activities that incorpo-

Table 14–7. SUBGROUPS OF JUVENILE RHEUMATOID ARTHRITIS

	POLYARTICULAR RHEUMATOID FACTOR–NEGATIVE	POLYARTICULAR RHEUMATOID FACTOR–POSITIVE	PAUCIARTICULAR TYPE I	PAUCIARTICULAR TYPE II	SYSTEMIC-ONSET
Per cent of JRA patients	20–25	5–10	35–40	10–15	20
Sex	90% girls	80% girls	90% girls	90% boys	60% boys
Age at onset	Throughout childhood	Late childhood	Early childhood	Late childhood	Through childhood
Joints	Any Multiple	Any Multiple	Few Large joints: knee, ankle, elbow	Few Large joints. hip girdle	Any Multiple
Sacroiliitis	No	Rare	No	Common	No
Iridocyclitis	Rare	No	30% chronic iridocyclitis	10–20% acute iridocyclitis	No
Rheumatoid factor	Negative	100%	Negative	Negative	Negative
Antinuclear antibodies	25%	75%	90%	Negative	Negative
HLA studies	?	HLA DR4	HLA DR5, DRW6, DRW8	HLA B27	?
Ultimate morbidity	Severe arthritis, 10%–15%	Severe arthritis, >50%	Ocular damage, 10% Polyarthritis, 20%	Subsequent spondylo arthropathy, ?%	Severe arthritis, 25%

(From Behrman, R., and Vaughan V. [1987]. *Nelson Textbook of Pediatrics,* 13th ed. Philadelphia, W. B. Saunders Company, p. 516.)

rate specific routines will help preserve function, maintain muscle strength, and prevent deformities. Morning tub baths and the application of moist hot packs will help lessen stiffness. Resting splints may be ordered to prevent flexion contractures and preserve functional alignment. Proper body alignment with regular change to the prone position (unless contraindicated) will facilitate comfort. Either no pillow or a small flat pillow is advocated. Measures to alleviate boredom are instigated.

Home Care. The patient is discharged with written instructions for home care. These are reviewed with the family to determine their level of understanding. A firm mattress or bed board is necessary to prevent joints from sagging. Age-appropriate tricycles and pedal cars promote mobility and exercise. Modifications in daily living such as elevation of toilet seats, installation of hand rails, Velcro fasteners, and so on, may be necessary. Swimming is an excellent form of exercise. Assist parents in planning nutritional meals. Weight gain is to be avoided, as it places further stress on the joints. Emphasize the importance of regular eye examinations. Unnecessary physical restrictions should be avoided, as these can lead to rebellion.

Encourage school attendance. Excess absence from school, particularly for nonspecific complaints, may suggest that the child is depressed or excessively preoccupied with the illness. In such cases the meaning of the illness to the child and family and its effect on daily life need to be explored. Parents need assistance in establishing limits. Consistent negative behavior in social situations can present more problems than the actual disability. Overindulgence and preferential treatment often compromise the child's potential for happiness and independence. Siblings of chronically ill children may resent the special attention received by the patient. They may be torn by loyalty to the brother or sister and their own need to be with others. Parents will need ongoing counseling and the services of various community resources. One resource is the Arthritis Foundation. The child may benefit from association with other arthritic children.

This disease is characterized by periods of remission and exacerbations. There is no known cure for JRA at this writing. Parents need assis-

tance in understanding the chronic nature of the disease and the potential for recurrence of signs and symptoms. Nurses can serve as advocates for the child, i.e., can help alleviate stress by recognizing the impact of the disease and by openly communicating with the child, the family, and other members of the health care team.

Nervous System

REYE SYNDROME

Description. Reye syndrome (RS) is a pediatric disease characterized by a nonspecific encephalopathy with fatty degeneration of the viscera. It mainly affects the liver and brain. The cause is unknown, although it is probably a mitochondrial disease. Mitochondria (*mitos,* thread + *chondros,* granule) are structures within the cytoplasm of cells. Damage to these structures impairs enzyme activity. This leads to hyperammonemia and fatty acidemia, which, along with other factors, are believed to account for brain swelling. The disease is triggered by a virus. Other controversial causes include genetic make-up, environmental factors, and the use of salicylates and phenothiazines. The American Academy of Pediatrics does not advise giving aspirin to children with influenza or varicella because this drug appears to be linked to Reye syndrome. The exact incidence of the disorder is unknown. Reye syndrome affects children under 18 years of age; most cases occur between the ages of 4 and 12 years, with peak incidence at ages 6 to 7 years. The younger the child, the higher the morbidity and fatality rates. Early diagnosis is crucial because of the rapid, life-threatening course of the disease.

Symptoms. The clinical picture is typical in that the child is recovering from a viral infection. Ninety per cent of the cases are preceded by an upper respiratory infection. This is generally influenza or chickenpox; however, other viruses have also been implicated. The recuperation is interrupted by general malaise; persistent vomiting, which may continue for 24 hours; and lethargy (Table 14–8). Diagnosis is based on the patient's history, symptoms, and laboratory data. Examples of the latter include liver function tests (SGOT,

Table 14–8. CLINICAL STAGING OF REYE SYNDROME

GRADE	SYMPTOMS AT TIME OF ADMISSION
I	Usually quiet, **lethargic** and sleepy, vomiting, laboratory evidence of liver dysfunction
II	Deep lethargy, **confusion**, delirium, combative, hyperventilation, hyperreflexic
III	Obtunded, **light coma**, ± seizures, decorticate rigidity, intact pupillary light reaction
IV	Seizures, deepening coma, **decerebrate rigidity**, loss of oculocephalic reflexes, fixed pupils
V	Coma, loss of deep tendon reflexes, respiratory arrest, fixed dilated pupils, **flaccidity/decerebrate** (intermittent); isoelectric EEG

(From Behrman, R., and Vaughan, V. [1987]. *Nelson Textbook of Pediatrics,* 13th ed. Philadelphia, W. B. Saunders Company, p. 841.)

SGPT, LDH), serum ammonia levels, blood glucose levels, and prothrombin times. Elevated serum liver assays and *increased serum ammonia* levels are indicative of the disorders. Metabolic acidosis and respiratory alkalosis may also be present. Liver biopsy may be done if the diagnosis is questionable. A CT scan may be ordered to rule out a brain tumor. The prognosis depends on the severity of the illness. Most survivors recover completely; however, some suffer complications of neurological sequelae.

Treatment and Nursing Care

The patient is admitted to the intensive care unit (ICU). Treatment is supportive. Of particular priority is preventing brain insult, as the disease process in most other organs is reversible. Fluid management in conjunction with treatment of increased intracranial pressure (ICP) is crucial. Electroencephalograms are performed until stabilization is seen. Medications include osmotic diuretics (such as mannitol), sedatives, and the barbiturates. Appropriate therapy for secondary infection is also instituted. Treatment programs are currently in a state of transition, with variations

subject to controversy. The nursing care for patients with increased ICP is summarized on page 259. This is assumed by ICU nurses during the acute stage of the disease. Important aspects include elevating the patient's head to 30 degrees. The neck should not be compressed. Consider all procedures in terms of their effect on the child's ICP. Nursing care is performed gently to reduce agitation. Anticipate and prepare for seizures. If the child is comatose, consider nursing measures to reduced secondary effects. Evaluate respiratory status frequently. Be on the alert for drug incompatibilities and avoid overhydration. Observe the patient for bleeding. A hypothermia pad may be used to prevent temperature elevations, which increase the demand for cerebral oxygen.

The rapid course of this disease is extremely frightening. Parents need information and reassurance. There is usually guilt. Family members may blame themselves for not recognizing the seriousness of the infection. Other children in the home may also be ill. Address parental concerns and prepare them for how the child looks, particularly if procedures with additional equipment have been introduced since their last visit. Provide parents with a comfortable place to sleep. Assess family coping skills and refer family members to a chaplain, social service, Reye Foundation, and so on. When patients awaken, they may be reserved, disoriented, and fearful of their environment. They may not recall any of the events surrounding hospitalization. Informing parents of this decreases apprehension.

BRAIN TUMORS

Description. Brain tumors are the second most common type of neoplasm in children (the first is leukemia). The majority of childhood tumors occur in the cerebral hemispheres. The etiology of these tumors is unknown. They occur most commonly in school age children. Diagnosis is difficult because of the insidious onset. Metastatic tumors of the brain are rare in children. A synopsis of brain tumors in children is listed in Table 14–9.

Symptoms. The signs and symptoms are directly related to the location and size of the tumor. Most tumors create increased ICP with the hallmark symptoms of headache, vomiting, drowsi-

Table 14–9. SYNOPSIS OF CHILDHOOD BRAIN TUMORS

TUMOR	PEAK AGE*	CHARACTERISTICS
Cerebellar astrocytoma (11% of all brain tumors)	6–14 yr	Grows slowly, cystic tumor, very high rate of cure with surgery (90%)
Medulloblastoma (20% of all brain tumors)	2–6 yr	Rapid growing, highly malignant, occurs more often in boys Treatment: surgery, craniospinal irradiation, chemotherapy Prognosis: much improvement in recent years
Glioma of brain stem (10%–20% of all brain tumors)	6–10 yr	Slow growing, cannot be removed by surgery, affects cerebral pathways, cranial nerves Treatment: site radiation to shrink tumor, chemotherapy, surgery Prognosis: poor
Ependymoma (8–10% of all brain tumors)	5–6 yr	Tumors grow at various speeds; because of location invades vital centers, obstructs flow of cerebrospinal fluid Treatment: partial surgical removal, radiation of entire cerebrospinal axis Prognosis: poor but related to age, location, and grade of tumor

ness, and seizures. Early morning headache relieved by vomiting may indicate a brain tumor. *Nystagmus* (constant jerky movements of the eyeball), *strabismus,* and *decreased vision* may be evidenced. *Papilledema* (edema of the optic nerve) may be seen. Other symptoms include ataxia, head tilt, behavioral changes, and cerebral enlargement, particularly in infants. Disturbances in vital signs are noticeable when the tumor presses on the brain stem.

Treatment and Nursing Care

Treatment is multidisciplinary and should take place at a hospital with appropriate support. In general, nursing care falls into several phases. These are diagnosis, preoperative care, postoperative care, radiation therapy and chemotherapy, and convalescence. The objectives for each area are specific but also overlap. One pervading theme is the continual emotional support for the child and family during this taxing ordeal. Diagnosis is determined by clinical manifestations, laboratory tests, and MRI and CT scans. At times the pathologist must perform special tests on the excised tissue. This results in a "waiting period" that increases the anxiety levels of the entire family. Myelograms may be done postoperatively to check for spinal metastasis.

Nursing care parallels the phase of treatment. Preoperative emphasis is placed on careful explanations of various procedures and on familiarizing the patient and family with the recovery room and ICU and with hospital personnel. Of importance is the fact that the patient will have the head shaved at the incision site. The nurse anticipates anxiety and provides empathy and support. The size of the postoperative dressing should be carefully explained. Applying a similar dressing to a doll may be helpful.

The postoperative care is that given the critically ill child. Student nurses may assist but are not expected to assume full responsibility. Adjuncts to care may include the use of a hypothermia blanket or a mechanical respirator. Parents must be prepared for the appearance of the child following surgery. The patient may be unconscious for a while or there may be facial edema. In supporting the family, several common issues may need to be addressed. These are the fear of pain, truthfulness versus withholding facts, feelings of helplessness and guilt, and concerns about the future. In addition, the fear of loss is always present.

Depending on the circumstances, supportive care for the terminally ill child and for the family may be necessary. Oncology support groups are particularly helpful. The families identify with one another and share common concerns.

Radiation treatment requires preparation. The radiologist outlines the areas to be treated. These marks should not be washed off. Small doses of radiation are given over a period of weeks. Determine what the radiologist has told the patient. Provide support to the child, who may feel that she or he will be burned. Advise that the child will be alone in the room but will retain voice contact. Tour the facility with the patient. Recognize physical symptoms of fear such as dry mouth, pupillary dilation, trembling, and clinging. Tape or lotion should not be placed on the skin prior to or during radiation to help prevent burns. Untoward effects of treatment may begin about the end of the first week. Headaches, anorexia, nausea and vomiting, diarrhea, and general lethargy may ensue. More severe effects include leukopenia, decrease in platelets, skin breakdown, and hair loss. Reassure the family that the hair will grow back but that it may be a different color or texture. Medication may be prescribed to help alleviate symptoms. Nutritious foods in small quantities should be offered. Provide a pleasant environment, one that is free of odors, sounds, and sights that might induce nausea.

Chemotherapy regimens vary somewhat. The child and family are prepared for the possible side effects of medications. This is done initially by the physician in charge of treatment. Ongoing education by nurses is important, as distraught parents can incorporate only so many facts. The nurse stresses the importance of return visits to monitor bone marrow depression and other parameters. Children need to know that the medicine is designed to make them feel better but that they may feel sicker at first. The nurse observes the sleeping child who has experienced nausea and vomiting frequently. The patient is positioned to avoid aspiration. Prolonged vomiting may be an indication that the medicine should be withheld or reduced. When therapy is being administered on an outpatient basis, careful instruction of parents or guardians is paramount.

The period of convalescence is punctuated by frequent clinic visits that are anxiety-provoking.

"Will the blood tests be all right?" "He's lost so much weight." "I hope he won't have to go back on medication." Some parents have to commute long distances to medical facilities. These problems involve all aspects of care of the chronically ill child. Many nurses try to maintain contact with discharged patients by mail, reunions at the clinic, and involvement in cancer camps. The community health nurse and school nurse become significant persons upon discharge. It is important that the child maintain adequate nutrition and hydration. The child is assisted in relating to a new body image. This may be augmented by the use of caps, wigs, or head scarfs. Residual effects depend on the type and extent of the tumor. It is not unusual for information such as the death of a loved child to filter back to persons who were directly involved with care. This always creates grief, which must be dealt with by the medical persons involved (see page 70).

Special Topics

OVERVIEW OF EMOTIONAL AND BEHAVIORAL DISORDERS

Growing up can be painful even under the best circumstances. It is difficult for the child in the early school years to live up to so many rapidly developing standards. Guilt and anxiety develop. Finger sucking, nail biting, excessive fears, stuttering, and conduct problems are reflections of nervous tension. Disorders that may or may not be traced to emotional problems include constipation, diarrhea, stomach aches, dermatitis, obesity, frequent urination, enuresis, and the common cold. The current trend toward prevention by identification of risk factors and intervention is a major goal of children's mental health services. The term *psychosomatic* has come to refer to the bodily dysfunctions that seem to have an emotional as well as an organic basis. Each person has a different potential for coping with life. Truancy, lying, stealing, failure in school, and a crisis such as death or divorce of parents are but a few of the difficulties that may require the services of the child guidance clinic.

The first psychiatric clinic for children in the

United States was established in Chicago in 1909 to serve delinquents. The basic staff of the modern child guidance clinic is composed of a psychiatrist, a psychologist, and a social worker; frequently, a pediatrician is also a member of the staff. Usually the child guidance clinic provides both diagnostic and treatment services. It may be part of a hospital, a school, a court, or a public health or welfare service, or it may be an independent agency.

The various psychiatric specialties may be confusing to the average person. A *psychiatrist* is a medical doctor who has specialized in mental disorders. The *psychoanalyst* is usually a psychiatrist but may be a psychologist (lay analyst); all psychoanalysts have advanced training in psychoanalytic theory and practice. The *clinical psychologist* should have a doctorate of philosophy in clinical psychology from a recognized university. Many work in the school system with children, teachers, and families in an attempt to prevent or resolve problems.

There are also emotionally disturbed children who require the type of care provided in residential treatment centers. Their home situations may be such that they can respond to therapy only with a complete change of environment. In both areas the total situation to which the child reacts needs to be treated rather than just the individual patient. Short-term residential care in the general hospital (preadolescent unit) is a newer adjunct to therapy. The length of stay varies from about 2 weeks to 2 months. Most of these children have not responded well to individual outpatient therapy.

Nursing Care

For nurses to work effectively with the disturbed child, they must first understand the types of behavior considered within a normal range, as the two are so intimately related. They are valuable members of the health care team in that they work closely with the hospitalized child and the long-term patient in particular. They keep a careful record of behavior and note the relationship with members of the family. Such notations are meaningful to the physician, who is as concerned with preventing problems from arising as with treating them. Is 4 year old Janice wetting the bed? What about Bobby who continually bangs his head against the crib during naptime? What does Allan do in the playroom? Is he sitting alone in a corner? Does he hit the other children? Is he constantly in motion? Does Eric seem indifferent to your attempts to establish rapport with him? Is there a physical cause for his behavior? Each action in itself might be considered well within the normal limits of behavior, but when carried to extremes, such actions may interfere with the child's experience of and reaction to reality and should be investigated further. Nurses should bear in mind that behavior one might describe as "bratty" may be interpreted very differently by persons skilled in understanding deeper levels of personality. They should feel free to discuss the conduct problems of patients with other members of the staff and should not consider these problems a threat to their own abilities.

One might ask where else the nurse sees such children. Wherever the children are—in the home, in nursery school, in residential institutions, at child health conferences, in special clinics, in the doctor's office. Perhaps they are her or his own children. Everyday, everywhere, children are trying to cope with stress. Many succeed and grow stronger. Many do not.

When parents request direction from nurses, they should encourage them to seek help from their family physician or pediatrician or from a community mental health center. If the child is in school, the services of the school psychologist may prove valuable. Some churches employ counselors who are available free of charge to parishioners. The nurse should support organizations concerned with mental health, vote on issues that are pertinent to the welfare of children in the community, and offer services when they are needed.

ATTENTION-DEFICIT HYPERACTIVITY DISORDER

The term *attention-deficit hyperactivity disorder* (ADHD) refers to a developmentally inappropriate degree of gross motor activity, impulsivity, and inattention in the school or home setting (Greenhill, 1990). Boys are affected more frequently than girls. Boys have more behavioral problems and girls more frequent academic underachievement.

According to the Diagnostic and Statistical Manual of Mental Disorders (American Psychiatric Association, 1987), for this diagnosis to be made, the child must have at least eight of the criteria set forth in the manual. Examples of these criteria include:

1. Often fidgets with hands or feet or squirms in seat
2. Has difficulty remaining seated when required to do so
3. Is easily distracted by extraneous stimuli
4. Often blurts out answers to questions before they have been completed
5. Has difficulty playing quietly
6. Often interrupts or intrudes on others
7. Often does not seem to listen to what is being said to him or her

Other criteria may be found in the manual. The student can begin to see that a child with these characteristics may have difficulties in school and in social situations. Other criteria include onset before age 7 years, duration of at least 6 months, and the absence of criteria that might indicate a pervasive developmental disorder (autism, mental retardation).

Treatment and Nursing Care

Children with ADHD should be managed by a multidisciplinary team of nurse, physician, social worker, psychologist, and special education teacher. Parents need support and should be referred to support groups. Family counseling may be warranted.

The cause of these difficulties is not thoroughly understood. Proponents of biochemical factors suggest that hyperactive children have a total lack or diminished amount of norepinephrine, a neurotransmitter present in the brain. Others attribute the problem to an alteration of the reticular activating system of the midbrain that causes the child to react to every stimulation in the environment rather than to selected ones. Newer evidence indicates that genetic factors may play an important role. These disorders have also been linked to fetal alcohol syndrome and lead toxicity.

The specific medications used for the treatment of behavior problems in ambulatory patients are listed in Table 14–10. They are believed to act directly on the reticular activating system and/or to stimulate the release of norepinephrine from the brain stem. Although the use of drugs to modify behavior in children is controversial, extensive experience has demonstrated their effectiveness, particularly in children with disorders of attention, activity, and organization. There is no evidence that these drugs are addictive; abuse is unlikely since the effect on the patient is opposite to that produced in persons without the problem.

Table 14–10. STIMULANT MEDICATIONS FOR ATTENTION-DEFICIT DISORDERS

DRUG	DAILY DOSAGE	SIDE EFFECTS
Dextroamphetamine (Dexedrine) 5 mg tablets (also long-acting tablets)	2.5–20 mg	Anorexia, weight loss, insomnia, emotional lability or oversensitivity, tics, growth delays
Methylphenidate* (Ritalin) 5 mg, 10 mg, 15 mg tablets	5–40 mg	Similar to dextroamphetamine
Pemoline† (Cylert) 18.75 mg, 37.5 mg, 75 mg tablets	18.75–112.5 mg	Insomnia, anorexia, abdominal pain, nausea, headache, dizziness, drowsiness, depression

*Primarily used because of rapid and predictable onset and relatively few side effects.
†Rarely used.

More controversial therapies include diet (particularly elimination of food additives, such as preservatives and artificial flavors and colors) and the use of megavitamins.

Initially, a careful medical history and neurological examination are indicated. Intelligence and psychological tests may aid in determining the specific assets and liabilities of the child, so that an individual learning plan can be outlined. Many schools today have special learning disability classes in which the children are helped to establish self-discipline by consistent controls, elimination of distractions, and recognition and appreciation of accomplishments. These methods are reinforced by the thoughtful nurse when such a child is hospitalized.

A priority in the care of these patients is a careful nursing admission history, a most useful tool in dealing with children with problems of this nature. Nurses observe the patient's behavior alone and in interaction with the family. They document what they see but do not analyze; for example, "Eric threw four crayons on the floor," not "Eric appeared distraught and misbehaved this morning." Careful attention is given to the child's attitude toward school. Other responsibilities might include dietary counseling if ordered, education in parenting, and assisting with screening and psychological tests. Functions pertinent to the nurse's work setting might also include referral to appropriate agencies, and assessing the home and school environments.

Listening to the child and the parents and providing support are particularly important. If the child is hyperactive, opportunities for gross motor play and screaming to externalize feelings, which must be encouraged at home, are limited in the hospital. The use of puppets, finger paints, and singing may be employed to offset this imbalance. One nurse each shift is assigned to a particular child to provide continuity of care. Nursing care plans should include both short- and long-term goals.

When medications are necessary, the child and the family must understand the reasons for their use and their possible side effects. Periodic evaluation by the physician is essential. It is helpful if a behavior chart is kept and is submitted to the doctor before prescriptions are renewed. The child

with a learning disability should not become a "sacrificial lamb" to the educational process, and the emphasis on education should not be disproportionate to the child's innate capabilities. Personal growth and self-esteem are emphasized. Parents should be aware that other opportunities exist that can be adjusted to the child's abilities.

References

American Psychiatric Association (1987). *Diagnostic Criteria from DSM-III-R*, 3rd ed. Washington, D.C., American Psychiatric Association.

Behrman, R., and Vaughan, V. (1987). *Nelson Textbook of Pediatrics*, 13th ed. Philadelphia, W. B. Saunders Company.

Cleland, B. (1983). *Constant Carbohydrate Diet*. Iowa City, Ia., The University of Iowa Hospitals and Clinics, Dietary Department.

Greenhill, L. (1990). Attention-deficit hyperactivity disorder in children. *In* Garfinkel, B., Carlson, G., and Weller, E. (eds.). *Psychiatric Disorders in Children and Adolescents*. Philadelphia, W. B. Saunders Company, pp. 149–191.

Bibliography

Baren, M. (1989). The case for Ritalin: A fresh look at the controversy. *Contemp. Pediatr.* 6:16–28.

Brimhall, C., and Esterly, N. (1990). Uninvited guests: Six infestations of childhood. *Contemp. Pediatr.* 7:18–57.

Clark, L., and Plotnick, L. (1990). Insulin pumps in children with diabetes. *J. Pediatr. Health Care* 4:3–10.

Grimes, D., and Woolbert, L. (1990). Facts and fallacies about streptococcal infection and rheumatic fever. *J. Pediatr. Health Care* 4:186–192.

Kaplan, E. (1987). The startling comeback of rheumatic fever. *Contemp. Pediatr.* 4:20–34.

Lipman, T., DiFazio, D., Meers, R., and Thompson, R. (1989). A developmental approach to diabetes in children: Birth through preschool. *Am. J. Matern./Child Nurs.* 14:255–259.

Lipman, T., DiFazio, D., Meers, R., and Thompson, R. (1989). A developmental approach to diabetes in children: School age—adolescence. *Am. J. Matern./Child Nurs.* 14:330–332.

Schiffrin, A. (1987). Management of childhood diabetes. *Pediatr. Ann.* 16:694–710.

Shiminski-Maher, T. (1990). Brain tumors in childhood: Implications for nursing practice. *J. Pediatr. Health Care* 4:122–130.

Skyler, J. (1987). Etiology and pathogenesis of insulin dependent diabetes mellitus. *Pediatr. Ann.* 16:682–691.

Tattersall, R. (1987). Psychosocial aspects of diabetes in childhood and adolescence. *Pediatr. Ann.* 16:728–740.

Travis, L., Brouhard, B., and Schreiner, B. (1987). *Diabetes in Children and Adolescents*. Philadelphia, W. B. Saunders Company.

STUDY QUESTIONS

1. Describe the terms *major* and *minor criteria* in rheumatic fever.
2. Ginny, age 10 years, is admitted with possible appendicitis. What observations made by the nurse will be useful in establishing or ruling out this diagnosis?
3. Mildred, age 68, has Type II diabetes and takes Orinase twice a day. Her grandchild Melinda, who is 8 years old, has Type I diabetes and is on insulin injections twice daily. Differentiate between the two forms of diabetes.
4. Melinda spends Wednesday with her grandmother (see above). Devise a day's meal plan for the two. Give rationale for modifications if necessary.
5. What factors would you consider when determining whether 8 year old Melinda is ready to administer her own insulin? What would your instructions to her include?
6. Melinda has joined the school softball team and practices twice a week after school. How will this affect her diabetes? What factors would you consider when providing anticipatory guidance to Melinda and her parents in regard to this new activity?
7. What structures are affected in Legg-Calvé-Perthes disease?
8. List several mannerisms that may indicate nervous tension in a child.
9. Kurt, age 12 years, is hospitalized with a diagnosis of a fractured ulna and radius. While you are taking his medical history, his mother states, "Kurt has always been superactive, and this has gotten him into a lot of trouble." Discuss the implications of her statement. What additional data would you want to obtain in order to determine, plan, and implement his nursing care?
10. Matthew, age 7 years, has a brain tumor. He wishes to go to cancer camp. How would you assist the family to prepare Matt for camp? Discuss both physical and psychological considerations.

CHAPTER 15 _____

Chapter Outline

GENERAL CHARACTERISTICS
PHYSICAL, MENTAL, EMOTIONAL, AND SOCIAL
  DEVELOPMENT
    Biological Development
    Sexuality
    Psychosocial Development
    Cognitive Development
SPECIAL NEEDS
    Peer Relationships
    Career Plans
    Responsibility
    Emotional Needs
    Daydreams
    Heterosexual Relationships
PARENTING
HEALTH EDUCATION AND GUIDANCE
    Nutrition
    Nursing Care
    Personal Care
    Dental Care

Objectives

Upon completion and mastery of Chapter 15, the
student will be able to
- Define the vocabulary terms listed.
- Identify two major developmental tasks of
  adolescence.
- List three characteristics of the adolescent that
  predispose to certain accidents and suggest
  methods of prevention for each.
- Summarize the nutritional requirements of the
  adolescent and give two factors that may
  contribute to dietary deficiencies in this age
  group.
- Discuss three methods of anticipatory guidance
  for a 15 year old girl just beginning to date.
- Describe three ways an adolescent can be given
  responsibility.
- Explain three ways parents can be assisted in the
  skills of parenting adolescents.
- Discuss three theories of adolescent personality
  development.

THE ADOLESCENT

Terms

androgen (419)
asynchrony (420)
estrogen (419)
gender (417)
identity (417)
intimacy (417)
menarche (420)

General Characteristics

Adolescence is defined as the period of life that begins with the appearance of secondary sex characteristics and ends with cessation of growth and emotional maturity. The term comes from the word *adolescere*, meaning to "grow up." For purposes of clarification, adolescence is often divided into early, middle, and late periods, as the teenager of 13 years varies a great deal from the 18 year old. Middle adolescence appears to be the time of greatest turmoil for most families. Perhaps one of the most characteristic features of adolescence is its uncertainty. It is a period of life that lasts a comparatively long time in our culture and involves a great number of adjustments.

Life is never dull when there are adolescents in the family. The adolescents' surge toward independence becomes more and more pronounced, making it practically impossible for them to get along with parents, who represent authority. When adolescents submit to their wishes, they feel humiliated and childish. If they revolt, con-

flicts arise within the family. Parents and teenagers have to weather the storm together and try to come up with solutions that are relatively satisfactory to all.

Numerous other factors also account for the restlessness of youth. Their bodies are rapidly changing, and they experience intense sexual drives. They want to be accepted by society, but are not sure how to go about it. Adolescents question life and search to find what psychologists term their *sense of identity:* "Who am I?" "What do I want?" This is followed by the *intimacy* stage in which teenagers must learn to avoid emotional isolation. They must face the fear of rejection in shared activities such as sports, in close friendships, and in sexual experiences. The older adolescent thinks about the future and is generally idealistic. Jean Piaget and other investigators indicated that it is at this time that the final stages of abstract reasoning, logic, and other symbolic forms of thought are reached, bringing about an increased sophistication in moral reasoning (Fig. 15–1).

These facts sound complicated in themselves, but they are intensified by a world that is constantly changing. Even adults are confused by the rapid pace of living and the many advances in technology. The feminist movement has challenged the traditional roles of men and women in society. *Gender roles* are becoming less well defined in some households, which is likely to create changes in the ways in which parents act as models for their children. Many adolescents are living in single parent homes or with working relatives where little, if any, supervision is avail-

SIGMUND FREUD considers adolescence as the time of the last identifiable stage of psychosexual development: the genital stage. During this stage, the individual's identity takes its final form and, in place of narcissistic self-love, love for others and altruistic behavior develop. Although the influence of peers and parents is as strong as it was during earlier stages, peers and parents still play an important role in providing love and realistic direction for the individual.

ERIK ERIKSON holds self-definition and self-esteem as central concerns for the individual during adolescence. As a result of physical changes, powerful sexual impulses, conflicting choices and possibilities, and confusion in the roles expected of him by parents and peers, the adolescent is confronted with an identity crisis. He must incorporate his new physical and sexual attributes into a new self-concept. He also must generate an orientation and a goal that will give him a sense of unity and purpose so that he can make a vocational choice that will best match his view of himself. Finally, he must integrate into his self-understanding the expectations and perceptions that others have of him.

▲ **FIGURE 15–1**

Some major theoretical views regarding personality development of adolescents. (From Hoffman, L. W., Paris, S. G., and Schell, R. (1988). *Developmental Psychology Today*, 5th ed. New York, CRM/Random House. Reproduced with permission of McGraw-Hill, Inc.)

able. Studies indicate that marked adolescent turmoil is actually less normal than was previously believed and that, in fact, many teenagers show indications of psychiatric distress.

Beall and Schmidt (1984) have developed a Youth Adaptation Rating Scale (YARS) to identify life events of adolescents that contribute to stress (Tables 15–1 and 15–2). In their survey, students described the severity of several life events by ranking each item from 0 to 5, with 0 being not stressful. A ratio value was then determined (figures in parentheses). Six ethnic categories were

identified and sampled, as well as five communities of different sizes. A surprising result was that no significant differences existed between the ethnic groups or the adolescents from communities of different sizes.

There is no one, perfect way to guide adolescents. However, recognizing their needs is a beginning. Adolescents' reactions are individual; one must realize that, in contrast to the stereotyped descriptions that abound, adolescence takes many forms in a free society. A great deal depends on the culture and experience a particular adolescent has as he or she is growing up. All experts in teenage guidance agree on the importance of keeping lines of communication open in the family and on the need to listen to and observe verbal and nonverbal cues for help. Amazingly enough, most children come through the period of adolescence with flying colors and relatively few scars, perhaps because each generation learns to live with the insecurities of its era, never having known any other.

Table 15–1. CATEGORIES FOR DESCRIBING DEGREES OF ADAPTATION IN THE YARS

5 Critical event in the life of a teenager. Very stressful. This would require a major change in one's life. Totally demanding.

4 Semicritical event. Stressful. This would require changing one's life to adjust to the differences it would make.

3 Moderately critical. This event causes stress, but one could take it without too great a change in living.

2 Semimoderate. Stress is evidenced, but one could adjust fairly easily to this event without too much strain mentally, emotionally, or physically.

1 Mild stress. Hardly any stress at all. One could make the changes that might be needed without much effort.

0 Not stressful at all. Probably no change would be required in order to adjust to this event.

(From Beall, S., and Schmidt, G. [1984]. *J. School Health* 54:197. Copyright 1984. American School Health Association, Kent, Ohio 44240.)

Table 15-2. YOUTH ADAPTATION RATING SCALE

☐ Graduation (.57)	☐ Going into debt (.72)
☐ Pet dies (.55)	☐ Being stereotyped/discriminated against/having bad rumors spread about you (.70)
☐ Fights with parents (.67)	☐ Death of a close family member (.94)
☐ Getting pressure about having sex (.63)	☐ Death of a boyfriend/girlfriend/close friend (.94)
☐ Caught cheating or lying repeatedly (.73)	☐ Getting V.D. (.86)
☐ Getting a major illness/injury/car accident (.81)	☐ Getting someone pregnant/getting pregnant (.92)
☐ Becoming religious or giving up religion (.63)	☐ Taking finals/SAT test (.61)
☐ Referral to the principal's office (.47)	☐ Moving to a different town/school/making new friends (.67)
☐ Getting acne/warts (.45)	☐ Getting a car (.35)
☐ Trouble getting a date when it was not a problem before (.61)	☐ Trying to get a job/job interview (.49)
☐ Problems developed with teachers/employers (.59)	☐ Getting an award, office, etc. (.36)
☐ Making career decisions (college, majors, training, etc.) (.64)	☐ Making a team (drill, athletic, debate) (.44)
☐ Starting to go to weekend parties/rock concerts (.35)	☐ Getting married (.73)
☐ First day of school (.37)	☐ Getting beat up by parents (.86)
☐ Going on first date/starting to date (.53)	☐ Taking the driver's license test (.55)
☐ Death of a parent/guardian (.95)	☐ Getting a new addition to the family (.45)
☐ Not getting promoted to next grade (.76)	☐ Going to the dentist or doctor (.37)
☐ Getting caught using drugs (.86)	☐ Going to jail/reform school (.88)
☐ Getting attacked/raped/beat up (.84)	☐ Starting to use drugs (.82)
☐ Getting a ticket or other minor problems with law (.58)	☐ Getting braces (.45)
☐ Parents getting a divorce/separation (.83)	☐ Going on a diet (.41)
☐ Getting expelled/suspended (.71)	☐ Losing or gaining weight (.49)
☐ Fad pressure (.43)	☐ Changing exercise habits (.21)
☐ Breaking up with boy/girlfriend (.57)	☐ Pressure to take drugs (.71)
☐ Getting minor illness (cold, flu, etc.) (.30)	☐ Moving out of the house (.56)
☐ Arguments with peers/brothers/sisters (.46)	☐ Falling in love (.66)
☐ Starting to perform (speeches, presentations, musical or drama performances) (.60)	☐ Getting a bad haircut (.57)
☐ Getting fired from a job (.63)	☐ Getting glasses (.49)
	☐ Family member moving out (.47)
	☐ Getting a bad report card (.59)

(From Beall, S., and Schmidt, G. [1984]. *J. School Health,* 54:197. Copyright 1984. American School Health Association, Kent, Ohio, 44240.)

Physical, Mental, Emotional, and Social Development

BIOLOGICAL DEVELOPMENT

Preadolescence is a short period immediately preceding adolescence. In girls it comprises the years 10 to 13 and is marked by rapid changes in the structure and function of various parts of the body. It is distinguished by *puberty*, the stage at which the reproductive organs become functional and secondary sex characteristics develop. Both sexes produce male hormones, *androgens,* and female hormones, *estrogens,* in comparatively equal amounts during childhood. At puberty the hypothalamus of the brain signals the pituitary gland to stimulate other endocrine glands—the adrenals and the ovaries or testes—to secrete their hormones directly into the blood stream in differing proportions (more androgens in boys and more estrogens in girls).

The age at which puberty takes place varies and is about two years earlier in girls than in boys. It is preceded by spurts in height and weight in both sexes. One's general appearance tends to be awkward, i.e., long-legged and gangling; this growth characteristic is termed *asynchrony* because different body parts mature at different rates. The sweat glands are very active, and greasy skin and acne are common. Both sexes mature earlier and grow taller and heavier than in past generations (Fig. 15–2).

The onset of menstrual periods (menarche) occurs in the United States at an average age of 12.5 years, with a normal range of 10 to 16 years (Vaughan and Litt, 1990). Secondary sex characteristics become more apparent prior to the menarche. Fat is deposited in the hips, thighs, and breasts, causing them to enlarge. Growth of the external genitals also takes place. Hair develops in the pubic area and underarms. The body reaches its final measurements about 3 years from the onset of puberty. At this time the ends of the long bones knit securely to their shafts, and further growth can no longer take place.

Although breast cancer is rare in adolescents, this is a time when girls are aware of their bodies, and breast self-examination should be taught. Various informational pamphlets describing the procedure are available through the American Cancer Society.

The first sign of puberty in boys is usually the enlargement of the testes, which begins between

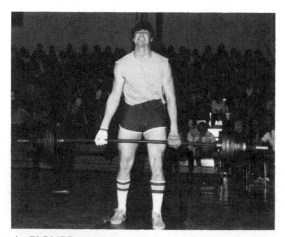

▲ FIGURE 15–2

Young people today mature earlier than in past generations and are also taller and heavier. Many develop high levels of physical competence.

10 and 13 years of age. Nocturnal emissions begin occurring after this; some sources indicate approximately 1 year afterward. The production of sperm begins between 13.5 and 14.5 years of age. Complete fertility is not present at this time, but impregnation is possible. The genitals enlarge. Hair develops in the pubic and axillary areas and finally on the face. Voice changes are also noticeable.

The American Cancer Society recommends that boys examine their testes during or after a hot bath or shower. Each testicle is examined using the index and middle fingers of both hands on the underside of the testicle and the thumbs on the top of the testicle. The testicles are gently rolled between the thumb and fingers. Testicular self-examinations are performed once a month. If a lump is discovered, it should be reported immediately.

NURSING BRIEF ▷ ▷ ▷ ▷ ▷ ▷ ▷ ▷
Although young girls are often taught breast self-examination, young boys are seldom instructed in examination of the testes.

SEXUALITY

Sexuality defines those characteristics that make each of us either female or male. A person's sexuality is affected by psychological, biological, and social factors. Because the adolescent is in a period of growth, the various factors of sexuality may be in conflict. The adolescent is not prepared for the responsibility of having a child and yet is biologically capable of reproduction. The number of teenagers giving birth rose in 1988 for the second year after declining in the 1970s and early 1980s. Sexual activity continues to increase. In a study conducted in 1989, 55 per cent of the 677 adolescents in grades 7 through 9 surveyed were sexually active (Orr and colleagues, 1989).

During this period the adolescent has an increased need to learn about sexuality. Values must be clarified and decision-making skills evaluated. The adolescent may be told that not making a decision about sexual activity is indeed making a decision. Although parental involvement in sex education is encouraged, parents often postpone until adolescence, or defer to others, the educating of their children. Consequently the adolescent receives information from peers, the media, and other sources that may be incorrect or biased.

Because the adolescent may receive incorrect information about the body, misconceptions should be identified and teaching should be done regarding menstruation, pregnancy, sexually transmitted diseases, and contraception. Most adolescents do not want to become pregnant and yet many do not use contraceptives. Adolescents cite the following reasons for not using contraceptives: they thought they could not conceive; they had not expected to have intercourse; they felt that using contraceptives interfered with sexual spontaneity, making the sexual act seem too planned (Castiglia, 1990). Clearly, this points to a lack of understanding.

Adolescents have fears and concerns that are specific to their sexuality. The girl who is the tallest person in her class is often just as concerned as the boy who is the shortest. Adolescent girls are also concerned about when to wear a bra and when they will begin their menstrual period and take on the characteristics of a woman. Adolescent boys may be worried because they may not have the height and strength of their peers. There is a wide age range for the physical changes that take place during puberty and the adolescent needs to be reassured that he or she is normal. An excellent time to teach normal growth and development to the developing adolescent is at the time of assessment. Nurses can talk about concerns as they examine each part of the child's body. Because there is such a wide variation in the age at which each child develops, nurses should point out to adolescents that they are exactly where they should be at their particular stage of sexual development.

Sex education in public schools tends to concentrate on the physiology of sex, on the reproductive systems, and on sexually transmitted disease and is usually less informative about the psychological and value aspects of sexuality and the facts concerning contraception. Few adolescents can talk freely with their parents about sex, in particular their own sexual behavior and problems. However, sexual values, attitudes, and information are conveyed in less conscious ways by role modeling. In this way parents serve as an initial source of sex role learning for their daughters and sons. In their sexuality and intimacy, adolescents reflect society's new openness about sexual matters and are inclined to see sexual behavior as a matter of personal choice rather than of morality or law. Like most adults, most adolescents do not condone promiscuity. Rather, some evaluate a specific sexual behavior within the framework of the relationship between the people engaging in it (Schell and Hall, 1983).

Homosexuality. Homosexual experiences in adolescence are not uncommon. This experimentation is not a positive prediction of one's sexual preference as an adult but may be merely a desire to explore alternative lifestyles. Conversely, however, most homosexuals report having had homosexual experiences during adolescence (Levine and colleagues, 1983). Homosexuality, while no longer classified as a disease, is nonetheless subject to great controversy. Whether or not one is homosexual, unspoken suspicions during adolescence can create anxiety and turmoil for the young person and the family. In some cultures, such as the Vietnamese, physical contact between peers of the same sex is common. "It is not unusual to see boys walking hand in hand while just displaying friendship" (Ching, 1984).

PSYCHOSOCIAL DEVELOPMENT

Adolescents are in a period of transition from childhood to adulthood (Table 15–3). Erikson identifies the major task of this group as identity versus role confusion. At this time the children must determine who they are, where they are going, and how they are getting there. This should not imply that adolescents wait until this stage to develop individuation. During the toddler period the child is first challenged with issues of autonomy which, if accomplished, will make the adolescent task less of a challenge.

Adolescents want to be people in their own right, and they "try on" different roles. Self-concept (one's view of oneself) fluctuates during this time and is molded by demands of parents, peers, teachers, and so on. Although gaining self-concept is an ongoing process, adolescence can be a time of particular challenge to the child's view of the self.

As adolescents move toward independence they begin to separate from the family. This separation

Table 15–3. GROWTH TASKS BY DEVELOPMENTAL PHASE

TASKS	EARLY: 10 TO 13 YEARS	MID: 14 TO 16 YEARS	LATE: 17 YEARS AND OLDER
Independence	Emotionally breaks from parents and prefers friends to family	Ambivalence about separation	Integration of independence issues
Body image	Adjustment to pubescent changes	"Trying on" different images to find real self	Integration of a satisfying body image with personality
Sexual drives	Sexual curiosity; occasional masturbation	Sexual experimentation; opposite sex viewed as sex object	Beginning of intimacy and caring
Relationships	Unisexual peer group; adult crushes	Begin heterosexual peer group; multiple adult role models	Individual relationships more important than peer group
Career plans	Vague and even unrealistic plans ⟶		Specific goals and specific steps to implement them
Conceptualization	Concrete thinking ⟶ Fascinated by capacity for thinking ⟶		Ability to abstract
Value system	Drop in superego; testing of moral system of parents	Self-centered	Idealism; rigid concepts of right and wrong. Other-oriented; asceticism

See accompanying text for further information on tasks.
(From Levine, M., et al. [1983]. *Developmental-Behavioral Pediatrics.* Philadelphia, W. B. Saunders Co.)

does not have to be achieved through deviance and rebellion in the context of peer group influence (Vaughan and Litt, 1990). Peer influences dominate decisions that relate to style of dress, but parents still hold sway over moral decisions

> In adolescence dependency creates hostility. Parents who foster dependence invite unavoidable resentment. Wise parents make themselves increasingly dispensable. Their language is sprinkled with such statements as "The choice is yours." "You decide about that." "If you want to." "It's your decision." "Whatever you choose is fine with me."
>
> *Haim Ginott* (1971)

and those that determine employment (Brittain, 1967). Parents are often ambivalent about letting go. Disagreements with parents often revolve around dating, the family car, money, chores, school grades, choice of friends, smoking, sex, and the use of social drugs. Parental values and morals are questioned, particularly if parents do not practice what they preach. Adults who associate with teenagers should try to create an atmosphere of interest and understanding. A caring environment that sets limits is essential. Adolescence is a little like being on a roller coaster. Parents, nurses, and other adults who interact with adolescents should be reminded not to take the ride with the child. Rather, they should remain objective, calm, understanding, and loving.

Americans are multicolored, multicultural, and multilingual. The value of independence as a goal

COGNITIVE DEVELOPMENT

Piaget's theory of cognitive development holds that development is systematic, sequential, and orderly. Early adolescents are still in the concrete phase of thinking. They take things literally. If asked by the nurse, "Have you ever slept with anyone?" a young teenage girl may not perceive this to have anything to do with a vaginal infection or sex. By midadolescence the ability to think in abstract terms has increased. Piaget terms this the stage of formal operations. Older adolescents can see a situation from many viewpoints and can imagine or organize unseen or unexperienced possibilities. The failure to develop formal thoughts is cited by some as connected to the failure to

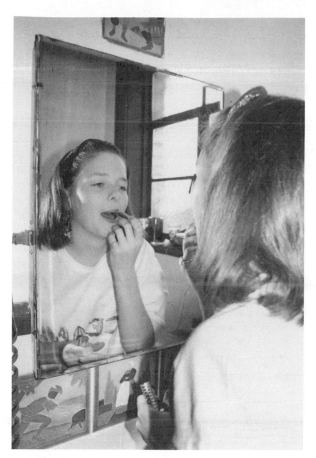

▲ **FIGURE 15–3**

The teenager's self-esteem is influenced by how far body image deviates from the mythical "body ideal." (Courtesy of Vickie Ashwill.)

of maturational and emotional development may not be adopted by all. Many immigrants and Americans of Asian/American background come from societies that are patriarchal and highly structured and have distinct social roles. The good of the family takes precedence over personal goals. The protection of family image and neighborhood reputation is very important. The Chinese do not recognize the period of adolescence. There is no word for it in their language. Chinese children grow up in a society that offers little choice for mobility. A period of rebellion or need to find identity is incongruent with their system (Brown, 1983). Nurses must be aware of different cultures and examine their own biases.

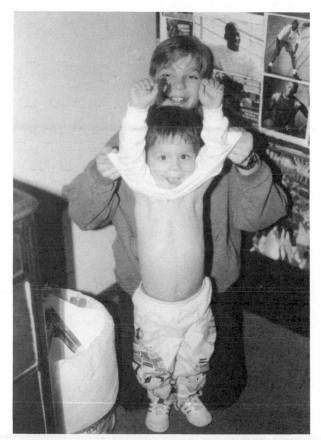

▲ **FIGURE 15–4**

Stereotypical roles are beginning to change. The male adolescent should be prepared to assume child care duties just as women have in the past.

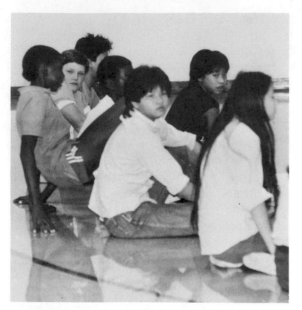

▲ **FIGURE 15–5**

Understanding ethnic and cultural variations among teenagers is important in assessment and planning.

develop a high level of moral reasoning. Adolescents who have developed both are most likely to evidence a high degree of morality and consistency in their behavior.

Special Needs

PEER RELATIONSHIPS

Adolescent peer groups vary in number, interests, social background, and structure. They may consist of small groups of the same sex or both sexes, and in late adolescence of small groups of couples. The young person may belong to one or several groups. The peer group serves as a mirror for "normality" and helps determine where one fits in. It is vitally important in helping the adolescent define the self. Acceptance by one's friends helps decrease the loneliness and sense of loss many teenagers experience on the road to adulthood (Fig. 15–6).

The social norms and pressures exerted by the group may cause problems. The selection of friends and allegiance to them may bring about confrontations within the family. Parents need help in understanding that the teenager's exaggerated conformity is a necessary process to moving away from dependence and obtaining approval from persons outside the nuclear family. Failure to develop social competence may produce feelings of inadequacy and low self-esteem.

Nurses can assist the family by their support and by educating them in the dynamics of this age group. They can direct them to such groups as peer helpers (for the adolescent) and community educational programs sponsored by various agencies. Organizations such as Parents Without Partners might be another avenue. Nurses must also remember that teenagers who do not belong to the dominant system, e.g., those from differing cultural, social, or economic backgrounds, may see themselves as being quite different from their friends. In such cases the utilization of family networks may prove helpful.

CAREER PLANS

Some adolescents enter high school with a definite idea of what they would like to do. Many, however, are unsure of what they want. In order to choose a career that he or she is best suited for, the teenager must first know the self and believe he has choices. What particularly interests him? What is she good at? What are the shortcomings?

By this time the boy or girl has already taken some rather definite steps toward a goal. Completing high school, choice of high school curriculum, and grades determine eligibility for college entrance or preparation for a specific vocation. Parents should observe the interests of their children and encourage them to take advantage of their particular talents. Whenever possible, a teenager should investigate various fields by talking to people who are involved in them. Valuable information also can be obtained by career exploration, which is available at most colleges, and by pamphlets from professional organizations, the government, and other sources. The school guidance counselor administers aptitude tests as an additional guide and can work with the teenager to expose the child to as wide a selection of careers as possible. The final decision must be made by the adolescent. If persons are to be happy in their

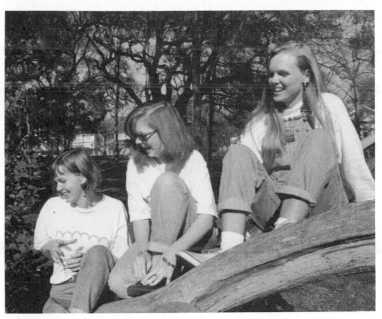

▲ **FIGURE 15–6**

The peer group is often the adolescent's "safety net" in the search for independence and identity. (Courtesy of Vickie Ashwill.)

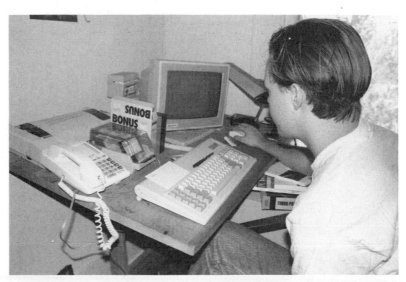

▲ **FIGURE 15–7**

The adolescent lives in a highly technical world that challenges the mind and offers a vast selection of careers. (Courtesy of Vickie Ashwill.)

work, they must choose it of their own free will, not because the parents expect them to follow in their footsteps.

As a result of the feminist movement, more types of work are open to young women. Many are selecting careers that will support an independent lifestyle, although they may choose to marry. Women also make up a larger proportion of the work force and are being introduced to more nontraditional jobs. Nevertheless, teenagers face more unemployment than adults, and young women experience a higher rate of unemployment than young men.

The job market today is extremely competitive and almost nonexistent for those without skills or education; unemployment is high among minority groups, and in some geographic locales. The causes for this are multifold, but the results are often feelings of hopelessness and decreased self-esteem in the individual. Productive employment of young people needs to fit into their total framework of life and also offer an opportunity for personality growth. Some constructive aspects of employment include helping build self-esteem, promoting responsibility, testing new skills, constructively channeling energies, providing money for increased independence, engaging young persons in interactions with adults, and allowing them to assume an active rather than a passive role. In contrast, when adolescents are forced to take a job because of economic or personal pressures, they may have to drop out of school. With few skills and no experience, they may remain locked in low level employment. This is often perpetuated from one generation to another.

RESPONSIBILITY

Young people look forward to challenges. Parents must watch for ways that they may free their children to take on new responsibilities. Even routine jobs can be made more inspiring if youths are taught to see them in relation to their overall objective. Astronauts have a certain amount of dull routine to their jobs; so do doctors, nurses, and scientists. They are able to accept routine tasks because they contribute to the effectiveness of the entire project. Young adolescents must also

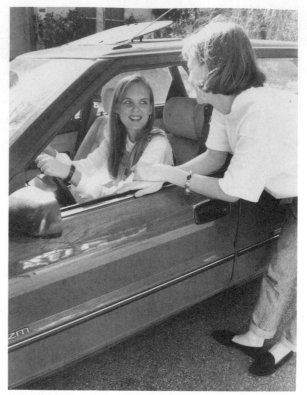

▲ FIGURE 15–8

With new independence comes responsibility. (Courtesy of Vickie Ashwill.)

be taught the value of money. An allowance helps them learn management. If money is simply handed out as requested, it is more difficult to develop a sense of responsibility regarding finances. Allowances should be increased from time to time to comply with the age and needs of the teenager.

Middle and older adolescents who have jobs can be taught the use of a checkbook and a savings account. Many find satisfaction in being able to purchase their own clothes. If a boy or girl buys an old car, he or she will soon discover it takes money to run and repair it. Experiences such as this provide valuable lessons in finance. A common way of earning money among younger teenagers is babysitting. Many boys and girls begin to babysit at about 12 or 13 years of age. Babysitting courses are valuable, as these young people need to be prepared for this important responsibility.

EMOTIONAL NEEDS

Teenagers worry a lot. They are able to talk about fears that are not too intimate, such as school examinations, how they will look with this or that type of haircut, and so on. They need assistance, nevertheless, in getting in touch with their feelings and in sorting out confused feelings. Adults must provide a confidential, accepting atmosphere in order to foster quality communication. One of the more difficult aspects of communicating with adolescents is their fluctuating attitudes. They may vary from unconcern about deadlines to panic. They may wish to please but be overly critical of themselves and their own performance. They may try to control others by overtalkativeness and a desire to demonstrate competence. Physical symptoms such as stomach aches, dizziness, headaches, and insomnia surface and disappear periodically. Anxiety over future events, the possibilities of injury, relationships with peers, and meeting expectations of others are also prevalent. Teenagers often experience their parents' pain and feel tremendously responsible for the family's burdens and failures. For many, the image of what a family should be is derived from television. Adolescents who have lifetime handicaps, alcoholic parents, physical or mental illness, or other serious problems such as poverty need the support of the medical community and other community resources. Bizarre behavior may signal a call for long overdue help.

DAYDREAMS

Adolescents spend a lot of time daydreaming, in the solitude of their rooms or during a biology lecture. Most of this is normal and natural for this age group. Daydreaming is usually considered harmless if the young person continues usual active pursuits. It also serves several purposes. Adolescence is a lonely, in-between age; daydreaming helps fill the void. Acting out imaginatively what will be said or done in various situations prepares teenagers to deal with others, so that when confronted with real situations they are better able to cope. Daydreams are also a valuable safety valve for the expression of strong feelings.

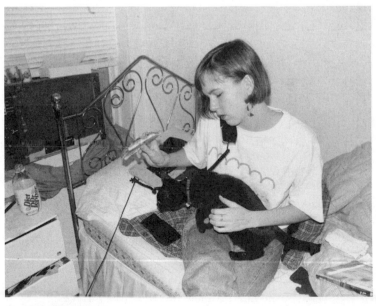

▲ FIGURE 15–9

The telephone is the teenager's link to the world and peer support. (Courtesy of Vickie Ashwill.)

HETEROSEXUAL RELATIONSHIPS

Adolescents need to meet and become acquainted with members of the opposite sex. This may begin by admiration from afar, which is accompanied by daydreams as the young person attempts to attract the attention of the object of her or his concentration. Competition and rivalry may be keen. The person may date a number of people or merely one. Dates may be frequent or sporadic.

The adolescent's cultural background has an influence on patterns of dating. Conflict often arises when the teenager wants to be independent and quickly adopt American norms of dating while parents insist on strict traditional values. This is particularly noticeable with daughters.

Dating represents one of the early social decision points of growing up. As such, it may serve as a battleground for the struggle for independence. Parental opposition is often based on unspoken fears of rejection and the adolescent's increased sexual experience and/or pregnancy. Parents may respond by imposing strict restrictions in regard to curfews, chaperones, use of the car, and so on. When these problems are not discussed openly with the young person, the adolescent may react by rebelling, by sexual acting out, or by other means designed to test injunctions of control, rather than out of a desire for the sexual act itself.

Parenting

It is difficult at times for parents to cope with adolescents. The shift that has occurred in parenting philosophy, from the rigid rules of discipline, to permissiveness, to the current middle-of-the-road position, leads to confusion. Some parents are unsure of their own opinions and may hesitate to exert authority. Others refuse to change any of their beliefs to accommodate youth. The teenager who is the subject of heavy concentrations of parental attention can become overanxious. Mothers have a particular problem because they have to find substitute satisfactions for the loss of a dependent child. As adolescents mature, they become more secure and are able to develop a new and more satisfactory relationship with parents.

Foster and associates define the task of the parent of an adolescent as "to provide security and reliability through clear, reasonable limits and communication of expectations for acceptable behavior" (Foster and colleagues, 1989). Adolescence may be one of the greatest parenting challenges. Parents need to be reassured that all parents make mistakes with their children. This may be an excellent time for parents to role model for their children the ability to say, "I'm sorry," or "I made a bad decision." Parents should be encouraged to know their children's friends and parents, become involved in their school and activities, and keep open lines of communication. The parent must

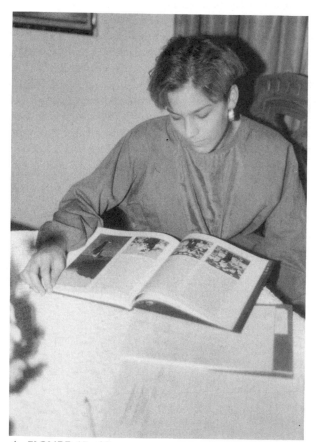

▲ **FIGURE 15–10**

Study time may become an issue between teenagers and their parents. Parental expectations of children should be realistic and should encourage a child to take responsibility for learning. Accepting the consequences of failure to do this can be a growth experience for the adolescent.

allow the teenager to make mistakes and assume the responsibility for individual actions. Parents who are experiencing difficulties in parenting may be referred for professional help.

Health Education and Guidance

NUTRITION

Teenagers are growing rapidly; therefore, they need foods that provide for the increase in height, body-cell mass, and maturation. Dietary deficiencies are more apt to occur at this age because of this acceleration and because eating patterns become more irregular. Adolescents require adequate intake of nutrients and calories regardless of chronological age.

The most noticeable changes in the adolescent's eating habits are skipping meals, increased between-meal snacks, and increased eating out. Breakfast and lunch are often omitted. Part-time jobs, school activities, and socialization may result in the teenager's eating little or nothing during the day and then catching up in the evening. Fast food restaurants are inexpensive and quick for the busy adolescent. These foods tend to be high in calories, fat, protein, sugar, and sodium, and low in fiber. Most fast food chains have added salad bars and other more "healthy" foods, which is to be commended. These appeal to the diet-conscious teenage girl and to vegetarians. Carbonated drinks often replace milk, resulting in low intakes of calcium, riboflavin, and vitamins A and D. The few fruits and vegetables eaten provide insufficient fiber.

Nutritional research pertaining to this age group is still meager, partly because studies must account not only for age but also for physical maturity. Minerals most apt to be in inadequate supply in the adolescent diet are calcium and iron. *Zinc* is known to be essential for growth and sexual maturation and is therefore of great importance in adolescence. The retention of zinc increases especially during the growth spurt, leading to more efficient use of sources of this nutrient in the diet (Krause and Mahan, 1984). Good sources of zinc include meat, liver, eggs, and seafood, particularly oysters. Sources for vegetarians include nuts, beans, wheat germ, and cheese. The importance of *calcium* lies in its key role in bone formation. In both boys and girls the recommended dietary allowance (RDA) for calcium increases from 800 mg at age 10 years to 1200 mg during the growth spurt. The primary source of calcium is dairy products. The need for *iron* is increased in both sexes at this time. This increased need is due primarily to increases in muscle mass and blood volume in boys and to a lesser degree in girls. A menstruating woman loses 15 to 30 mg of iron per cycle. Iron absorption varies in individuals. Good sources of iron include liver, poultry, fish, dried beans, vegetables, egg yolk, and enriched breads.

Sports and Nutrition. The best training diet is one that contains foods from each of the basic four food groups in sufficient quantities to meet energy demands and nutrient requirements. There is no evidence that eating large amounts of special foods or nutrients is beneficial in terms of athletic performance. Protein supplements are not necessary and could even be harmful. Sweat losses must be replaced by drinking small amounts of fluid during the workout. Thirst is the best guide for intake. Carbohydrates should not be used as the sole energy source, as they are stored for relatively short spans in the body. Sodium and potassium replacement usually will be met by eating a well-balanced diet. Caffeine and alcohol deplete body water and are to be avoided. Anabolic steroids, used by some athletes to gain weight and increase strength, are detrimental to bone growth. Iron is particularly necessary for female athletes, who may be borderline or deficient in their intake of this mineral. On the day of the event, the athlete is advised to eliminate roughage, fats, and gas-forming foods.

NURSING CARE

Adolescent girls have special nutritional needs. They have fewer caloric requirements than boys do. There is a concern with body image that may lead to anorexia or bulimia. The nurse should emphasize that "skipping meals" can lead to decrease in essential nutrients. Encourage physical exercise to maintain body weight, as well as nu-

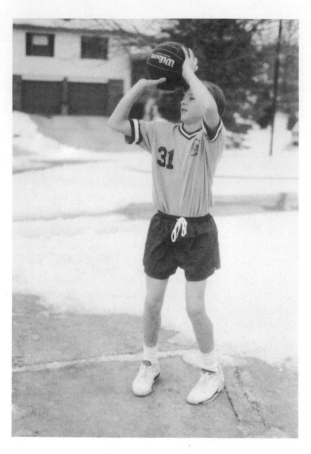

▲ FIGURE 15–11

The adolescent should be involved in some type of activity that involves exercise. Many teenagers choose organized sports.

tritious foods that are low in calories, e.g., skim milk, fruits. The adolescent should avoid high-calorie fast foods. Besides salad bars, many fast food chains have added grilled and high fiber foods to their menu.

Many adolescent boys are concerned with their body image and body building. They should have a well-balanced diet with increased calories. Part of the dietary requirement is proper hydration without supplements. Overeating can lead to adult obesity.

Adolescents who are obese will need guidance in weight reduction. They should be instructed to

▲ Eat a variety of foods low in calories and high in nutrients
▲ Eat less fat and fewer fatty foods
▲ Eat less sugar and sweets
▲ Drink less alcohol

▲ Eat more fruits, vegetables, and whole grains
▲ Increase physical activity

Physical Examination. The prevention of illness in this age group, as in all others, is of primary importance. Yearly physical examinations are recommended for healthy adolescents. In reality, this is often obtained as a requirement for the young person to enter a certain sport. Locker room physical examinations can vary greatly in their thoroughness. Immunizations need to be reviewed and updated. Rubella titer should be obtained in all girls. Those found to lack protective levels should be immunized regardless of any history of previous infection or immunizations. The young woman is instructed to avoid pregnancy for at least 2 months after immunization.

The American Academy of Pediatrics currently recommends that a second dose of the measles vaccine be given at 11 to 12 years of age. It is further recommended that college entrants and persons starting employment in medical facilities have two doses or other evidence of measles immunity (documented physician diagnosis or laboratory evidence of immunity) (Markowitz and Orenstein, 1990).

Many other screening programs are conducted in the schools and community. Deficits of vision and hearing, scoliosis, or high blood pressure may be detected.

A menstrual history and gynecological examination should be a routine part of the assessment of the adolescent girl. In sexually active teenagers, screening for common sexually transmitted diseases (STDs) should be done (Green and Haggerty, 1990).

PERSONAL CARE

Sleep. Sleep requirements vary from individual to individual. Adolescents may obtain the 8 hours generally suggested but often at irregular hours. Many young people who are employed have to work very late hours, particularly in the summer months. This necessitates sleeping later in the morning. Another trend is for the young person who has worked long hours during the day to try to make up for lost time after work. It would seem that adolescents are either sleeping all the time or burning the candle at both ends! Complaints of fatigue are heard more often at home than elsewhere. The nurse should advise parents to become aware of the young person's sleep patterns. Crankiness, frustration, impatience, accident proneness, and other such behaviors may be precipitated by lack of sleep. The teenager needs a bed with a firm mattress, preferably in a room of her or his own.

Exercise. Exercise has many benefits. One does not have to participate actively in sports per se to derive the benefits from a brisk walk, bike ride, or swim. Many teenagers are not athletes by choice but can benefit from a less sedentary life style. These patterns, when carried over into adulthood, contribute to good health.

Personal Hygiene. Personal hygiene information is necessary at this time when the body changes of puberty require more frequent bathing and the use of deodorants. Hair removal, menstrual hygiene, and cosmetics in general are topics regarding which the nurse can help the young person sort out the various claims of reliability for products and procedures. Ear piercing should be performed by an experienced person. The skin around the point of insertion of the earring is inspected regularly for signs of infection. Swapping of earrings is discouraged.

Clothing. Clothing is of great interest to the adolescent. Peer influence and the media have a high impact on fashion. How adolescents dress may indicate the peer group they belong to. Dress varies from very contemporary to conservative, depending on the particular teenager's preferences. Much of this is just fun and provides a good entry for conversation with this age group. The power of television advertising in regard to clothes sales and other commercial messages may be explored.

Safety. The chief hazard to the adolescent is the automobile. Road accidents kill and cripple teenagers at alarming rates. Many schools today offer driver training courses as an integral part of the educational program. Students learn how to drive and what responsibilities accompany it; however, this does not assure compliance. Preventing motor vehicle accidents is of utmost importance to every community. Adolescents who ride motorcycles, motor scooters, or motorbikes should know the rules of the road and should wear special safety equipment, such as helmets, for protection.

Although most adolescents know how to swim, accidents occur from diving into unsafe areas and the use of alcohol or drugs while playing in the water. Both accidental and deliberate morbidity and mortality caused by firearms continue to be a major concern during the adolescent period. The adolescent's feeling of "it couldn't happen to me" plagues this group in handling firearms. Gang-related injuries and deaths are often related to the use of firearms. Gun control continues to be controversial. At the very least, control must be stringent for this age group, and respect and safety for the use of firearms must be taught.

DENTAL CARE

The prevalence of tooth decay has decreased substantially over the past few years. This is believed to be due to the widespread use of fluorides, including community fluoridation, and the use of dental products containing fluorides. Teenagers nonetheless are at risk for dental caries because of inadequate dental maintenance and frequent snacking on sucrose-containing candies and beverages. When dental hygiene is neglected, the period of greatest tooth decay in the permanent teeth is from ages 12 to 18 years. Lack of oral hygiene (inadequate brushing, flossing, and rinsing, particularly after meals) fosters the accumulation of plaque and food debris. Missing, aching, or decayed teeth contribute to poor nutrition. Young people with unattractive teeth may suffer from feelings of low self-esteem. Healthy white teeth are synonymous with popularity and sex appeal according to media hype. A visit to the dentist twice a year is out of reach for many financially strapped young persons. For others it is a low family financial priority. There is a need for more school dental programs and other innovative measures to reach a major proportion of our society. Dental insurance, while helpful, is generally available only for fully employed persons.

References

Beall, S., and Schmidt, G. (1984). Development of a youth adaptation scale. *J. School Health* Vol. 54.

Brittain, C. (1967). An exploration of the bases of peer-compliance and parent-compliance in adolescence. *Adolescence* 2:445–458.

Brown, B. (1983). Growing up healthy: The Chinese experience. *Pediatr. Nurs.*, July-Aug.

Castiglia, P. (1990). Adolescent mothers. *J. Pediatr. Health Care*, Sept.-Oct., pp. 262–264.

Ching, C. (1984). Vietnamese in America: A case study in cross-cultural health education. *Health Values*, May–June.

Foster, R., Hunsberger, M., and Anderson, J. (1989). *Family-Centered Nursing Care of Children*. Philadelphia, W. B. Saunders Company.

Ginott, H. (1971). *Between Parent and Teenager*. New York, Avon Books.

Green, M., and Haggerty, R. (1990). *Ambulatory Pediatrics*. Philadelphia, W. B. Saunders Company.

Krause, M., and Mahan, L. (1984). *Food, Nutrition, and Diet Therapy*. Philadelphia, W. B. Saunders Company.

Levine, M., Carey, W., Crocker, A., and Gross, R. (1983). *Developmental-Behavioral Pediatrics*. Philadelphia, W. B. Saunders Company.

Markowitz, L., and Orenstein, W. (1990). Measles vaccines. *Pediatr. Clin. North Am.*, pp. 603–625.

Orr, D., Wilbrandt, M., Brack, C., Rauch, S., and Ingersoll, G. (1989). Reported sexual behaviors and self-esteem among young adolescents. *Am. J. Dis. Child.*, 143:86–90.

Schell, R., and Hall, E. (1983). *Developmental Psychology Today*, 4th ed. New York, Random House.

Vaughan, V., and Litt, I. (1990). *Child and Adolescent Development*. Philadelphia, W. B. Saunders Company.

Bibliography

Behrman, R., and Kliegman, R. (1990). *Nelson Essentials Of Pediatrics*. Philadelphia, W. B. Saunders Company.

Braden, W. (1989). History and definition of adolescence. *In* Brown, E., and Hendee, W. (eds.). Adolescent Health: Synopsis of the First Annual American Medical Association Congress on Adolescent Health. *Am. J. Dis. Child.* 143:466–467.

Erikson, E. (1965). *Challenge of Youth*. Garden City, New York, Anchor Books.

Erikson, E. (1968). *Identity, Youth, and Crisis*. New York, W. W. Norton & Company.

Freiberg, K. (1987). *Human Development: A Life-Span Approach*. Boston, Jones and Bartlett Publishers.

Gortmaker, S., Walker, D., Weitzman, M., and Sobol, A. (1990). Chronic conditions, socioeconomic risks, and behavioral problems in children and adolescents. *Pediatrics* 85:267–276.

Irwin, C. (1989). Risk taking behaviors in the adolescent patient: Are they impulsive? *Pediatr. Ann.* 18:122–133.

Jack, M. (1989). Personal fable: A potential explanation for risk-taking behavior in adolescents. *J. Pediatr. Nurs.* 4:334–338.

Mott, S., James, S., and Sperhac, A. (1990). *Nursing Care of Children and Families*. Redwood City, Cal., Addison-Wesley.

Smith, K., Turner, J., and Jacobsen, R. (1987). Health concerns of adolescents. *Pediatr. Nurs.* 13:311–315.

Whaley, L., and Wong, D. (1987). *Nursing Care of Infants and Children*. St. Louis, C. V. Mosby Company.

STUDY QUESTIONS

1. Define the following: preadolescence; puberty; menstruation; menarche; self-image.
2. Identify the physiological changes that occur during puberty and adolescence.
3. Pedro and Maria are each beginning to establish a sense of identity. What does this mean? How may this development be reflected in their behavior?

4. Do you think that you were well prepared for the changes that took place at puberty? How might you have been helped to meet this adjustment more satisfactorily?

5. At what age do you think heterosexual relationships should begin? What anticipatory guidance is required to adequately prepare young persons for this event?

6. Plan a day's menu for 15 year old Susan and 17 year old Ron. What are their nutritional requirements in terms of calories, protein, calcium, and iron?

7. Janet is 18 and a freshman in college. She has not yet selected a major field of study because she is not sure what she wants to do. What information would you need to know about Janet to guide her in this decision?

8. Alice, age 16 years, spends a great deal of her time daydreaming. Of what value is this to her? How can it be detrimental?

9. Identify the common anxieties and fears of adolescents and suggest ways in which they might try to conceal them.

10. What are the advantages of special clinics for teenagers? Discuss the particular "needs" that such facilities try to meet.

CHAPTER 16 _____

Chapter Outline

NURSING GOALS IN THE CARE OF THE
  HOSPITALIZED ADOLESCENT
LYMPHATIC SYSTEM
  Hodgkin Disease
DIGESTIVE SYSTEM
  Obesity
  Anorexia Nervosa
  Bulimia
THE BLOOD
  Infectious Mononucleosis
SKELETAL SYSTEM
  Scoliosis
  Sports Injuries
THE SKIN
  Acne Vulgaris
REPRODUCTIVE SYSTEM
  Dysmenorrhea (Primary)
  Sexually Transmitted Diseases
    Overview
    Gonorrhea
    Nongonococcal Urethritis (NGU)
    Syphilis
    Genital Herpes
  Adolescent Pregnancy
MALADAPTIVE REACTIONS TO THE STRESS OF
  ADOLESCENCE
  Depression and Suicide
  Substance Abuse
    Teenage Alcoholism
    Children of Alcoholics
    Marijuana

Objectives

Upon completion and mastery of Chapter 16, the
student will be able to

- Differentiate between the illness and
  hospitalization of an adolescent and that of a
  younger child.
- List and define the more common disorders of
  adolescents.
- Discuss the nursing goals for the hospitalized
  adolescent.
- Develop a nursing care plan for the adolescent
  receiving chemotherapy.
- Formulate a nursing care plan designed to help a
  16 year old girl with scoliosis adjust to
  confinement in a Risser cast, including nursing
  goals to prevent physical complications.
- Detail the special needs of teenagers with
  sexually transmitted disease.
- Contrast anorexia nervosa and bulimia.
- List three ways of preventing sports injuries.

DISORDERS OF THE ADOLESCENT

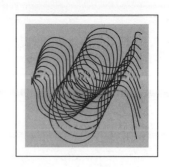

Terms

Adolescence is a relatively healthy period. Most health problems occurring at this time are not life-threatening but are of particular significance to the developing adolescent. A current area of interest in this age group is a focus on identifying the adolescent at risk for coronary heart disease as an adult.

Motor vehicle and other types of accidents are a major threat to life during adolescence and lead mortality rate lists for this age group. Suicide is also on the rise among young people. The adolescent who is handicapped or has a chronic disease may face numerous social problems at this time, as he or she works to achieve independence and make life choices. The number one cause of death, excluding accidents and violence, is cancer. The types of cancer most often seen are leukemia, lymphoma, Hodgkin disease, and bone and genital cancers.

Nursing Goals in the Care of the Hospitalized Adolescent

Early Teens. In caring for the adolescent, it is important that nursing plans be oriented to the patient's age. Illness during the early teens, approximately 12 to 15 years of age, is seen mainly as a threat to body image. There is a narcissistic concern about height, weight, and sexual development. Patients are aware of heightened body sensations and often have numerous physical complaints. Intense relationships with members of one's own sex are prevalent; they precede heterosexual involvement.

According to Vaughan and Litt (1990), early adolescence is a time of self-consciousness, which results both in the increased empathy that comes from understanding the perspective of another person and in increasing self-centeredness. The young adolescent is less overwhelmed by the enforced dependency of illness and is more concerned with physical appearance, function, and mobility.

Midadolescence. During midadolescence, approximately 15 to 18 years of age, teenagers are anxious about their ability to appeal to the opposite sex and to meet sex role expectations. Physical growth is practically complete. The peer group assumes greater importance in determining acceptability and behavior. This period often begins with group dating, followed by "going together." These relationships are no longer narcissistic reflections but begin to show signs of mutual caring, affection, and responsibility. During midadolescence the emancipation struggle within the family, although erratic, is at its peak. This is disturbing not only to the child but also to parents, who must relinquish much of their control and allow a certain amount of testing by their offspring. They may also experience a real sense of loss. Hospitalization is least tolerated by this age group. The dependency and decreased control of life when hospitalized conflict with their strong drive for independence.

Late Adolescence. Late adolescence, from approximately 17 to 22 years, is mainly concerned with the task of education, career, marriage, children, community, and style of life. The dating partner becomes the person of primary importance. Although hospitalization may pose the threat of postponement of career and future plans, hospitalization at this time is better tolerated; the older adolescent sees the family as a support system and can tolerate dependence.

ADJUSTMENT TO ILLNESS

The adolescent has many intellectual strengths, including the ability to think abstractly and to solve problems. Adolescents can understand the implications of their disease both in the present and in the future and are capable of participating in decisions related to treatment and care. The nurse who recognizes these skills and encourages their practice will help patients gain confidence in their intellectual abilities, thus increasing their sense of independence and self-esteem.

When hospitalization is necessary, it generates anxiety in proportion to the patient's past experiences and available strengths. The nature and treatment of the illness, the hospital environment, and the quality of support received from the medical staff, family, and peers all contribute toward adjustment. How the illness is perceived is also a major factor, sometimes more so than the seriousness of the condition.

Roommate Selection. Roommate selection, although frequently overlooked, is extremely important for this age group. Most children's hospitals have a separate unit for adolescents, and community hospitals may designate a particular wing for this age group. Many children's hospitals have a recreation room set aside for adolescents,

with games, music, and other diversions they enjoy. When special areas for teenagers are not available, they should be placed with someone near their age or in a private room where friends can visit without disturbing other patients and families. Avoid placing teenagers next to confused or disoriented, dying, or severely debilitated patients, because seeing the severely ill may increase their own stress.

Admission to the Unit. Upon arrival in the unit, introduce the patient to the staff, review routines, including any specific rules, and provide an information booklet. Repeat the information periodically and have the teenager verbalize understanding of it. Acquaint new patients with the mechanics of the unit, e.g., how to raise and lower the bed and use the call system, television, and intercom. Help them locate bathroom, kitchen, and recreational facilities. Teenagers need a bedside telephone. Explain the dialing system. They generally prefer their own clothes; however, most adolescent units keep scrub pants and tops in the unit, and the teenager usually prefers wearing these to conventional hospital garb.

The health assessment of the adolescent should include a complete psychosocial history as well as a physical examination. It is important that the adolescent be involved in the interviewing process. Some parents dominate the conversation and the child should be allowed and encouraged to take part in the admission interview. Some nurses prefer to interview the parent and child separately as well as together. It may be difficult to obtain all this information in emergency situations, but it definitely should be completed within 24 hours of admission. Such information is invaluable to the staff in anticipating behavior, identifying unmet health needs, planning care, assessing unhealthy reactions to adolescence, and determining just how the illness will affect the patient's maturation.

Communication. Keep patients informed about what to expect. This includes personnel they will be seeing and tests that will be done in the near future. Avoid childlike explanations. Allow time for questions and for patients to express their feelings. The physician should discuss with the patient just what is wrong and what can be expected of therapy. When this is not predictable, uncertainty should be shared honestly, while emphasizing that everyone is working together for the best possible outcome. This is more complex when the prognosis is poor; therefore, frequent staff conferences are needed to facilitate communication among professionals. The prognosis is shared with the patient and the family in almost all situations.

Surgery. Surgical patients need preoperative information. This includes such matters as what if any area of the body is to be shaved, why this needs to be done, and the likelihood of enemas, dietary restrictions, and medications. When possible, a visit to the recovery room is made to orient patients to postoperative surroundings. They are prepared in advance for waking up surrounded by life support systems, bandages, casts, traction or other apparatus following surgery. Also, it is important to explain to patients and the family the type of feedback system employed by the hospital immediately thereafter so that they are kept informed of progress. The inclusion of family and the sharing of feelings and ideas are extended throughout the period of confinement.

Pain. Adolescents are able to describe the location, intensity, and duration of pain. They may also verbalize the need for pain medication. Regression, withdrawal, depression, anorexia, and aggression are a few of the reactions seen in adolescents. Teenagers are advised of expected discomfort from procedures and surgery. Comfort measures should be implemented, including analgesics. The nurse should be alert for nonverbal cues of discomfort. Teenagers who have had surgery are often very cautious in the immediate postoperative period.

Staff expectations should not exceed what adolescents can do. As patients begin to take an interest in their surroundings, encourage self-care, ambulation, and socialization. Teenagers progress more slowly than their younger counterparts, and there is often a gap between how the adolescent perceives progress and how the staff perceives it. It is unlikely, however, that the exuberant teenager will succumb to a life of bed rest if given an alternative!

Behavioral Considerations. Skillful management of adolescent behavior is achieved best through careful selection of nursing staff members. The nurses working with young people must be *flexible*. Often their patients will compete for attention, so nurses must try to be as fair and impartial as possible and set limits on their behavior. Adolescents may also try to split or come between staff members. It is difficult to know how to handle the patient who instigates trouble, argues, or uses profanity. Personnel need frequent staff meetings where they can air their concerns and develop awareness about their own reactions to certain aspects of behavior in their patients. The nurse's role should be that person to whom the patient can relate in time of need. Working with this age group is a unique experience that carries its own rewards. The nurse who understands this and who is knowledgeable about the developmental and psychosocial considerations of adolescence will contribute greatly to the patient's adjustment and recovery.

COMMUNICATION ALERT ▶ ▶ ▶ ▶ ▶
Problems of confidentiality may arise between the adolescent and nurse if the nurse is not clear on this issue. Incidents that could be harmful or that the nurse can and should take action on must be communicated to other health care workers and sometimes to the family. The nurse must tell the child, "I will be with you and support you, but I must tell the doctor and your parents about your thoughts of suicide." Nurses should never say they will "keep a secret" when they have no intention of doing so.

Issues of Confidentiality and Legality. Respecting the confidentiality of the teenager is important in establishing trust. In general, information should not be divulged or shared without the patient's consent. Many problems can be avoided if the confidentiality of the relationship is clearly defined during initial meetings. At this time nurses explain to teenagers that there are two conditions that they are obligated to report: if they plan to harm themselves or if they plan to harm someone else. One guideline offered by a leading authority on medical ethics is to break confidentiality only if (1) there is a high likelihood of serious physical harm to someone, and (2) there is a clear and likely benefit from intervening (Frost, 1987).

Patient records must be carefully monitored to avoid loss or observation by unauthorized personnel. The nurse must avoid giving any private information about the teenager to telephone callers or visitors.

The *emancipated minor* is a term that generally refers to adolescents less than 18 years of age who are no longer under their parents' authority. Married minors or minors in the military are automatically considered emancipated and may give consent for medical treatment for themselves and their children. The *mature minor doctrine* recognizes that individuals mature at different rates. In most parts of the United States the young adolescent may receive medical assistance for certain conditions without parental awareness, e.g., sexually transmitted diseases, contraception, pregnancy, abortion, and drug abuse. These laws are designed to afford the young person immediate medical help without fear of reprisal. However, they are subject to controversy. All states allow minors to obtain treatment in life-threatening situations when legal guardians are not available. As laws vary from state to state, the nurse must keep informed about policies and legislation within her practice state. Such information is usually available from the local medical or nursing association office.

Chronic Illness. Chronic illness during this period of life is in direct opposition to developmental needs. Specific programs that foster feelings of security and independence within the limits of the situation are essential. Behavior problems are lessened when patients can verbalize specific concerns with persons sensitive to their problems. If they feel rejected by and different from peers, they may be prone to depression. To be in school and to be considered one of the group are important. Hospital school programs enable teenagers to keep pace with their classmates and to achieve their educational goals. Recreational programs are also helpful in combating boredom and providing outlets for tension. Nurses need to help patients to accept the body with all its strengths and imperfections. They must develop an awareness of the teenager's particular fears of forced dependence, bodily invasion, mutilation, rejection, and loss of face, especially within the peer group. The nurse should anticipate a certain amount of reluctance to adhere to hospital regulations, which reflects the adolescent's need for self-determination. Recognizing this as an asset rather than a liability enables the nurse to respond in a constructive manner.

Developmental Disabilities. The adolescent who has a developmental disability that affects the intellect or ability to cope faces some rather unique difficulties. He or she is often overprotected, unable to break away from supervision, and deprived of necessary peer relationships. The pubertal process with its emerging sexuality becomes a worrisome concern for parents and may precipitate a family crisis. It is becoming more common for hospitals to provide an interdisciplinary team that works to meet the needs of the adolescents and their families.

Home Care. Adolescents with both acute and chronic health needs are increasingly being cared for at home. Home health care agencies, public school districts, and community agencies work together to meet the physical and psychosocial needs of the patient. *Respite* care for parents provides for a helper to come into the home to relieve parents of the responsibility of caring for the child for brief periods of time. This enables the parents to shop, transact business affairs, or simply take a much needed vacation.

One mother whose 13 year old daughter had a severe developmental disability (cerebral palsy, blindness, mental retardation) offered these suggestions for the health care worker assisting in the home. (1) Observe how the parents interact with the child. (2) Do not wait for the child to cry out for attention, as the youngster may be unable to communicate in this way. (3) Watch for facial expression and body language. (4) Post signs above the bed denoting special considerations, such as never position on left side, do not feed with plastic spoon, and so on. (5) Listen to the parents and observe how they attend to the physical needs of the youngster. (6) Do not be afraid to ask questions or discuss apprehensions you may feel concerning your ability to care for the child. (7) Be attuned to the needs of other children in the home. (8) Be creative in exploring avenues for socialization, as these teenagers are seldom invited to birthday or slumber parties. (9) Explore community facilities and support groups that might be of benefit to the family.

Lymphatic System

HODGKIN DISEASE

Description. Hodgkin disease is a malignancy of the lymph system that primarily involves the lymph nodes. It may metastasize to the spleen, liver, bone marrow, lungs, or other parts of the body. The predominant cell affected is the Reed-Sternberg, which contains two nuclei and is diagnostic of the disease. Hodgkin disease is rare before 5 years of age, but the incidence increases during adolescence and early adulthood. It is twice as common in boys as in girls.

Symptoms. The presenting symptom is generally a painless lump along the cervical area of the neck. It occurs in older children and adolescents who are past the time when infections in this area are common. Occasionally, nodes of the supraclavicular, axillary, and inguinal areas are primary sites. Characteristically, there are few other manifestations. The swelling is generally first noted by the patient or the parents. In more advanced cases there may be low-grade fever, anorexia, weight loss, night sweats, general malaise, rash, and itching of the skin. Blood counts may be nonspecific. Diagnosis is confirmed by x-ray studies, CT scan, and lymphangiogram. A laparotomy may be performed to determine the stage of the disease. At this time the spleen may be removed, and biopsies of the liver, accessible nodes, and bone marrow are performed. The stages in Hodgkin disease are defined as follows:

Stage I   Disease restricted to single site or localized in a group of lymph nodes. Asymptomatic.
Stage II   Two or more lymph nodes in the area or on the same side of the diaphragm.
Stage III   Involves lymph node regions on both sides of the diaphragm, involvement of adjacent organ or spleen.
Stage IV   Diffuse disease, least favorable prognosis.

Treatment. Well-established treatment regimens are now utilized to combat this illness. Both radiation therapy and chemotherapy are used in accordance with the clinical stage of the disease. The prognosis is favorable for remission. Cure is primarily related to the stage of the disease at diagnosis.

Nursing Care

Nursing care is mainly directed to the symptomatic relief of the side effects of radiation and chemotherapy (Nursing Care Plan 16–1). Education of the patient and family is paramount, as most patients will be cared for in the home. A common side effect of radiation is malaise. The teenager tires easily and may be irritable and anorectic. The skin in the treated area may be sensitive and should be protected against exposure to sunlight and irritation. During treatment, the skin should not be exposed to sunlight. After treatment, a sun-blocking agent containing PABA should be used to prevent burning. The attending physician may prescribe an ointment to relieve itching of the skin. Nothing should be applied to the treatment area without the recommendation of the doctor. There may be diarrhea after abdominal radiation. The patient *does not* become radioactive during or after therapy.

Following splenectomy the patient faces the long-term risk of serious infection. This is explained to the parents and teenager. Elevations of temperature need to be monitored carefully. There may also be infection with little or no fever as a result of masking by certain medications. In such cases throat cultures may need to be taken as well as cultures of blood, urine, sputum, or stool. Instruct parents or the adolescent to feel free to call the clinic, particularly if there is a change in the condition or if they are apprehensive or confused about symptoms. Medication readjustments should not be attempted unless specifically advised by the physician. Emotional support of the teenager should be age-appropriate. Nurses must be prepared in particular for periods of anger, which may be directed at them. Suitable exercise, such as the use of a punching bag, allows for safe direction of anger. Routine use will help prevent unnecessary build-up of tension. Activity in general is regulated by the patient. The physician will advise the patient if special precautions are necessary.

CARE PLAN 16–1

THE ADOLESCENT RECEIVING CANCER CHEMOTHERAPY

Nursing Diagnosis	Goals/Outcome Criteria	Nursing Intervention
Knowledge deficit, related to prevention of infection due to myelosuppression	Child will understand disease and treatment and remain free of infection Child will remain free of infection as evidenced by temperature between 36.5 and 37.6°C (97.7 and 99.6°F) and intact skin and mucous membranes	Instruct patient about body's immune system and immunotherapy as age-appropriate; use visual aids Monitor WBC and interpret blood values at patient's level of understanding Place patient in private room, avoid crowds, practice proper handwashing and good personal hygiene, monitor .temperature Observe mouth and perianal area for infection Use soft toothbrush, Water-pik, soothing mouthwashes Limit exposure to direct sunlight
Hemorrhage, potential for, related to platelet deficit from bone marrow suppression	Child will not hemorrhage Child will show no signs of bleeding, as evidenced by stable vital signs and absence of hematuria, petechiae, and ecchymosis	Observe for hematuria, hematemesis, melena, epistaxis, petechiae, ecchymosis Increase fluid intake Use local measures if necessary to control bleeding Monitor platelet counts and assist patient in types of safe activity when count is low
Nutrition, alterations in, related to stomatitis, nausea, and vomiting	Child will maintain nutritional status Child will not lose weight and will eat 60% of diet	Inspect mouth daily for ulcerations Serve bland, moist, soft diet Apply local anesthetics to ulcerated areas before meals Monitor weight Alert patient to expected reactions to treatment protocol Give antiemetic prior to onset of nausea and vomiting Suggest appropriate relaxation techniques

CARE PLAN 16–1 *Continued*

THE ADOLESCENT RECEIVING CANCER CHEMOTHERAPY

Nursing Diagnosis	Goals/Outcome Criteria	Nursing Intervention
Self-concept; disturbance in body image, related to moon face, hair loss; patient may have amputation	Child will maintain positive self-concept Child will discuss feelings concerning body changes	Allow teenager to ventilate feelings Provide continuity of care Utilize wigs, scarfs, eyebrow pencil, false eyelashes; stress hair loss is temporary Suggest clothing that will minimize body changes and enhance appearance Assess level of knowledge concerning situation Have patient draw self-portrait: "How I see myself, how others see me" Discuss this
Self-concept, disturbance in self-esteem, independent/dependence tasks	Child will maintain independence Child will participate in care of self, as evidenced by giving self bath, feeding self, and ambulating outside room	Involve patient in decision-making as age appropriate; denial of this will increase noncompliance Set appropriate limits on disruptive behavior Avoid overprotection, overattention, overanxiety Encourage peers to visit, phone, send cards
Social isolation related to interrupted schooling, rejection by peers	Child will maintain contact with support system Child will show signs of contact with support system, as evidenced by friends visiting and calling and verbalizing plans that involve peers	Provide opportunity for "rap" sessions with peers Encourage letter writing, phone calls Suggest cancer camp Respect privacy with adolescent visitors Contact spiritual advisor, church youth groups, etc.

Continued on following page

CARE PLAN 16–1 *Continued*

THE ADOLESCENT RECEIVING CANCER CHEMOTHERAPY

Nursing Diagnosis	Goals/Outcome Criteria	Nursing Intervention
Fear of death related to treatment or nature of disease	Child will express fears, anxiety, and concern regarding death Child will establish trusting relationship in which child will feel free to express fears regarding disease and possibility of death	Convey empathic understanding of patient's and family's worries, fears, and doubts Determine patient's perception of diagnosis, e.g., "What are your concerns?" Ascertain response of family/significant others to patient's concerns Support "hope" by clarifying, and by educating patient about, the disease and side effects Develop listening skills, be alert for nonverbal cues of anxiety Avoid discounting the patient by statements such as "I know exactly how you feel," "You shouldn't feel that way," or by changing the subject Draw "strongest feeling I've had today" Discuss

Digestive System

OBESITY

Description. Obesity, or *overnutrition*, is the accumulation of excess body fat. It is the most common nutritional disorder in Western society today, and its treatment record is dismal. Obesity is difficult to define during adolescence because of height and age variations within this age group. Some definitions include a body weight 20 per cent or more over ideal body weight based on weight tables and triceps skinfolds exceeding 85 per cent (Behrman and Kliegman, 1990). Weight for height measurements may be confusing and result in a muscular child being labeled as obese. An increase in lean body mass and fat is characteristic of this age group; therefore, one must know what stage of puberty the teenager is in and

whether or not she or he has completed the growth spurt.

Weight gain may occur at any age but appears most frequently in the first year of life, at 5 to 6 years of age, and during adolescence. Most children stay plump during puberty and then return to their normal size.

Self-Concept. Obesity becomes particularly significant during adolescence, when feelings of inadequacy are pronounced. Obese adolescents are concerned about their appearance but are unable to conform to the standards of the group. They are often the subject of cruel ridicule. For instance, overweight males frequently appear to have developed breasts, white striae may appear on the abdomen, and the penis appears disproportionately small. Obese teenagers date less and may feel rejected, unattractive, and unloved. Accompanying the mental anxieties are the more obvious physical handicaps. They may be unable to participate in sports or other school activities and are more accident prone. Their choice of careers is more limited.

Causes. There are many theories concerning the causes of obesity. In reality, the etiology is very complex. The onset of obesity can be traced to excess food, reduced physical activity, or both. Contrary to popular belief, obesity due to abnormal function of the glands is rare. Genetic studies have shown that there is an increased incidence of obesity in twins, even though they may have been raised in separate homes. Children born to obese parents are more likely to become obese. However, environmental factors such as ethnic diet, family eating practices, and psychological factors are also operating, making it difficult to isolate these from genetic factors.

The risk of obesity persisting into adulthood increases with a more advanced onset (adolescence vs. infancy) and severity of obesity (Behrman and Kliegman, 1990). The longer the adolescent is overweight, the more difficult it is to overcome the problem. This phenomenon is described as the "set point" theory. The set point is defended by the channeling of energy to maintain a certain rather narrow range of body weight (Pipes, 1989). The only way to break the chain is to decrease intake and increase the amount of energy used through activity.

Prevention. The prevention of obesity in children is important. The earlier in life this begins the better. Identification of the infant or child at risk is necessary while the child is still under parental control, and before eating and activity patterns are firmly established. Breast feeding is desirable for infants, in that sufficient quantities of milk are obtained and there is less chance of overfeeding. Solid foods should be delayed until 6 months of age. Mothers should be informed that a baby's food requirements diminish greatly as growth slows at about the first year. Overfeeding should be discouraged, as "fat babies are not necessarily healthy babies." Parents should be told that a crying baby does not necessarily mean that the infant is hungry.

Parents should foster activities that promote freedom of movement and exercise during the first few years of life. If there are any questions concerning weight gain, these should be voiced during well-baby conferences.

During the school years nutritious snacks rather than junk foods should be kept in the home. Television viewing should be restricted and walking and other exercise encouraged. Parents need to promote participation in a regular exercise program. Sound nutritional practices are of particular importance during puberty when there is an increase in fat cells. The teenager is capable of assuming responsibility for what she or he eats. If a weight problem exists at this time, remember, "Unlike adults, a reasonable goal is not always weight loss but may be just a slowing down of the weight gain or maintenance of body weight until linear growth occurs" (Neumann, 1983).

Helping the child feel good about the self by encouragement, praise, and support is essential. The depressed young person may turn toward food as an outlet for emotions. Be generous and specific with your praise. Sprinkle your conversation with such comments as, "I knew you could do it." "That's quite an improvement." "You made it look easy." "I couldn't have done better myself." This type of positive approach may help the child or young person feel better about the self and decrease the need to overeat.

Treatment and Nursing Care

Dieting is difficult. When the problem begins in early childhood, a person is faced with a lifetime of fighting calories. This is complicated by the fact that food is readily available in the United States, and advertisers bombard the public with tempting treats. Parents must be keenly interested in helping their child to control the weight if the diet is to be successful. Sometimes it is necessary for the entire family to go without some of the richer dishes. They should refrain from buying cookies and cakes, and fresh fruits should be substituted as between-meal snacks. The nurse should emphasize the fact that diets must be carefully planned and based on accurate nutrition information. Adolescents are apt to go on diets that they invent themselves and that are dangerous to their health. Whenever such a major satisfaction as eating is denied, it must be replaced with something equally satisfying and rewarding, such as new social activities, hobbies, friends, or sports.

Behavior modification techniques show promise, although their long-term value has not yet been established. This approach helps a person identify and control poor eating patterns. Such techniques include eating only at the table, using a smaller plate, eating only at specific times, recording food intake and feelings at the time of eating, and so on. A point system or system of rewards is established upon initiation of this technique. Groups such as Weight Watchers, Overeaters Anonymous, or diet workshops, although helpful, are frequented mostly by adults. A few parents accompany their teenagers and participate themselves.

Support groups for adolescents are more acceptable. These are usually found in teenage clinics, schools, and specialized summer camps. Diet pills are not recommended. Their long-term effectiveness is minimal and the potential for misuse by the teenager is high. Jejunoileal bypass has many complications and is seldom advised unless the child is morbidly obese. The long-term consequences of these procedures have yet to be established.

The nurse interested in helping teenagers in weight reduction can play an important role. Many nurses are or have been personally involved with losing weight and know how frustrating this can be. Motivating the adolescent requires ingenuity and patience. A sense of hope must be instilled and the adolescent must be involved in the treatment plan. Positive parent involvement seems to increase the chances of the teenager's being successful. Failure is almost certain if the parent is committed to weight reduction and the child is not. Nurses should approach the obese adolescent in a nonthreatening way. They should try to recognize achievements and increase the adolescent's self-esteem. The basic dignity of the individual should always be foremost. Family therapy may be necessary to alleviate tension and promote understanding; nurses can assist in the referral process. They can also be the source of contact for a registered dietitian.

ANOREXIA NERVOSA

Description. Anorexia nervosa is an eating disorder characterized by self-imposed starvation due to the relentless pursuit of thinness and the mor-

bid fear of fatness. This includes varying degrees of emaciation and is accompanied by medical and psychiatric problems (Goldbloom & Garfinkel, 1990). The disorder occurs primarily in girls and affects about 1 per cent of American teenagers. The adolescent sees herself as being fat even in stages of advanced emaciation (Fig. 16–1). The term anorexia is misleading since many patients do not suffer from a lack of appetite. Instead they experience intense hunger, which they deny or satisfy by eating binges. A combination of factors may cause the disease, including genetic or physiological predisposition, sociocultural influences, and impaired psychological development.

Patients with anorexia come from model middle

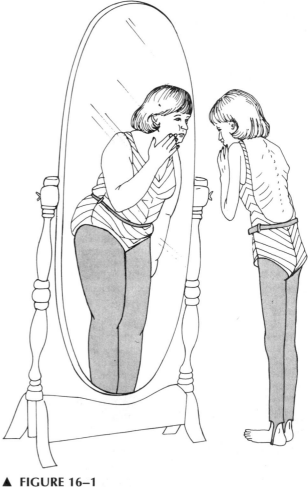

▲ **FIGURE 16–1**

Patients with eating disorders often have a disturbance in self-image.

to upper class families. They have average to superior intelligence and are generally overachievers who expect to be perfect in all areas. Their emerging sexuality is very threatening to these young women. They experience anxiety and guilt over fancied or real fear of intimacy.

Some theorists believe that families of these young people are dysfunctional. They may exhibit such behaviors as overprotectiveness, rigidity, lack of privacy, and inability to resolve conflicts. In addition, the patient's illness may serve to maintain family balance, as the parents focus on the needs of the child and thus avoid other internal conflicts.

Symptoms. Early signs and symptoms may be vague and in retrospect may be seen to have begun with a diet. Table 16–1 lists early signs and symptoms of the disease. As the patient's weight drops, her sense of being overweight rises. Despite lack of intake, the patient has a great deal of energy and may exercise strenuously to reduce. The onset can often be pinpointed to the young girl's inability to wear some of her clothes or to life changes such as a move, parental divorce, or the death of a relative or close friend. Upon physical examination some of the following conditions may be evident: dry skin, amenorrhea, lanugo hair over the back and extremities, cold intolerance, low blood pressure, abdominal pain, and constipation. Electrolyte imbalance may be noticeable in the patient who induces vomiting or uses laxatives or diuretics.

Teenagers with anorexia experience feelings of helplessness, lack of control, low self-esteem, and depression. Socialization with peers diminishes. Mealtime becomes a family battleground. The patient feels guilty and may go on an eating binge, which is followed by self-induced vomiting as the fear of gaining weight returns. Persistent vomiting can cause erosion of the enamel of the teeth and eventually cause tooth decay. The perception of body image becomes increasingly disturbed and there is a lack of self-identity. The young person remains egocentric and unable to resolve normal adolescent tasks. The relentless pursuit to be thin may lead to shoplifting of laxatives and other associated items. Although eating less, the anorectic patient is preoccupied with food and its preparation. Hunger is denied. The patient complains of bloating and abdominal pain after small amounts of food are ingested.

Treatment and Nursing Care

The treatment of anorexia is complex and involves several modalities. A brief period of hospitalization may be necessary to correct electrolyte imbalance, establish minimal restoration of nutrients, and stabilize the patient's weight. Therapies include psychotherapy, behavioral therapy, drug therapy, and family therapy. Nasogastric feedings and total parenteral nutrition are usually used only when other means have failed because they are only a temporary answer to a much larger problem. They do not reflect normal eating patterns.

The nurse can play an important role in ensuring that the atmosphere is relaxed and nonpunitive. Some hospitals now have units that specialize in eating disorders. Continued follow up after discharge from the unit is essential. Nurses working with adolescents in any capacity need to be alert to the symptoms of this disease, as lack of recognition is one of the biggest obstacles to treatment. Young people need to be educated as to its seriousness. Educational materials, referral sources, and counseling are available from the National Association of Anorexia Nervosa and Associated Disorders. Encouragement and support from self-help groups are also valuable.

Prognosis. The prognosis for patients with anorexia nervosa is uncertain. Most patients gain weight in the hospital regardless of the type of

Table 16–1. SIGNS AND SYMPTOMS OF ANOREXIA NERVOSA
Changing weight loss goals
Dieting that increases dissatisfaction with appearance of body
Dieting that leads to social isolation
Amenorrhea
Vomiting
Misuse of laxatives, diuretics, and diet pills

(From Garfinkel, B. D., Carlson, G. A., and Weller, E. B. [1990]. *Psychiatric Disorders in Children and Adolescents.* Philadelphia, W. B. Saunders Company.)

Table 16–2. COMPARISON OF ANOREXIA NERVOSA AND BULIMIA NERVOSA

FACTOR	ANOREXIA	BULIMIA
Age range	10 to 25 years (mean, 13 years)	Older, average 18 years
Weight	Fear of normal weight	Many are of normal weight or overweight prior to onset, wider weight fluctuations
Impulse control	Normal to slight variations	More prone to substance abuse, shop-lifting
Vomiting	Varies	More prevalent
Starvation	Yes	Seldom
Severity	More severe	Usually not as devastating

therapy. This may not, however, predict future success. About half of treated patients continue to have problems and experience below-normal weight or wide fluctuations in their weight. Menstrual irregularities persist and overall psychological, social, and sexual functioning is impaired (Comerci, 1990). Complications include gastritis, cardiac arrhythmias, inflammation of the intestine, kidney problems, and others. Deaths do occur, particularly in untreated persons. Table 16–2 compares anorexia with bulimia and Table 16–3 presents complications of anorexia and bulimia.

BULIMIA

Description. Bulimia, or compulsive eating, is now recognized by the Diagnostic and Statistical Manual of Mental Disorders as a separate eating disorder. It is estimated that approximately 4 to 5 per cent of adolescent and young women and 0.5 per cent of young men are affected by this disease (Comerci, 1990). Bulimics binge periodically, usually on easily accessible high-caloric food items. These episodes are generally carried out in private. They may be followed by self-induced vomiting or the use of cathartics. The person is aware that eating is out of control. Binging periods are followed by feelings of dejection, guilt, and self-deprecation. (See Table 16–2 for a comparison summary of anorexia and bulimia.) The principles of nursing care are similar to those mentioned for the anorectic patient. Table 16–3 summarizes complications, causes, and treatments of bulimia as well as anorexia.

The Blood

INFECTIOUS MONONUCLEOSIS

Description. Infectious mononucleosis is a global disease caused by a herpes-type Epstein-Barr (EB) virus. It occurs chiefly in older children and adults, its peak incidence being in persons between 17 and 25 years of age or earlier in low socioeconomic groups. Studies suggest that the organism is transmitted by oral contact and also by eating utensils; however, its communicability is considered low. The incubation period is from 2 to 6 weeks.

Symptoms. Symptoms vary from mild to moderately severe and may last for several weeks. They include low-grade fever, sore throat, headache, fatigue, skin rash, and general malaise. The cervical glands of the neck enlarge. Splenomegaly develops in approximately half the patients. Liver involvement with mild jaundice occurs in a small number of persons and requires bed rest until serum bilirubin levels return to normal. Diagnosis is confirmed by the examination of peripheral blood. There is lymphocytosis and the presence of atypical lymphocytes. Rising titer of antibody to EB virus is also indicative; the *Monospot* test is rapid, can detect the infection earlier than the heterophile antibody test, and is now widely used. Complications, although uncommon, include rupture of the spleen, secondary pneumonia, neurological manifestations, and heart involvement.

Table 16–3. BIOLOGICAL COMPLICATIONS OF ANOREXIA NERVOSA AND BULIMIA NERVOSA

	FREQUENCY	CAUSE	TREATMENT
CARDIOVASCULAR CHANGES			
Bradycardia	Common	Starvation	Weight restoration
Hypotension	Common	Starvation, fluid depletion	Weight restoration
Arrhythmias	Infrequent	Usually provoked by exercise in starvation; may be due to hypokalemia	Weight restoration or potassium supplements
Cardiomyopathy	Rare	Emetine toxicity from ipecac	Stop the ipecac
CENTRAL NERVOUS SYSTEM CHANGES			
Nonspecific EEG changes	Common	Starvation	Weight restoration
Reversible cortical atrophy	Uncommon	Starvation	Weight restoration
RENAL/ELECTROLYTE CHANGES			
Hypokalemia	Common	Loss of potassium from multiple routes (vomiting, diarrhea, and diuretics)	Prevent purging; may need a potassium supplement
		Salt restriction and water intoxication (to meet weight goals)	Well-balanced diet with appropriate amount of fluids
Increased blood urea nitrogen	Uncommon	Dehydration	Rehydration
Hypochloremic metabolic alkalosis	Common	Purging	Prevent purging
Edema	Common	Not clearly understood	Elevate feet for 1 hour three times a day; avoid salt; do not use diuretics
GASTROINTESTINAL CHANGES			
Parotitis	Common	Mechanical trauma; starvation	Stop binges and vomiting
Early satiety	Common	Delayed gastric emptying	Domperidone, 20 mg, three times a day
Gastric dilatation	Rare	Rapid refeeding	Avoid oral feeding; use intravenous feeding
Constipation	Common	Starvation; reliance on laxatives	Use diet: emphasis on dietary bulk, fruits, and vegetables and try to avoid laxatives
Dental caries	Common	Acidic nature of vomitus	Dental consultation
Hyperamylasemia	Common in bulimia	Salivary ± pancreatic hypersecretion	Prevent purging
Gastric rupture	Rare	Bingeing	Surgery
Superior mesenteric artery syndrome	Rare	Weight loss	Weight restoration

Table continued on following page

Table 16–3. BIOLOGICAL COMPLICATIONS OF ANOREXIA NERVOSA AND BULIMIA NERVOSA *Continued*

	FREQUENCY	CAUSE	TREATMENT
MUSCULOSKELETAL CHANGES			
Myopathy	Uncommon	Starvation; hypokalemia; emetine myotoxicity of ipecac	Weight restoration; stop ipecac abuse
Osteoporosis and pathologic fractures	Rare	Starvation	Weight restoration
NEUROENDOCRINE CHANGES			
Decreased serum triiodothyronine and increased reverse triiodothyronine	Common	Starvation	Weight restoration
Hypercortisolism	Common	Starvation	Weight restoration
Primary or secondary amenorrhea	Infrequent	Low weight; emotional stress	Restore weight to 90% of average
Hypothermia	Infrequent	Low weight	Weight restoration
Cortisol escape from dexamethasone suppression	Common	Unknown	Weight restoration
Prepubertal luteinizing and follicle-stimulating hormone	Common	Starvation	Weight restoration
HEMATOLOGIC CHANGES			
Anemia	Infrequent	Bone marrow hypoplasia; due to starvation	Weight restoration; may need iron
Thrombocytopenia	Rare	Starvation	Weight restoration
Hypercholesterolemia	Common	Unknown	Balanced diet
Hypercarotenemia	Infrequent	Ingestion of high carotene foods	Balanced diet
DERMATOLOGIC CHANGES			
Dry, cracking skin	Common	Dehydration, loss of subcutaneous fat	Weight restoration
Lanugo hair development	Common	Unknown	Weight restoration
Callus on dorsum of hand	Common	Friction against teeth in inducing vomiting	Stop vomiting

(From Garfinkel, B. D., Carlson, G. A., and Weller, E. B. (1990). *Psychiatric Disorders in Children and Adolescents.* Philadelphia, W. B. Saunders Company.)

Treatment and Nursing Care

Treatment is supportive because the disease is self-limiting. An antipyretic is given to reduce fever and discomfort. An initial period of rest or restricted activities is usually needed. Gargling with warm saline and sucking throat lozenges are useful for pharyngitis. Adequate fluid intake is necessary, in particular of bland, cool liquids that are not irritating to the throat. Smoking should be discouraged. There is no special diet. Isolation is not necessary. The patient is alerted to signs of secondary infection. Steroid hormones are given when complications arise. Activities are increased in accordance with the diminution of fever and fatigue. The patient with an enlarged spleen is cautioned to avoid heavy lifting, trauma to the abdomen, and vigorous athletics until splenomegaly subsides. Severe abdominal pain is unusual except in the presence of splenic rupture and requires immediate attention. The teenager with mononucleosis may be discouraged and depressed. The teenager worries about job, school work, and the ability to continue extracurricular activities of importance. Open communications with school officials and classmates will help alleviate some of the anxieties. The prognosis in mononucleosis is good. It is no longer considered a prolonged debilitating disease. Many cases go unrecognized. Researchers are currently searching for a vaccine to prevent the disease.

Skeletal System

SCOLIOSIS

Description. Scoliosis is the term used to describe an S-shaped curvature of the spine. It is the most prevalent of the three skeletal abnormalities shown in Figure 16–2. To say that 4 to 8 per cent of school age and adolescent children are affected is somewhat misleading because not all these children will need treatment. All scoliotic curves are not progressive and may require only periodic evaluation. During adolescence scoliosis is more common in girls. Untreated progressive scoliosis may lead to back pain, fatigue, disability, and heart and lung complications. Skeletal deteriora-

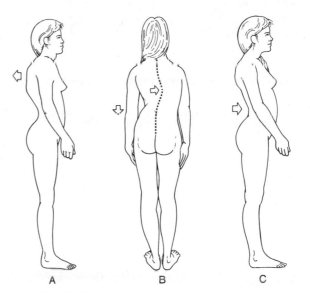

▲ FIGURE 16–2

Postural defects.

Figure	Term	Definition
A	Kyphosis	Hunchback, outward curvature of spine
B	Scoliosis	S-shaped curvature of spine
C	Lordosis	Curved spine, forward tilt to pelvis

(From Foster, R., Hunsberger, M., and Anderson, J. J. (1989). *Family-Centered Nursing Care of Children.* Philadelphia, W. B. Saunders Company.)

tion does not stop with maturity and may be aggravated by pregnancy.

Causes. There are two types of scoliosis—functional and structural. Functional scoliosis is usually caused by poor posture and not by spinal disease. The curve is flexible and easily correctable. Structural or fixed scoliosis is due to changes in the shape of the vertebrae or thorax and is a result of disease. It is usually accompanied by rotation of the spine. The patient cannot correct the condition voluntarily, i.e., by standing straighter.

Structural scoliosis has many causes. Some of these are *congenital,* e.g., meningomyelocele; *paralytic,* e.g., cerebral palsy; *traumatic;* and *spinal irritation from tumors.* About 70 to 80 per cent of cases of scoliosis are *idiopathic* (cause unknown). Current evidence indicates a genetic susceptibility transmitted as an autosomal-dominant trait with incomplete penetrance. A person who has sco-liosis has a one in three chance of having children with the condition (DeRosa, 1990). Familial sco-liosis is classified according to age of onset as infantile (birth to 3 years), juvenile (4 to 10 years), and adolescent (10 years to maturity). In the United States, the most common form of familial (genetic) scoliosis occurs during adolescence.

Treatment

Treatment is aimed at correcting the curvature and preventing further scoliosis. Curves up to 20 degrees do not require treatment but are carefully followed. Curves between 20 and 40 degrees re-quire a brace. The child is usually required to wear the brace for 23 hours a day. Some experts seem to think the same effect can be obtained from wearing the brace fewer hours. The *Milwaukee* brace (Fig. 16–3) exerts pressure on the chin, pelvis, and convex (arched) side of the spine. It is worn over a T-shirt. The child is also involved in an active exercise program. Electrical stimulation had been thought at one time to be a way to

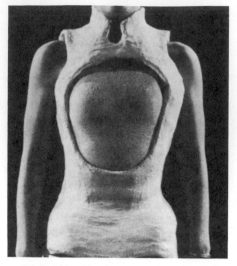

▲ **FIGURE 16–4**

Localizer cast. (From Rothman R., Simeone, F. (1975). *The Spine*. Philadelphia, W. B. Saunders Company.)

prevent progression of scoliosis. Several studies have shown this to be ineffective, and this treat-ment is currently controversial. Curvatures greater than 40 degrees will most likely require surgical intervention in the form of a spinal fusion. This is sometimes done in stages. A Harrington rod, Dwyer instrument, or Luque wires may be in-serted for immobilization during the time required for the fusion to become solid. A Risser localizer cast may be applied sometime postoperatively (Fig. 16–4). This is not always used, but when it is, it is worn for 6 to 9 months and changed according to the physician's procedure.

Nursing Care

Community Nursing. The management of sco-liosis begins with *screening* (Fig. 16–5). This is done in junior high school or preferably middle school. It should also be a part of every yearly physical given to prepubescent youngsters. Camp nurses also need to be aware of symptoms. Early recog-nition is of utmost importance in detecting mild cases amenable to nonsurgical treatment.

Screening in the school system is usually done by the school nurse. Students are prepared for screening by explaining the purpose of the pro-

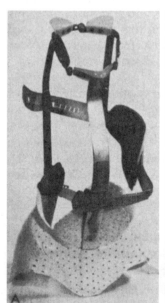
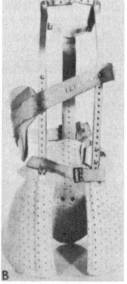

▲ **FIGURE 16–3**

Milwaukee brace; *(A)* front and *(B)* back views. (From Tachdjian, M. (1972). *Pediatric Orthopedics*. Philadel-phia, W. B. Saunders Company.)

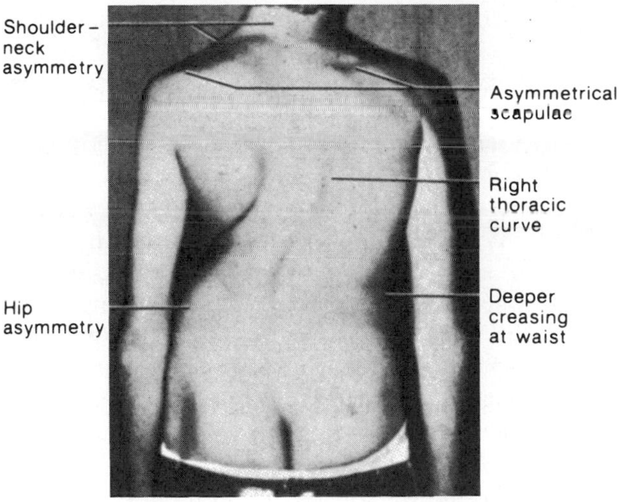

Shoulder–neck asymmetry

Asymmetrical scapulae

Right thoracic curve

Hip asymmetry

Deeper creasing at waist

▲ **FIGURE 16–5**

Screening procedure for scoliosis. (From Foster, R., Hunsberger, M., and Anderson, J. J. (1989). *Family-Centered Nursing Care of Children*. Philadelphia, W. B. Saunders Company.)

cedure and by reassuring them that it merely entails observation of the back while standing and while bending forward. Students need to know that it is simple, quick, and painless and that privacy will be afforded. They are instructed to wear clothing that is easy to remove, such as a pullover top. Boys disrobe to the waist, girls generally to the bra. No slip or undershirt should be worn. The procedure consists of examining the spine from the front, side, and back while the student stands erect and then to observe the back as he or she bends forward. One looks initially for general body alignment and *asymmetry* (lack of proportion). In scoliosis, one shoulder may be higher than the other, a scapula may be prominent, the arm-to-body spaces may be unequal, or a hip may protrude; one arm may appear longer than the other when the person bends forward. Sometimes the patient complains of a "crooked back," uneven hemline, and difficulty in fitting clothes. Fourth grade boys are especially lordotic; therefore, developmental patterns at various ages must be considered. Referrals are made as indicated. Because of the familial tendencies of this condition, brothers and sisters of patients should be examined. Community understanding of scoliosis will benefit those who must obtain further treatment.

Hospital Care. Nursing care for hospitalized patients coincides with treatment programs. Patients may be admitted overnight for a cast change or may require more extensive correction by spinal fusion. The nurse's knowledge of preadolescent and adolescent developmental tasks is imperative, because therapy often conflicts with this.

Basic cast care is described on page 137. The adolescent in a body cast has many adjustments to make as a result of its weight and the restrictions it makes on mobility. Ambulation is difficult, as is sleeping. Modifications must be made in bathing, shampooing, dressing, and eating, and these can be frustrating. Teenagers are concerned about how they look in the cast, and clothes made especially for them are a morale booster.

Preoperative Care. The usual preoperative preparation of the patient is necessary for spinal fusion. It is important that the nurse evaluate and document the patient's neuromuscular status at this time so that it may be used as a basis for comparison after the procedure. All four extremities are observed for color, temperature, capillary filling, edema, sensation, and motion. The nurse explains to the patient that breathing exercises and frequent change of position are necessary to prevent heart and lung complications. If postoperative log-rolling is anticipated, it can be practiced before surgery or, when possible, the patient may watch the procedure being done on another patient.

Postoperative Care. Much of the postoperative nursing care is directly related to combating the physical results of immobilization. The body systems become sluggish owing to inactivity. This is evidenced in the gastrointestinal tract by anorexia, irregularity, and constipation. Allowing the adolescent to select foods with the aid of the dietitian is helpful in improving appetite. Increasing fluid intake will reduce constipation; laxatives and enemas are sometimes required as supplemental aids. Juices, gelatin, cola drinks, soup, and noncarbonated beverages will promote kidney function. Limit milk and milk products to prevent the formation of renal calculi. Cardiopulmonary complications are avoided by frequent change of position, exercise, and allowing the patient to do as much for the self as possible. Range of motion exercises will help maintain muscle tone. Activities to stimulate mental awareness are of equal importance. Emotional reaction to confinement should be anticipated. In particular, the patient fears for safety.

When pins and wires are used, their sites are inspected daily to detect redness, heat, drainage, and slippage. Such symptoms are reported immediately, as the danger of bone infection is great. Instructions for home care are begun early in treatment. These should be written and their importance should be carefully explained.

NURSING BRIEF ▷ ▷ ▷ ▷ ▷ ▷ ▷ ▷
Insertion of a Harrington rod or other metal device will delay a patient at an airport security scanner, as the metal activates the alarm. A note can be obtained from the physician, which can be used as a clearance for air travel.

SPORTS INJURIES

A high percentage of adolescents of both sexes participate in athletic activities. Authorities disagree about what constitutes a good sports physical examination; however, they are unanimous about the necessity for precompetition medical examinations. The American Academy of Pediatrics recommends that a complete physical examination be given at least every other year during adolescence and that sports-specific examinations

be given for those involved in strenuous activity on entry into junior or senior high school. Such examinations should be updated by an annual questionnaire. The family history and an orthopedic screening are important in identifying risk factors.

Prevention. Several factors help prevent sport injuries. Some of these are an adequate warm-up and cool-down period; year-round conditioning; careful selection of activity according to physical maturity, size, and skill necessary; proper supervision by adults; safe, well-fitting equipment; and avoidance of participation when in pain. Proper diet and fluids are also necessary. A few of the more common injuries are listed in Table 16–4. The nurse plays an important role in educating and directing parents to sources of accurate information to ensure that the physical, emotional, and maturational levels of the adolescent are appropriate for the activity. Parents are encouraged to inquire about the capabilities of personnel and availability of emergency services prior to the beginning of the competition.

Considerations for Female Athletes. Irregular menses and amenorrhea are relatively common with heavy exercise. This may be due to a decrease in the percentage of body fat. Weight loss, thinness, and physical and emotional stress may also precipitate such irregularities. It is suggested that girls who stop menstruating for 2 months or more and those who menstruate irregularly be examined. Amenorrhea that is exercise induced can be confused with pregnancy by the teenager. While breast injuries are not common, sports bras in several styles are available that provide protection as well as support.

The Skin

ACNE VULGARIS

Description. Acne is an inflammation of the sebaceous glands and hair follicles in the skin. At puberty, owing to hormonal influence, the sebaceous follicles enlarge and secrete increased amounts of a fatty substance called *sebum*. Genetic factors and stress are also thought to play a part. The course of acne may be brief or prolonged

Table 16–4. SELECTED SPORTS INJURIES

TYPE	COMMENT
Concussion	Any blow to the head followed by alterations in mental functioning should be treated as a possible concussion. Observe carefully for sequelae.
"Stingers" or "burners"	A common neck injury when a player hits another with his head in such sports as football or rugby. It is due to brachial plexus trauma. Feels like an "electrical jolt." Usually mild, disappears suddenly. Restrict sports activity until symptoms disappear. Reassess protective gear.
Injured knee ligaments	Usually a result of stress on the knee. Can be potentially serious. Should be evaluated by an experienced trainer or physician. May require arthroscopy.
Sprain or strained ankle	May injure growth plate. X-rays important in adolescents.
Muscle cramps	Due to injury, alterations in blood flow, electrolyte deficiencies. Important to warm up before activity. Ensure fluid intake is adequate.
Shin splints	Pain and discomfort in lower leg due to repeated running on a hard surface such as concrete, which should be avoided; use well-fitting shoes. Decrease inflammation by rest.

(lasting 10 or more years). Premenstrual acne in girls is not uncommon. The principal lesions include comedones, papules, and nodulocystic growths.

A *comedo* (pleural, *comedones*) is a plug of keratin, sebum, and bacteria. Keratin is a protein substance that is the main constituent of epidermis and hair. There are two types of comedones, open and closed. In the open comedo, or blackhead, the surface is darkened by melanin. Closed comedones, or whiteheads, are responsible for the inflammatory process of acne. With continued build-up the walls of the follicle rupture, releasing their irritating content into the surrounding skin. A pustule may appear when this develops near the exterior. This process occurs no matter how carefully the teenager washes, because surface bacteria are not involved in the pathogenesis. Acne is usually seen on the chin, cheeks, and forehead. It can also develop on the chest, upper back, and shoulders. It usually is more severe in winter.

Treatment

The basic treatment of acne has changed considerably over the past few years. It is no longer felt that certain foods trigger the condition; therefore, chocolate, peanuts, and cola drinks are not restricted unless the patient is convinced of a correlation between a specific item and the condition. A regular, well-balanced diet is encouraged. Patients who are not taking tetracycline or vitamin A benefit from sunshine. General hygienic measures of cleanliness, rest, and avoidance of emotional stress may help prevent exacerbations.

The physician may prescribe the use of a special soap such as Fostex. Excessive cleansing of the skin can be harmful, however, since it irritates and chaps the tissues. Squeezing pimples serves to rupture intact lesions and causes local inflammation. The topical preparations recommended include benzoyl peroxide gels, such as Benzagel, PanOxyl, or Desquam X, which act to dry and peel the skin and suppress fatty acid growth, and vitamin A acid (Retin-A), which aids in the elimination of keratinous plugs. Vitamin A acid can increase sensitivity to the sun, so precautions should be taken when it is used. Tetracycline or erythromycin may be given in conjunction with topical medications in more serious cases. Monilial vaginitis is a secondary complication sometimes seen with the use of these drugs and should be explained to the unsuspecting female teenager.

Accutane (13-cis-retinoic acid) is now being utilized for patients with severe pustulocystic acne who have been unable to benefit from other types of treatment. It has many side effects, thus the patient requires careful monitoring. **It is not prescribed during pregnancy or to those at any risk for pregnancy because of the possibilities of fetal deformity.** The long-term effects of this medication have not been established. *Dermabrasion* (planing of the skin to minimize scarring) is done selectively, as it is not always successful.

Acne is very distressing to the adolescent, particularly when the face is extensively involved. Sometimes even a minimal problem is seen as disastrous when it happens before an important event. The self-conscious young person feels different and embarrassed. The nurse who is attuned to the feelings of individuals can provide understanding support. Although the teenager is educated to assume responsibility for her or his regimen, inclusion of the parents helps prevent conflict surrounding it.

Reproductive System

DYSMENORRHEA (PRIMARY)

Description. *Primary dysmenorrhea*, or painful menstruation, refers to pain associated with the menstrual cycle in the absence of organic pelvic disease. It is distinguished from *secondary dysmenorrhea* in which the patient may have an underlying condition such as endometriosis, pelvic inflammatory disease, ovarian cysts, adhesions, or congenital abnormalities. *Mittelschmerz* refers to midcycle pain during ovulation. For many years dysmenorrhea was thought to be psychological. It is now recognized that painful menses results from myometrial stimulation by prostaglandins E and F

produced in the endometrium (Litt, 1990). The concentration of these prostaglandins is higher in women suffering from dysmenorrhea than in controls.

Prevalence and Symptoms. About two thirds of postpubescent teenagers in the United States experience some degree of dysmenorrhea. Approximately 10 per cent are incapacitated from 1 to 3 days per month. Dysmenorrhea is the greatest single cause of lost school and work days in women. Its onset is usually before age 20 years. Symptoms include cramping, abdominal discomfort, and leg aches. Systemic symptoms such as nausea, vomiting, dizziness, diarrhea, backache, and headache may occur. Dysmenorrhea is graded from mild to severe. *Premenstrual tension syndrome* (PMS) is more common in adults than in teenagers. Although the symptoms may overlap with those of dysmenorrhea, weight gain, breast tenderness, irritability, and insomnia are also seen. PMS does not generally occur before ovulatory cycles begin.

Treatment and Nursing Care

Although psychological factors are no longer considered the sole determinant for dysmenorrhea, one must nevertheless consider a holistic approach to this disorder. Principles of menstrual hygiene need to be reviewed with the adolescent. Factors that may aggravate the condition include lack of exercise, poor posture, lack of sleep, constipation, and unbalanced meals. Improving the health status of patients is always a consideration of care. The perceptive nurse will also recognize that "cramps" in a young girl are often a mask for other concerns and will intervene accordingly. A warm beverage, aspirin or acetaminophen, and the application of a heating pad to the lower abdomen may be sufficient. When these measures fail, a thorough history and pelvic examination by a gynecologist should be performed to rule out organic disorders. Patients with dysmenorrhea who are also in need of contraception may be candidates for combination (estrogen-progesterone) oral contraceptives. Patients with severe discomfort will benefit from the use of prostaglandin inhibitors such as Motrin, Anaprox, and Ponstel. These medications decrease myometrial contractions. Some side effects that the nurse must be aware of include gastric irritation (pain, nausea, and vomiting), headache, pruritus, and fluid retention.

SEXUALLY TRANSMITTED DISEASES

Overview

Sexually transmitted disease (STD) is the general name given to infections that are spread through direct sexual activity (Table 16–5). The term replaces the term "venereal disease," which was used in the past. The two most common types of STD are gonorrhea and chlamydial infection; however, over 20 other diseases are now considered to be prevalent. Some of these are syphilis, scabies, pediculosis pubis, herpes progenitalis, genital warts, pelvic inflammatory disease, cytomegalovirus, and AIDS (acquired immune deficiency syndrome). Gonorrhea occurs far more frequently than syphilis, but the effects of untreated syphilis are more debilitating. One may contract both diseases at the same time. Each can be transmitted by a pregnant woman to her unborn child, causing serious problems in the fetus such as blindness, birth defects, and death.

The first written record of STDs appears in the Bible in about 1500 B.C. It was thought that with the advent of penicillin STDs would be eradicated, but there has been a widespread resurgence. The incidence of STDs among teenagers has been rising more rapidly than that of the general population (Brown, 1989).

The reasons for this resurgence are many: cultural, economic, social, and moral factors are intertwined. Specific reasons cited include changing values and lifestyles of society; an increase in sexual contact, particularly in the middle and upper classes; the increase in the mobility of society and surges in population; the reluctance of many persons to seek medical help (particularly adolescents); inadequate education about the diseases; widespread apathy among professionals; social equality of the sexes; and the change in common methods of contraception. The occurrence of a sexually transmitted disease in a prepubertal pa-

tient should always prompt investigation into the possibility of sexual abuse of the child.

The incidence of AIDS continues to increase, and public awareness of spread through sexual contact is a priority in prevention. Since persons with human immunodeficiency virus (HIV) infection may remain asymptomatic for many years, they may unknowingly spread the disease. Infants may acquire the disease perinatally.

NURSING CARE

Regardless of how one may feel about the changes in society and sexual permissiveness, they must be recognized and dealt with when one is a medical professional (Nursing Care Plan 16–2). For nurses to be of help to teenagers with a sexually transmitted disease, they must create an environment in which the teenagers will feel at ease. What adolescents need at this point is support of self-esteem, which nurses are able to provide through listening and through a nonjudgmental attitude.

Approach. The nurse approaches the patient with sensitivity. The nurse must recognize that the teenager is embarrassed and in need of privacy, especially during examinations. Girls are often afraid of and always nervous about a pelvic examination. This is true even when their outward manner may seem otherwise. Careful explanations are needed. The patient is draped appropriately and the nurse remains during the examination to provide reassurance. The findings are discussed with the patient and questions are encouraged. Most teenagers need help in being drawn out and will not readily ask questions even when they do not understand.

The reporting of sexual contacts required by law is an emotionally charged topic that often prevents patients from seeking help. The person who is assured of confidentiality and who has been treated in a dignified manner is more apt to cooperate. Girls who are sexually active must be taught to take responsibility for their own health and are encouraged to request a gonorrhea culture as a routine part of their physical examination. This is of particular importance if they suspect that their partner has an STD. Medical attention

Table 16–5. SEXUALLY TRANSMITTED DISEASE SUMMARY

DISEASE	CLINICAL PRESENTATION	THERAPY	COMPLICATIONS AND SEQUELAE	TEACHING
NONGONOCOCCAL URETHRITIS (NGU)	Men usually have dysuria, urinary frequency, and mucoid-to-purulent urethral discharge. Some men have asymptomatic infections Female sexual partners of men with NGU are likely to have mucopurulent cervicitis (MPC)	Doxycycline, 100 mg orally 2 times a day for 7 days **OR** Tetracycline, 500 mg orally 4 times a day for 7 days	Urethral strictures Prostatitis Epididymitis The organisms that cause NGU may be transmitted to female sexual partners, resulting in mucopurulent cervicitis, pelvic inflammatory disease, and other adverse outcomes	Understand how to take any prescribed oral medications. If tetracycline is prescribed, take it 1 hour before or 2 hours after meals and avoid dairy products, antacids, iron or other mineral-containing preparations, and sunlight. Return for evaluation if symptoms persist or recur after treatment. Refer sexual partner(s) for examination and treatment. Avoid sex until patient and partner(s) are cured. Use condoms to prevent future infections
GONORRHEA	When symptomatic, men usually have dysuria, frequency, and purulent urethral discharge. When symptomatic, women may have abnormal vaginal discharge, abnormal menses, dysuria, or abdominal pain. In both sexes, but particularly in women, infection may be asymptomatic. Anorectal and pharyngeal infections may be symptomatic or asymptomatic	Ceftriaxone, 250 mg IM once **PLUS** Doxycycline, 100 mg orally 2 times a day for 7 days	Women with untreated gonorrhea may develop pelvic inflammatory disease and are at risk for its sequelae. Men are at risk for urethral stricture, epididymitis, and infertility. Newborns born to women with untreated infection are at risk for scalp abscess at the site of fetal monitors, ophthalmia neonatorum, rhinitis, disseminated infection, or anorectal infections. Untreated persons are at risk for disseminated gonococcal infection (e.g., septicemia, arthritis, dermatitis, disseminated gonococcal infection (DG), meningitis, and endocarditis)	Understand how to take any prescribed oral medications. If tetracycline is prescribed, take it 1 hour before or 2 hours after meals and avoid dairy products, antacids, iron or other mineral-containing preparations, and sunlight. Return for evaluation if symptoms persist or recur after treatment. Refer sexual partner(s) for examination and treatment. Avoid sex until patient and partner(s) are cured. Use condoms to prevent future infections
GENITAL WARTS	Present as single or multiple soft, fleshy, papillary or sessile, painless growths around the anus, vulvovaginal area, penis, urethra, or perineum. Subclinical infection, particularly of the cervix, may occur and is best recognized by colposcopy	The goal of treatment is removal of exophytic warts and the amelioration of signs and symptoms, not the eradication of human papillomavirus (HPV). Cryotherapy with liquid nitrogen (or cryoprobe for external genital/perianal warts) *Alternative Treatments for External Genital/Perianal/Vaginal Warts:* (1) Podophyllin, 10%–25% in compound tincture of benzoin, (2) Trichloroacetic acid, 80%–90% **NOTE:** For women with cervical warts, dysplasia must be excluded before treatment is begun. Management should therefore be carried out in consultation with an expert	Most anogenital warts are thought to be caused by HPV type 6 or 11. Other types (principally 16, 18, and 31) have been associated with genital dysplasia and carcinoma. All women with anogenital warts should have an annual Pap smear, and atypical, pigmented, or persistent warts should be biopsied. Lesions may enlarge and produce tissue destruction. Giant condyloma may simulate carcinoma, yet be histologically benign In pregnancy, warts enlarge and are extremely vascular. Rarely, they may obstruct the birth canal, necessitating cesarean section. HPV can cause laryngeal papillomatosis in infants	Return for weekly or biweekly treatment and follow-up until lesions have resolved. Women should have annual Pap smears. Partners should be examined for warts. Abstain from sex or use condoms during therapy. Using condoms may help prevent future infections

Table 16–5. SEXUALLY TRANSMITTED DISEASE SUMMARY *Continued*

DISEASE	CLINICAL PRESENTATION	THERAPY	COMPLICATIONS AND SEQUELAE	TEACHING
HERPES GENITALIS	Single or, more commonly, multiple vesicles appear anywhere on the genitalia. Vesicles spontaneously rupture to form shallow ulcers that may be very painful. Because the vesicular phase may be missed, especially in women, genital ulcers may be the initial presentation. Lesions resolve spontaneously without scarring. The first occurrence is termed *initial infection or first clinical episode* (mean duration, 14–21 days). Subsequent, usually milder, occurrences are termed *recurrent infections* (mean duration of lesions, 8–12 days). The interval between clinical episodes is termed *latency*. Viral shedding may occur intermittently during latency	No known cure exists. Systemic acyclovir treatment of acute disease may reduce symptoms and signs of herpes episodes and may accelerate healing but does not eradicate the infection nor affect subsequent recurrences *First Clinical Episode— Genital:* Acyclovir, 200 mg orally 5 times daily for 7 to 10 days or until clinical resolution occurs *First Clinical Episode— Herpes Proctitis:* Acyclovir, 400 ml orally 5 times daily for 10 days or until clinical resolution occurs *Recurrent Episodes:* Acyclovir, 200 mg orally 5 times daily for 5 days initiated within 2 days of onset **OR** Acyclovir, 800 mg orally 2 times a day for 5 days *Suppression of Recurrent Genital Herpes Infection:* Continuous treatment reduces the frequency or severity of active disease in at least 75% of patients with frequent (at least 6 per year) recurrences. Dosage must be individualized for each patient: Acyclovir, 200 mg orally 2 to 5 times daily, **OR** Acyclovir, 400 mg orally 2 times daily **NOTE:** Topical therapy with acyclovir is substantially less effective than therapy with the oral drug	Aseptic meningitis may occur during the first clinical episode. Initial acquisition of HSV infection during pregnancy increases the likelihood of maternal to infant transmission; women with recurrent infection infrequently transmit the virus to the neonate during vaginal delivery. Neonatal herpes ranges in severity from clinically inapparent infection to local infections of the eyes, skin, or mucous membranes to severe disseminated infection that may involve the central nervous system	Keep involved area clean and dry. Since both initial and recurrent lesions shed virus, patients should abstain from sex while symptomatic. An undetermined but presumably small risk of transmission also exists during asymptomatic intervals. Condoms may offer some protection. The risk of fetal infection should be explained to all patients. Nonpregnant women should be reassured that genital herpes does not affect their ability to have children and that, in the great majority of cases, delivery can be performed vaginally. Pregnant women should make their clinicians/obstetricians aware of any history of herpes. Genital herpes (and other diseases causing genital ulcers) has been associated with increased risk of acquiring HIV infection
SYPHILIS	*Primary:* The classic chancre is painless, indurated, and located at the site of exposure. All genital ulcers should be suspected to be syphilitic *Secondary:* Patients may have a highly variable skin rash, mucous patches, condylomata lata, lymphadenopathy, or other signs *Latent:* Patients are without clinical signs	Primary, secondary, or early syphilis of less than 1 year's duration: Benzathine penicillin G, 2.4 million units IM, in one dose. Syphilis of indeterminate length or of more than 1 year's duration: Benzathine penicillin G, 7.2 million units total, administered as 2.4 million units IM given 1 week apart for 3 consecutive weeks	Both late syphilis and congenital syphilis are preventable complications upon prompt diagnosis and treatment of early syphilis. Sequelae of late syphilis includes neurosyphilis (although neurosyphilis may occur at any stage), cardiovascular syphilis (thoracic aortic aneurysm, aortic valve disease), and localized gumma formation.	Return for follow-up blood studies as indicated (usually 3 and 6 months after therapy). Follow-up may be of longer duration or at more frequent intervals. Understand the importance of returning for follow-up treatment or taking oral medications correctly, if prescribed. Refer sexual partner(s) for evaluation and treatment. Avoid sexual activity until patient and partner(s) are cured.

Table continued on following page

Table 16–5. SEXUALLY TRANSMITTED DISEASE SUMMARY *Continued*

DISEASE	CLINICAL PRESENTATION	THERAPY	COMPLICATIONS AND SEQUELAE	TEACHING
SYPHILIS *Continued*	*Neurosyphilis:* Neurosyphilis may be asymptomatic. If symptomatic, a variety of neurological symptoms and signs occurs, including lightning pains, ataxia, bladder disturbances, confusion, and obtundation	Neurosyphilis (Inpatient therapy recommended): Aqueous crystalline penicillin G, 12–24 million units per day, administered as 2–4 million units every 4 hours IV, for 10–14 days	Congenital syphilis affects multiple organ systems. In addition to stillbirth and intrauterine growth retardation, sequelae of congenital syphilis may include mucocutaneous, skeletal, hematological, central nervous system, and ocular involvement	Use condoms to prevent future infections. Understand the risks of syphilis during pregnancy. Pregnant women should be screened early in pregnancy. Syphilis (and other diseases causing genital ulcers) has been associated with an increased risk of acquiring HIV infection. HIV-infected patients treated for syphilis should be followed clinically and serologically at 1, 2, 3, 6, 9, and 12 months after treatment
HEPATITIS B	Clinical symptoms and signs are indistinguishable from other forms of hepatitis and may include various combinations of anorexia, malaise, nausea, vomiting, abdominal pain, dark urine, and jaundice. Skin rashes, arthralgias, and arthritis may also occur. Only 33–50% of acute infections are symptomatic. Acute infections may resolve, resulting in permanent immunity. In 5–10% of acute cases, infection is persistent, resulting in a chronic carrier state, which can be asymptomatic	No specific therapy is available for acute hepatitis B or for the chronic carrier state. Hepatitis B vaccine is recommended for persons at risk for acquiring HBV infection. HIV coinfection reduces the humoral response to the hepatitis B vaccine. Infants born to infected (i.e., HBsAg-positive) mothers should receive both hepatitis B immune globulin (HBIG) at birth and hepatitis B vaccine at birth, at 1 month, and at 6 months. Sexual partners of persons with acute hepatitis B should receive the hepatitis B vaccine, and should receive HBIG if seen within 14 days of the last exposure. Sexual partners of persons who are found to be chronic carriers of HBV should receive the hepatitis B vaccine. Before treatment, testing of sexual partners for susceptibility to HBV infection is recommended if it does not delay treatment beyond 14 days	Long-term sequelae include chronic persistent and chronic active hepatitis, cirrhosis, hepatocellular carcinoma, hepatic failure, and death. Rarely, acute infection may be fulminant with hepatic failure, resulting in death. Infectious chronic carriers may be asymptomatic. Infants infected at birth are at high risk of developing chronic hepatitis B infection	Although often asymptomatic, hepatitis B can be life-threatening and can cause serious complications. Hepatitis B is prevented by hepatitis B vaccine, which is both safe and highly effective. Persons at risk of exposure should be immunized with hepatitis B vaccine. Persons whose sexual partners have acute HBV infection should receive postexposure prophylaxis with hepatitis B vaccine, and HBIG if seen within 14 days of the last exposure. Persons whose sexual partners are found to be chronic carriers of HBV should receive the hepatitis B vaccine. All pregnant women should be screened for HBsAg during pregnancy to insure optimal management of the infant. Homosexually active men and parenteral drug users are at increased risk for both HBV and HIV infections. The frequency of clinical follow-up of persons with acute HBV infection is determined by symptomatology and the results of liver function tests. Use condoms to prevent sexual transmission to susceptible persons

Table 16–5. SEXUALLY TRANSMITTED DISEASE SUMMARY *Continued*

DISEASE	CLINICAL PRESENTATION	THERAPY	COMPLICATIONS AND SEQUELAE	TEACHING
HIV INFECTION AND AIDS	Persons with HIV infection may remain asymptomatic for many years. Most people who are infected with HIV will eventually develop symptoms related to their infection. The progression of symptoms associated with HIV extends from the initial acute stage of HIV infection to asymptomatic HIV infection to symptomatic HIV infection and finally to the full clinical syndrome of AIDS. Symptoms and signs associated with symptomatic HIV infection may include fatigue, poor appetite, unexplained weight loss, generalized lymphadenopathy, persistent diarrhea, fever, and night sweats. Other signs and symptoms specific to opportunistic diseases occur in patients with AIDS, such as purple to bluish skin lesions associated with Kaposi's sarcoma (KS), shortness of breath, and nonproductive cough resulting from *Pneumocystis carinii* pneumonia (PCP), and glossitis, dysphagia, and retrosternal pain associated with oral and esophageal candidiasis	Although no vaccine or cure is available for HIV infection or AIDS, the development of treatment therapies, including antiviral agents, immunomodulators, and others, is progressing rapidly. For persons with HIV infection, zidovudine (ZDV, formerly called AZT) may be effective in delaying the clinical conditions of HIV disease. Aerosol pentamidine as well as trimethoprim-sulfamethoxazole has been shown to be effective in preventing *Pneumocystis carinii* pneumonia. These drugs have serious side effects and require careful monitoring by knowledgable clinicians. For persons in whom AIDS has been diagnosed, standard therapy consists of antiretroviral therapy, infection prophylaxis, and treating opportunistic diseases aggressively as they occur	While most persons with HIV infection eventually will develop some symptoms related to their infection, some remain asymptomatic for 10 or more years. About 30–50% of infants born to HIV-infected women are infected with HIV. The prognosis for these infants is poor, but therapeutic advances are being made. Treatment trials are under way for pregnant women with HIV infection	Individuals initiating a sexual relationship should be counseled about sexual practices that reduce the risk of HIV transmission. Sexual partners should be informed of HIV seropositivity. Sexual practices should be limited to those that do not permit any exchange of blood, semen, or vaginal secretions. Condoms should be used consistently. Persons should not inject illicit drugs. Drug users should enroll or continue in a drug treatment program. If drug-use practices continue, needles and syringes should never be shared. If sharing does occur, cleaning the "works" with bleach may decrease the risk of HIV transmission. Alcohol and other drugs that are not injected may result in carelessness in practicing safer sex. Women of childbearing age who may be at risk for HIV infection should be counseled about the risks of perinatal transmission and about contraception options. Pregnant women with known or suspected HIV infection should promptly notify their physicians to ensure optimal management of the pregnancy. STD causing genital ulcers has been associated with an increased risk of acquiring or transmitting HIV infection. Persons with HIV infection should be skin-tested for tuberculosis

(Adapted from STD Treatment Guidelines [1989]. *Quality Assurance Guidelines for STD Clinics, and Subsequent Updates.* U.S. Department of Health and Human Services, Public Health Service, Division of STD/HIV Prevention, Centers for Disease Control, Atlanta.)

should be sought immediately even if they are menstruating. Young people need to be made aware of the fact that sex with only one partner does not eliminate the risk, as this person may have had contact with others; the partner has to have one sexual experience with only one infected person to transmit the disease.

Sexual experimentation, lack of education, and lack of caution make adolescents highly susceptible to STDs. Goals of care should include reducing

CARE PLAN 16–2

PREVENTION AND TREATMENT OF STD IN THE ADOLESCENT

Nursing Goals:

To provide anticipatory guidance concerning sexuality at a level that the child or young person can comprehend throughout developmental cycle

To prevent infection

To identify early symptoms and provide prompt treatment if infection occurs

To prevent sequelae

Assessment	Nursing Intervention
Children under 12	Provide age-appropriate instruction concerning sexuality. Also explore expected patterns that might occur before next visit. Suspect sexual abuse
Puberty and adolescence	Review structure and function of reproductive systems. Review personal hygiene. Discuss values and decision-making, possible sexual behavior and consequences, prevention of pregnancy and STDs
Self-concept: anticipate evidence of fear, embarrassment, anger, and decreased self-esteem upon suspicion of infection	Create nonjudgmental atmosphere, listen, assess level of knowledge, observe nonverbal behavior, establish confidentiality
	Provide privacy when assisting with pelvic or genital examination. Provide appropriate draping of patient
	Realize anger is often a mask for depression, grief; do not take personally
Skin and hair	It is not uncommon to see skin rashes, crabs (pubic lice) or scabies (mites)
	Clothing is disinfected by washing in hot water.
Sexual partners	Determine sex preference. Investigate and direct to treatment. Persons with multiple sexual partners, homosexuals, persons with new partners, and those with history of prior STD are at particular risk
Sexual intercourse	Advise to abstain during treatment and to use condom to prevent reinfection
Medication	Advise to take all of prescribed medication. If patient is on tetracycline, advise to take 1 hour before or 2 hours after meals (on empty stomach) and to avoid dairy products, antacids, iron, and sunlight
Compliance with treatment	Stress importance of follow-up, routine Pap smears
Sequelae	Discuss possible complications of specific disorders such as birth defects, infertility, etc.

the patient's fear, obtaining a thorough history, and developing a trusting relationship. If a therapeutic relationship develops between the adolescent and the nurse, then preventive teaching can take place.

The percentage of patients hospitalized with STDs is small because of adequate outpatient treatment measures. Diagnosed cases are isolated. Nevertheless, because of the insidious nature of these disorders, nurses must practice scrupulous techniques of handwashing when assisting with vaginal and rectal examinations on new admissions and when handling equipment such as rectal thermometers and douche nozzles. Hands should be kept away from the face to prevent gonorrheal conjunctivitis.

An illness of this nature, which affects the reproductive organs, is a serious threat to the self-image and creates a great deal of anxiety. The nurse has to assess the person's level of knowledge and provide information at that level. Many young people have little knowledge of their bodies and their developing sexuality. Others have mild to deep-seated emotional problems that need to be addressed. They may be using sex as an escape from reality, to express hostility or rebellion, or to call attention to themselves. They may be involved in relationships they no longer desire, so they need help in formulating positive attitudes toward themselves. They also need help understanding their behavior and that of others. In particular, adolescents need to learn that they are responsible for their own actions if they choose to be sexually active.

The prevention of STDs is everyone's concern and demands individual initiative and responsibility. Nurses must keep themselves informed about the latest techniques in diagnosis and treatment. Education of the public, particularly young people, is paramount. Nurses who work in settings frequented by teenagers can distribute some of the many excellent health pamphlets available. Structured courses in sex education should include presentations on STDs (there are also excellent audiovisual aids) and discussions on how one establishes healthy sexual behavior patterns. The community health or school nurse is involved in case finding and referral. Delays due to fear of disclosure are tragic. Legislation has now been enacted in all 50 states that permits physicians to treat infected minors without first obtaining parental consent.

Gonorrhea

Description. The major rise in the incidence of STDs is attributed to gonorrhea. The infectious agent that causes this highly communicable disease is *Neisseria gonorrhoeae*, anaerobic bacteria that penetrate the mucous membrane surfaces that line the genital tract, rectum, and mouth. They thrive in warm, moist areas of the body and can also survive in the tissues around the eyes of the newborn infant and in the immature vulvar tissues of prepubescent girls. They quickly die outside the human body. The common names for this disease include "GC," "clap," "a dose," "strain," or "the drip."

Symptoms. The symptoms in men appear within 3 to 5 days after sexual contact with an infected person (although some men are asymptomatic). The germs invade the urethral canal, causing a painful burning sensation during urination. Pus that gradually becomes thin and watery is discharged from the penis. Increased burning, urinary frequency, and urgency are signs of bladder infection. The disease may spread to the prostate gland, seminal vesicles, and testes. The scrotum when inflamed is hard, swollen, painful, and heavy. Scarring of the tubules and of the epididymides can result in permanent sterility. The disease can be transmitted by homosexual practices in both male and female patients. Anal gonorrhea is increasing in prevalence and causes no symptoms.

Eighty to ninety per cent of women with gonorrhea are asymptomatic; therefore, they may spread the infection without knowing it. Those who have symptoms experience mild burning or smarting in the genital area, with or without discharge. When discharge is present, it is of a light yellow, purulent nature. There may be slight inflammation and swelling of Bartholin glands, which makes sitting or walking painful. The patient may also complain of a feeling of pelvic heaviness and discomfort in the abdomen. Anal itching and urinary symptoms may prevail. After one or more menstrual periods, the disease may invade the reproductive organs—including the fallopian tubes and ovaries—or may spread to the pelvis, causing pelvic inflammatory disease. Scar tissue may cause sterility. Adhesions of the abdomen and fibroids may also occur. The incidence of gonococcemia appears to be increasing in association with pimple-like lesions on the extremities that were once seldom seen. In both sexes arthritis, endocarditis, and death may occur if gonorrhea is untreated.

TREATMENT

The diagnosis of gonorrhea is based on medical history, symptoms, and laboratory test results. In men, a smear of the discharge from the penis is taken with a cotton swab and transferred to a special culture plate or bottle where the organisms are grown for identification. The physician may want to take separate cultures a week or two apart. In women, the doctor usually takes a culture from within the vagina. Fluorescent-tagged antibody methods are the most accurate laboratory tests in women. Procedures are simple and painless and the results are confidential. If the patient is a minor, he or she can still receive free, confidential treatment without parental consent from the city or state health department or most physicians. If the test results are positive, sexual contacts are traced so that they may be treated before complications arise.

Current treatment includes the administration of one dose of ceftriaxone (Rocephin) IM and oral doxycycline (Vibramycin) for 7 days. Other antibiotics may be used if the patient is allergic to Rocephin or the organism is sensitive to penicillin. Research is under way to develop a vaccine to prevent gonorrhea.

Nongonococcal Urethritis (NGU)

Nongonococcal urethritis, also known as "Cinderella disease," is an inflammation of the urethra, which carries urine from the bladder. The incidence of NGU is increasing at epidemic rates, particularly among young college students and single whites from the upper and middle classes. In many cases *Chlamydia trachomatis* has been cited as the organism responsible for the infection. The symptoms include painful urination and a watery mucoid discharge. In women the disease may be asymptomatic. When untreated, the infection can cause sterility. It can also be transmitted to the newborn infant during birth and cause eye infections and pneumonia. NGU is at present diag-

nosed by the process of elimination. A culture of the discharge is examined for gonococci; if none are present, a diagnosis of NGU is made. Treatment consists of the administration of tetracycline or ceftriaxone (Rocephin). If tetracycline is prescribed, advise the patient to take it 1 hour before or 2 hours after meals and to avoid dairy products, antacids, iron, and sunlight. The patient is instructed to return for evaluation 4 to 7 days after therapy is finished, or earlier if symptoms recur. Sexual relations are to be avoided until patient and partners are cured. Condoms should be used to prevent further infection. It is important to educate the public to the seriousness of this infection, as the symptoms may be minimal.

Syphilis

Description. Syphilis, also known as "lues," causes destruction throughout the body. It was also a major cause of stillbirths, prematurity, and neonatal infection before the use of penicillin. The disease is caused by the spirochete *Treponema pallidum,* a spiral organism that reproduces rapidly in warm, moist areas of the body and quickly invades other tissues and organs. The organisms enter the body during coitus or through cuts or other breaks in the skin and mucous membranes. The incubation period is usually 3 weeks but may be anywhere from 7 to 90 days.

Symptoms. The symptoms of syphilis occur in three stages: primary, secondary, and tertiary (third). The primary stage consists of the appearance of a painless sore called a *chancre* (pronounced "shanker"), which appears where the spirochete enters the body—upon genital, anal, or oral membranes. The chancre resembles a pimple, which ulcerates and forms a crater-like depression. It is highly infectious. In women the chancre may go unnoticed when it is located around the cervix or in the vagina. It disappears without treatment in about 6 weeks. During this time the serologic blood test is negative, but the organism can be identified by examination of the scrapings from the sore under the darkfield microscope. Although the chancre disappears, the destructive work of the spirochete continues as it invades various body systems.

The symptoms of secondary syphilis vary among individuals and can begin from 6 weeks to

6 months after the infection. A rose-colored skin rash may be evident. Wartlike lesions called mucous patches, or *condylomata lata*, may also appear on the skin and mucous membranes. These are highly infectious. *Alopecia* (the loss of hair) may occur, usually in patches. The patient complains of general malaise, sore throat, and fever. The lymph glands may swell. Symptoms subside and reappear intermittently. If left untreated, the disease enters a latent period, in which there are no symptoms, that may last for many years. The disease remains contagious during the first 2 years, after which it is generally not communicable. Serological tests are positive.

The tertiary stage occurs after the fourth year. The disease is noninfectious at this time but very serious. The spirochetes attack the heart, blood vessels, brain, and spinal cord, in any of which the infection can cause death. Insanity and blindness can result. There is destruction of bone tissue and severe crippling or paralysis.

Transmission to Fetus and Neonate. A mother who has syphilis can infect her unborn child. A serological test (called VDRL, for Venereal Disease Research Laboratories) is performed at the first prenatal visit. This has been successful in preventing *congenital syphilis*. Some physicians repeat this later in pregnancy to detect syphilis contracted after the original test. When the result is positive, the mother is treated with penicillin, which effectively permeates the placenta regardless of the stage of pregnancy and protects the fetus. If the syphilitic mother is untreated, abortion, stillbirth, or congenital syphilis may result. Young unwed mothers and their babies are in jeopardy, particularly when early prenatal care is neglected. Case finding in adults is furthered by means of preemployment physicals, required by many companies, and by preinduction physicals by the armed services. The adolescent who has been raped and is at risk may need prophylactic treatment.

Genital Herpes

Herpes simplex virus type II is a sexually transmitted infection of the genitals. Its frequency among teenagers appears to be increasing. Five to ten per cent of cases are caused by herpes simplex virus type I. Type I virus is isolated most frequently

from lesions above the umbilicus, whereas type II is generally isolated from genital lesions (Green and Haggerty, 1990). In men the herpetic blisters or ulcers appear on the glans penis, prepuce, or penile shaft. In women the vulva and vagina may be involved, but the cervix is the primary site. Recurrence of herpes is common. The incubation period is from 5 to 10 days, and the lesions may persist from 3 to 6 weeks. The infection can be extremely painful, especially if the urethra and bladder are involved. The virus can be identified by tissue culture (Tzanck test). Systemic symptoms include fever, headache, malaise, and anorexia. Patients should be advised to abstain from sex while symptomatic, as both initial and recurring lesions shed high concentrations of the virus.

The administration of acyclovir may reduce signs and symptoms and aid in healing, but it does not cure the disease. Continuous treatment reduces the frequency and severity of attacks. Topical therapy is not as effective as systemic administration.

Sitz baths, heat lamps, and local compresses of Burow solution may also bring relief. Herpes simplex virus type II, which can be fatal to the newborn infant, is acquired from the mother during passage through the birth canal. Overwhelming infection involving many of the body systems occurs. A cesarean section is performed on mothers known to have this virus.

Herpes is thought to be a predisposing factor in cancer of the cervix. Regular follow-up Papanicolaou smears will detect early carcinoma.

Adolescent Pregnancy

Approximately 1.1 million girls aged 15 through 19 years become pregnant each year. Of this number, an estimated 84 per cent did not intend to get pregnant. Teenage mothers are more likely than others to not finish school, to be unemployed, to have low birth weight babies, and to lack parental skills (U.S. Department of Health and Human Services, 1990). In addition, these young women are at risk of developing complications of pregnancy and to have repeated pregnancies in their adolescent years.

First-intercourse experiences among young people are characterized by the absence of effective contraception. For the pregnant girl, concerns of body image become blurred, education is interrupted, and she may be separated from sources of support, such as her peer group. The father's studies may also be interrupted, he may become locked in low-paying employment, and he may face responsibilities for which he is ill prepared. Parenting classes, which provide guidance and support, and continued education regarding the normal processes of child growth and development are vital for these young people and for the health and welfare of their children.

There is growing evidence that comprehensive programs for the pregnant teenager and her baby, especially those that emphasize continued schooling, are associated with fewer repeat pregnancies. Methods of contraception should be clarified to the adolescent who is at risk, even though there may be no guarantee that they will be put to use. Many teenagers prefer to postpone intercourse. It is important that they understand that a choice exists and that delay is acceptable. Awareness of the responsibility of parenting together with decision making skills can aid in the lowering of the number of teenage pregnancies.

NURSING BRIEF ▷ ▷ ▷ ▷ ▷ ▷ ▷ ▷

A major problem for teenagers is that they receive mixed messages from society about sexuality.

Maladaptive Reactions to the Stress of Adolescence

DEPRESSION AND SUICIDE

Description. Suicide is one of the leading causes of death among persons aged 15 to 19 years. It ranks second as a cause of death for adolescents and college students. The incidence increases during the spring. Completed suicide is more common in boys than in girls, but girls make more attempts. Many adolescent suicides are not intended but are cries for help. The risk of death increases when there is a definite plan of action, the means is readily available (e.g., pills, guns), and the person has few resources for help and support.

Symptoms. Adolescents who do not have so-

cially acceptable ways to express their frustrations may turn their anger and hostility inward. Their self-esteem is low and they feel trapped, rejected, and abandoned. Although each experience is individual, a group of teenagers who had attempted suicide had these common feelings: emptiness and loss, inability to experience pleasure, lack of concentration, confusion, inability to make decisions, and ideas of no meaning or purpose to life. Physical problems revolved around eating and sleeping disturbances. Patients experienced lack of appetite and insomnia or the reverse, in which they slept all day. Hyperactivity was yet another symptom. Behavioral problems surfaced; these included a drop in school grades, truancy, running away, promiscuity, and other forms of acting out (Fig. 16–6). Alcoholism and substance abuse were significant contributing factors, as were the breakdown of family ties and the pressure to succeed. Some felt that their own expectations and those of others significant to them were too high.

Over half of suicide attempts are directly preceded by conflict with parents, ranging from misunderstanding to long-term, deep-seated problems. Some teenagers are loners, isolated from their peers and family, and unable to communicate

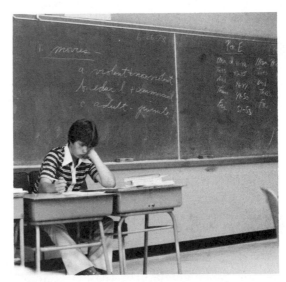

▲ **FIGURE 16–6**

A drop in school grades may be a signal of inner turmoil.

their distress. Since the symptoms are difficult to distinguish from healthy adolescent reactions to stress, they may go unrecognized. However, if the manifestations are uncharacteristic and interfere with the person's ability to function on a daily basis, further investigation is imperative. In assessing the situation, questions to the patient must be very direct and specific. "Are you planning to kill yourself? How? When?" Determine what coping skills the adolescent has used in the past to solve problems. If the person has made previous serious suicide attempts, the current suicidal situation should be considered more dangerous.

Depression is not always a negative experience. *Often it is a reaction to a real or fancied loss.* Although it is painful, it can lead to growth. Withdrawal is frustrating to those close to the young person, and they experience a feeling of helplessness. It is futile to bombard the person with platitudes such as "Cheer up," and "Nothing can be that bad." Instead, the nurse accepts adolescents where they are and helps them to look at and externalize their feelings. Ask them how you can help. Remain available to the client. Activities that promote physical exercise provide "hostility outlets" and are very therapeutic. Some days nurses may not feel very effective and need to retreat. They nevertheless assure the young person that they will return. This helps lessen feelings of desertion. It is important that the nurse keep in touch with his or her feelings to avoid burnout. As teenagers begin to feel more secure, they will reach out and progress at their own rate.

Adults are startled and disturbed when a 15 year old boy or girl takes his or her life. Many adults view adolescence as a carefree time and forget the painful circumstances that surrounded their own young lives. Suicide is unacceptable in Judeo-Christian society, and many persons find it difficult to console the grieving family, who carry a heavy burden of guilt, anger, and sorrow. Self-help groups for survivors are available in most cities. The nurse needs assistance in identifying feelings toward the patient who expresses suicidal intentions.

It is usually better if the responsibility for a suicidal patient is shared by as many people as possible. A combined effort indicates to the young person that others care and are interested and ready to help. It is also beneficial for the team in

that concerns can be discussed and grief shared should the suicidal intent be carried out. In the hospital the nurse is often the person most accessible and least threatening to the patient. Frequent brief visits provide surveillance and also serve to break destructive thought chains. The nurse must realize how sensitive the patient is to other people's reactions, and should not add to the patient's guilt.

Treatment

Treatment is multidimensional. When possible, individual, group, and family therapy are provided in an outpatient setting such as a community mental health agency. Group therapy seems to be especially helpful for adolescents. The adolescent mental health or behavioral unit of a hospital provides a structured environment with peers. It has the additional advantages of separating the adolescent from the stressful surroundings and providing support and protection.

Crisis intervention is required for acute and repeated episodes. Other voluntary services such as hotlines, drop-in centers, runaway houses, and free clinics focus on the immediate needs of the patient and are usually accepted by troubled youngsters. Unfortunately, there are not enough of these resources. Professionals need to be alert for warning signals of destructive behavior so that prompt intervention can be instigated; this might include earlier consideration of placement in a foster home. Community training courses for parenthood are becoming more popular and may provide another means of alleviating the complex problem of teenager suicide.

SUBSTANCE ABUSE

The problem of substance abuse is serious and complex and of great magnitude. Government efforts to control the supply and distribution of dangerous drugs have generally failed. Adult society, through its widespread acceptance of self-administered pills and alcohol, has compounded the problem; in particular, the drinking patterns of teenagers appear to directly reflect those of their parents and the community.

Numerous reasons have been cited as to why adolescents resort to drug use. Some reasons cited are curiosity; peer pressure; rebellion; the need to escape from loneliness, boredom, or family problems; and the desire to become more sociable and to relax. Teenagers differ from the adult in a preference for *polypharmacy* (use of several drugs together), a sense of invulnerability, and a delay in psychosocial maturation with chronic drug use. Drug-seeking behavior may include stealing—shoplifting in particular—dealing in drugs, sexual promiscuity, and prostitution. In addition, a disproportionately high number of suicides are related to substance abuse. Sex-related differences have narrowed, particularly in the use of alcohol (more girls are experimenting with drugs and alcohol in their teens).

Four levels of substance abuse have been established: experimentation, controlled use, abuse, and dependence. Although there is often a fine line between control and abuse, frequency may be a major signal. This is especially true when accompanied by inappropriateness, e.g., "getting stoned" at the weekend party versus on the way to school. There are two kinds of dependence, *psychological* and *physical.* People become hooked on the drug, and in addition to psychological dependence they experience physical withdrawal symptoms. Most substances can lead to psychological dependence but not all will cause physical dependence. *Tolerance* develops when a user's body gets accustomed to certain drugs. The person must then increase the dosage each time to get the same effect.

Table 16–6 summarizes the characteristics of some of the more commonly abused drugs by adolescents.

NURSING BRIEF ▷ ▷ ▷ ▷ ▷ ▷ ▷ ▷
It has recently been estimated that over 2 million people are now using cocaine on a regular basis. "Crack" is a popular form that can be extremely addictive.

Teenage Alcoholism

Alcohol abuse is the number one drug problem of American teenagers and even children.

Experimentation with alcohol has traditionally been accepted as a normal part of growing up. Although all states have legal drinking ages of 21 years, these have not prevented teenagers from drinking. The first drinking experience generally occurs about the age of 12 years. The amount and frequency of drinking increase with age, peaking around ages 18 to 22 years.

The American Medical Association, the American College of Physicians, the American Psychiatric Association, and other professional bodies have accepted the concept of alcoholism as a disease for some time. This unfortunately has not been true of the general public. Many people still consider the alcoholic a derelict or moral degenerate, who does not have enough "will power" to control her or his drinking. Others consider it a laughing matter. Nurses dealing with adolescents need to emphasize the fact that alcoholism is a disease with established criteria and that it is treatable.

Alcohol is a mind-altering drug that works as a depressant. Because of the small size of the ethyl alcohol molecule, alcohol begins to oxidize immediately and is absorbed into the stomach and small intestine virtually unchanged. It is carried by the blood to the liver, which is not able to handle large amounts. The excess is pumped back into the circulation in relatively pure form. It reaches every part of the body, including the brain, and eventually returns to the liver. This process continues until the alcohol is completely oxidized. Alcohol has no food value but contains calories, which account for the weight gain seen in some persons.

Excessive consumption over a period of time can cause problems such as vomiting, diarrhea, ulcers, cirrhosis of the liver, pancreatitis, and brain damage. Although teenagers are seldom impressed by these remote consequences, the abusive effects on immature body systems are being seen earlier. This is particularly significant because a substantial number of alcoholics are preadolescents whose smaller bodies are affected more quickly by the drug. Studies have shown that even a low concentration of alcohol in the blood is a factor in teenage accidents. As the weight of the person is an important factor in the effect of the drug, adults should not allow small children to sample their drinks.

Alcohol dependence adversely affects the mental health of adolescents. Although the scope of the problem cannot be covered here, a few facts bear mentioning. Alcoholism prevents the teen-

Table 16–6. LONG-TERM EFFECTS, TOLERANCE, DEPENDENCE, ADULTERATION, AND METHODS OF ADMINISTRATION OF SUBSTANCES ADOLESCENTS ABUSE

| SUBSTANCE | LONG-TERM EFFECTS | TOLERANCE | DEPENDENCE | | ADULTERATION OR SUBSTITUTION | METHOD OF ADMINISTRATION |
			Psychologic	Physical		
Alcohol	Blackouts; behavioral changes; ↑ accidents; homocide, suicide; gastritis; peptic ulcer; alcoholic hepatitis; fatty liver; pancreatitis	Yes	Yes	Yes	No	Ingested
Ampheta-mine, other stimulants	Weight loss, insomnia, anxiety, paranoia, hallucinations. Skin abscesses and amphetamine psychosis following injections	Yes	High	Yes	More than 90% of speed is adulterated with caffeine, asthma medications, PCP, LSD, strychnine, sugars	Ingested, injected
Tobacco	↑ risk of chronic bronchitis, heart disease, and cancer. Oral cancer with smokeless tobacco	Yes	Yes	Yes	No	Smoke inhaled, snuff "dipped," chewed
Cocaine, crack	Nasal perforation with snorting, weight loss, insomnia, anxiety, paranoia, hallucinations, soft tissue abscesses with injections	Yes	High	Yes, especially following smoking or injection	Local anesthetics, sugars, PC	Snorted, smoked, ingested, injected
Inhalants (solvents, gasoline, etc.)	Liver damage with toluene, trichloroethylene, gasoline; anemia with tetraethyl lead; leukemia with benzene; kidney damage with trichloroethylene	Yes, especially with toluene	Yes	Yes	None	Sniffing rags soaked with the compound, inhaling fumes through the mouth
LSD, other hallucino-gens	Flashbacks, pronounced personality changes, ↑ risk of chronic psychosis	Yes, cross-tolerance with mescaline, DMT, and psilocybin	Degree unknown	No	Sold as tablets, in liquids, in microdots in many colors. Often adulterated with or substituted for other drugs	Ingested, injected, sniffed
Marijuana, hashish	Great variety involving several body systems. ↓ motivation	Yes	Degree unknown	No	With phencyclidine (PCP)	Smoke inhaled, ingested

Table continued on following page

Table 16–6. LONG-TERM EFFECTS, TOLERANCE, DEPENDENCE, ADULTERATION, AND METHODS OF ADMINISTRATION OF SUBSTANCES ADOLESCENTS ABUSE *Continued*

SUBSTANCE	LONG-TERM EFFECTS	TOLERANCE	DEPENDENCE Psychologic	DEPENDENCE Physical	ADULTERATION OR SUBSTITUTION	METHOD OF ADMINISTRATION
PCP and PCP analogues	Personality disorders, flashbacks, catatonia, neuropsychological disturbances, increased risk of schizophrenia	Yes	High	Degree unknown	Often added to other drugs or advertised as other drugs	Ingested, injected, smoked
Opioids	↓ motivation, antisocial behavior, crime to support habit, skin abscess, endocarditis, osteomyelitis, nephritis, hepatitis, HIV, amenorrhea	Yes	Yes	Yes	Quinine, sugar	Ingested, injected, subcutaneous (skin-popping), intravenous

(Modified from Jones, R. L. K. [1983]. Substance abuse. *In* Shearin R. B. (ed.): *Handbook of Adolescent Medicine*. Kalamazoo, MI, Upjohn Company, pp. 133–152.)

ager from working out crucial developmental tasks. Self-deception replaces self-esteem. Normal feelings of inadequacy, which are first masked by the drug, are then intensified by it. Social awkwardness is concealed, retarding growth in this area. Sexual inhibitions are lowered; thousands of unmarried adolescents are bearing children each year. Research shows that girls who drink heavily before pregnancy is detected and during pregnancy run a greater risk of having smaller or deformed babies. Sexual performance decreases with continued use, which can be shattering to the adolescent's emerging sexuality. Serious emotional problems may be camouflaged by alcohol use and abuse.

TREATMENT

Although the exact cause of alcoholism is unknown, several theories have been proposed. Investigations have revealed that genetics may play a part, as may biochemical, nutritional, psychological, and sociological factors.

Treatment programs vary. Alcoholics Anonymous (AA), a worldwide, nonprofit organization, has had the highest success rate. Its approach is based on abstinence "one day at a time" with the help of a higher power. Its leaders are recovered alcoholics who offer group counseling and answering services throughout the world. In the United States, AA's number is listed in the local telephone directory. AA programs for young people are available in some cities; however, as these programs are not as developed, young alcoholics are also welcomed at regular adult meetings. The concept of alcoholism as a family disease has been well established. Two programs closely related to Alcoholics Anonymous are Al-Anon and Alateen. Their inclusion in any treatment program for the adolescent is important. Al-Anon offers guidance to nonalcoholic family members who have their own problems resulting from living with the disease and teaches them how changes in their attitudes best help the alcoholic. Alateen, a fellowship for teenage sons and daughters of alcoholics, provides a setting in which youngsters can exchange experiences and learn to cope with their problems that may be related to the drinking adult in their family.

Many communities also have public and private alcoholism rehabilitation centers. As the magnitude of the problem has increased and more mon-

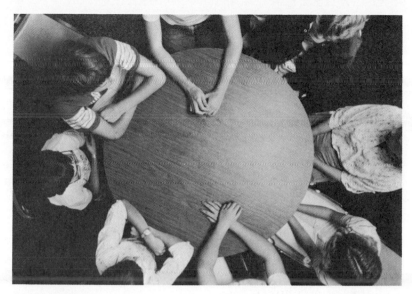

▲ **FIGURE 16–7**

Support groups with peers are an important therapeutic modality for adolescents with various addictions and/or mental health problems.

ies have become available, general hospitals are establishing detoxification units and counseling for these patients. One such model program is dedicated to 13 to 19 year old alcohol users. It consists of eight weeks in a residential treatment setting with a typical day of school, structured activities, and therapy. Parents attend weekly sessions and participate in group family therapy. One year of continuing care is available to patients and family after primary treatment. Other kinds of help include family therapy, alcohol clinics, and the use of physicians specializing in the disease. Often a patient will use AA in combination with other treatment modalities.

PREVENTION AND NURSING GOALS

The prevention of alcohol and other types of substance abuse begins by helping expectant parents develop good parenting skills. It is vitally important that children learn to feel good about themselves very early in life. They need adults they can trust and who serve as good role models. As orderly development proceeds, the growing child learns to interact with others and develops a sense of identity. A positive self-image and feelings of self-worth help adolescents fine tune

their adaptive coping skills. In time, they can rely on their own problem-solving abilities and, it is hoped, will not need chemicals to deal with the complexities of life. Nurses in their various settings can contribute to this process. They can also educate their clients about the seriousness of substance abuse.

Although it is generally true that problem drinkers cannot be helped unless they want to be, more *intervention* is now being done. Most adolescents involved in substance abuse do not choose to enter treatment but are coerced by family members or the juvenile justice system. Although this is a controversial issue, clinical experience in substance abuse treatment settings has shown that many adolescents become interested in treatment and make behavioral changes after they have been required to enter a treatment program.

NURSING CARE

The nurse's view of the disease and how he or she responds during a crisis may significantly affect the adolescent. Assessment of the patient includes finding out what particular alcoholic beverage was taken and what has happened to the patient since its consumption. Behavior and mood, level of consciousness, vital signs, pupil size, and any gastrointestinal disturbance are noted. The patient is placed on the side to prevent aspiration of fluids. Time is the only way to sober the patient, and the amount of time it takes depends on the patient's body weight and the amount of alcohol consumed.

The treatment plan of abstinence is especially difficult for adolescents, whose developmental patterns for conformity are at their peak. The motivational phase of treatment has the goal of establishing in the adolescent both a sense of self-worth and a commitment of self-help. The rehabilitative phase requires the readiness to substitute dependence on the self for dependence on alcohol.

Children of Alcoholics

Until recently, very little attention has been given to children of alcoholics. This trend is changing, and support groups such as Adult Children of Alcoholics are more numerous. This discussion concerns young children of alcoholics, although unresolved issues are similar in adults. Pediatric nurses are in an excellent position to recognize and intervene in cases in which physical or emotional neglect exists because of parental alcoholism. These problems stem from the fact that the parents are preoccupied with the disease. It is not unusual for both parents to be users.

Children of alcoholics are often very confused by the unpredictability of family life. They do not understand why their needs are not being met. In some families there is a role reversal, with the child being forced to act maturely and make decisions ordinarily assumed by a parent. Often these children feel that they are responsible for the disruptive environment. They are at high risk for physical abuse, including sexual abuse. Children of alcoholics are also strong candidates for developing alcoholism as adults. Role models are distorted or lacking. A parent may try to cover up for the drinking partner by lying to employers and relatives but may punish the child for the same behavior. The child may become isolated from peers while trying to avoid embarrassment at home. Four predominant coping patterns of these children are flight, fight, the perfect child, and the "super coper" or "family savior." This last child

becomes the family comforter and frequently works to provide income.

Early recognition of and intervention for children of alcoholics are paramount. The nurse with heightened awareness of alcoholism can expand admission observations and nursing history. Some clues that may or may not be related to this problem include refusal to talk about family life, poor school grades or overachievement, unusual need to please, fatigue, passive or acting-out behavior, or maturity beyond the child's years. Treatment is multifold. One immediate priority is to teach the child how to get help in an emergency and to put the youngster in touch with someone from the extended family, school, or another suitable agency. Cultural diversities need to be incorporated in treatment plans.

Marijuana

Marijuana, also known as "pot" or "grass," is a drug found in the plant *Cannabis sativa*, which grows wild in almost any temperate climate. The dried tops and leaves are usually chopped up like tobacco and rolled and smoked in cigarettes known as "joints." Marijuana produces a state of relaxation when smoked or eaten. The drug quickly enters the blood stream and acts on the nervous system. The physical effects include tachycardia and reddening of the eyes. Patients may also experience an acute increase in appetite ("the munchies").

The psychological effects vary with the individual. The patient may feel excited or depressed. There may be distortions in the sense of time, perceptions of color, and hearing. Memory and reaction time are impaired. The inexperienced user may develop "pot panic" and paranoia.

The active ingredient of marijuana is tetrahydrocannabinol (THC), which is primarily metabolized by the liver. The drug is fat soluble and can accumulate for long periods of time in the body. There has been an increase in potency in THC in the past years, leading to more side effects. The young person who smokes a great deal is at greater risk than the adult who smokes occasionally. Marijuana should not be used by those with seizure disorders, as it is known to cause convulsions in animals and interferes with anticonvulsant medication. Cardiopulmonary and endocrine problems have also been cited (Neinstein, 1984). Driving an automobile while under the influence of the drug is extremely hazardous.

Nothing in this drug causes a person to go to the "harder" drugs, but the *personality of the user* may lead to use of other drugs. Studies show that users also tend to drink alcohol and smoke cigarettes more than nonusers; alcohol is often used along with pot. The Marijuana Tax Act of 1937 made possession of the drug a criminal offense. In spite of this it has been widely available. More information is required to determine the long-term consequences of use of marijuana.

References

Behrman, R., and Kligman, R. (1989). *Nelson Essentials of Pediatrics.* Philadelphia, W. B. Saunders Company.

Brown, H. (1989). Recognizing STDs in adolescents. *Contemp. Pediatr.* 6:17–36.

Comerci, G. (1990). Eating disorders: Anorexia nervosa and bulimia nervosa. *In* Green, M., and Haggerty, R. (eds.). *Ambulatory Pediatrics.* Philadelphia, W. B. Saunders Company, pp. 490–500.

DeRosa, G. (1990). Musculoskeletal disorders. Congenital, developmental, and nontraumatic. *In* Green, M., and Haggerty, R. (eds.). *Ambulatory Pediatrics.* Philadelphia, W. B. Saunders Company, pp. 333–347.

Frost, N. (1987). Ethical dilemma: How far can confidentiality stretch? *Contemp. Pediatr.* 4:55–64.

Goldbloom, D., and Garfinkel, P. (1990). Eating disorders: Anorexia nervosa and bulimia nervosa. *In* Garfinkel, P., Carlson, G., and Weller, E. (eds.). *Psychiatric Disorders in Children and Adolescents.* Philadelphia, W. B. Saunders Company, pp. 106–119.

Green, M., and Haggerty, R. (1990). *Ambulatory Pediatrics.* Philadelphia, W. B. Saunders Company.

Litt, I. (1990). Adolescent health care. *In* Green, M., and Haggerty, R. (eds.). *Ambulatory Pediatrics.* Philadelphia, W. B. Saunders Company, pp. 123–135.

Neinstein, L. (1984). *Adolescent Health Care.* Baltimore, Urban and Schwarzenberg.

Neumann, C. (1983). Obesity in childhood. *In* Levine, M., Carey, W., Crocker, A., and Gross, R. (eds.). *Developmental-Behavioral Pediatrics.* Philadelphia, W. B. Saunders Company, pp. 536–551.

Pipes, P. (1989). *Nutrition in Infancy and Childhood.* St. Louis, Times Mirror/Mosby College Publishing.

U.S. Department of Health and Human Services. (1990). *Healthy People 2000* (DHHS Publication No. (PHS) 91-50213). Washington, D.C., U.S. Government Printing Office.

Vaughan, V., and Litt, I. (1990). *Child and Adolescent Development.* Philadelphia, W. B. Saunders Company.

Bibliography

Atton, A., and Tunnessen, W. (1988). Acne update: Help your patients help themselves. *Contemp. Pediatr.* 5:18–50.

Behrman, R., and Vaughan, V. (1987). *Nelson Textbook of Pediatrics.* 13th ed. Philadelphia, W. B. Saunders Company.

Beach, R. (1989). Menstrual cramps need not be a "curse." *Contemp. Pediatr.* 6:41–54.

Blythe, M. (1990). Sexually transmitted diseases. *In* Green, M., and Haggerty, R. (eds). *Ambulatory Pediatrics.* Philadelphia, W. B. Saunders Company, pp. 201–218.

Castiglia, P. (1990). Adolescent fathers. *J. Pediatr. Health Care* 4:311–313.

Foster, R., Hunsberger, M., and Anderson, J. (1989). *Family-Centered Nursing Care of Children.* Philadelphia, W. B. Saunders Company.

Goldenring, J., and Cohen, E. (1988). Getting into adolescent heads. *Contemp. Pediatr.* 5:75–90.

Halikas, J. (1990). Substance abuse in children and adolescents. *In* Garfinkel, B., Carlson, G., and Weller, E. (eds.). *Psychiatric Disorders in Children and Adolescents.* Philadelphia, W. B. Saunders Company, pp. 210–234.

Joffe, A. (1990). Too little, too much: Eating disorders in adolescents. *Contemp. Pediatr.* 7:114–135.

Jones, M., and Bonte, C. (1990). Conceptualizing community interventions in social service needs of pregnant adolescents. *J. Pediatr. Health Care* 4:193–201.

Moore, D. (1988). Body image and eating behavior in adolescent girls. *Am. J. Dis. Child.* 142:1114–1118.

Pfeffer, C. (1989). Spotting the red flags for adolescent suicide. *Contemp. Pediatr.* 6:59–70.

Robinson, D., and Greene, J. (1988). The adolescent alcohol and drug problem: A practical approach. *Pediatr. Nurs.* 14:305–310.

Rolfes, S., and DeBruyne, L. (1990). *Life Span Nutrition: Conception Through Life.* St. Paul, West.

U.S. Department of Health and Human Services (1990). *Sexually Transmitted Diseases Summary.* Washington, D.C., U.S. Government Printing Office.

STUDY QUESTIONS

1. Kelly is a 15 year old girl who is receiving chemotherapy for bone cancer. She has a small reddened area surrounding her fingernail. She states, "Oh, that's nothing." What instructions would you give to Kelly? Provide the rationale for these instructions.
2. The year-end class picnic is in another week. Kelly has a new swim suit and is very excited about the event. Her prothrombin count is low today. What counseling will Kelly require? Explain.

3. Mrs. Pizinger's son Larry wants to join the high school swimming team. What health factors need to be considered in investigating this possibility?

4. Janice Nichols is a 15 year old patient with scoliosis. She is hospitalized and in a Risser body cast. Identify the nursing measures required to maintain the integrity of Janice's skin. State the rationale for each measure.

5. List two developmental tasks of the adolescent. How does immobilization interfere with these? Suggest nursing interventions to help the patient cope with confinement.

6. Eighteen year old Margaret has anorexia nervosa. Define this condition and its cause. What approach would you take when meeting Margaret for the first time? Discuss the reasons for your approach.

7. Pedro is a very obese 13 year old. His favorite foods are french fries and Coca-Cola. What nutritional principles would you teach Pedro? How does "being fat" affect Pedro's psychosocial development?

8. Mike DesRosiers, age 17, is a star basketball player. His coach has informed his mother that lately Mike seems unusually tired. His mother says that he has had a sore throat for several weeks. After examination by a physician a diagnosis of mononucleosis is made. What laboratory test would support this diagnosis? Outline the nursing management for this condition.

9. Mel, who is 15, discloses to you that he has a friend who thinks he has "clap." What knowledge do you need in order to discuss this with Mel? What immediate suggestions might you offer?

APPENDICES

APPENDIX A

COMMONLY USED PEDIATRIC DRUGS

DRUG	ROUTE AND FORM*	DOSAGE AND FREQUENCY*	SOME INDICATIONS FOR USE	NURSING CONSIDERATIONS
Achromycin (tetra-cycline)	O, IM, IV Tablets, capsules, syrup	Children over 8 years:—O: 25–50 mg/kg/24 hr divided q 6 hr; IM: 15–25 mg/kg/24 hr divided q 8–12 hr; IV: 10–20 mg/kg/24 hr divided q 12 hr	Broad-spectrum anti-biotic	Diarrhea, limit in children under 8 years to avoid staining and pitting of the teeth, photosensitivity, gastric distress, superimposed infection Do not give with milk or antacids Take careful history to determine allergies Give 1 hr before meals
Adrenalin, Sus-phrine (epineph-rine)	SC, IM, inhalation Ampules, vials	In acute asthmatic attack—children—SC: 0.01/mg/kg/dose, repeat prn q 20 min, 2 times	Antispasmodic for use in patients with asthma Local hemostat in surgery	Causes blood pressure to rise; use with caution in cardiac patients Massage well after injection Do not use discolored solution
Aminophylline (theophylline ethylenediamine)	O, IV Oral solution, tablets, enteric-coated tablets, extended-release tablets, rectal suppository (rare)	O: 1–9 years: 20 mg/kg/24 hr divided q 6 hr; 9–16 years: 16 mg/kg/24 hr divided q 6 hr IV: Loading dose: 6 mg/kg one dose only; 1–9 years: 1 mg/kg/24 hr; 9–12 years: 0.9 mg/kg/24 hr Therapeutic range is 10–20 µg/ml	Bronchodilator used in asthma, chronic bronchitis, and apnea and bradycardia in premature infants	Food delays absorption of oral form Extended-release capsules or enteric-coated tablets should not be crushed or chewed Usually administered IV over 30 minutes IV solution incompatible with most other drugs Observe for irritability, headache, nausea, vomiting, restlessness
Amoxicillin (Amoxil, Larotid)	O Capsules, oral suspension, pediatric drops	20–40 mg/kg 24 hr divided q 8 hr	Broad-spectrum antibiotic	Hypersensitivity may cause anaphylactic reaction Shake suspension well
Ampicillin (Omnipen, Penbritin, Amcill)	O, IM, IV Capsules, oral suspension, pediatric drops	50–100 mg/kg/24 hr divided q 6 hr (O), 100–200 mg/kg/24 hr divided q 4 hr, q 6 hr (IM) (IV)	Septicemia, meningitis	May cause agranulocytosis, rash, stomatitis, contraindicated in patients with a history of hypersensitivity to penicillins; take on empty stomach Reconstituted should be used within 1 hr

DRUG	ROUTE AND FORM*	DOSAGE AND FREQUENCY*	SOME INDICATIONS FOR USE	NURSING CONSIDERATIONS
Aspirin (acetylsalicylic acid)	O, R Tablets, suppositories	Infants and children— O: 30–65 mg/kg/24 hr divided q 4–6 hr prn	High fever, general malaise, rheumatic fever, relief of itching	Do not use in children with chickenpox or influenza-like symptoms Ringing in ears, GI upsets, disturbance in acid-base balance of body Keep out of reach of children
Ceclor (Cefaclor)	O Capsules, suspension	20–40 mg/kg/24 hr divided q 8–12 hr	Antibiotic	Determine allergy to penicillins or cephalosporins Refrigerate/shake suspension well Observe for superinfections or diarrhea
Dilantin (phenytoin)	O, IM, IV Tablets, capsules, suspension, solution for injection	As anticonvulsant— infants and children—O: 3–8 mg/kg/24 hr divided q 12 hr	Anticonvulsant for seizures, epilepsy	Confusion, slurred speech, blood dyscrasias, ataxia, rash, nausea, vomiting Give with at least a half glass of water with or after meals to minimize gastric distress Avoid abrupt withdrawal Instruct patients to adhere strictly to prescribed dosage routine, call physician if skin rash develops, stress good oral hygiene to prevent gingivitis
Erythromycin (Pediamycin, Ilotycin) Erythromycin estolate (Ilosone)	O, IV Tablets, drops, suspension, ampules	Infants and children— O: 30–50 mg/kg/24 hr divided q 6 hr; IV: 10–20 mg/kg/24 hr divided q 6 hr	Rheumatic fever prophylaxis Useful if child is sensitive to penicillin	GI irritation, rash Administer punctually to maintain blood levels Take careful history to determine allergies
Ferosol, Fer-in-Sol (ferrous sulfate)	O Tablets, capsules, syrup, elixir, drops	For prophylaxis: 0.5– 1 mg/kg/24 hr, single or divided doses For treatment: 6 mg/ kg/24 hr divided into 3 doses	Iron deficiency anemia	GI distress, diarrhea, constipation Administer after meals or use coated tablets Administer oral liquid through straw to avoid discoloration of teeth Keep out of reach of children; overdose may be fatal As oral iron products tend to interfere with the absorption of oral tetracycline antibiotics, these products should not be taken within 2 hr of each other
Glucagon	SC, IM, IV Ampules	0.025 mg/kg; may repeat in 20 min	Emergency treatment of severe hypoglycemia reactions in diabetes	Rare; when the patient responds give supplemental carbohydrate to restore liver glycogen and prevent secondary hypoglycemia, particularly important for juvenile diabetics who may not have as great a response in blood glucose levels as adults
Imferon (iron dextran)	IM Solution for injection	Dose calculated by formula using weight of child + hemoglobin	Iron deficiency anemia; used when oral administration is unsatisfactory or impossible	Arthralgias, anaphylactoid reactions, rash, itching Test dose of 0.5 ml should be given on first day Use "Z" track technique, inject deeply, observe for tissue staining

Table continued on following page

DRUG	ROUTE AND FORM*	DOSAGE AND FREQUENCY*	SOME INDICATIONS FOR USE	NURSING CONSIDERATIONS
Ipecac syrup	O Syrup	Emetic (for children older than 1 year): 15 ml by mouth in single dose; may repeat once in 20 min Expectorant: 1–2 ml taken with glass of water	To induce vomiting in poisoning As expectorant for croup	Follow with water Always order by complete name (other preparations are toxic) Store in dry, cool place Do not give to unconscious patients Do not induce vomiting for poisoning with substances such as petroleum distillates, strong alkali or acid, or strychnine
Isuprel (isoproterenol hydrochloride)	Sublingual, R, IV Inhalation, tablets, vials, mist	By nebulizer; pressurized mist, 1:400, 3–4 times a day	Bronchodilator in treatment of asthma, bronchitis	Tachycardia, flushing of skin, restlessness Use with care in patients with heart complications Elicit child's cooperation
Keflex (cephalexin)	O Capsules, tablets, suspension	Infants and children— O: 25–50 mg/kg/24 hr divided q 6 hr	Antibiotic, antibacterial	Contraindicated in patients with known allergies to cephalosporin group of antibiotics Observe for rash, diarrhea Evaluate glycosuria with Tes-Tape to avoid false-positive tests
Keflin (cephalothin sodium)	IM, IV Ampules	Infants and children— IM, IV: 80–160 mg/kg/24 hr q 4 hr	Broad-spectrum antibiotic for most infections, particularly of urinary tract or by resistant staphylococci	Anaphylaxis, diarrhea Rotate injection sites, chart exact site Administer punctually to maintain blood levels
Lanoxin (digoxin)	O, IV, IM Tablets, elixir, solution for injection	Individualized regimens; consult pharmacopeia	Frequently used for neonates and children with heart conditions	Check apical pulse before administering If anorexia, dizziness, or irregular or slow heartbeat develops, withhold additional doses and consult physician
Mycostatin (nystatin)	O, topical Tablets, suspension, powder, ointment, vaginal tablets	Suspension, O, and topical: neonates— 100,000 units, q 6 hr, swabbed in mouth; children— 400,000–600,000 units q 6 hr	Antifungal antibiotic for thrush, diaper rash, other types of skin lesions caused by Candida albicans	GI distress Virtually nontoxic, well tolerated by all age groups
Oxacillin sodium (Prostaphlin)	O, IM, IV Capsules, solutions for injection	Infants and children— O: 50–100 mg/kg/24 hr divided q 6 hr	Mild to moderate infections of skin, soft tissues, or upper respiratory tract and resistant staphylococcal infections	See Penicillin G Take careful history to determine allergies Chart exact site of IM injection Administer punctually to maintain blood levels Give oral preparations 1–2 hr before meals

DRUG	ROUTE AND FORM*	DOSAGE AND FREQUENCY*	SOME INDICATIONS FOR USE	NURSING CONSIDERATIONS
Pancreatic enzymes (Cotazym, Viokase)	O Granules, tablets, capsules	Individualized dosage regimens	Aid to digestion in cystic fibrosis	Contraindicated in persons hypersensitive to beef or pork products May be taken with water or milk or sprinkled on foods
Penicillin G (benzyl penicillin G) (Pentids)	O, IM, IV Many forms and preparations	Older children— 25,000–50,000 units/kg/24 hr divided into 4–6 doses	Antibiotic used for many types of infection	Take careful history to determine allergies May cause anaphylactic reactions Many other warnings—consult pharmacopeia Chart exact site of injection, administer on time
Phenergan (promethazine hydrochloride)	O, R, IM, IV Tablets, syrup, ampules, vials, suppositories	Children—O: 0.125 mg/kg/24 hr divided into half dose at bedtime and quarter doses every 6 hr of the remaining day; IM, IV: 1 mg/kg every 4–6 hr	As treatment for nausea, vomiting, or motion sickness or as antihistamine	Causes drowsiness When giving IM, aspirate carefully before injecting Rotate injection sites IV rarely used
Phenobarbital (Luminal)	O, IM Tablets, capsules, elixir, solution for injection	Status epilepticus: 15–20 mg/kg (IV) over 10 to 15 min Sedation: 2 mg/kg/24 hr q 8 hr (O)	CNS depressant, epilepsy, convulsions associated with high fever	May be habit-forming; avoid sudden withdrawal, reactions uncommon with small doses
Povan (pyrivinium pamoate)	O Tablets, suspension	5 mg/kg single dose	Anthelmintic used in treating pinworms	Colors stools red, nausea, vomiting Avoid chewing tablets—will stain teeth Not for aspirin-sensitive patients
Ritalin (methylphenidate hydrochloride)	O	Patients over 3 years; 5 mg (O) before breakfast and lunch	CNS stimulant, used in treatment of attention-deficit disorder	Nervousness, weight loss, anorexia, insomnia Last dose is given several hours before bedtime Contraindicated in convulsive disorders
Rocephin (ceftriaxone sodium)	IM, IV	Neonates—50 mg/kg/ 24 hr as single dose; infants, children 50–75 mg/kg/24 hr divided q 12 hr; over 12 years: 1–2 g daily or in divided doses q 12 hr *Note:* In meningitis the dosage is increased	Antibiotic	Determine allergy to penicillins or cephalosporins Observe IV site for vein irritation Watch for signs of superinfection or diarrhea
Slo-Phyllin (theophylline)	O, R Tablets, elixir, suppositories	Dose has wide range and is adjusted according to weight of child	Bronchodilator used for asthmatics and patients with chronic bronchitis	Nausea, vomiting, irritability, convulsions Contraindicated in patients with peptic ulcers, diabetes, hypertension Monitor vital signs

Table continued on following page

DRUG	ROUTE AND FORM*	DOSAGE AND FREQUENCY*	SOME INDICATIONS FOR USE	NURSING CONSIDERATIONS
Solu-Medrol (methylprednisolone sodium succinate)	O, IM, IV, R, topical	O: 0.4–1.67 mg/kg/24 hr in 3–4 divided doses IM: 0.03–0.2 mg/kg 1–2 times per day IV: 1.6 mg/kg/24 hr q 6 hr R: 0.5–1 mg/kg/24 hr Topical: apply a thin film 1–2 times/24 hr	Corticosteroid with anti-inflammatory, immunosuppressant, and metabolic actions	Oral should be taken with food to reduce GI irritation Inject IM deep into muscle, do not use deltoid muscle Incompatible with aminophylline Do not alter dosage or stop drug abruptly Monitor for signs and symptoms of corticosteroid overdosage Should not be immunized with live viruses Observe for signs of infection
Staphcillin (methcillin sodium)	IM, IV Solution for injection	Infants and children— 200–400 mg/kg/24 divided q 4 hr IV, q 6 hr IM	Treatment of respiratory and skin infections caused by susceptible organisms Form of penicillin	Superimposed infections, blood changes, nausea, vomiting, diarrhea Use with care in patients with allergies (especially to other penicillins), may cause anaphylactic reactions Administer punctually; chart exact site of IM injection
Sulfadiazine (a sulfonamide)	O, SC, IV Tablets, suspension solution for injection	Infants and children— O, IV: 120–150 mg/kg/24 hr divided into 4–6 doses	Rheumatic fever prophylaxis, urinary tract infections, meningococcal meningitis	Record intake and output Sore throat, fever, and rash may indicate blood dyscrasia, report immediately Crush tablets if large Report oliguria, hematuria Observe for mouth sores
Tylenol, Liquiprin, Tempra (acetaminophen)	O Tablets, drops, syrup, elixir	Infants and children— O: 20–40 mg/kg/24 hr divided q 4–6 hr prn	Analgesic and antipyretic	See label In general, do not use for more than a few days unless under care of a physician Keep away from children; overdose may cause liver failure; contact poison control center immediately for advice
Ventolin, Proventil (albuterol)	O, inhalation Tablets, extended-release tablets, solution for nebulization	O: 2–6 years: 0.1 mg/kg/24 hr in 3 divided doses (maximum dose 2 mg 3 times/24 hr); 6–12 years: 2 mg 3–4 times/24 hr (maximum of 24 mg/24 hr) Inhalation: under 12 years: 1–2 inhalations 4 times/24 hr; over 12 years: 1–2 inhalations 4–6 times/24 hr Note: Not recommended for children under 12 years	Bronchodilator used to relieve bronchospasms of asthma, bronchitis, and cystic fibrosis	Do not crush coated tablets Monitor pulse and respiratory response to medication Teach use and care of inhaler Inhaler should not be used more frequently than prescribed Notify physician if condition worsens

DRUG	ROUTE AND FORM*	DOSAGE AND FREQUENCY*	SOME INDICATIONS FOR USE	NURSING CONSIDERATIONS
Zinacef (cefuroxine sodium)	IM, IV	Over 3 months: 50–100 mg/kg/24 hr divided q 6–8 hr *Note:* In meningitis the dosage is increased	Antibiotic	Determine allergy to penicillins or cephalosporins IM injection is painful for about 5 min

*IM = intramuscular injection, IV = intravenous injection, O = oral, R = rectal, SC = subcutaneous, prn = as needed.

(Adapted from Behrman, R., and Vaughan, V. [1987]. *Nelson Textbook of Pediatrics,* 13th ed. Philadelphia, W. B. Saunders Company, and Bindler, R. M., and Howry, L. B. [1991]. *Pediatric Drugs and Nursing Implications.* Norwalk, Conn., Appleton & Lange.)

NOTE: **This table serves only as a quick reference and should not replace the use of a more detailed reference.**

APPENDIX B

Nanda-approved nursing diagnoses

This list represents the NANDA† approved nursing diagnoses for clinical use and testing (1990).

PATTERN 1:   EXCHANGING

1.1.2.1	Altered nutrition: More than body requirements
1.1.2.2	Altered nutrition: Less than body requirements
1.1.2.3	Altered nutrition: Potential for more than body requirements
1.2.1.1	Potential for infection
1.2.2.1	Potential altered body temperature
1.2.2.2	Hypothermia
1.2.2.3	Hyperthermia
1.2.2.4	Ineffective thermoregulation
1.2.3.1	Dysreflexia
*1.3.1.1	Constipation
1.3.1.1.1	Perceived constipation
1.3.1.1.2	Colonic constipation
*1.3.1.2	Diarrhea
*1.3.1.3	Bowel incontinence
1.3.2	Altered urinary elimination
1.3.2.1.1	Stress incontinence
1.3.2.1.2	Reflex incontinence
1.3.2.1.3	Urge incontinence
1.3.2.1.4	Functional incontinence
1.3.2.1.5	Total incontinence
1.3.2.2	Urinary retention
*1.4.1.1	Altered (specify type) tissue perfusion (renal, cerebral, cardiopulmonary, gastrointestinal, peripheral)
1.4.1.2.1	Fluid volume excess
1.4.1.2.2.1	Fluid volume deficit
1.4.1.2.2.2	Potential fluid volume deficit
*1.4.2.1	Decreased cardiac output
1.5.1.1	Impaired gas exchange
1.5.1.2	Ineffective airway clearance
1.5.1.3	Ineffective breathing pattern
1.6.1	Potential for injury
1.6.1.1	Potential for suffocation

1.6.1.2	Potential for poisoning
1.6.1.3	Potenital for trauma
1.6.1.4	Potential for aspiration
1.6.1.5	Potential for disuse syndrome
†1.6.2	Altered protection
1.6.2.1	Impaired tissue integrity
*1.6.2.1.1	Altered oral mucous membrane
1.6.2.1.2.1	Impaired skin integrity
1.6.2.1.2.2	Potential impaired skin integrity

PATTERN 2:   COMMUNICATING

2.1.1.1	Impaired verbal communication

PATTERN 3:   RELATING

3.1.1	Impaired social interaction
3.1.2	Social isolation
*3.2.1	Altered role performance
3.2.1.1.1	Altered parenting
3.2.1.1.2	Potential altered parenting
3.2.1.2.1	Sexual dysfunction
3.2.2	Altered family processes
3.2.3.1	Parental role conflict
3.3	Altered sexuality patterns

PATTERN 4:   VALUING

4.1.1	Spiritual distress (distress of the human spirit)

PATTERN 5:   CHOOSING

5.1.1.1	Ineffective individual coping
5.1.1.1.1	Impaired adjustment
5.1.1.1.2	Defensive coping
5.1.1.1.3	Ineffective denial
5.1.2.1.1	Ineffective family coping: Disabling
5.1.2.1.2	Ineffective family coping: Compromised
5.1.2.2	Family coping: Potenital for growth
5.2.1.1	Noncompliance (specify)
5.3.1.1	Decisional conflict (specify)
5.4	Health-seeking behaviors (specify)

PATTERN 6:   MOVING

6.1.1.1	Impaired physical mobility
6.1.1.2	Activity intolerance

6.1.1.2.1	Fatigue
6.1.1.3	Potential activity intolerance
6.2.1	Sleep pattern disturbance
6.3.1.1	Diversional activity deficit
6.4.1.1	Impaired home maintenance management
6.4.2	Altered health maintenance
*6.5.1	Feeding self-care deficit
6.5.1.1	Impaired swallowing
6.5.1.2	Ineffective breast feeding
†6.5.1.3	Effective breast feeding
*6.5.2	Bathing/hygiene self-care deficit
*6.5.3	Dressing/grooming self-care deficit
*6.5.4	Toileting self-care deficit
6.6	Altered growth and development

Pattern 7:   Perceiving

*7.1.1	Body image disturbance
*7.1.2	Self-esteem disturbance
7.1.2.1	Chronic low self-esteem
7.1.2.2	Situational low self-esteem
*7.1.3	Personal identity disturbance
7.2	Sensory/perceptual alterations (specify) (visual, auditory, kinesthetic, gustatory, tactile, olfactory)
7.2.1.1	Unilateral neglect
7.3.1	Hopelessness
7.3.2	Powerlessness

PATTERN 8:   KNOWING

8.1.1	Knowledge deficit (specify)
8.3	Altered thought processes

PATTERN 9:   FEELING

*9.1.1	Pain
9.1.1.1	Chronic pain
9.2.1.1	Dysfunctional grieving
9.2.1.2	Anticipatory grieving
9.2.2	Potential for violence: Self-directed or directed at others
9.2.3	Post-trauma response
9.2.3.1	Rape-trauma syndrome
9.2.3.1.1	Rape-trauma syndrome: Compound reaction
9.2.3.1.2	Rape-trauma syndrome: Silent reaction
9.3.1	Anxiety
9.3.2	Fear

*Categories with modified label terminology.
†New diagnostic categories approved 1990.

RECOMMENDATIONS FOR PREVENTIVE PEDIATRIC HEALTH CARE

RECOMMENDATIONS FOR PREVENTIVE PEDIATRIC HEALTH CARE
Committee on Practice and Ambulatory Medicine

Each child and family is unique; therefore, these **Recommendations for Preventive Pediatric Health Care** are designed for the care of children who are receiving competent parenting, have no manifestations of any important health problems, and are growing and developing in satisfactory fashion. **Additional visits may become necessary** if circumstances suggest variations from normal. These guidelines represent a consensus by the Committee on Practice and Ambulatory Medicine in consultation with the membership of the American Academy of Pediatrics through the Chapter Presidents. The Committee emphasizes the great importance of **continuity of care** in comprehensive health supervision and the need to avoid **fragmentation of care.**

A **prenatal visit** by first-time parents and/or those who are at high risk is recommended and should include anticipatory guidance and pertinent medical history.

	INFANCY							EARLY CHILDHOOD					LATE CHILDHOOD					ADOLESCENCE[2]			
AGE[3]	2–3 d[1]	By 1 mo	2 mo	4 mo	6 mo	9 mo	12 mo	15 mo	18 mo	24 mo	3 y	4 y	5 y	6 y	8 y	10 y	12 y	14 y	16 y	18 y	20y+
HISTORY																					
Initial/Interval	●	●	●	●	●	●	●	●	●	●	●	●	●	●	●	●	●	●	●	●	●
MEASUREMENTS																					
Height and Weight	●	●	●	●	●	●	●	●	●	●	●	●	●	●	●	●	●	●	●	●	●
Head Circumference	●	●	●	●	●	●	●	●	●	●											
Blood Pressure											●	●	●	●	●	●	●	●	●	●	●
SENSORY SCREENING																					
Vision	S	S	S	S	S	S	S	S	S	S	S	O	O	O	O	S	O	O	S	O	O
Hearing	S	S	S	S	S	S	S	S	S	S	S	O	O	S[4]	S[4]	S[4]	O	S	S	O	S
DEVELOPMENTAL/ BEHAVIORAL ASSESSMENT[5]	●	●	●	●	●	●	●	●	●	●	●	●	●	●	●	●	●	●	●	●	●
PHYSICAL EXAMINATION[6]	●	●	●	●	●	●	●	●	●	●	●	●	●	●	●	●	●	●	●	●	●
PROCEDURES[7]																					
Hereditary/Metabolic Screening[8]	●—————→																				
Immunization[9]		●	●	●	●	←———	●	●	←———	●			←———	←———					←———		
Tuberculin Test[10]							←———	●					●———					●———			
Hematocrit or Hemoglobin[11]		←—————————→				●		←—————————→					←—————————→					←—————————→			
Urinalysis[12]		←—————————→						←—————————→					←—————————→					←—————————→			
ANTICIPATORY GUIDANCE[13]	●	●	●	●	●	●	●	●	●	●	●	●	●	●	●	●	●	●	●	●	●
INITIAL DENTAL REFERRAL[14]											●										

1. For newborns discharged in 24 hours or less after delivery.
2. Adolescent-related issues (eg, psychosocial, emotional, substance usage, and reproductive health) may necessitate more frequent health supervision.
3. If a child comes under care for the first time at any point on the schedule, or if any items are not accomplished at the suggested age, the schedule should be brought up to date at the earliest possible time.
4. At these points, history may suffice: if problem suggested, a standard testing method should be employed.
5. By history and appropriate physical examination: if suspicious, by specific objective developmental testing.
6. At each visit, a complete physical examination is essential, with infant totally unclothed, older child undressed and suitably draped.
7. These may be modified, depending upon entry point into schedule and individual need.
8. Metabolic screening (eg, thyroid, PKU, galactosemia) should be done according to state law.
9. Schedule(s) per *Report of the Committee on Infectious Diseases,* 1991 Red Book, and current AAP Committee statements.

10. For high-risk groups, the Committee on Infectious Diseases recommends annual TB skin testing.
11. Present medical evidence suggests the need for reevaluation of the frequency and timing of hemoglobin or hematocrit tests. One determination is therefore suggested during each time period. Performance of additional tests is left to the individual practice experience.
12. Present medical evidence suggests the need for reevaluation of the frequency and timing of urinalyses. One determination is therefore suggested during each time period. Performance of additional tests is left to the individual practice experience.
13. Appropriate discussion and counseling should be an integral part of each visit for care.
14. Subsequent examinations as prescribed by dentist.

NB: **Special chemical, immunologic, and endocrine testing is** usually carried out upon specific indications. Testing other than newborn (eg, inborn errors of metabolism, sickle disease, lead) is discretionary with the physician.

Key: ● = to be performed   S = subjective, by history   O = objective, by a standard testing method

The recommendations in this publication do not indicate an exclusive course of treatment or serve as a standard of medical care. Variations, taking into account individual circumstances, may be appropriate.

AAP News, July 1991   RE9224

American Academy
of Pediatrics

NORMAL LABORATORY VALUES FOR CHILDREN—REFERENCE RANGES
Reference Ranges

Reference ranges are guides for judging health and disease. For many years, the method of defining the normal range was to make a series of measurements in healthy individuals and then calculate the mean and standard deviation of those measurements. By convention the normal range was defined as the mean ± 2 SD. This system does not work in most medical situations because the distribution of measurements does not fit a gaussian distribution. Most biologic measurements are skewed. A more appropriate normal distribution or reference range can be defined as the central 90 per cent (5th to 95th percentiles) of a group of measurements in normal individuals. This listing of reference ranges uses the measured or reasonable estimate of the central 90 per cent of a normal distribution of values. These ranges have proved to be clinically useful in . . . pediatric wards and clinics.

Test and Specimen	Reference Range		Reference Range International Units
Albumin		*g/dL*	*g/L*
Serum	Premature:	3.0—4.2	30—42
	Newborn:	3.6—5.4	36—54
	Infant:	4.0—5.0	40—50
	Thereafter:	3.5—5.0	35—50
CSF	10—30 mg/dL		100—300 mg/L
Urine, *Qualitative*	<20 mg/dL		<200 mg/L
Quantitative	<80 mg/d		<80 mg/d
Ammonia Nitrogen, Resin or Enzymatic		*µg/N/dL*	*µmol/L*
Serum or plasma (Na-heparin)	Newborn	90—150	64—107
	0—2 wk:	79—129	56—92
	> 1 mo:	29—70	21—50
	Thereafter:	15—45	11—32
Urine, 24 hr	500—1200 mg/d		36—86 mmol/d
Amphetamine	Therap. conc. 20—30 ng/mL		150—220 nmol/L
Serum plasma (heparin, EDTA)	Toxic conc.: > 200		> 1500
Amylase (*Beckman; BMD*)			
Serum	Newborn: 5—65 U/L		Same
	>1 yr: 25—125		Same
Urine, timed specimen	1—17 U/hr		Same
Anion Gap [Na − (Cl + CO₂)]	7—16 mmol/L		Same
Plasma (heparin)			
Anti-Deoxyribonuclease B Titer (Anti-DNAse Titer)	≤ 170 units		Same
Serum			
Antidiuretic Hormone (hADH, Vasopressin)	*Plasma*	*Plasma ADH*	*Plasma ADH*
Plasma (EDTA)	*mOsmol/kg*	*pg/mL*	*ng/L*
	270—280:	<1.5	Same
	280—285:	<2.5	
	285—290:	1—5	
	290—295:	2—7	
	295—300:	4—12	
Anti-Streptolysin-O Titer (ASO titer)	≤166 Todd Units		
Serum	170—330 Todd Units in school-aged children		

Test and Specimen	Reference Range	Reference Range International Units
Base Excess Whole blood (heparin)	*mmol/L* Newborn: $(-10)-(-2)$ Infant: $(-7)-(-1)$ Child: $(-4)-(+2)$ Thereafter: $(-3)-(+3)$	Same
Bicarbonate Serum	Arterial: 21–28 mmol/L Venous: 22–29	Same
Bile Acids, Total Serum, fasting Serum, 2 hr postprandial Feces	0.3–2.3 μg/mL 1.8–3.2 μg/mL 120–225 mg/d	0.3–2.3 mg/L 1.8–3.2 mg/L 120–225 mg/d

Bilirubin

	Premature mg/dL	Full-Term mg/dL	μmol/L	
Total Serum Cord: 0–1 d: 1–2 d: 2–5 d: Thereafter:	<2.0 <8.0 <12.0 <16.0 <2.0	<2.0 <6.0 <8.0 <12.0 0.2–1.0	<34 <137 <205 <274 <34	<34 <103 <137 <205 3.4–17.1

Test and Specimen	Reference Range	Reference Range International Units
Total Urine *Total* Amniotic fluid	Negative 28 wk: <0.075 mg/dL (or ΔA_{450} <0.048) 40 wk: <0.025 mg/dL (or ΔA_{450} <0.02)	Negative <1.3 μmol/L (or ΔA_{450} <0.048) <0.43 μmol/L (or ΔA_{450} <0.02)
Conjugated (Direct) Serum	0–0.2 mg/dL	0–3.4 μmol/L
Bleeding Time (BT) Blood from skin puncture *Ivy* *Simplate (G D)*	Normal: 2–7 min Borderline: 7–11 min 2.75–8 min	Same
Blood Volume Whole blood (heparin)	M: 52–83 mL/kg F: 50–75 mL/kg	M: 0.052–0.083 L/kg F: 0.050–0.075 L/kg
C-Reactive Protein Serum	Cord: 10–350 ng/mL Adult: 68–8200	10–350 μg/L 68–8200

Calcium, Ionized (ICa)

Serum, plasma, or whole blood (heparin)	mg/dL	mmol/L
Cord:	5.0–6.0	1.25–1.50
Newborn, 3–24 hr:	4.3–5.1	1.07–1.27
24–48 hr:	4.0–4.7	1.00–1.17
Thereafter:	4.48–4.92	1.12–1.23
or	2.24–2.46 mEq/L	1.12–1.23

Calcium, Total

Serum	mg/dL	mmol/L
Cord:	9.0–11.5	2.25–2.88
Newborn, 3–24 hr:	9.0–10.6	2.3–2.65
24–48 hr:	7.0–12.0	1.75–3.0
4–7 d:	9.0–10.9	2.25–2.73
Child:	8.8–10.8	2.2–2.70
Thereafter:	8.4–10.2	2.1–2.55

Urine, 24 hr	*Ca in Diet*	mg/d	mmol/d
	Ca Free:	5–40	0.13–1.0
	Low to average:	50–150	1.25–3.8
	Average (20 mmol/d):	100–300	2.5–7.5

Test and Specimen	Reference Range	Reference Range International Units
CSF	2.1–2.7 mEq/L or 4.2–5.4 mg/dL	1.05–1.35 mmol/L 1.05–1.35 mmol/L
Feces	Avg.: 0.64 g/d	16 mmol/d
Carbamazepine Serum, plasma (heparin, EDTA); collect at trough conc.	Therap. conc.: 8–12 μg/mL Toxic conc.: >15	34–51 μmol/L >63

Carbon Dioxide, Partial Pressure (pCO_2)

Whole blood (heparin)	mmHg	kPa
Newborn:	27–40	3.6–5.3
Infant:	27–41	3.6–5.5
Thereafter, M:	35–48	4.7–6.4
F:	32–45	4.3–6.0

Test and Specimen	Reference Range		Reference Range International Units
Carbon Dioxide, Total (tCO₂)		*mmol/L*	Same
Serum or plasma (heparin)	Cord:	14–22	
	Premature:	14–27	
	Newborn:	13–22	
	Infant:	20–28	
	Child:	20–28	
	Thereafter:	23–30	
Catecholamines, Fractionated	Norepinephrine,		
Plasma (EDTA-sodium metabisulfite)	Supine:	100–400 pg/mL	591–2364 pmol/L
	Standing:	300–900	1773–5320
	Epinephrine,		
	Supine:	<70 pg/mL	<382 pmol/L
	Standing:	<100	<546
	Dopamine:	<30 pg/mL	<196 pmol/L
	(no postural change)		(no postural change)
Urine, 24 hr	Norepinephrine,	*μg/d*	*nmol/d*
	0–1 yr:	0–10	0–59
	1–2 yr:	0–17	0–100
	2–4 yr:	4–29	24–171
	4–7 yr:	8–45	47–266
	7–10 yr:	13–65	77–384
	Thereafter:	15–80	87–473
	Epinephrine,	*μg/d*	*nmol/d*
	0–1 yr:	0–2.5	0–13.6
	1–2 yr:	0–3.5	0–19.1
	2–4 yr:	0–6.0	0–32.7
	4–7 yr:	0.2–10	1.1–55
	7–10 yr:	0.5–14	2.7–76
	Thereafter:	0.5–20	2.7–109
	Dopamine,	*μg/d*	*nmol/d*
	0–1 yr:	0–85	0–555
	1–2 yr:	10–140	65–914
	2–4 yr:	40–260	261–1697
	Thereafter:	65–400	424–2611
Catecholamines, Total Free		*μg/d*	Same
Urine, 24 hr	0–1 yr:	10–15	
	1–5 yr:	15–40	
	6–15 yr:	20–80	
	Thereafter:	30–100	
Cerebrospinal Fluid Pressure	70–180 mm water		Same
CSF			
Cerebrospinal Fluid Volume	Child: 60–100 mL		0.006–0.10 L
CSF	Adult: 100–160		0.1–0.16
Chloral Hydrate	As Trichloroethanol:		
Serum	Therap. conc.: 2–12 μg/mL		13–80 μmol/L
	Toxic conc.: >20		>134
Chloride		*mmol/L*	
Serum or plasma (heparin)	Cord:	96–104	Same
	Newborn:	97–110	
	Thereafter:	98–106	
CSF	118–132 mmol/L		Same
Urine, 24 hr		*mmol/d*	Same
	Infant:	2–10	
	Child:	15–40	
	Thereafter:	110–250	
	(varies greatly with Cl intake)		
Sweat		*mmol/L*	Same
	Normal (homozygote):	0–35	
	Marginal:	30–60	
	Cystic fibrosis:	60–200	
	Increases by 10 mmol/L during lifetime		
Cholesterol, Total		*mg/dL*	*mmol/L*
Serum or plasma (EDTA or heparin)	Cord:	45–100	1.17–2.59
	Newborn:	53–135	1.37–3.50
	Infant:	70–175	1.81–4.53
	Child:	120–200	3.11–5.18

Test and Specimen	Reference Range		Reference Range International Units
Cholesterol, Total			
Serum or plasma (EDTA or heparin) *(Continued)*	Adolescent:	120–210	3.11–5.44
	Adult:	140–310	3.63–8.03
	Recommended (desirable) range for adults:	140–250	3.63–6.48
Clotting Time, Lee-White, 37° C			
Whole blood (no anticoagulant)	Glass tubes: 5–8 min (5–15 min at RT) Silicone tubes: about 30 min prolonged		Same
Coagulation Factor Assays			
Plasma (citrate)			
Factor I, see *Fibrinogen*			
Factor II	0.5–1.5 U/mL or 60–150% of normal		0.5–1.5 kU/L 60–150 AU
Factor IV, see *Calcium*			
Factor V	0.5–2.0 U/mL or 60–150% of normal		0.5–2.0 kU/L 60–150 AU
Factor VII	65–135% of normal		65–135 AU
Factor VIII	60–145% of normal		60–145 AU
Factor VIII antigen	50–200% of normal		50–200 AU
Factor IX	60–140% of normal		60–140 AU
Factor X	60–130% of normal		60–130 AU
Factor XI	65–135% of normal		65–135 AU
Factor XII	65–150% of normal		65–150 AU
Whole blood (citrate or oxalate)			
Factor XIII (*Fibrin Stabilizing Factor, FSF*)	Minimal hemostatic level: 0.02–0.05 U/mL or 1–2% of normal		20–50 U/L or 1–2 AU
Complement Components			
Plasma (EDTA)			
Total hemolytic complement activity	75–160 U/mL or >33% of plasma CH_{50}		75–160 kU/mL >0.33 of plasma CH_{50}
Total complement decay rate (functional)	~10–20%		~0.10–0.20 (fraction of decay rate)
	Deficiency: >50%		0.50 (fraction of decay rate)
Copper		μg/dL	μmol/L
Serum	Birth-6 mo:	20–70	3.14–10.99
	6 yr:	90–190	14.13–29.83
	12 yr:	80–160	12.56–25.12
	Adult, M:	70–140	10.99–21.98
	F:	80–155	12.56–24.34
Erythrocytes (heparin)	90–150 μg/dL		14.13–23.55 μmol/L
Urine, 24 hr	15–30 μg/d		0.24–0.47 μmol/d
Coproporphyrin			
Urine, 24 hr	34–234 μg/d		51–351 nmol/d
Feces, 24 hr	<30 μg/g dry wt 400–1200 μg/d		<45 nmol/g dry wt 600–1800 nmol/d
Cortisol		μg/dL	nmol/L
Serum or plasma (heparin)	Newborn:	1–24	28–662
	Adults, 0800 hr:	5–23	138–635
	1600 hr:	3–15	82–413
	2000 hr:	≤50% of 0800 hr	Fraction of 0800 hr: ≤0.50
Cortisol, Free		μg/d	nmol/d
Urine, 24 hr	Child:	2–27	5.5–74
	Adolescent:	5–55	14–152
	Adult:	10–100	27–276
Creatine Kinase			
(CK, CPK; 30 °C)		U/L	
Serum	Newborn:	68–580	Same
Total	Adult, M:	12–70	
	F:	10–55	
	Ambulatory,		
	M:	25–90	Same
	F:	10–70	
	Higher after exercise		
Isoenzymes	Fraction 2 (MB) <5% of total		Fraction of total: <0.05

Test and Specimen	Reference Range		Reference Range International Units	
Creatinine	*mg/dL*		*μmol/L*	
Serum or plasma	Cord:	0.6–1.2	53–106	
Jaffe, kinetic or enzymatic	Newborn:	0.3–1.0	27–88	
	Infant:	0.2–0.4	18–35	
	Child:	0.3–0.7	27–62	
	Adolescent:	0.5–1.0	44–88	
	Adult, M:	0.6–1.2	53–106	
	F:	0.5–1.1	44–97	
Jaffe, manual	0.8–1.5 mg/dL		70–133 μmol/L	
Amniotic fluid	After 37 wk gestation: >2.0 mg/dL		After 37 wk gestation: >180 μmol/L	
Urine, 24 hr	*mg/kg/d*		*μmol/kg/d*	
	Infant:	8–20	71–180	
	Child:	8–22	71–195	
	Adolescent:	8–30	71–265	
	Adult:	14–26	124–230	
	or: *mg/d*		*mmol/d*	
	M:	800–2000	7–18	
	F:	600–1800	5.3–16	
Creatinine Clearance (Endogenous)	Newborn: 40–65 mL/min/1.73 m²			
Serum or plasma and urine	<40 yr, M: 97–137			
	F: 88–128			
	Decreases ~6.5 mL/min/decade			
Digoxin	*ng/mL*		*nmol/L*	
Serum, plasma (heparin, EDTA); collect at least 12 hr after dose	Therap. conc.,			
	CHF:	0.8–1.5	1–1.9	
	Arrhythmias:	1.5–2.0	1.9–2.6	
	Toxic conc.,			
	Child:	>2.5	>3.2	
	Adult:	>3.0	>3.8	

Dihydrotestosterone (DHT)
Serum

		ng/dL			*nmol/L*	
Prepubertal:		<3.5			<0.12	
Pubertal	*M*	*F*		*M*	*F*	
stage I:	<10	<10		<0.34	<0.34	
II:	<20	<15		<0.7	<0.5	
III:	<35	<25		<1.2	<0.86	
IV–V:	<75	<25		<2.6	<0.86	
Adult:	30–85	4–22		1.03–2.92	0.14–0.76	

Eosinophil Count
Whole blood (EDTA or heparin); capillary blood

50–350 cells/mm³ (μL)   50–350 × 10⁶ cells/L

Erythrocyte Count (RBC Count)	*millions of cells/mm³ (μL)*		× 10¹² cells/L	
Whole blood (EDTA)	Cord blood:	3.9–5.5	Same	
	1–3 d (cap.):	4.0–6.6		
	1 wk:	3.9–6.3		
	2 wk:	3.6–6.2		
	1 mo:	3.0–5.4		
	2 mo:	2.7–4.9		
	3–6 mo:	3.1–4.5		
	0.5–2 yr:	3.7–5.3		
	2–6 yr:	3.9–5.3		
	6–12 yr:	4.0–5.2		
	12–18 yr, M:	4.5–5.3		
	F:	4.1–5.1		
	18–49 yr, M:	4.5–5.9		
	F:	4.0–5.2		

Erythrocyte Sedimentation Rate (ESR)	*mm/hr*			
Whole blood (EDTA)	Child:	0–10	Same	
Westergren, modified	Adult: M, <50 yr:	0–15		
	F, <50 yr:	0–20		
Wintrobe	Child:	0–13		
	Adult, M.	0–9		
	F.	0–20		
ZETA	41–54%		41–54 AU	

Erythropoietin
Serum

	Reference Range	International Units
RIA	<5–20 mU/mL	<5–20 U/L
Hemagglutination	25–125	25–125
Bioassay	5–18	5–18

Test and Specimen	Reference Range		Reference Range International Units
Estradiol		*pg/mL*	*pmol/L*
Serum or plasma (heparin or EDTA)	M, pubertal		
	stage I:	2–8	7–29
	II:	11	40
	III:	>20	>73
	Adult, M:	8–36	29–132
	F, pubertal		
	stage I:	0–23	0–84
	II:	0–66	0–242
	III:	0–105	0–385
	IV:	20–300	73–1101
	Follicular:	10–90	37–330
	Midcycle:	100–500	367–1835
	Luteal:	50–240	184–881
		μg/d	*nmol/d*
Urine, 24 hr	Adult, M:	0–6	0–22
	F:		
	Follicular:	0–3	0–11
	Ovulatory peak:	4–14	15–51
	Luteal:	4–10	15–37
Estrogens, Total		*pg/mL*	*ng/L*
Serum	Child:	<30	Same
	M:	40–115	
	F, cycle—days		
	1–10 d:	61–394	
	11–20 d:	122–437	
	21–30 d:	156–350	
	Prepubertal:	≤40	
		μg/d	*μg/d*
Urine, 24 hr	Child:	<10	Same
	Adult, M:	5–25	
	F, Preovulation:	5–25	
	Ovulation:	28–100	
	Luteal peak:	22–80	
	Pregnancy:	<45,000	
	Postmenopausal:	<10	
Ethanol	Toxic conc.: 50–100 mg/dL		11–22 mmol/L
Whole blood (oxalate), serum	Depression of CNS: >100		>22
Ethosuximide	Therap. conc.: 40–100 μg/mL		280–700 μmol/L
Serum, plasma (heparin, EDTA); collect at trough conc.	Toxic conc.: >150		>1060
Fat, Fecal		*g/d*	*g/d*
Feces, 72 hr	Infant, breast-fed:	<1	Same
	0–6 yr:	<2	
	Adult:	<7	
	Adult (fat-free diet):	<4	
	Coefficient of fat absorption (%)		*Absorbed fraction*
	Infant, breast-fed:	>93	>0.93
	Infant, formula-fed:	>83	>0.83
	>1 yr:	≥95	≥0.95
Fatty Acids, Nonesterified (Free)	Adults: 8–25 mg/dL		0.30–0.90 mmol/L
Serum or plasma (heparin)	Children and obese adults: <31		<1.10
Ferric Chloride Test	Negative		Negative
Urine, fresh random			
Ferritin		*ng/mL*	*μg/L*
Serum	Newborn:	25–200	Same
	1 mo:	200–600	
	2–5 mo:	50–200	
	6 mo–15 yr:	7–140	
	Adult, M:	15–200	
	F:	12–150	
Fibrinogen	Newborn: 125–300 mg/dL		1.25–3.00 g/L
Whole blood (Na citrate)	Adult: 200–400		2.00–4.00
Folate			
Serum	Newborn: 7.0–32 ng/mL		15.9–72.4 nmol/L
	Thereafter: 1.8–9		4.1–20.4
Erythrocytes (EDTA)	150–450 ng/mL cells		340–1020 nmol/L cells

Test and Specimen	Reference Range			Reference Range International Units	
Follicle Stimulating Hormone (hFSH)		*mU/mL*			
Serum or plasma (heparin)		*(IRP-2-hMG)*		*IU/L*	
	Birth–1 yr, M:	<1–12		Same	
	F:	<1–20			
	1–8 yr, M:	<1–6			
	F:	<1–4			
	9–10 yr, M:	<1–10			
	F:	2–8			
	11–12 yr, M:	2–12			
	F:	3–11			
	13–14 yr, M:	3–15			
	F:	3–15			
		mU/mL		*IU/L*	
	Adult, M:	4–25		Same	
	F,				
	Premenopause:	4–30		Same	
	Midcycle peak:	10–90			
	Pregnancy: Low to undetectable				
Galactose					
Serum	Newborn: 0–20 mg/dL			0–1.11 mmol/L	
	Thereafter: <5			<0.28	
Urine	Newborn: ≤60 mg/dL			≤3.33 mmol/L	
	Thereafter: <14 mg/d			<0.08 mmol/d	
Glucose		*mg/dL*		*mmol/L*	
Serum	Cord:	45–96		2.5–5.3	
	Premature:	20–60		1.1–3.3	
	Neonate:	30–60		1.7–3.3	
	Newborn,				
	1 d:	40–60		2.2–3.3	
	>1 d:	50–90		2.8–5.0	
	Child:	60–100		3.3–5.5	
	Adult:	70–105		3.9–5.8	
Whole blood (heparin)	Adult:	65–95		3.6–5.3	
CSF	Adult:	40–70		2.2–3.9	
Urine					
Quantitative, enzymatic	<0.5 g/d			<2.8 mmol/d	
Qualitative	Negative			Negative	
Glucose, 2 hr Postprandial	<120 mg/dL			<6.7 mmol/L	
Serum	Diabetes: see *Glucose Tolerance Test, Oral*				
Glucose Tolerance Test		*mg/dL*		*mmol/L*	
(GTT), Oral		*Normal*	*Diabetic*	*Normal*	*Diabetic*
Serum	Fasting:	70–105	>115	3.9–5.8	>6.4
Dose, Adult: 75 g	60 min:	120–170	≥200	6.7–9.4	≥11
Child: 1.75 g/kg	90 min:	100–140	≥200	5.6–7.8	≥11
of ideal weight up to	120 min:	70–120	≥140	3.9–6.7	≥7.8
maximum of 75 g					
Growth Hormone (hGH, Somatotropin)		*ng/mL*		*µg/L*	
Serum or plasma (EDTA, heparin)	Cord:	10–50		Same	
Fasting, at rest	Newborn:	10–40			
	Child:	<5			
	Adult, M:	<5			
	F:	<8			
Hematocrit (HCT, Hct)	*% of packed red cells*			*Volume fraction*	
Whole blood (EDTA)	*(V red cells/V whole blood × 100)*			*(V red cells/V whole blood)*	
Calculated from MCV and	1 d (cap):	48–69		0.48–0.69	
RBC (electronic	2 d:	48–75		0.48–0.75	
displacement or laser)	3 d:	44–72		0.44–0.72	
	2 mo:	28–42		0.28–0.42	
	6–12 yr:	35–45		0.35–0.45	
	12–18 yr, M:	37–49		0.37–0.49	
	F:	36–46		0.36–0.46	
	18–49 yr, M:	41–53		0.41–0.53	
	F:	36–46		0.36–0.46	
Hemoglobin (Hb)		*g/dL*		*mmol/L*	
Whole blood (EDTA)	1–3 d (cap):	14.5–22.5		2.25–3.49	
	2 mo:	9.0–14.0		1.40–2.17	
	6–12 yr:	11.5–15.5		1.78–2.40	
	12–18 yr, M:	13.0–16.0		2.02–2.48	
	F:	12.0–16.0		1.86–2.48	

Test and Specimen	Reference Range		Reference Range International Units
Hemoglobin (Hb)			
Whole blood (EDTA)*(Continued)*	18–49 yr, M:	13.5–17.5	2.09–2.71
F:		12.0–16.0	1.86–2.48
Serum or plasma (heparin, ACD, EDTA)	<10 mg/dL		<1.55 µmol/L
	<3 mg/dL with butterfly set-up and 18 g needle		<0.47 µmol/L with butterfly set-up and 18 g needle
Urine, fresh random	Negative		Negative
Hemoglobin, glycosylated			Fraction of Hb
Whole blood (heparin, EDTA, or oxalate)			
Electrophoresis	5.6–7.5% of total Hb		0.056–0.075
Column	6–9% of total Hb		0.06–0.09
HPLC	HbA$_{1a}$ 1.6% total Hb		0.016
	HbA$_{1b}$ 0.8		0.008
	HbA$_{1c}$ 3.6		0.03–0.06
Hemoglobin A			
Whole blood (EDTA, citrate, or heparin)	>95%		Fraction of Hb: >0.95
Hemoglobin F		*% HbF*	*Mass fraction HbF*
Whole blood (EDTA)	1 d:	63–92	0.62–0.92
Alkali denaturation (White)	5 d:	65–88	0.65–0.88
	3 wk:	55–85	0.55–0.85
	6–9 wk:	31–75	0.31–0.75
	3–4 mo:	<2–59	<0.02–0.59
	6 mo:	<2–9	<0.02–0.09
	Adult:	<2	<0.02
17-Hydroxyprogesterone (17-OHP)		*ng/mL*	*nmol/L*
Serum	M,		
	Pubertal stage I:	0.1–0.3	0.3–0.9
	Adult:	0.2–1.8	0.6–5.4
	F,		
	Pubertal stage I:	0.2–0.5	0.6–1.5
	Follicular:	0.2–0.8	0.6–2.4
	Luteal:	0.8–3.0	2.4–9.0
	Postmenopausal:	0.04–0.5	0.12–1.5
Immunoglobulin A (IgA)		*mg/dL*	*mg/L*
Serum	Cord:	0–5	0–50
	Newborn:	0–2.2	0–22
	1/2–6 mo:	3–82	30–820
	6 mo–2 yr:	14–108	140–1080
	2–6 yr:	23–190	230–1900
	6–12 yr:	29–270	290–2700
	12–16 yr:	81–232	810–2320
	Thereafter:	60–380	600–3800
Immunoglobulin D (IgD)	Newborn: None detected		None detected
Serum	Thereafter: 0–8 mg/dL		0–0.44 µmol/L
Immunoglobulin E (IgE)	M: 0–230 IU/mL		0–230 kIU/L
Serum	F: 0–170		0–170
Immunoglobulin G (IgG)		*mg/dL*	*g/L*
Serum	Cord:	760–1700	7.6–17
	Newborn:	700–1480	7–14.8
	1/2–6 mo:	300–1000	3–10
	6 mo–2 yr:	500–1200	5–12
	2–6 yr:	500–1300	5–13
	6–12 yr:	700–1650	7–16.5
	12–16 yr:	700–1550	7–15.5
	Adults:	600–1600	6–16
	(higher in blacks)		(higher in blacks)
Immunoglobulin M (IgM)		*mg/dL*	*mg/L*
Serum	Cord:	4–24	40–240
	Newborn:	5–30	50–300
	1/2–6 mo:	15–109	150–1090
	6 mo–2 yr:	43–239	430–2390
	2–6 yr:	50–199	500–1990
	6–12 yr:	50–260	500–2600
	12–16 yr:	45–240	450–2400
	Thereafter:	40–345	400–3450
	Results vary with std. preparation		
Insulin (12 hr Fasting)	Newborn: 3–20 µU/mL		3–20 mU/L
Serum or plasma (no anticoagulant)	Thereafter: 7–24		7–24

Test and Specimen	Reference Range		Reference Range International Units	
Iron				
Serum		μg/dL		μmol/L
	Newborn:	100–250		17.90–44.75
	Infant:	40–100		7.16–17.90
	Child:	50–120		8.95–21.48
	Thereafter, M:	50–160		8.95–28.64
	F:	40–150		7.16–26.85
	Intoxicated child:	280–2550		50.12–456.5
	Fatally poisoned child:	>1800		>322.2
Iron-Binding Capacity, Total (TIBC)				
Serum	Infant: 100–400 μg/dL			17.90–71.60 μmol/L
	Thereafter: 250–400			44.75–71.60
17-Ketogenic Steroids (17-KGS)				
Urine, 24 hr		mg/d		μmol/d
	0–1 yr:	<1.0		<3.5	(Conversion based
	1–10 yr:	<5		<17	dehydroepi-
	11–14 yr:	<12		<42	androsterone,
	Thereafter, M:	5–23		17–80	M.W. 288)
	F:	3–15		10–52	
Ketone Bodies				
Serum, random urine *Qualitative*	Negative			Negative
Serum *Quantitative*	0.5–3.0 mg/dL			5–30 mg/L
17-Ketosteroids (17-KS), Total				
Zimmermann reaction		mg/d		μmol/d
Urine, 24 hr	14 d–2 yr:	<1		<3.5	(Conversion based
	2–6 yr:	<2		<7	on dehydroepi-
	6–10 yr:	1–4		3.5–14	androsterone,
	10–12 yr:	1–6		3.5–21	M.W. 288)
	12–14 yr:	3–10		10–35	
	14–16 yr:	5–12		17–42	
	Thereafter,				
	M, 18–30 yr:	9–22		31–76	
	M, >30 yr:	8–20		28–70	
	F:	6–15		21–52	
	Decreases with age			Decreases with age	
Lactate				
Whole blood (heparin)		mmol/L		mmol/L
	Venous:	0.5–2.2		Same
	Arterial:	0.5–1.6		
	Inpatients,			
	Venous:	0.9–1.7		
	Arterial:	<1.25		
Lead				
Whole blood (heparin)		μg/dL		μmol/L
	Child:	<30		<1.45
	Adult:	<40		<1.93
	Acceptable for industrial exposure:	<60		<2.90
	Toxic:	≥100		≥4.83
Urine, 24 hr	<80 μg/L			<0.39 μmol/L
Leukocyte Differential Count				
Whole blood (EDTA)		%		Number fraction
Myelocytes		0		0
Neutrophils—"bands"		3–5		0.03–0.05
Neutrophils—"segs"		54–62		0.54–0.62
Lymphocytes		25–33		0.25–0.33
Monocytes		3–7		0.03–0.07
Eosinophils		1–3		0.01–0.03
Basophils		0–0.75		0–0.0075
		Cells/mm³ (μL)		× 10⁶ cells/L
		0		0
		150–400		150–400
		3000–5800		3000–5800
		1500–3000		1500–3000
		285–500		285–500
		50–250		50–250
		15–50		15–50
Lysergic Acid Diethylamine				
Plasma (EDTA)	After hallucinogenic dose:			After hallucinogenic dose:
	0.005–0.009 μg/mL			15.5–27.8 nmol/L
Urine	0.001–0.050 μg/mL			3.1–155 nmol/L

Test and Specimen	Reference Range		Reference Range International Units	
Magnesium	*mEq/L*		*mmol/L*	
Serum	Newborn, 2–4 d:	1.2–1.8	0.6–0.9	
	5 mo–6 yr:	1.4–1.9	0.7–1.0	
	6–12 yr:	1.4–1.7	0.7–0.8	
	12–20 yr:	1.4–1.8	0.7–0.9	
	Adult:	1.3 2.1	0.6 1.0	
Mean Corpuscular Hemoglobin	*pg/cell*		*fmol/cell*	
(MCH)	Birth:	31–37	0.48–0.57	
Whole blood (EDTA)	1–3 d (cap.):	31–37	0.48–0.57	
	1 wk–1 mo:	28–40	0.43–0.62	
	2 mo:	26–34	0.40–0.53	
	3–6 mo:	25–35	0.39–0.54	
	0.5–2 yr:	23–31	0.36–0.48	
	2–6 yr:	24–30	0.37–0.47	
	6–12 yr:	25–33	0.39–0.51	
	12–18 yr:	25–35	0.39–0.54	
	18–49 yr:	26–34	0.40–0.53	
Mean Corpuscular Hemoglobin	*% Hb/cell or*		*mmol*	
Concentration (MCHC)	*g Hb/dL RBC*		*Hb/L RBC*	
Whole blood (EDTA)	Birth:	30–36	4.65–5.58	
	1 3 d (cap.):	29–37	4.50–5.74	
	1–2 wk:	28–38	4.34–5.89	
	1–2 mo:	29–37	4.50–5.74	
	3 mo–2 yr:	30–36	4.65–5.58	
	2–18 yr:	31–37	4.81–5.74	
	>18 yr:	31–37	4.81–5.74	
Mean Corpuscular Volume (MCV)	μm^3		*fL*	
Whole blood (EDTA)	1–3 d (cap):	95–121	Same	
	0.5–2 yr:	70–86		
	6–12 yr:	77–95		
	12–18 yr, M:	78–98		
	F:	78–102		
	18–49 yr, M:	80–100		
	F:	80–100		
Niacin (Nicotinic Acid)	0.4–1.5 mg/d		2.43–12.17 μmol/d	
Urine, 24 hr				
Occult Blood				
Feces, random	Negative (<2 mL blood/d in ~100–200 g stool)		Negative	
Urine, random	Negative		Negative	
Osmolality				
Serum	Child, Adult: 275–295 mOsmol/kg H_2O			
Urine, random	50–1400 mOsmol/kg H_2O, depending on fluid intake. After 12 hr fluid restriction: >850 mOsmol/kg H_2O			
Urine, 24 hr	≈300–900 mOsmol/kg H_2O			

Test and Specimen	% NaCl (g/dl)	% Hemolysis	NaCl (g/L)	Hemolyzed fraction
Osmotic Fragility Test (RBC Fragility)				
Whole blood (heparin)	0.30	97–100	3.0	0.97–1.00
pH 7.4, 20 °C	0.35	90–99	3.5	0.90–0.99
	0.40	50–95	4.0	0.50–0.95
	0.45	5–45	4.5	0.05–0.45
	0.50	0–6	5.0	0.00–0.06
	0.55	0	5.5	0.00
	% NaCl (g/dL)	*% Hemolysis*	*NaCl (g/L)*	*Hemolyzed fraction*
Sterile incubation at 37 °C	0.20	95–100	2.0	0.95–1.00
	0.30	85–100	3.0	0.85–1.00
	0.35	75–100	3.5	0.75–1.00
	0.40	65–100	4.0	0.65–1.00
	0.45	55–95	4.5	0.55–0.95
	0.50	40–85	5.0	0.40–0.85
	0.55	15–70	5.5	0.15–0.70
	0.60	0–40	6.0	0.00–0.40
	0.65	0–10	6.5	0.00–0.10
	0.70	0–5	7.0	0.00–0.05
	0.85	0	8.5	0.00

Test and Specimen	Reference Range	Reference Range International Units
Oxygen, Partial Pressure (*p*O₂)	*mm Hg*	*kPa*
Whole blood (heparin), arterial	Birth: 8–24	1.1–3.2
	5–10 min: 33–75	4.4–10.0
	30 min: 31–85	4.1–11.3
	>1 hr: 55–80	7.3–10.6
	1 d: 54–95	7.2–12.6
	Thereafter: 83–108	11–14.4
	(Decreases with age)	
Oxygen Saturation		Fraction saturated:
Whole blood (heparin), arterial	Newborn: 40–90%	0.40–0.90
	Thereafter: 95–99%	0.95–0.99
Paraldehyde	μ*g/mL*	μ*mol/L*
Serum, plasma (heparin, EDTA)	Therap. conc.,	
	Sedation: 10–100	75–750
	Anesthesia: >200	>1500
	Toxic conc.: 20–40	150–300
	Lethal conc.: >50	>375
Partial Thromboplastin Time (PTT)		
Whole blood (Na citrate)		
Nonactivated	60–85 s (Platelin)	Same
Activated	25–35 s (differs with method)	
pH		*H⁺ concentration:*
Whole blood (heparin), arterial	Premature (48 hr): 7.35–7.50	31–44 nmol/L
	Birth, full term: 7.11–7.36	43–77
	5–10 min: 7.09–7.30	50–81
	30 min: 7.21–7.38	41–61
	>1 hr: 7.26–7.49	32–54
	1 d: 7.29–7.45	35–51
	Thereafter: 7.35–7.45	35–44
	Must be corrected for body temperature	
Urine, random	Newborn/neonate: 5–7	0.1–10 μmol/L
	Thereafter: 4.5–8	0.01–32 μmol/L
	(average ≃ 6)	(average ≃ 1.0 μmol/L)
Stool	7.0–7.5	31–100 nmol/L
Phenacetin	Therap. conc.: 1–20 μg/mL	5.6–110 μmol/L
Plasma (EDTA)	Toxic conc.: 50–250	280–1400
Phenobarbital	μ*g/mL*	μ*mol/L*
Serum, plasma (heparin, EDTA); collect at trough conc.	Therap. conc.: 15–40	65–170
	Toxic conc.,	
	Slowness,	
	ataxia,	
	nystagmus: 35–80	150–345
	Coma with	
	reflexes: 65–117	280–504
	Coma without	
	reflexes: >100	>430
Phenylalanine	*mg/dL*	*mmol/L*
Serum	Premature: 2.0–7.5	0.12–0.45
	Newborn: 1.2–3.4	0.07–0.21
	Thereafter: 0.8–1.8	0.05–0.11
	mg/d	μ*mol/d*
Urine, 24 hr	10 d–2 wk: 1–2	6–12
	3–12 yr: 4–18	24–110
	Thereafter: trace–17	trace–103
Phenylpyruvic Acid, Qualitative	Negative by FeCl₃ test	Negative by FeCl₃ test
Urine, fresh random		
Phenytoin	Therap. conc.: 10–20 μg/mL	40–80 μmol/L
Serum, plasma (heparin, EDTA); collect at steady-state trough conc.	Toxic conc.: >20	>80
Phosphatase, Alkaline (*p*-nitrophenyl phosphate)		
Serum	*U/L*	
SKI method; 30°C	Infant: 50–155	Same
	Child: 20–150	
	Adult: 20–70	
Bowers and McComb, 30°C	25–90 U/L	Same

Test and Specimen	Reference Range	Reference Range International Units
Phospholipids, Total Serum or plasma (EDTA)	*mg/dL* Newborn: 75–170 Infant: 100–275 Child: 180–295 Adult: 125–275	*g/L* 0.75–1.70 1.00–2.75 1.80–2.95 1.25–2.75
Phosphorus, Inorganic Serum	*mg/dL* Cord: 3.7–8.1 Premature (1 wk): 5.4–10.9 Newborn: 4.3–9.3 Child: 4.5–6.5 Thereafter: 3.0–4.5	*mmol/L* 1.2–2.6 1.7–3.5 1.4–3.0 1.45–2.1 0.97–1.45
Plasma Volume Plasma (heparin)	M: 25–43 mL/kg F: 28–45	M: 0.025–0.043 L/kg F: 0.028–0.045
Platelet Count (Thrombocyte Count) Whole blood (EDTA)	$\times 10^3/mm^3$ *(μL)* Newborn: 84–478 (After 1 wk, same as adult) Adult: 150–400	$\times 10^9/L$ Same
Potassium Serum	*mmol/L* Newborn: 3.9–5.9 Infant: 4.1–5.3 Child: 3.4–4.7 Thereafter: 3.5–5.1	*mmol/L* Same
Plasma (heparin)	3.5–4.5 mmol/L	Same
Urine, 24 hr	2.5–125 mmol/d varies with diet	Same
Progesterone Serum	*ng/mL* M, Pubertal stage I: 0.11–0.26 Adult: 0.12–0.3 F, Pubertal stage I: 0–0.3 II: 0–0.46 III: 0–0.6 IV: 0.05–13.0 Follicular: 0.02 0.9 Luteal: 6.0 30.0	*nmol/L* 0.35–0.83 0.38–1 0–1 0–1.5 0–2 0.16–41 0.06–2.9 19–95
Protein Serum, *Total*	*g/dL* Premature: 4.3–7.6 Newborn: 4.6–7.4 Child: 6.2–8.0 Adult, Recumbent: 6.0–7.8 ~0.5 g higher in ambulatory patients	*g/L* 43.0–76.0 46.0–74.0 62.0–80.0 60.0–78.0 ~5 g higher in ambulatory patients
Urine, 24 hr *Total*	1–14 mg/dL 50–80 mg/d (at rest) <250 mg/d after intense exercise	10–140 mg/L 50–80 mg/d <250 mg/d after intense exercise
CSF, *Total* *Column*	Lumbar: 8–32 mg/dL	80–320 mg/L
Turbidimetry	*mg/dl* Lumbar, Premature: 40–300 Newborn: 45–120 Child: 10–20 Adolescent: 15–20 Thereafter: 15–45	*mg/L* 400–3000 450–1200 100–200 150–200 150–450
Prothrombin Time (PT) Whole blood (Na citrate) *One-stage (Quick)*	In general: 11–15 s (varies with type of thromboplastin) Newborn: prolonged by 2–3 s	Same Same
Two-stage modified (Ware and Seegers)	18–22 s	Same

Test and Specimen	Reference Range	Reference Range International Units
RBC Count, see *Erythrocyte Count*		
Red Cell Volume Whole blood (heparin)	M: 20–36 mL/kg F: 19–31	M: 0.020–0.036 L/kg F: 0.019–0.031
Renin (Renin Activity, Plasma; PRA) Plasma (EDTA)	*ng/mL/h* 0–3 yr: <16.6 3–6 yr: < 6.7 6–9 yr: < 4.4 9–12 yr: < 5.9 12–15 yr: < 4.2 15–18 yr: < 4.3 *Normal sodium diet:* Supine: 0.2–2.5 Upright: 0.3–4.3 *Low sodium diet:* Upright 2.9–24	*μg/L/h* Same
Reticulocyte Count Whole blood (EDTA, heparin, or oxalate)	Adults: 0.5–1.5% of erythrocytes or 25,000–75,000/mm³ (μL)	0.005–0.015 (number fraction) 25,000–75,000 × 10⁶/L
Capillary	*%* 1 d: 0.4–6.0 7 d: <0.1–1.3 1–4 wk: <0.1–1.2 5–6 wk: <0.1–2.4 7–8 wk: 0.1–2.9 9–10 wk: <0.1–2.6 11–12 wk: 0.1–1.3	*Number fraction* 0.004–0.060 <0.001–0.013 <0.001–0.012 <0.001–0.024 0.001–0.029 <0.001–0.026 0.001–0.013
Riboflavin (Vitamin B₂) Urine, random, fasting	*μg/g creatinine* 1–3 yr: 500–900 4–6 yr: 300–600 7–9 yr: 270–500 10–15 yr: 200–400 Adult: 80–269	*μmol/mol creatinine* 150–270 90–180 81–150 60–120 24–81
Salicylates Serum, plasma (heparin, EDTA); collect at trough conc.	Therap. conc.: 15–30 mg/dL Toxic conc.: >30	1.1–2.2 mmol/L >2.2
Sediment Urine, fresh random *Casts*	Hyaline: occasional (0–1) casts/hpf RBC: not seen WBC: not seen Tubular epithelial: not seen Transitional and squamous epithelial: not seen	Same
Cells	RBC: 0–2/hpf WBC, Males: 0–3/hpf Females and children: 0–5/hpf Epithelial: few; more frequent in newborn Bacteria, unspun: no organisms/oil immersion field spun: <20 organisms/hpf	Same
Sedimentation Rate, see *Erythrocyte Sedimentation Rate*		
Sickle Cell Tests *Sodium Metabisulfite* *Dithionite Test* Whole blood (EDTA, heparin, or oxalate)	Negative Negative	
Sodium Serum or plasma (heparin)	*mmol/L* Newborn: 134–146 Infant: 139–146 Child: 138–145 Thereafter: 136–146	*mmol/L* Same

Test and Specimen	Reference Range		Reference Range International Units	
Sodium *(Continued)*				
Urine, 24 hr	Adult:	40–220 (diet-dependent)	Same	
	Full-term, 7–14 d old neonates have Na clearance of ~ 20% of adult values.			
Sweat		10–40	Same	
		Cystic fibrosis, >70		

Somatomedin C
Plasma (EDTA)

Vary with laboratory, e.g., Nichols Institute

	U/mL		*U/L*	
	M	F	M	F
0–2 yr:	0.10–0.72	0.10–1.7	100–720	100–1700
3–5 yr:	0.12–1.5	0.15–2.3	120–1500	150–2300
6–10 yr:	0.19–2.2	0.44–3.6	190–2200	440–3600
11–12 yr:	0.22–3.6	1.50–6.9	220–3600	150–6900
13–14 yr:	0.79–5.5	0.81–7.4	790–5500	810–7400
15–17 yr:	0.76–3.3	0.59–3.1	760–3300	590–3100
18–64 yr:	0.34–1.9	0.45–2.2	340–1900	450–2200

Endocrine Sciences

Cord:		0.25–0.66	250–660	
0–1 yr:		0.17–0.62	170–620	
1–5 yr:		0.14–0.94	140–940	
6–12 yr:		0.87–2.06	870–2060	
13–17 yr:		1.35–3.00	1350–3000	
18–25 yr:		0.92–2.06	920–2060	
Thereafter:		0.70–2.04	700–2040	

Specific Gravity

Urine, random	Adult: 1.002–1.030	Same
	After 12 hr fluid restriction: >1.025	
Urine, 24 hr	1.015–1.025	

Testosterone, Total
Serum

	ng/dL	*nmol/L*
Prepubertal,		
M:	1.6–11.6	0.06–0.40
F:	1.6–11.6	0.06–0.40
Adult,		
M:	302–842	10.47–29.19
F:	17–57	0.59–1.98

Theophylline
Serum, plasma (heparin, EDTA)

	μg/mL	*μmol/L*
Therap. conc.,		
Bronchodilator:	8–20	44–110
Prem. apnea:	6–13	33–72
Toxic conc.:	>20	>110

Thiamine (Vitamin B₁)

Serum	0–2.0 μg/dL	0.0–75.4 nmol/L

Urine, acidify with HCl

	μg/g creatinine	*μmol/mol*
1–3 yr:	176–200	75–85
4–6 yr:	121–400	52–170
7–9 yr:	181–350	77–149
10–12 yr:	181–300	77–128
13–15 yr:	151–250	64–107
Thereafter:	66–129	28–55

Thrombin Time

Whole blood (Na citrate)	Control time ± 2 s when control is 9–13 s	Same

Thyroid Stimulating Hormone (hTSH)
Serum or plasma (heparin)

	μU/L	*mU/L*
Cord:	3–12	Same
Newborn:	3–18	
Thereafter:	2–10	

Test and Specimen	Reference Range		Reference Range International Units	

Thyroxine, Total (T_4)
Serum

		μg/dL	nmol/L	
Cord:		8–13	103–168	
Newborn:		11.5–24	148–310	
(lower in low birth weight infants)				
Neonate:		9–18	116–232	
Infant:		7–15	90–194	
1–5 yr:		7.3–15	94–194	
5–10 yr:		6.4–13.3	83–172	
Thereafter:		5–12	65–155	
Newborn screen				
(filter paper):		6.2–22	80–284	

**Tourniquet Test
(Capillary Fragility)**

<5–10 petechiae in 2.5 cm circle on forearm (halfway between systolic and diastolic pressure for 5 min); 0–8 petechiae in 6 cm circle (50 torr for 15 min); 10–20 petechiae in 5 cm circle (80 mm Hg)   Same

Triglycerides (TG)
Serum, after ≥12 hr fast

	mg/dL		g/L	
	M	F	M	F
Cord blood:	10–98	10–98	0.10–0.98	0.10–0.98
0–5 yr:	30–86	32–99	0.30–0.86	0.32–0.99
6–11 yr:	31–108	35–114	0.31–1.08	0.35–1.14
12–15 yr:	36–138	41–138	0.36–1.38	0.41–1.38
16–19 yr:	40–163	40–128	0.40–1.63	0.40–1.28
20–29 yr:	44–185	40–128	0.44–1.85	0.40–1.28

Recommended (desirable) levels for adults:
    Male: 40–160 mg/dL
    Female: 35–135

Recommended (desirable) levels for adults:
    Male: 0.40–1.60 g/L
    Female: 0.35–1.35

Triiodothyronine, Free
Serum

	pg/dL	pmol/L
Cord:	20–240	0.3–3.7
1–3 d:	200–610	3.1–9.4
6 wk:	240–560	3.7–8.6
Adult (20–50 yr):	230–660	3.5–10.0

Triiodothyronine, Total (T_3-RIA)
Serum

	ng/dL	nmol/L
Cord:	30–70	0.46–1.08
Newborn:	75–260	1.16–4.00
1–5 yr:	100–260	1.54–4.00
5–10 yr:	90–240	1.39–3.70
10–15 yr:	80–210	1.23–3.23
Thereafter:	115–190	1.77–2.93

Urea Nitrogen
Serum or plasma

	mg/dL	mmol urea/L
Cord:	21–40	7.5–14.3
Premature (1 wk):	3–25	1.1–9
Newborn:	3–12	1.1–4.3
Infant/Child:	5–18	1.8–6.4
Thereafter:	7–18	2.5–6.4

Uric Acid
Serum
Phosphotungstate

	mg/dL	μmol/L
Newborn:	2.0–6.2	119–369
Adult, M:	4.5–8.2	268–488
F:	3.0–6.5	178–387

Uricase

Child:	2.0–5.5	119–327
Adults, M:	3.5–7.2	208–428
F:	2.6–6.0	155–357

Urine Volume
Urine, 24 hr

	mL/d	L/d
Newborn:	50–300	0.050–0.300
Infant:	350–550	0.350–0.500
Child:	500–1000	0.500–1.000
Adolescent:	700–1400	0.700–1.400
Thereafter, M:	800–1800	0.800–1.800
F:	600–1600	0.600–1.600
(varies with intake and other factors)		

Test and Specimen	Reference Range	Reference Range International Units
Valproic Acid Serum, plasma (heparin, EDTA); collect at trough conc.	Therap. conc.: 50–100 μg/mL Toxic conc.: >100	350–700 μmol/L >700
Vanillylmandelic Acid **(Vanilmandelic Acid)** Urine, 24 hr	*mg/d* Newborn: <1.0 Infant: <2.0 Child: 1–3 Adolescent: 1–5 Thereafter: 2–7 or: 1.5–7 μg/mg creatinine	*μmol/d* <5.0 <10.1 5–15 5–25 10–35 or: 0.86–4 mmol/mol creatinine
Vitamin A Serum	*μg/dL* Newborn: 35–75 Child: 30–80 Thereafter: 30–65	*μmol/L* 1.22–2.62 1.05–2.79 1.05–2.27
Vitamin B₁, see *Thiamine*		
Vitamin B₂, see *Riboflavin*		
Vitamin B₆ Plasma (EDTA)	3.6–18 ng/mL	14.6–72.8 nmol/L
Vitamin B₁₂ Serum	Newborn: 175–800 pg/ml Thereafter: 140–700	129–590 pmol/L 103–517
Vitamin C Plasma (oxalate, heparin, or EDTA)	0.6–2.0 mg/dL	34–113 μmol/L
Vitamin D₂, 25-Hydroxy Plasma (heparin)	Summer: 15–80 ng/mL Winter: 14–42	37–200 nmol/L 34–105
Vitamin D₃, 1,25-Dihydroxy (Calcitriol) Serum	25–45 pg/mL	60–108 nmol/L
Vitamin E Serum	5.0–20 μg/mL	11.6–46.4 μmol/L
Zinc Serum	70–150 μg/dL	10.7–22.9 μmol/L

(From Behrman, R., and Vaughan, V. [1987]. *Nelson Textbook of Pediatrics.* 13th ed. Philadelphia, W. B. Saunders Company.)

APPENDIX E

Universal precautions

The U.S. Department of Health and Human Services, CDC (Centers for Disease Control), in Atlanta, Georgia, issued "Recommendations for Prevention of HIV Transmission in Health-Care Settings," known as "CDC Guidelines."

Human immunodeficiency virus (HIV), which causes acquired immune deficiency syndrome (AIDS), is transmitted through sexual contact and exposure to infected blood or blood components and perinatally from mother to neonate. HIV has been isolated from blood, semen, vaginal secretions, saliva, tears, breast milk, cerebrospinal fluid, amniotic fluid, and urine and is likely to be isolated from other body fluids, secretions, and excretions. However, epidemiological evidence has implicated only blood, semen, vaginal secretions, and possibly breast milk in transmission.

The increasing prevalence of HIV increases the risk that healthcare workers will be exposed to blood from patients infected with HIV, especially when blood and body fluid precautions are not followed for all patients. The CDC emphasizes the need for healthcare workers to consider *all* patients as potentially infected with HIV or other blood-borne pathogens (e.g., hepatitis B). Healthcare workers are defined as persons, including students and trainees, whose activities involve contact with patients or with blood or other body fluids from patients in a healthcare setting.

Recent studies indicate that the incubation period for AIDS may be as long as 5 to 7 years after exposure, therefore the use of *universal precautions* in all areas in which body fluids are encountered is advisable.

SUMMARY OF UNIVERSAL PRECAUTIONS IN CDC GUIDELINES

1. All healthcare workers should routinely use appropriate barrier precautions to prevent skin and mucous membrane exposure when contact with blood or other body fluids of any patient is anticipated.
   - ▲ *Gloves* should be worn for touching blood and body fluids, mucous membranes, or nonintact skin of all patients; for handling items or surfaces soiled with blood or body fluids; and for performing venipuncture and other vascular access procedures. Gloves should be changed after contact with *each* patient.
   - ▲ *Masks* and *protective eyewear* or *face shields* should be worn during procedures that are likely to generate droplets of blood or body fluids.
   - ▲ *Gowns* or *aprons* should be worn during procedures that are likely to generate splashes of blood or body fluids.
2. Hands and other skin surfaces should be *washed immediately* and *thoroughly* if contaminated with blood or body fluids.

3. All healthcare workers should take precautions to prevent injuries caused by needles, scalpels, and other sharp instruments. To prevent needlestick injuries, needles should *not* be recapped, bent, broken, removed from disposable syringes, or otherwise manipulated by hand. After sharp items are used, they should be placed in nearby *puncture-resistant containers* for disposal or, in the case of large-bore reusable needles, for transport to the reprocessing area.

4. To minimize the need for emergency mouth-to-mouth resuscitation, mouthpieces, resuscitation bags, or other ventilation devices should be availble for use in areas in which the need for resuscitation is predictable.

5. Healthcare workers who have exudate (oozing) lesions or weeping dermatitis (inflammation of the skin) should refrain from all direct patient care and from handling patient-care equipment until the condition resolves.

6. Pregnant healthcare workers should be especially familiar with precautions to minimize the risk of HIV transmission and should strictly adhere to such precautions.

PRECAUTIONS FOR INVASIVE PROCEDURES

The following precautions for invasive procedures, combined with the preceding *universal precautions*, are recommended as the minimum precautions for invasive procedures on *all* patients.

Invasive procedures include surgical entry into tissues, cavities, or organs; repair of major traumatic injuries, cardiac catheterization, and angiographic procedures; vaginal or cesarean deliveries or other invasive obstetric procedures during which bleeding may occur; or the manipulation, cutting, or removal of any oral or perioral tissues during which the potential for bleeding exists.

1. All healthcare workers who participate in invasive procedures must routinely use appropriate barrier precautions to prevent skin and mucous membrane contact with blood or other body fluids of *all* patients.

▲ *Gloves* and *surigical masks* must be work for all invasive procedures.

▲ *Protective eyewear* or *face shields* should be worn for procedures that commonly result in the generation of droplets, splashing of blood or other body fluids, or the generation of bone chips.

▲ *Gowns* or *aprons* made of materials that provide an effective barrier should be worn during invasive procedures likely to result in the splashing of blood or other body fluids.

▲ All healthcare workers who perform or assist in *vaginal* or *cesarean deliveries* should wear *gloves* and *gowns* when handling the placenta or the infant until blood and amniotic fluid have been removed from the infant's skin and should wear *gloves during postdelivery care of the umbilical cord*.

2. If a glove is torn or a needlestick or other injury occurs, the glove should be removed and a new glove used as promptly as patient safety permits. The needle or other instrument involved in the incident should also be removed from the sterile field.

IMPLEMENTION OF PRECAUTIONS

The CDC Guidelines state that employers of healthcare workers should ensure that policies exist for

1. *Initial orientation and continuing education and training* of all healthcare workers on the epidemiology, modes of transmission, and prevention of HIV and other blood-borne infections *and the need for routine use of universal precautions for all patients.*

2. *Provision of equipment and supplies* necessary to minimize the risk of infection with HIV and other blood-borne pathogens.

3. *Monitoring adherence to recommended protective measures.* When monitoring reveals a failure to follow recommended precautions, counseling, education, or retraining should be provided, and, if necessary, appropriate disciplinary action should be considered.

NATIONAL RESOURCE

Centers for Disease Control
AIDS Activity
Building 6, Room 274
1600 Clifton Rd, NE
Atlanta, GA 30333
(404) 639-2891

Services Provided:

▲ national surveillance
▲ printed materials
▲ listing of HIV test sites
▲ publishers of *Morbidity & Mortality Weekly Report* (MMWR)

APPENDIX F

GROWTH CHARTS

GIRLS: BIRTH TO 36 MONTHS
PHYSICAL GROWTH
NCHS PERCENTILES*

NAME _____ RECORD # _____

*Adapted from: Hamill PVV, Drizd TA, Johnson CL, Reed RB, Roche AF, Moore WM: Physical growth: National Center for Health Statistics percentiles. AM J CLIN NUTR 32:607-629,1979. Data from the Fels Research Institute, Wright State University School of Medicine, Yellow Springs, Ohio.

© 1980 ROSS LABORATORIES

DATE	AGE	LENGTH	WEIGHT	HEAD C.
	BIRTH			

DATE	AGE	LENGTH	WEIGHT	HEAD C.

GIRLS: BIRTH TO 36 MONTHS
PHYSICAL GROWTH
NCHS PERCENTILES*

NAME＿＿＿＿＿＿＿＿＿＿＿＿＿＿＿＿＿＿＿　RECORD #＿＿＿＿＿＿

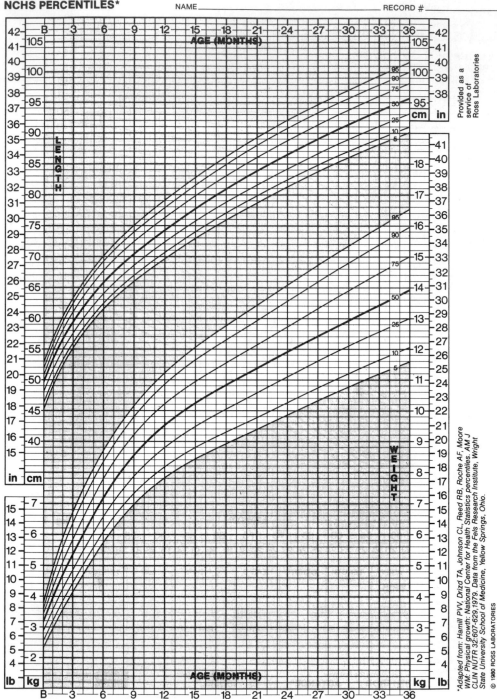

Provided as a service of Ross Laboratories

*Adapted from: Hamill PVV, Drizd TA, Johnson CL, Reed RB, Roche AF, Moore WM: Physical growth: National Center for Health Statistics percentiles. AM J CLIN NUTR 32:607-629,1979. Data from the Fels Research Institute, Wright State University School of Medicine, Yellow Springs, Ohio.

© 1980 ROSS LABORATORIES

BOYS: BIRTH TO 36 MONTHS
PHYSICAL GROWTH
NCHS PERCENTILES*

NAME_____   RECORD #_____

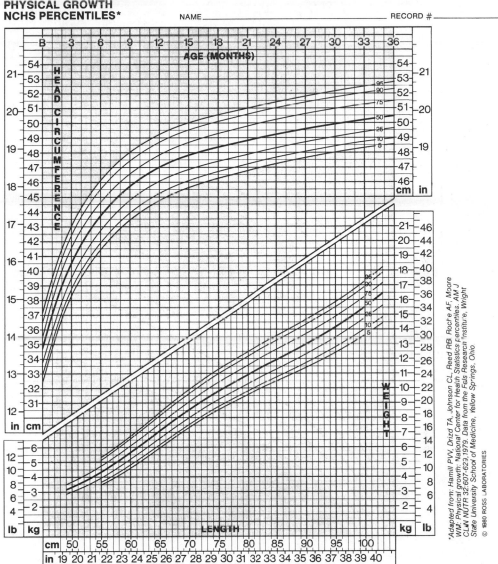

*Adapted from: Hamill PVV, Drizd TA, Johnson CL, Reed RB, Roche AF, Moore WM: Physical growth: National Center for Health Statistics percentiles. AM J CLIN NUTR 32:607-629,1979. Data from the Fels Research Institute, Wright State University School of Medicine, Yellow Springs, Ohio

© 1980 ROSS LABORATORIES

DATE	AGE	LENGTH	WEIGHT	HEAD C.
	BIRTH			

DATE	AGE	LENGTH	WEIGHT	HEAD C.

BOYS: BIRTH TO 36 MONTHS
PHYSICAL GROWTH
NCHS PERCENTILES*

NAME_____ RECORD #_____

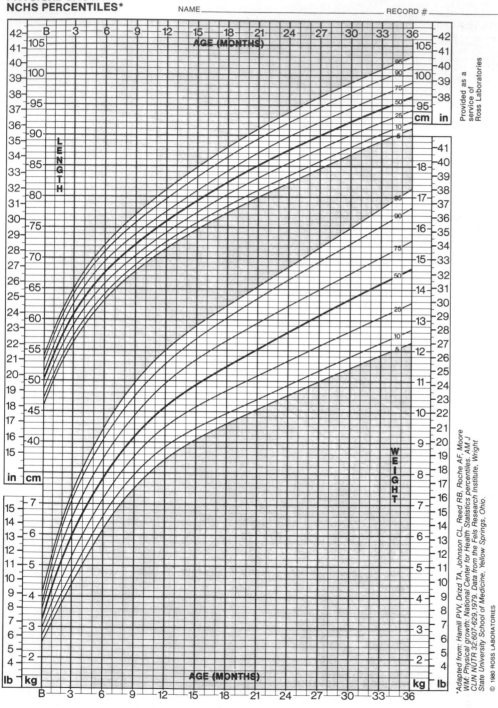

Provided as a service of Ross Laboratories

*Adapted from: Hamill PVV, Drizd TA, Johnson CL, Reed RB, Roche AF, Moore WM: Physical growth: National Center for Health Statistics percentiles. AM J CLIN NUTR 32:607-629,1979. Data from the Fels Research Institute, Wright State University School of Medicine, Yellow Springs, Ohio.

© 1980 ROSS LABORATORIES

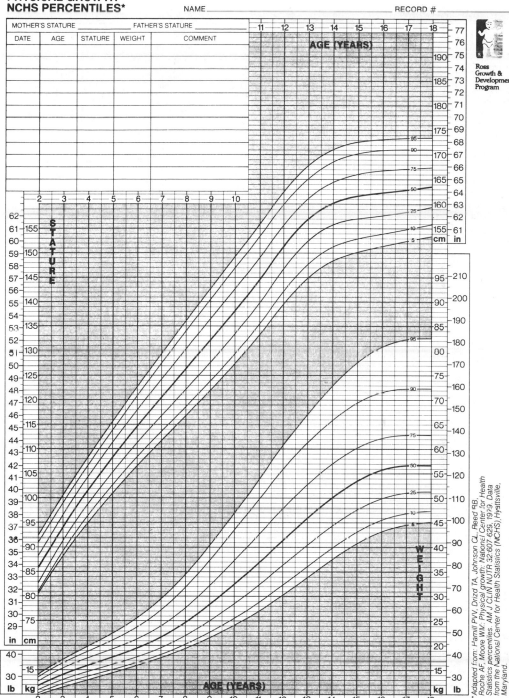

GIRLS: 2 TO 18 YEARS
PHYSICAL GROWTH
NCHS PERCENTILES*

NAME _____   RECORD # _____

Ross
Growth &
Development
Program

*Adapted from: Hamill PVV, Drizd TA, Johnson CL, Reed RB, Roche AF, Moore WM: Physical growth: National Center for Health Statistics percentiles. AM J CLIN NUTR 32:607-629, 1979. Data from the National Center for Health Statistics (NCHS), Hyattsville, Maryland.

© 1982 Ross Laboratories

GIRLS: PREPUBESCENT
PHYSICAL GROWTH
NCHS PERCENTILES*

NAME_____ RECORD #_____

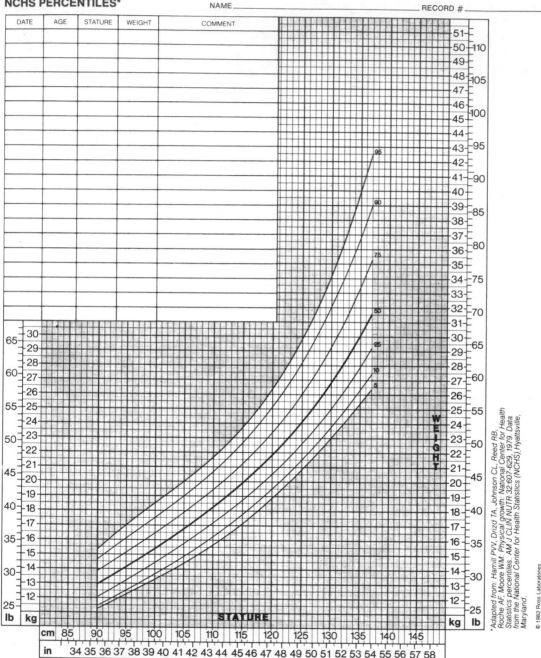

DATE	AGE	STATURE	WEIGHT	COMMENT

*Adapted from: Hamill PVV, Drizd TA, Johnson CL, Reed RB, Roche AF, Moore WM: Physical growth: National Center for Health Statistics percentiles. AM J CLIN NUTR 32:607-629, 1979. Data from the National Center for Health Statistics (NCHS), Hyattsville, Maryland.

© 1982 Ross Laboratories

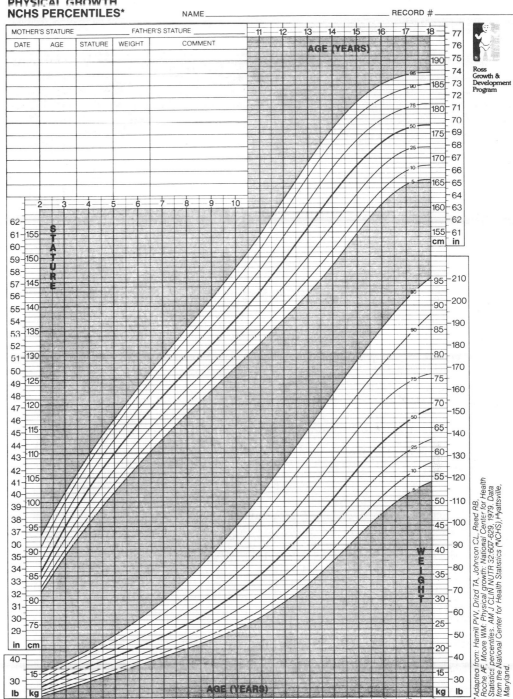

BOYS: 2 TO 18 YEARS
PHYSICAL GROWTH
NCHS PERCENTILES*

NAME _____   RECORD # _____

MOTHER'S STATURE _____		FATHER'S STATURE _____		
DATE	AGE	STATURE	WEIGHT	COMMENT

Ross
Growth &
Development
Program

*Adapted from: Hamill PVV, Drizd TA, Johnson CL, Reed RB, Roche AF, Moore WM. Physical growth: National Center for Health Statistics percentiles. AM J CLIN NUTR 32:607-629, 1979. Data from the National Center for Health Statistics (NCHS), Hyattsville, Maryland.

© 1982 Ross Laboratories

BOYS: PREPUBESCENT
PHYSICAL GROWTH
NCHS PERCENTILES*

NAME _____   RECORD # _____

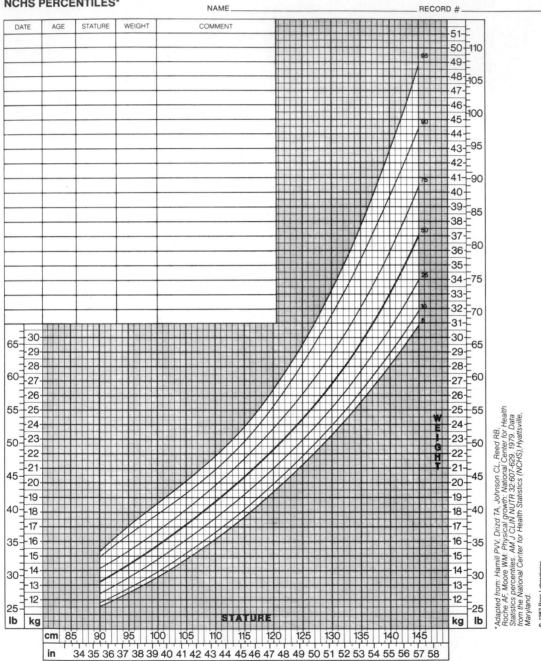

DATE	AGE	STATURE	WEIGHT	COMMENT

STATURE

*Adapted from: Hamill PVV, Drizd TA, Johnson CL, Reed RB, Roche AF, Moore WM: Physical growth: National Center for Health Statistics percentiles. AM J CLIN NUTR 32:607-629, 1979. Data from the National Center for Health Statistics (NCHS), Hyattsville, Maryland.

© 1982 Ross Laboratories

APPENDIX G

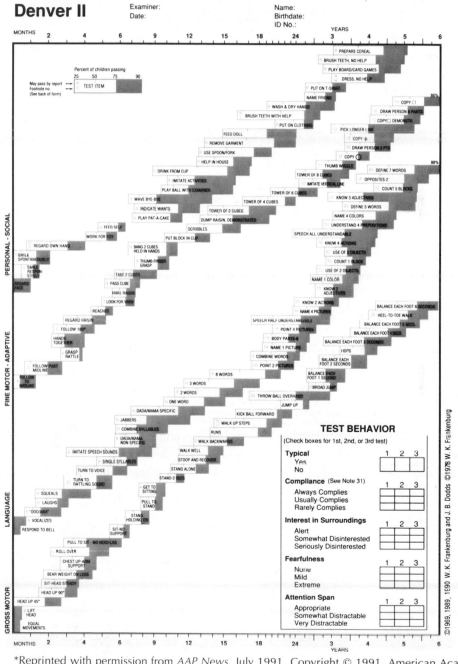

DENVER DEVELOPMENTAL SCREENING TEST—II

Denver II

Examiner:
Date:

Name:
Birthdate:
ID No.:

*Reprinted with permission from *AAP News*, July 1991. Copyright © 1991, American Academy of Pediatrics.

DIRECTIONS FOR ADMINISTRATION

1. Try to get child to smile by smiling, talking or waving. Do not touch him/her.
2. Child must stare at hand several seconds.
3. Parent may help guide toothbrush and put toothpaste on brush.
4. Child does not have to be able to tie shoes or button/zip in the back.
5. Move yarn slowly in an arc from one side to the other, about 8" above child's face.
6. Pass if child grasps rattle when it is touched to the backs or tips of fingers.
7. Pass if child tries to see where yarn went. Yarn should be dropped quickly from sight from tester's hand without arm movement.
8. Child must transfer cube from hand to hand without help of body, mouth, or table.
9. Pass if child picks up raisin with any part of thumb and finger.
10. Line can vary only 30 degrees or less from tester's line. ⎿/
11. Make a fist with thumb pointing upward and wiggle only the thumb. Pass if child imitates and does not move any fingers other than the thumb.

12. Pass any enclosed form. Fail continuous round motions.
13. Which line is longer? (Not bigger.) Turn paper upside down and repeat. (pass 3 of 3 or 5 of 6)
14. Pass any lines crossing near midpoint.
15. Have child copy first. If failed, demonstrate.

When giving items 12, 14, and 15, do not name the forms. Do not demonstrate 12 and 14.

16. When scoring, each pair (2 arms, 2 legs, etc.) counts as one part.
17. Place one cube in cup and shake gently near child's ear, but out of sight. Repeat for other ear.
18. Point to picture and have child name it. (No credit is given for sounds only.)
    If less than 4 pictures are named correctly, have child point to picture as each is named by tester.

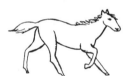

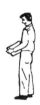

19. Using doll, tell child: Show me the nose, eyes, ears, mouth, hands, feet, tummy, hair. Pass 6 of 8.
20. Using pictures, ask child: Which one flies?... says meow?... talks?... barks?... gallops? Pass 2 of 5, 4 of 5.
21. Ask child: What do you do when you are cold?... tired?... hungry? Pass 2 of 3, 3 of 3.
22. Ask child: What do you do with a cup? What is a chair used for? What is a pencil used for? Action words must be included in answers.
23. Pass if child correctly places and says how many blocks are on paper. (1, 5).
24. Tell child: Put block **on** table; **under** table; **in front of** me, **behind** me. Pass 4 of 4. (Do not help child by pointing, moving head or eyes.)
25. Ask child: What is a ball?... lake?... desk?... house?... banana?... curtain?... fence?... ceiling? Pass if defined in terms of use, shape, what it is made of, or general category (such as banana is fruit, not just yellow). Pass 5 of 8, 7 of 8.
26. Ask child: If a horse is big, a mouse is __? If fire is hot, ice is __? If the sun shines during the day, the moon shines during the __? Pass 2 of 3.
27. Child may use wall or rail only, not person. May not crawl.
28. Child must throw ball overhand 3 feet to within arm's reach of tester.
29. Child must perform standing broad jump over width of test sheet (8 1/2 inches).
30. Tell child to walk forward, ⚬══⚬══⚬══► heel within 1 inch of toe. Tester may demonstrate. Child must walk 4 consecutive steps.
31. In the second year, half of normal children are non-compliant.

OBSERVATIONS:

APPENDIX H

GLOSSARY

acrocyanosis. Peripheral blueness of the hands and feet, which is normal in newborn infants.

AIDS. Acquired immune deficiency syndrome, characterized by depression of the immune system and opportunistic infection. Seen in neonates and infants who live in high risk populations and in children with hemophilia and other conditions who have received contaminated blood products.

amniocentesis. A needle is placed into the uterus of an expectant mother to obtain a specimen of amniotic fluid for analysis. This is done to determine possible damage to the fetus by Rh incompatibility, to determine Down syndrome, and for other tests.

angioma. A tumor, usually benign, which is made up chiefly of blood and lymph vessels.

animism. A period of cognitive development in which the child attributes life to inanimate objects.

anorexia nervosa. A syndrome most often seen in adolescent girls, characterized by an extreme form of poor appetite or self-starvation. Although its onset may be acute, the underlying emotional problem develops over a relatively long period of time.

Apgar scoring chart. A standardized chart used to evaluate the condition of the neonate immediately after delivery. Five objective signs are evaluated: heart rate, respiration, muscle tone, reflexes, and color.

aplastic anemia. Anemia caused by deficient red blood cell production because of bone marrow dysfunction.

arthroscopy. Direct visualization of a joint by means of an arthroscope.

ascariasis. Roundworm infestation.

asynchrony. Lack of concurrence in time. The appearance of a growing child may be gangling because of asynchrony of growth, i.e., different body parts maturing at different rates.

atelectasis. Incomplete expansion of the lungs at birth or a collapse after expansion due to mucous plug, tumor, pressure from organs, and other causes.

atresia. A congenital anomaly in which a normal opening is absent, e.g., atresia of the esophagus.

autism. A type of mental illness in which the child becomes absorbed in the self, excluding reality.

autoimmunity. A condition in which antibodies are produced against the body's own tissues.

autonomy. Functioning independently, self-control.

barrier technique. A method of medical asepsis using various types of isolation.

bleb. An irregularly shaped elevation of the epidermis: a blister or bulla.

bonding. Attachment, the process whereby a unique relationship is established between two people. Used in conjunction with parent-newborn infant ties.

bone marrow transplant. Transplantation of bone marrow from one person to another. Currently used to treat aplastic anemia and leukemia.

booster injection. Administration of a substance to renew or increase the effectiveness of a prior immunization injection, e.g., a tetanus booster.

Bradford frame. A special oblong frame made of one inch pipe, covered with canvas strips, and supported by blocks to raise it from the mattress. The canvas strips are movable; thus the patient can urinate and defecate without moving the spine.

Broviac catheter. A central venous line used in small children who require total parenteral or continuous intravenous infusion.

Bryant traction. A type of traction apparatus commonly used for toddlers suffering from a fractured femur. Vertical suspension is used. Child may not weight more than 30 to 32 pounds.

bulimarexia. A neurotic disorder seen in female adolescents and young women who wish to remain thin. Characterized by overeating and induced vomiting, fasting, and use of purgatives (synonym, bulimia).

café-au-lait spots. Light brown patch spots on the skin characteristic of neurofibromatosis (condition of tumors of various sizes on peripheral nerves).

cardiac decompression. Heart failure.

catecholamines: A group of compounds, including epinephrine and dopamine, that have a marked effect on nervous, cardiovascular, and other systems.

celiac syndrome. An inability to absorb fats, which results in malnutrition, vitamin deficiency, foul bulky stools, and a distended abdomen.

cephalocaudal. The orderly development of muscular control, which proceeds from head to foot and from the center of the body to the periphery.

cerebral palsy. A term used to describe a group of nonprogressive disorders that affect the motor centers of the brain.

cerumen. Ear wax.

chickenpox. A communicable disease of childhood, also known as varicella. It is caused by a virus and is characterized by successive crops of macules, papules, vesicles, and crusts.

chordee. A congenital anomaly in which a fibrous strand of tissue extends from the scrotum of the penis, preventing urination with the penis in the normal elevated position. Commonly associated with hypospadias.

chromosome. A DNA-containing structure found in the nuclei of plant and animal cells, responsible for the transmission of hereditary characteristics.

chronic ulcerative colitis. A serious chronic inflammatory disease of the large intestine.

circumcision. The surgical removal of the foreskin of the penis.

cleft lip and palate. Congenital anomalies due to failure of the embryonic structures of the face to unite. Characterized by an opening in the upper lip or palate.

clubfoot. A congenital orthopedic anomaly, characterized by a foot that has been twisted inward or outward.

coarctation of the aorta. A constriction of the aortic arch or of the descending aorta.

comedo. A skin lesion caused by a plug of keratin, sebum, and bacteria; there are two types, blackheads and whiteheads.

congenital anomaly. A malformation present at birth.

craniosynostosis. Premature closure of the cranial sutures that produces a head deformity and damage to the brain and eyes; also called craniostenosis.

cretinism. A congenital defect in the secretion of the thyroid hormones, characterized by physical and mental retardation.

Crohn's disease. Regional enteritis. Inflammation is most often found in the anus and ileum.

cryptorchidism. Failure of the testicles to descend into the scrotum.

cystic fibrosis. A generalized disorder of the exocrine glands, especially the mucous and sweat glands. The lungs and pancreas in particular are involved.

cystic hygroma. A lymphangioma most frequently seen in the neck and the axillae.

DDST. Denver Developmental Screening Test. Assesses the developmental status of a child during the first 6 years of life in five areas: personal, social, fine motor adaptive, language, and gross motor activities.

deciduous teeth. Baby teeth.

Denis Browne splint. Two separate footplates attached to a crossbar and fitted to a child's shoes, used in the correction of clubfeet.

diaphoresis. Profuse sweating.

disseminated intravascular coagulation (DIC). A secondary disease characterized by abnormal overstimulation of the coagulation process.

DNA (deoxyribonucleic acid). A complex protein believed to be the storehouse of hereditary information. It is present in the chromosomes of cell nuclei.

Down syndrome. A form of mental retardation caused by chromosomal defects; formerly known as mongolism.

Duchenne muscular dystrophy. A genetically determined progressive muscular disorder.

ductus arteriosus, patent. A congenital anomaly in which the opening between the aorta and the pulmonary artery fails to close after birth.

dyscrasia. A disease that is usually undefined and associated with blood disorders.

dysfunctional. Inadequate, abnormal.

eczema. An inflammation of the skin, frequently associated with an allergy to food protein or environment.

egocentrism. A kind of thinking in which a child has difficulty seeing anyone else's point of view; this self-centering is normal in young children.

empyema. Pus, especially in the chest cavity.

encephalitis. An inflammation of the brain.

encopresis. The passage of stools in a child's underwear or other inappropriate places after the age of 4 years. Some children display concurrent behavioral problems.

enuresis. Abnormal inability to control urine; may be due to organic, allergic, or psychological problems.

epilepsy. A convulsive disease, characterized by seizures and loss of consciousness.

epispadias. A congenital anomaly in which the urethral meatus is located on the upper (dorsal) surface of the penis.

erythroblastosis fetalis. Physiological hemolytic anemia due to blood incompatibility. Associated with babies born of Rh-positive fathers and Rh-negative mothers.

Ewing sarcoma. Endothelioma that occurs in long bones and in flat bones such as pelvis, ribs, and scapulae.

family APGAR. Screening test that reveals how a member of the family perceives its function.

fontanels. Openings at the point of union of skull bones, often referred to as "soft spots."

foreskin. The fold of loose skin covering the end of the penis; also called prepuce.

fulminating. Occurring rapidly; usually said of a disease.

gavage. Feeding the patient by means of stomach tube or with a tube passed through the nose, pharynx, and esophagus into the stomach.

genetics. The study of heredity.

geographic tongue. Unusual patterns of papilla formation and denuded areas on the tongue.

glioma. Sarcoma involving the support tissue or glial cells of the brain.

glucometer. A meter used to measure blood glucose.

hemangioma. A benign tumor of the skin, consisting of blood vessels.

hemophilia. A hereditary disease, characterized by an abnormal tendency to bleed.

Henoch-Schönlein purpura. An allergic purpura seen in children generally between the ages of 2 and 8 years. Can be caused by medication, insect bites, or other factors.

Hickman catheter. A tiny rubber catheter that is inserted into a chest vein to establish a long- or short-term central venous line. Used mainly in adults and teenagers. See *Broviac catheter*.

Hirschsprung disease. Megacolon; enlargement of the colon without evidence of mechanical obstruction. There is a congenital absence of ganglionic cells in the distal segment of the colon.

holism. An approach to caring for a child that recognizes and adapts to the physical, intellectual, emotional, and spiritual natures; a way of relating to the patient as a whole or biopsychosocial individual rather than just a person with an ailment.

hyaline membrane disease. Respiratory distress often seen in premature babies, in which a membranous substance lines the alveoli of the lungs, preventing the exchange of gases.

hydrocele. An abnormal collection of fluid surrounding the testicles, causing the scrotum to swell.

hydrocephalus. A congenital anomaly, characterized by an increase of cerebrospinal fluid of the ventricles of the brain, which results in an increase in the size of the head and in pressure changes in the brain.

hypercapnia. Increased amount of carbon dioxide in the blood.

hypernatremia. Excess sodium in the blood.

hypokalemia. Potassium deficit in the blood.

hypospadias. A developmental anomaly in which the urethra opens on the lower surface of the penis.

imperforate anus. A congenital anomaly in which there is no anal opening.

impetigo. An infectious disease of the skin, caused by staphylococci or streptococci.

incarcerated. Confined, constricted.

incest. Sexual activities among family members. Often seen in father-daughter relationships, less frequent in mother-son or sibling relationships.

infant mortality. The ratio between the number of deaths of infants less than one year of age during any given year and the number of live births occurring in the same year.

infanticide. The killing of an infant.

infectious mononucleosis. A generalized disease causing enlargement of the lymph tissues throughout the body. The number of mononuclear leukocytes in the blood is increased. It occurs mainly in older children and adolescents.

interatrial septal defect. An abnormal opening between the right and left atria of the heart. Blood that contains oxygen is forced from the left to the right atrium.

intertrigo. A chafe of the skin that occurs when two skin surfaces come together.

interventricular septal defect. An opening between the right and left ventricles of the heart. Blood passes directly from the left to the right ventricle.

intussusception. The slipping of one part of an intestine into another part just below it, often noted in the ileocecal region.

in vitro fertilization. Test tube fertilization in which the ripe ovum is collected and fertilized in vitro (glass) with sperm collected from a man. The embryo is then transferred to the woman's uterus.

karyotype. The chromosomal makeup of a normal body cell.

kernicterus. A grave form of jaundice of the neonate, accompanied by brain damage.

kwashiorkor. Extreme protein malnutrition seen in infants and children living in poverty.

laryngotracheobronchitis. Inflammation of the larynx, trachea, and bronchi.

Legg-Calvé-Perthes disease. Inadequate blood supply to the head of the femur, characterized by pain in the hip joint; also called "flat hip."

Lonalac. Low salt formula.

lupus erythematosus. A chronic inflammatory disease of collagen or connective tissue that may be life-threatening.

Meckel diverticulum. A congenital blind pouch, sometimes seen in the lower part of the ileum. A cord may continue to the umbilicus, or a fistula may open at the umbilicus. An intestinal obstruction may occur if the cord becomes strangulated. Corrected by surgery.

meconium. The first stool of the newborn; a mixture of amniotic fluid and secretions of the intestinal glands.

meconium ileus. A deficiency of pancreatic enzymes in the intestinal tract of the fetus in which the meconium becomes excessively sticky and adheres to the intestinal wall, causing obstruction. Occasionally seen in babies born with cystic fibrosis.

megacolon. See *Hirschsprung disease.*

meningocele. A congenital anomaly, caused by a protrusion of the *meninges* or membranes through an opening in the spinal column.

meningomyelocele. A congenital anomaly, characterized by a protrusion of the *membranes* and *spinal cord* through an opening in the spinal column.

microcephaly. A congenital anomaly in which the head of the newborn infant is abnormally small.

miliaria. Prickly heat; inflammation of the skin caused by sweating.

mongolism. See *Down syndrome.*

Moro reflex. When newborn infants are jarred, they will draw the legs up and fold the arms across the chest in an embrace position.

mucoviscidosis. See *Cystic fibrosis*.

multifactorial. The result of many factors, such as a disease resulting from the combined action of several conditions.

murmur. A sound heard when listening to the heart, caused by blood leaking through openings that have not closed before birth, as they normally do.

muscular dystrophy. Wasting away and atrophy of muscles. There are several forms, all having some common characteristics.

mutation. A change in genetic material.

nevus (pl. *nevi*): A congenital discoloration of an area of the skin, such as a strawberry mark or mole.

Niemann-Pick disease. A hereditary disease in which there is a disturbance in the metabolism of lipids (substances resembling fats), causing physical and mental retardation.

nuchal. Pertaining to the neck.

omphalocele. A herniation of the abdominal contents at the umbilicus.

ophthalmia neonatorum. Acute conjunctivitis of the newborn infant, often caused by the gonococci of gonorrhea, venereal disease.

orthopnea. A disorder in which the patient has to sit up in order to breathe.

Osgood-Schlatter disease. Tendinitis of the knee, seen in adolescents and adults who participate in sports.

osteochondroma. Benign tumor composed of cartilage and bone.

osteogenesis imperfecta. A congenital bone disease in which the bones fracture easily.

osteosarcoma. The malignant bone tumor most frequently encountered in children.

otitis media. Inflammation of the middle ear.

paraphimosis. Impaired circulation of the uncircumcised penis due to improper retraction of the foreskin.

patent ductus arteriosus. One of the most common cardiac anomalies, in which the ductus arteriosus fails to close. Blood continues to flow from the aorta into the pulmonary artery.

pectus excavatum. A variation in the normal configuration of the chest in which the lower portion of the sternum is depressed.

phenylketonuria (PKU). An inborn error of metabolism causing retardation; the body is unable to utilize phenylalanine, an amino acid.

phimosis. A tightening of the prepuce of the uncircumcised penis.

pica. Abnormal appetite, or compulsive ingestion of nonfood substances such as paint, clay, or crayons.

poliomyelitis. An acute infectious disease of the brain stem and spinal cord.

polydactyly. A developmental anomaly characterized by the presence of extra fingers or toes.

prehension. Use of hands to pick up small objects; grasping.

pyloric stenosis. A congenital narrowing of the pylorus of the stomach due to an enlarged muscle.

rapport. Harmonious relationship.

rectal prolapse. A dropping or protrusion of the mucosa of the rectum through the anus.

retrolental fibroplasia. Blindness usually found in preterm infants that is associated with oxygen concentrations and in which the blood vessels of the retina become damaged.

Reye syndrome. Acute encephalopathy with fatty degeneration of the liver, characterized by fever and impaired consciousness.

rhabdomyosarcoma. Extremely malignant neoplasm originating in skeletal muscle.

rickets. A disease of the bones, caused by lack of calcium or vitamin D.

rooting reflex. The infant turns the head toward anything that touches the cheek, as a means of reaching food.

roseola. Self-limited infection manifested by high fever followed by maculopapular rash. The child appears well otherwise and usually remains active.

rubella. German measles.

rubeola. Measles.

scoliosis. Lateral curvature of the spine.

scurvy. A disease caused by the lack of vitamin C in the diet and characterized by joint pains, bleeding gums, loose teeth, and lack of energy.

shunt. A bypass.

sickle cell anemia. A disease associated with an inherited defect in the synthesis of hemoglobin.

SIDS. Sudden infant death syndrome. The sudden and unexpected death of an apparently healthy infant, typically occurring between the ages of 3 weeks and 5 months, and not explained by careful postmortem studies; called also *crib* or *cot death*.

Snellen Alphabet Chart. A device used to measure near and far vision; a variation is the Snellen E chart.

spina bifida. A congenital defect in which there is an imperfect closure of the spinal canal.

talipes equinovarus. See *Clubfoot*.

Tay-Sachs disease: A degenerative, fatal brain disease caused by a lack of hexosaminidase A in all body tissues. Seen mostly in Eastern European Jews and genetically transmitted.

tetralogy of Fallot. A congenital heart defect involving pulmonary stenosis, ventricular septal defect, dextroposition of the aorta, and hypertrophy of the right ventricle.

thalassemia. A hereditary blood disorder in which the patient's body cannot produce sufficient hemoglobin.

thrush. An infection of the mucous membranes of the mouth or throat caused by the fungus *Candida*.

tinea. A contagious fungus infection: ringworm.

torticollis. Wryneck; a condition in which the head inclines to one side because of a shortening of either sternocleidomastoid muscle.

TPN. Total parenteral nutrition. Providing for all nutritional needs by administration of liquids into the blood; used in life-threatening conditions. Also called hyperalimentation.

tracheoesophageal fistula. The esophagus, instead of being an open tube from the throat to the stomach, is closed at some point. A fistula between the trachea and the esophagus is common.

truncus arteriosus. A single arterial trunk leaves the ventricular portion of the heart and supplies the pulmonary, coronary, and systemic circulations.

truncus arteriosus. A single arterial trunk leaves the ventricular portion of the heart and supplies the pulmonary, coronary, and systemic circulations.

turgor. Elasticity of the skin.

tympanometry. Measurement of mobility of the tympanic membrane of the ear and estimation of middle ear pressure.

varicella. Chickenpox.

variola. Smallpox.

ventriculography. X-ray examination of the ventricles of the brain following the injection of air into the ventricles.

vernix caseosa. A cheeselike substance that covers the skin of a newborn infant.

volvulus. A twisting of the loops of the small intestine, causing obstruction.

wheal. Large, slightly raised red or blistered area of skin; may itch.

Wilms tumor. A malignant tumor of the kidneys.

zygote. A fertilized egg.

INDEX

Note: Page numbers in *italics* indicate figures; those followed by t indicate tables.